Handbook of
Learning Disabilities

Handbook of
Learning Disabilities

Edited by

H. Lee Swanson
Karen R. Harris
Steve Graham

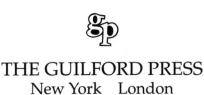

THE GUILFORD PRESS
New York   London

© 2003 The Guilford Press
A Division of Guilford Publications, Inc.
72 Spring Street, New York, NY 10012
www.guilford.com

Printed in the United States of America

Last digit is print number: 9 8 7 6 5 4 3 2

Library of Congress Cataloging-in-Publication Data

Handbook of learning disabilities / edited by H. Lee Swanson, Karen R. Harris, Steve Graham.
        p. cm.
Includes bibliographical references and index.
    ISBN 1-57230-851-6 (hard)
    1. Learning disabilities—Handbooks, manuals, etc.   2. Learning disabled children—Education—United States—Handbooks, manuals, etc. I. Swanson, H. Lee, 1947–   II. Harris, Karen R.   III. Graham, Steven, 1950–
LC4704 .H364 2003
371.92'6—dc21   2002015272

To my mentors: Annette Tessier, Bill Watson, and Barbara Keogh.
—H. L. S.

To Donald Deshler, Barbara Keogh, and Bernice Wong—
very broad shoulders to stand on indeed.
—K. R. H.

To Lamoine Miller, a wonderful mentor and colleague, who took a
chance on a raw young man from Georgia; I am forever grateful.
—S. G.

About the Editors

H. Lee Swanson, PhD, is Distinguished Professor and holds an endowed chair at the University of California, Riverside. He did his doctoral studies at the University of New Mexico and his postdoctoral work at the University of California, Los Angeles. Dr. Swanson was recently awarded a large U.S. Department of Education grant, which provides support for a longitudinal study of working memory in children with and without math disabilities. He served as Editor of *Learning Disability Quarterly* for 10 years, and also has published over 200 articles, 13 books, and 30 chapters.

Karen R. Harris, PhD, is Distinguished Scholar–Teacher and Professor of Special Education at the University of Maryland, College Park. She has taught kindergarten and fourth-grade students, as well as elementary and secondary students with ADHD, learning disabilities, and behavioral/emotional difficulties. Dr. Harris's research focuses on theoretical and intervention issues in the development of academic and self-regulation strategies among students with ADHD, learning disabilities, and other challenges. Author of over 100 scholarly publications, she is Editor of the *Journal of Educational Psychology* and Codirector of the federally funded Center for Accelerating Student Learning in collaboration with Vanderbilt and Columbia Universities. She is also a past president and Awards Committee Chair of the Division for Research of the Council for Exceptional Children.

Steve Graham, PhD, is Professor of Special Education at the University of Maryland, College Park. He received his doctoral degree from the University of Kansas. Following the completion of his doctorate, he was a member of the special education faculties at Auburn University and Purdue University. Dr. Graham's research has focused primarily on identifying the factors that contribute to the development of writing difficulties; the development and validation of effective procedures for teaching planning, revising, and the mechanics of writing to struggling writers; and the use of technology to enhance writing performance and development. One outcome of this focus has been the development of an instructional approach to writing, known as Self-Regulated Strategy Development (SRSD), which provides a powerful way to assist students in the development of higher-level cognitive processes involved in written language, the capability to monitor and manage their own writing, and positive attitudes about themselves as writers. Dr. Graham is the author of more than 150 scholarly publications and coauthor of several books.

Contributors

Robert D. Abbott, PhD, Department of Educational Psychology, College of Education, University of Washington, Seattle, Washington

Gary Adams, PhD, Department of Special Education, George Fox University, Newberg, Oregon

Stephanie Al Otaiba, PhD, Department of Special Education, Florida State University, Tallahasee, Florida

Dagmar Amtmann, PhD, Center for Technology and Disability Studies, University of Washington, Seattle, Washington

Scott Baker, PhD, Eugene Research Institute, University of Oregon, Eugene, Oregon

Roderick W. Barron, PhD, Department of Psychology, University of Guelph, Guelph, Ontario, Canada

Barbara D. Bateman, PhD, JD, Department of Special Education, University of Oregon, Eugene, Oregon

Nancy J. Benson, PhD, Population Health Sciences Program, The Hospital for Sick Children, Toronto, Ontario, Canada

Virginia W. Berninger, PhD, Department of Educational Psychology, College of Education, University of Washington, Seattle, Washington

Patricia Greig Bowers, PhD, Department of Psychology, University of Waterloo, Waterloo, Ontario, Canada

Deborah L. Butler, PhD, Department of Educational Psychology and Special Education, University of British Columbia, Vancouver, British Columbia, Canada

Douglas Carnine, PhD, National Center to Improve the Tools of Educators, University of Oregon, Eugene, Oregon

Laurie E. Cutting, PhD, Kennedy Krieger Institute and Departments of Developmental Cognitive Neurology and Education, Johns Hopkins University, Baltimore, Maryland

Martha Bridge Denckla, MD, Kennedy Krieger Institute and Department of Developmental Cognitive Neurology, Johns Hopkins University, Baltimore, Maryland

Donald D. Deshler, PhD, Center for Research on Learning, University of Kansas, Lawrence, Kansas

Batya Elbaum, PhD, Department of Education and Psychology, University of Miami, Coral Gables, Florida

Carol Sue Englert, PhD, College of Education, Michigan State University, East Lansing, Michigan

Jack M. Fletcher, PhD, Department of Pediatrics, Center for Academic and Reading Skills, University of Texas–Health Science Center at Houston, Houston, Texas

Steven R. Forness, EdD, Department of Psychiatry and Biobehavioral Science, University of California, Los Angeles, California

Douglas Fuchs, PhD, Department of Special Education, Vanderbilt University, Nashville, Tennessee

Lynn S. Fuchs, PhD, Department of Special Education, Vanderbilt University, Nashville, Tennessee

David C. Geary, PhD, Department of Psychological Services, University of Missouri, Columbia, Missouri

Russell Gersten, PhD, Instructional Research Group, Long Beach, California

Steve Graham, PhD, Department of Special Education, University of Maryland, College Park, Maryland

Daniel P. Hallahan, PhD, Curry School of Education, University of Virginia, Charlottesville, Virginia

Karen R. Harris, PhD, Department of Special Education, University of Maryland, College Park, Maryland

Cynthia M. Herr, PhD, Department of Special Education, University of Oregon, Eugene, Oregon

George W. Hynd, EdD, Department of Special Education and Psychology and Center for Clinical and Developmental Neuropsychology, University of Georgia, Athens, Georgia

Galit Ishaik, BS, Department of Psychology, University of Waterloo, Waterloo, Ontario, Canada

Joseph R. Jenkins, PhD, Department of Special Education, College of Education, University of Washington, Seattle, Washington

Kenneth A. Kavale, PhD, Division of Special Education, College of Education, University of Iowa, Iowa City, Iowa

Maureen W. Lovett, PhD, Brain and Behavior Program, The Hospital for Sick Children, and Departments of Pediatrics and Psychology, University of Toronto, Toronto, Ontario, Canada

G. Reid Lyon, PhD, Child Development and Behavior Branch, National Institute of Child Health and Human Development, Bethesda, Maryland

Charles MacArthur, PhD, School of Education, University of Delaware, Newark, Delaware

Virginia A. Mann, PhD, Department of Cognitive Science, School of Social Sciences, University of California, Irvine, California

Troy Mariage, PhD, College of Education, Michigan State University, East Lansing, Michigan

Margo A. Mastropieri, PhD, Graduate School of Education, George Mason University, Fairfax, Virginia

Kristen N. McMaster, PhD, Department of Educational Psychology, Vanderbilt University, Nashville, Tennessee

Carlin J. Miller, MEd, Center for Clinical and Developmental Neuropsychology, University of Georgia, Athens, Georgia

Devery R. Mock, MA, Curry School of Education, University of Virginia, Charlottesville, Virginia

Robin D. Morris, PhD, Department of Psychology, Georgia State University, Atlanta, Georgia

Jeff Munson, PhD, Program Project on Autism, University of Washington, Seattle, Washington

Rollanda E. O'Connor, PhD, Department of Instruction and Learning, School of Education, University of Pittsburgh, Pittsburgh, Pennsylvania

Wendy H. Raskind, PhD, Department of Medicine and Multidisciplinary Learning Disability Center, University of Washington, Seattle, Washington

Leilani Sáez, MA, Graduate School of Education, University of California, Riverside, California

Juliana Sanchez, MEd, Center for Clinical and Developmental Neuropsychology, University of Georgia, Athens, Georgia

Jean B. Schumaker, PhD, Center for Research on Learning, University of Kansas, Lawrence, Kansas

Thomas E. Scruggs, PhD, Graduate School of Education, George Mason University, Fairfax, Virginia

Bennett A. Shaywitz, MD, Departments of Pediatrics and Neurology, Yale University School of Medicine, New Haven, Connecticut

Sally E. Shaywitz, MD, Department of Pediatrics, Yale University School of Medicine, New Haven, Connecticut

Linda S. Siegel, PhD, Department of Educational and Counseling Psychology and Special Education, University of British Columbia, Vancouver, British Columbia, Canada

Deborah L. Speece, PhD, Department of Special Education, University of Maryland, College Park, Maryland

H. Lee Swanson, PhD, Graduate School of Education, University of California, Riverside, California

Jennifer B. Thomson, PhD, Department of Educational Psychology, College of Education, University of Washington, Seattle, Washington

Sharon Vaughn, PhD, Department of Special Education, University of Texas at Austin, Austin, Texas

Joanna P. Williams, PhD, Department of Human Development, Teachers College, Columbia University, New York, New York

Bernice Y. L. Wong, PhD, Faculty of Education, Simon Fraser University, Burnaby, British Columbia, Canada

Naomi Zigmond, PhD, Department of Instruction and Learning, School of Education, University of Pittsburgh, Pittsburgh, Pennsylvania

Preface

Research on learning disabilities (LD) has become a major scientific endeavor across several academic disciplines, including psychology and education. This research has provided scientifically based models for practice in several areas across both special and general education, such as those in the areas of instruction and methodology included in this text. Thus, the purpose of this book was to chronicle the major findings that have emerged in the field of LD over the past 20 years. In extensive discussions, we identified programmatic research programs that have been and continue to be well recognized over this time period. This handbook covers a wide range of topics in LD. Selection of authors was based upon a number of factors, the most important of which being whether the research programs were programmatic and well represented in scientific journals.

We are grateful to Chris Jennison at The Guilford Press for his tremendous support through all phases of this project, and to his colleague Laura Patchkofsky, who handled the production details, including chapter author coordination, with exemplary skill and enthusiasm. We are also thankful to Crystal Howard for monitoring the progress of all chapters (submission, revisions, and follow-up). We are most grateful, however, to all contributors for their willingness to undertake this difficult and challenging task; we thank them for making this undertaking not only doable, but enjoyable.

H. LEE SWANSON
KAREN R. HARRIS
STEVE GRAHAM

Preface

Contents

Part I. Foundations and Current Perspectives

Part II. Causes and Behavioral Manifestations

Part III. Effective Instruction

Part IV. Formation of Instructional Models

Part V. Methodology

Handbook of
Learning Disabilities

I
FOUNDATIONS AND CURRENT PERSPECTIVES

1

Overview of Foundations, Causes, Instruction, and Methodology in the Field of Learning Disabilities

H. Lee Swanson
Karen R. Harris
Steve Graham

The authors of the chapters in this *Handbook* review major theoretical, methodological, and instructional advances that have occurred in the field of learning disabilities (LD) over the last 20 years. The first, and only previous, comprehensive *Handbook on Research in Learning Disabilities* was published in 1986 and edited by Steven Ceci. This text was an important contribution to the field. Since that time, significant progress has been made in identifying and treating children and adults with LD. This volume captures major research programs that underlie these advances. Because of the diversity of subjects covered, the *Handbook* is divided into five sections.

Part I: Foundations and Current Perspectives

The foundations of and current perspectives in the field are the focus of the first section. Chapter 2 reviews some of the major research-based landmarks of the field. In this chapter, Hallahan and Mock divide the history of LD into five periods. The European Foundation period (1800 to 1920) is characterized by findings from clinical studies on brain injury and mental impairment. The U.S. Foundation period (1920 to 1960) is characterized as focusing on remediation and educational studies. The Emergent period (1960 to 1975) is characterized by the formation of organizations to advocate for children with LD. This period focuses on definitions of LD and intervention programs. Some of these intervention programs are still foundational to the field; others have been criticized and dismissed. The Solidification period (1975 to 1985) reflects a period of calm for the LD field. Researchers for the most part abandoned models of the past to focus on empirically validated applied research. Also during this time, key legislation was passed reiterating earlier definitions of the field. The Turbulent period (1985 to 2000) reflects an epidemic increase in the number of students identified with LD which in turn escalates the intensity of the unresolved issues. Although professional and governmental organizations put forward definitions, these definitions were not necessarily related to intervention practices. The authors also characterize the field as currently wrestling with postmodernism orientations.

In Chapter 3, Fletcher, Morris, and Lyon address the issues of classification, definition, and public policy. Their review concludes that classification research over the last 10 to 15 years provides little evidence to support IQ discrepancy definitions. The authors further review research suggesting that neither IQ scores nor an IQ discrepancy are relevant to treatment planning. They review some methodological measurement problems in subtype research. They conclude, however, that research on subtypes that are based on either achievement or processing skills do not suggest much as to evidence of subtype by treatment interactions. They further critique two models that have emerged in relationship to the classification of LD. One involves an intraindividual-differences approach that looks at discrepancies within the child, and the other focuses on a problem-solving model that focuses on a child's response to instruction. The authors do not see these two models as incompatible. They argue, however, that both models reflect confusion about different levels of classification and a failure to recognize that no single classification is suitable for all purposes. They argue that an intraindividual-differences perspective leads to excessive testing, which, in turn, does not have a strong relationship to treatment outcomes. They argue that the problem-solving model is not independent of classification issues or even the concept of intraindividual differences. Although the problem-solving model is less focused on within-child variation, it retains, according to the authors, the concept of "discrepancy" with environmental or social expectations. Furthermore, this discrepancy is relative to the expectations of a local context. In their research they emphasize the importance of a multivaried approach with both dependent and independent variables. They indicate that focusing on single variables are not helpful except beyond pilot data. Their classification research calls for an integrated model. They argue that for identification and eligibility purposes, LD should be conceptualized as unexpected, largely in the absence of response to adequate instruction, and a discrepancy should be a matter of not learning to expectations. They argue that as a goal to identify children for special education, test scores and ability discrepancies are not valid indicators. Furthermore, children should not be placed in special education without

evidence of failure to respond to quality instruction. They key is to measure children in multiple ways over multiple time periods.

In Chapter 4, Herr and Bateman analyze important legislative influences in the field. They suggest that some legislation and litigation have had a detrimental effect on the practices of evaluating students who are suspected of having LD. For example, they argue that the definition of LD as indicated by the Individuals with Disabilities Education Act (IDEA) has led to widespread misuse of standardized tests and discrepancy formulas. There are several important cases reviewed in their chapter, including *Corchado v. Board of Education of Rochester City School District* (2000). This case raised the issues of defining a learning disability. The implication of the court decision was that severe discrepancy between achievement and ability cannot be used as a litmus test of LD. The *Wrowley* case (1982), which recognized that free and appropriate education had to be tailored to individual capabilities, is detailed. An Indiana case (*Nein v. Greater Clark County School Corporation,* 2000) that follows the progress of one student identified in first grade as having a learning disability is also reviewed. In this case, the school district had failed to provide an appropriate education for a student with LD. Other court decisions (e.g., *Cleveland Heights-University Heights City School District v. Voss,* 1998) have challenged the expectation that parents must pay for private school education when public schools fail. Current cases focus on program effectiveness as measured by student progress.

In Chapter 5, Kavale and Forness evaluate how far the LD discipline has progressed from its historical foundations. Fundamental problems of definition have severely affected the LD discipline. They note that even though research has increased significantly within the field of LD, it lags behind in theory development. Although there have been a number of theories proposed, none fully explains the deficits experienced by the increasingly heterogeneous LD population. The scientific discipline of LD suffers because of a continued movement away from attempts to delineate the structure of LD. These authors note that while the discrepancy concept has precipitated many debates within the field, the real problem is that a discrepancy is viewed as equivalent to underachievement. Kavale and Forness do not see underachievement and LD as equivalent; they suggest that discrepancy might be better viewed as necessary but insufficient criteria for LD identification. They view the inclusion of low achievers within LD samples as undermining the scientific integrity of the field. One major difficulty within the field is that students identified by a social–political–economical notion of LD have little resemblance to the description offered within the scientific discipline. Kavale and Forness argue that the scientific discipline of LD should seek to provide a new formal definition that explicitly states what LD represents, based on several decades of accumulated understanding about its nature.

In Chapter 6, Gersten and Baker provide a review of literature on English-language learners with LD. English-language learners are disproportionately represented in special education. Some of the instructional issues in the ongoing research involve merging English-language development with academic instruction. Current reconceptualizations of LD in terms of paying attention to rates of learning growth and elimination of discrepancy models, as well as the dramatic increase in the number of English-language learners in schools, pose increasing problems for the field. Gersten and Baker note that determining rates of academic growth over time is a key criterion for determining LD, and early intervention is critical for English-language learners. Although research is fairly clear about some of the ingredients of effective reading intervention programs, their application to English-language learners is somewhat more complex. These authors highlight some of their attempts to synthesize the knowledge base on effective teaching with application to English-language learners. Recent research has focused on the transition into English-language instruction in grades 3 through 6. Gersten and Baker's research suggests that effective instructional principles build and use vocabulary as a curricular anchor. They discuss several means to reinforce vocabulary (effective use of visuals as well as paying attention to the cognitive and language demands).

In the final chapter of this section (Chapter 7), Zigmond focuses on effective service delivery models. She provides a review of research studies on the relative effectiveness of service delivery models for students with LD and other mild-to-moderate disabilities. She argues that data on the relative efficacy of one special education placement over another are scarce. Furthermore, some of this research is flawed because the studies fail to conform to rigorous standards of experimental research. Zigmond also argues that research focused on delivery models asks the wrong question. She concludes that what goes on in a particular setting makes the difference, not where the delivery of service occurs. Her work demonstrates that some instructional practices are easier to implement and more likely to occur in some settings than in others.

Part II: Causes and Behavioral Manifestations

The second section of the *Handbook* focuses on the causes and behavioral manifestations of LD. Leading researchers address their work and in some cases the work of others in the areas of attention (Chapter 8), speed and reading (Chapter 9), basic cognitive processing (phonological, semantic, orthographic processing abilities) (Chapter 10), memory (Chapter 11), problem solving (Chapter 12), language processes (Chapter 13), social cognition (Chapter 14), neurological correlates (Chapter 15), and genetic influences (Chapter 16). Each author was asked to consider the following questions when writing his or her chapter:

1. What is the operation definition of LD in your research program?
2. What theoretical models provide a framework for your research?
3. What findings have been consistently replicated in your laboratory, school context, and/or fieldwork?
4. What independent researchers have confirmed these findings?
5. How do students with LD differ from controls on the constructs under investigation?
6. What applications does your research have for practice?

In Chapter 8, Cutting and Denckla focus on the relationship between attention-deficit/hyperactivity disorder (ADHD) and LD. They study known genetic disorders (neurofibromatosis, Tourette syndrome) to understand brain–behavior relationships in children with ADHD and LD. They indicate that there is overwhelming evidence that the supply of attentional resources in children and adults with ADHD is not impaired. Rather, it is a deficit in the deployment or allocation of attention resources that characterizes ADHD samples. Over the last 12 years their research used the behavioral–neurogenetics approach to studying LD and ADHD. For example, they study neurofibromatosis, a common gene disorder. Mental retardation is rare in this population, although LD is reported in approximately 25 to 61% of children with this disability. This population has been found to have lower than expected performance on a variety of language tasks (many related to phonological processing). When compared to children with reading disabilities, many processing deficits were similar, such as slow naming and poor phonic segmentation. Comparisons of LD and ADHD to children with Tourette syndrome have also yielded similar processing characteristics. Cutting and Denckla find that characteristics of LD related to executive dysfunction are not particularly characteristic of pure Tourette syndrome, with the sole exception of cognitive slowing. Their findings on Tourette syndrome and ADHD yield several parallels: Both disorders show abnormal frontal lobe volumes and additional abnormalities in the subcortical structures. Their research has made several contributions to our understanding of the complex interrelationships between executive function, language, and academic skills.

In Chapter 9, Bowers and Ishaik review their research related to rapid naming and reading disabilities. There are three foci to their work: (1) independence of the contribution of rapid automatic naming (RAN) to reading from that of phonological awareness, memory span, and verbal ability; (2) association between orthographic processing and RAN; and (3) understanding the "why" of the association between RAN and reading. Their work suggests that measures of verbal working memory overlap considerably with phoneme deletion and sound pattern tasks and also demonstrates a strong relationships between RAN of letters

and sound deletion (a phonological awareness task). Rapid naming is associated not only with initial fluency but also with fluency gained after practice. Bowers and Ishaik suggest that RAN is more closely related to orthographic skill than to phonemic encoding. Their recent research has focused on subtyping by strengths and weaknesses of RAN as well as phonemic deletion skill. They suggest a double-deficit hypothesis in which children can vary in terms of difficulty on phonological skills, rapid naming skills, or both. The literature is unclear as to whether RAN measures represent domain general or domain specific processing speed, but it is clear that it makes an important contribution to reading.

In Chapter 10, Siegel outlines the normal course of development in reading and examines why poor readers fail to develop adequately. She provides a strong theoretical model for our understanding of basic cognitive processes. She argues that a focus on word recognition measures is fundamental to evaluating reading disabilities because these measures are a strong correlate of basic psychological processes. She states that definitions should be at the reading recognition level and that a cutoff below the 25th or 20th percentile contributes to the operationalization of the field. Reading problems are best conceptualized as a continuum with varying degrees of severity. Her research indicates that children with reading disabilities show remarkable homogeneity in cognitive profiles. Siegel finds that when reading disabilities are defined in terms of word recognition skills, all children with reading problems have deficits in phonological processing, working memory, and short-term memory and syntactic awareness. She also indicates there is no reliable evidence to indicate that IQ plays a cognitive role in development of reading skills. She provides an extensive review of five possible processes that underlie the development of reading skills in the English language. These processes involve phonology, syntax, working memory, semantics, and orthography. Siegel's research shows that difficulties in phonological processing are fundamental problems for children with reading disabilities and this problem continues to adulthood. She reports that there is no evidence to suggest that development of decoding skills is a result of specific instruction in grapheme–phoneme conversion rules. Siegel's research points to three processes critical in analysis of reading disabilities: those related to phonological, syntactic, and working memory processes.

In Chapter 11, Swanson and Sáez review memory research completed within the last 20 years on samples of children with LD. This research focuses primarily on the contribution of both short-term and working memory to academic performance. Deficits experienced by children with LD in the areas of reading and math are related to problems in the phonological loop and a speech-based representational system, as well as problems in the general executive system. The executive system focuses on the monitoring of information, focusing and switching attention, and activating representations from long-term memory. The research is couched within Baddeley's tripartite structure. The definition of LD used by Swanson and Sáez relies on cutoff scores (i.e., student performance below the 16th percentile in reading or math, with average IQ scores). Problems in the executive system are reviewed in terms of studies where researchers have manipulated the mental allocation of attention, focused on how children use strategies to inhibit irrelevant information, and focused on how children combine processing and storage demands. Problems in executive processing are described in terms of limitations in attentional capacity rather than processing strategies. Problems in the phonological system are reviewed in terms of a meta-analysis focusing on the recall of ordered information in which few resources from long-term memory are activated. Because short-term memory has less direct application to complex academic tasks, the remainder of the chapter considers the relationship between working memory and complex cognition. Practical applications for instruction are also provided, including four instructional principles.

In Chapter 12, Geary focuses on the diagnosis of arithmetic disabilities. He suggests that a score lower than the 20th or 25th percentile on a mathematics achievement test combined with low, average, or high IQ is a typical criterion for diagnosing arithmetic disabilities. He indicates, however, that this criterion is slippery because most children who meet this criterion in year 1 will not necessarily meet it in successive grades. His earlier cross-sectional research shows that most academically normal children gradually switch from counting to direct retrieval of an answer, whereas most children with arithmetic disabilities do not make such a transition. Geary also found that children with arithmetic disabilities did not necessarily differ from their academically normal peers in types of strategies used to solve simple arithmetic problems. Differences, however, were found in the percentage of retrieval and counting errors. These children's long-term memory representations of addition facts were incorrect. He provides a taxonomy of three general subtypes of mathematical disability: those related to procedural errors, semantic memory, and visual/spatial difficulties. In the review of literature, Geary delineates an inability to retrieve basic facts from long-term memory as a defining feature of arithmetic disabilities. When children with arithmetic disabilities retrieve arithmetic facts from long-term memory they commit more errors than do their academically normal peers and show error and reaction time patterns that often differ from those of younger academically normal children. The results of additional studies from his laboratory suggest that inhibitory mechanisms should be considered as potential contributors to retrieval errors.

In Chapter 13, Mann focuses on the relationship between language processes and reading disabilities. Moving away from the notion of discrepancy, she justifies a language-based approach. She indicates that orthography rests on the nature of the spoken language it transcribes. She also indicates that language processing skills and reading problems result when poor readers have problems with phoneme awareness, morpheme awareness, and three language skills: speech perception under difficult listening conditions; vocabulary, especially naming ability; and using the phonetic representation in linguistic short-term memory. Based on comparative studies (e.g., American and German instruction), Mann suggests that awareness of phonemes is enhanced by methods of instruction that direct a child's attention to the phonetic structure of words. Instructional experiences alone are not the only factor that account for failure to achieve phoneme awareness. Some of the factors relate to speech perception (i.e., the awareness of rhyme). Recent research has confirmed the relationship between speech perception and early reading skill.

In Chapter 14, Elbaum and Vaughn review research on self-concept. Self-concept is a multidimensional construct; therefore, the authors emphasize only those dimensions of self-concept especially relevant to students with LD. These areas include academic self-concept, social concept, and global self-worth. Their meta-analysis shows little reliable association between the self-concept of an individual with LD and educational placement. They conclude that educational placement is not an overriding determinant of self-concept, placing more importance on other factors such as individual teacher understanding and acceptance of students with disabilities. They also find that students with LD who have a low self-concept can benefit from appropriate interventions. They indicate a caveat in the literature, however, because students who have a low self-concept do not necessarily have low general self-perceptions. In addition, some students with LD have self-concept scores in the same range as do students without disabilities. Research indicates that there are several issues related to the measurement of self-concept, including those resulting from the poor theoretical foundation of a number of measures. Elbaum and Vaughn indicate that further research needs to be done on a longitudinal basis to investigate the extent to which LD students' self-concept changes as a function of academic progress.

In Chapter 15, Miller, Sanchez, and Hynd consider the neurological correlates of reading disabilities. Their research focuses on children characterized by difficulties in reading and spelling, including difficulties in segmentation, rapid and automatic recognition in decoding of single words, articulation, and anomia. During the last decade there has been consensus that a core component of reading disabilities is difficulty in phonological processing. These authors also report evidence of visual deficits in some people with reading disabilities. They review the neurobiological evidence done through postmortem, electrophysiological, family, and functional magnetic resonance imaging studies (fMRI), all pointing to a

clear disruption of the neurological system for language in individuals with dyslexia. Brain-based research in dyslexia has primarily focused on the planum temporale, gyral morphology of the perisylvian region, corpus colossum, and cortical abnormalities of the temporal–parietal region. Miller and colleagues state that the neural biological codes believed to underlie cognitive deficits in individuals with reading disabilities are centered on the left temporal–parietal region. Differences in the symmetry of the planum temporale have consistently been found in association with reading disabilities. Specifically, asymmetry of the planum temporale is due to a larger right plana. A reversal of normal pattern of left greater than right asymmetry has been found in individuals with developmental dyslexia. Although the core deficit in dyslexia appears to be phonological processing, they conclude that visual processing is also implicated. Their research indicates, however, that variability in the pattern of the plana symmetry or asymmetry is not a sufficient cause of severe reading disability or dyslexia. This is because such symmetry or reverse asymmetry in the plana also appears in the normative population. Although their review suggests that there is a strong heritability component in the reading process, many unknowns have yet to be explored. For example, although certain genes have been targeted as being involved in dyslexia, it is not known how these chromosomes cause manifestation of reading deficits. The authors also indicate that there has been little investigation of the genetic contributions to dyslexia in minority populations.

In the final chapter (Chapter 16) of this section, Thomson and Raskin focus on genetic influences on reading and writing disabilities. Their work has shown that phonological short-term memory has a genetic ideology, leading to an instructional program in which reading begins with precise representation of syllables and phonemes and spoken words. They review some of the Colorado twin study findings that support the existence of major gene effects on reading disabilities, although they indicate that the precise information about the mode of inheritance is less clear. Literature suggests localization of dyslexic gene sites (i.e., gene sites have been attributed to chromosome 1,

2, 6, 15, and 18). The authors review a variety of mathematical approaches developed to model the inheritance patterns of a trait in families. Thomson and Raskin examined nuclear families consisting of 409 individuals and found a genetic contribution to phonological decoding rate, in addition to the genetic contribution that is shared with phonological decoding accuracy. Their results also indicate that genes which contributed to nonword repetition account for the genetic basis of the digit-span score, but there is an additional genetic contribution to nonword repetition tasks not accounted for by measures of digit span. They indicate that future developments will focus on genotype/phenotype correlations, biological consequences of specific genetic changes, and intervention strategy guided by genetic profiles.

Part III: Effective Instruction

The third section includes chapters from leading researchers focusing on effective instruction in the areas of word skills (Chapter 17), reading comprehension (Chapter 18), mathematics (Chapter 19), writing (Chapter 20), spelling (Chapter 21), and science and social sciences (Chapter 22). The authors of these chapters were asked to address the following questions:

1. How are students with LD operationally defined?
2. What does research indicate are the most important components of instruction?
3. What behaviors or targets of instruction show the largest or weakest gains?
4. What is the magnitude of treatment outcomes (effect sizes)?
5. What evidence is provided on transfer and generalization?
6. What evidence is provided that students with LD respond similarly or differently from their counterparts under treatment conditions?
7. What are the principles of instruction that emerge from the research?
8. What are the results related to the transfer of findings to classroom practice?

In Chapter 17, Lovett, Barron, and Benson provide an overview of intervention research on word identification and decoding. Although developmental reading disabilities have been acknowledged for the past century it is only within the past 10–15 years that well-controlled studies have emerged. Lovett and colleagues have overcome previous methodological and measurement problems. They review previous studies on phonological processing and indicate there is limited knowledge on remediating "severe" forms of developmental dyslexia. Although advances in our understanding have been made regarding children in younger grades, mixed results and a range of outcomes exist among remediation studies with readers with severe disabilities and older children. Further difficulties relate to generalizations which implicate processes besides the phonological system. Lovett and colleagues review the extensive research program conducted at The Hospital for Sick Children in Toronto which specifically addresses issues of generalization and transfer of learning. They test two remedial programs, one focusing on direct instruction (phonological analysis and blending/direct instruction) and another on strategy training (word identification strategy training). Both procedures yield substantial changes in reading behavior when compared to control conditions. Results indicated that a combination of the two intervention programs enhanced generalization over either program in isolation. Their research focus has moved to enhancing reading fluency.

In Chapter 18, Williams provides a detailed review of her research on reading comprehension. She takes the position that regardless of the controversies about the nature and extent of the disability, instructional techniques recommended for students with LD are qualitatively different than those recommended for poor readers. Her research is based on the assumption that one should focus on school-identified groups because they are more ecologically representative settings yielding more useful results. Williams found in her earlier work that children with LD have difficulty producing a representation of information from their reading of text. She does not imply that they do not monitor; rather, their representation of a paragraph develops less adequately than in a child without disabilities. Her general principles of instruction attempt to externalize some of the steps of comprehension. Some of these principles make use of modeling strategies, sequencing tasks that reflect progression from easier to more difficult material, and provision for extensive practice and feedback. She has designed interventions related to theme identification to incorporate some goals of constructivism (integrating text meaning and concepts that are personally meaningful) as well as structured, direct instruction. In this instructional model, Williams makes use of teacher explanation and modeling, guided practice, and independent practice. Instruction is directed to focus on components of organization (e.g., theme identification via a series of questions that help the students generalize the theme to relevant life situations). The instructional sequence makes use of stories with single clear and accessible themes. She has analyzed her findings as a function of responsiveness to instruction. She found that for children in second and third grade no significant relationship emerges between nonresponders and special education status. Williams's current research focuses on various types of informational texts, such as single structure versus a compare–contrast structure.

In Chapter 19, Fuchs and Fuchs summarize their research on mathematical problem solving. They define students with math disabilities as having an intelligence test score of at least 90 and performance at least 1.5 standard deviations below the mean on a mathematics achievement test. Their work clearly shows that students with math disabilities lack a strong foundation in the rules of problem solving. Their research shows that it is necessary to have explicit instruction on transfer in order to draw the connection between novel and familiar problems. Fuchs and Fuchs indicate that additional work is needed to identify strategies for increasing the magnitude and range of problem-solving effects. Their work emphasizes the importance of process variables, by making the rules of problem solving explicit. To optimize the quality of providing effective explanation as well as continuing their work on strengthening transfer to real problem-solving tasks, they are presently identifying the cognitive correlates that underlie effective instruction.

In Chapter 20, Graham and Harris review

research on a model of strategy instruction referred to as self-regulated strategy development (SRSD). Their instructional model is designed to enhance students' strategic behaviors, self-regulation skills, content knowledge, and motivation for writing. An important goal of their program is to help students with LD develop more sophisticated approaches to composing by teaching powerful composition strategies for planning, composing, and revising, as well as self-regulation strategies critical to the writing process. Earlier research found that children have difficulty writing due to an inability to sustain the writing effort. Students with LD fail to access the knowledge they possess, and their difficulties in the mechanics of writing interfere with the process of generating content, leading to meager output. Graham and Harris indicate that gaps in writing knowledge are not limited to genre but also to other aspects of writing such as knowledge of how to write. They provide a meta-analysis of research using the SRSD model. The SRSD model has produced large effect sizes for students with and without LD, including strong positive effects on the quality, structure, and length of writing by students with LD. Although they raise questions about what components provide the largest effect sizes, the full SRSD model appears to be the most powerful related to measures of grammar, maintenance, and generalization. Graham and Harris's instructional model has a profound effect not only on students with LD but also on writers of poor, average, and good ability.

In Chapter 21, Berninger and Amtmann review 12 years of research on the prevention of spelling and writing problems. In their view of writing, this can be represented in a triangle that encompasses short-term memory, working memory, and long-term memory environments. They find that early intervention aimed at teaching handwriting or spelling to at-risk writers reduces the number of students who need to rely on computer technology to bypass low-level writing processes. They indicate that transcription skills differentiate good and poor readers. Their earlier work has shown that orthographic coding is directly related to handwriting and spelling in students who have dyslexia, as well as in those who have specific writing problems without any motor disabilities. They find that handwriting draws on orthographic coding but spelling draws on both orthographic and phonological coding. Berninger and Amtmann's recent research suggests that because phonological short-term memory is genetically constrained it may also apply to learning to spell. With young children, explicit training in the alphabetic principle in isolation and words in context leads to significant improvement in the spelling accuracy in young children's composition. They also review several instructional principles which influence both low-level and high-level spelling skills in the same lesson. They propose a model of writing which takes into consideration the transcription and executive functions. Developmentally, the executive function plays an increasing role in text generation and management of the writing processes. Berninger and Amtmann also provide an extensive review of research supporting use of computer technology. They indicate that computers can assist in writing beyond bypassing transcription problems (spelling).

In Chapter 22, Scruggs and Mastropieri review intervention research on science and social studies. They indicate that major educational decisions relative to science and social studies have been made without considering students with LD. Nevertheless, a substantial amount of research has been undertaken in science and social studies education for students with LD. The majority of their studies were conducted as true laboratory experiments or actual classroom and teacher applications. They present the argument that phonological processing deficits are related to some problems in comprehending science and social studies texts, but these processes are no more important than higher-order processes. Scruggs and Mastropieri characterize science and social studies education by two major models of instruction: constructivist–child-centered models and content-driven or textbook-based approaches. They note potential advantages to constructivist approaches. However, there is an overreliance on discoveries or insights into concept acquisition. Content-driven models typically emphasize breadth over depth of learning in the acquisition of factual material. Overall, their approach to facilitating content learning has in-

volved text-processing strategies, mnemonic strategies, elaborative integration, inquiry-oriented or activities-oriented instruction, and peer tutoring. They draw several conclusions for enhancing positive outcomes in instruction, including specifying instructional objectives, maximizing engagement through approaches such as opportunities to respond, enhancing concreteness and meaningfulness via mnemonic instructional strategies, and actively retrieving steps of a mnemonic strategy or reasoning through science problems and experiments, as well as the explicit provision of learning strategies. Current research focuses on developing appropriate tutoring materials with application to more complex subjects, such as high school chemistry.

Part IV: Formation of Instructional Models

The fourth section of this *Handbook* focuses on general instructional models. This section differs from the previous section due to the focus on models that would be considered general heuristics of effective instruction regardless of instructional domain. These chapters focus on research related to strategy instruction (Chapter 23), direct instruction (Chapter 24), cooperative learning (Chapter 25) and curriculum-based measurement models (Chapter 26). This section also addresses the influence of constructivist models on instructional outcomes (Chapter 27). The authors in this section were asked to consider the same seven questions listed in Part III.

In Chapter 23, Wong, Harris, Graham, and Butler provide a comprehensive overview of cognitive strategies instruction research in the field of LD. They define cognitive strategies as processes that the learner intentionally performs to influence learning. These models include self-control components as a way of planning and executing a strategy, as well as a way of monitoring and evaluating its effectiveness. Wong and colleagues organize their review by age level: children, adolescents, and young adults. They identify connecting themes or discernible commonalties among cognitive strategies instruction approaches. Strategies instruction for elementary grades includes research in the area of mnemonics, composition, and mathematics and strategy instruction for secondary students with LD. These authors also provide a comprehensive review of a strategic-content learning program that is focused on adults with LD. The key theme is that children who have difficulties learning need to be engaged in more extensive, structured, and explicit instruction to develop learning, performance, and self-regulation strategies. The authors indicate that many questions remain about strategies instruction, particularly the contributions of various components to the multicomponent models of strategies instruction.

In Chapter 24, Adams and Carnine provide an overview of their work on direct instruction. They define direct instruction as emanating from the foundational work of Engelmann and associates. In these programs, information about what the teacher needs to say and do is scripted within each curriculum program. They provide a meta-analysis of the relevant research on direct instruction that relates to students with LD and an effect-size index (a quantitative index) as a means for judging outcomes. Some of the important findings are that the effect sizes are larger in older than younger groups, effect sizes were larger in mathematics than reading, effect sizes were larger on criterion-related measures when compared to norm-referenced measures, and effect sizes were larger for studies implemented within a year period. Effect sizes decreased when interventions lasted over a year (Adams and Carnine attribute this to using multiple teachers affecting the fidelity of the implementation). However, regardless of the manipulations, they found effect sizes related to direct instruction were in the range of 0.73 to 1.26.

In Chapter 25, Jenkins and O'Connor provide a review of research on cooperative learning for students with LD. They define cooperative learning as instructional use of small groups so that students work together to maximize their own and each others' learning. They provide a comprehensive review of the experimental studies on cooperative learning for students with LD in the areas of mathematics, writing, and reading. They also address the application of cooperative learning to different forms of peer mediation, such as crossed age peer tutoring,

as well as mixed models (i.e., restructured and structural arrangements in a general class). Their work suggests that assistance provided by peers during cooperative learning may not be sufficient for students with LD. Sometimes students with LD have difficulty meeting the reading requirements of the group's work. Jenkins and O'Connor indicate that less than half of the students with LD (around 40%) successfully participate in cooperative groups. They also observe a significant side effect for using cooperative learning as an inclusion strategy. Their research clearly indicates that students with LD differ in their response to cooperative learning. The way teachers implement cooperative learning and the characteristics of the students themselves determine outcomes. Further, how the characteristics of students with LD are perceived by their classmates must be considered when using cooperative learning in a general education setting.

In Chapter 26, Fuchs, Fuchs, McMaster, and Al Otaiba focus on the link between treatment resisters (or nonresponders) and the application of curriculum-based measurement. Treatment resisters are children who are unresponsive to generally effective treatments. Fuchs and colleagues provide an extensive review of the literature regarding what nonresponsiveness to instruction entails. Previously, researchers have defined lack of responsiveness as related to the level of performance and the rate of growth. There are serious limitations to each of these definitions in isolation. They suggest a dual-discrepancy approach where attention is given to performance level and growth rate. The procedure requires an assessment of every child in every classroom weekly, evaluation of progress on a regular basis, formulation of interventions in general education classrooms for children identified as dually discrepant, and implementation of those procedures with fidelity. Within this context, nonresponders are identified as those who score 1 standard deviation below their average-achieving peers in performance level and slope (growth). However, it is important to realize that if a student's growth was similar to that of average students, even though the student performs poorly, the student would not be identified as a nonresponder. Likewise, a student who performed at a borderline level but made no growth would likely be identified as a nonresponder.

Fuchs and colleagues also indicate that validating the notion of discrepancy in terms of responsiveness to treatment may further validate the IQ-discrepant group. After examining this dual-discrepancy approach, they turn their attention to curriculum-based measurement (CBM). Generally, the procedure requires gathering samples of relatively broad skills, examining dimensions within the curriculum as reflected in weekly tests. Their repeated measurements and sampling differs markedly from typical classroom approaches in which teachers assess mastery of a single skill and move on to different or more difficult skills. Because CBM information is collected in a time series format, the researcher or teacher is able to calculate slopes or estimates for each individual as a means to describe growth and the effects of treatment. The goal is to describe individual trajectories of changes in academic performance.

In Chapter 27, Englert and Mariage investigate sociocultural models of special education interventions that focus on higher-order thinking skills. They focus on social constructivism as a theoretical model for designing and implementing instructional programs. Palincsar and Brown's early research provides a foundation for much of this work. The authors review three research programs that view students as a community of learners. Particular emphasis in each program is on teacher modeling and thinking aloud and providing strategies to be a successful learner. Teachers are viewed as providing an apprenticeship to students in cognitive activity. A key concept in these models is the "zone of proximal development." This is the distance between the level of performance obtained by the child in independent problem-solving activity and the level attained by the child in collaboration with others. This sociocultural model of learning suggests that instruction has to be situated in activities which promote transfer and generalization.

Part V: Methodology

The final section focuses on methodology. Research practice in LD today bears scant resemblance to that in the field of LD 20 years ago. Since the inception of the field, the body of knowledge concerning LD has been influenced by the sophistication of the research process. In this section authors identify how methodologies illuminate our understanding about the causes and/or correlates of LD. The areas covered include exploratory and confirmatory models (Chapter 28), single-subject and group-design models (Chapter 29), subtype analysis (Chapter 30), neuropsychological indices (Chapter 31), and qualitative research (Chapter 32). Research conducted by the author of each of these chapters exemplifies a particular methodological approach. The authors review their research using the targeted methodology with LD participants. In addition, these authors were asked to consider the following questions when writing their chapters:

1. What has this methodology told us about LD that is not apparent in other methodologies?
2. What are the strengths and limitations of this methodology?
3. How does this methodology complement or refine traditional comparisons (e.g., analysis of variance) found in the literature between students with LD and those without disabilities?
4. What part does context, error, and complexity play in the applications of these methods?
5. What variations exist within the methodological approach and why is a particular variation used in your research?

In Chapter 28, Abbott, Amtmann, and Munson provide an overview of exploratory and confirmatory methods in LD research. They describe current data management systems and limitations to traditional approaches of handling missing data. They discuss the use of methods that explore measurement structures in the context of new theories. These exploratory factor analysis procedures are useful in early stages of conceptualization. In their view, exploratory methods should be guided by theory as much as possible and performed so that Type 1 errors are tightly controlled. Confirmatory methods, in contrast, provide for comparison of consistency of data with competing models. Much of Abbott and colleagues' research has focused on the covariation of individual differences in growth. They often use confirmatory factor analysis and structural equation modeling to create a complete mapping of the theoretical constructs and the model of measurement error. They contrast structural equation modeling and traditional multiple analysis of variance (MANOVA) approaches. MANOVA depends on the type of correlation among dependent variables. If the multiple dependent measures are not indicated with latent variables, then a MANOVA is appropriate. However, if multiple dependent measures are indicated with other latent variables, then structural equation modeling is appropriate. Abbott and colleagues argue strongly that attention should be given to the fit of relevant competing theoretical models. They also outline new directions in confirmatory modeling of data. Besides the new software packages for a variety of statistical methods, innovations have been related to permutation-based tests.

In Chapter 29, Schumaker and Deshler focus on group and single-subject design for applied educational research. Several studies are reviewed that were conducted under the auspices of the Kansas University Center for Research and Learning. Challenges in designing effective intervention studies are reviewed. Schumaker and Deshler adopt standards to field-test their interventions that focus on application, usability, and generalizability. Particular attention is given to single-subject designs. The term "single subject" is a misnomer, because these designs involve multiple subjects. Single-subject design is particularly useful for students who are receiving intervention in a setting with a small number of students, and for close examination and development of intervention components and procedures. Because the focus is to develop interventions that create large changes in skills within a reasonable period, these designs are useful in assessing effectiveness. The designs are also useful in studying changes in growth, because all students can participate and act as a control as well as participate in the treatment conditions. Several of the designs used by Schumaker and Deshler are of a hybrid nature and manipulate setting, student, and sequences of behaviors taught. The Kansas

University researchers use group designs when attempting to compare the effects of an innovative instructional procedure to traditional instructional procedures. Several studies showing variations of single-subject designs are embedded within group design. Through these various designs, instructional methods for teaching a variety of strategies associated with general education courses are validated. Schumaker and Deshler also indicate the conditions in which rules of an experimental design must be considered within the context of the current school situation.

In Chapter 30, Speece reviews the empirical procedures of handling sample heterogeneity. She focuses on subtyping procedures known as cluster analysis. Part of the appeal of cluster analysis is that it is not a single method but encompasses a variety of approaches. Her analysis focuses primarily on hierarchical agglomerative methods in which the researcher starts with a participant (whether LD or non-LD) in his or her own cluster and then moves to successive iterations until all participants are in a single cluster. How the investigator decides at what point the hierarchy best reflects the true underlying structure of the data is discussed. Speece reviews the three major elements for designing and evaluating classification research: theory formulation, internal validity, and external validity. She reviews the difficulties with "distance" measures. She indicates that because of the uncertainty associated with statistical stopping rules, replication of a cluster structure is a requirement. Her own analysis indicates, however, that cluster analysis within the field of LD has been infrequent. Possible reasons for infrequent use include the complicated process for using hierarchical and ultra-agglomerate methods, the sheer amount of work involved, and the fact that the prior classification work has had little impact on research in reading disabilities. Speece presents a compelling argument that this is an appropriate tool in the classification of children experiencing learning problems.

In Chapter 31, Shaywitz and Shaywitz focus on the neurobiological indices of dyslexia. They define dyslexia as unexpected failure in reading among children and adults who otherwise possess levels of intelligence and motivation considered necessary for accurate fluent reading. Dyslexia is one of the most common neurological-based disorders affecting children with prevalence rates of 5 to 10% in clinics and about 17% in unselected population-based samples. The authors also argue that dyslexia is a persistent chronic condition that does not represent a transient developmental lag. Shaywitz and Shaywitz's results indicate that reading disability in young children as well as adults is due to a deficit in phonology. Shaywitz and Shaywitz's research further suggests that there are differences in the temporo–parieto–occipital brain regions between dyslexic and readers without impairment. They review the methodology related to functional brain imaging (positron emission tomography, fMRI, and magnetoencephalography). The converging evidence using functional brain imaging in adult readers with dyslexia shows failure in the left-hemisphere posterior brain system to function properly during reading. In recent studies, these researchers use fMRI to examine the functional organization of brain for reading and reading disability. They use a subtraction methodology to isolate brain–cognitive function relationships. Their findings indicate that sex differences exist in functional organization of the brain for language. In general, there is evidence of relatively greater right-hemisphere involvement for females than for males. Their research has focused on the brain regions where previous research has implicated reading and language. They find activation patterns related to phonological analysis. For example, on nonword rhyming tasks, individuals with dyslexia experience a disruption of the posterior system that involves the posterior superior temporal gyrus (also known as Wernicke's area, the angular gyrus, and the striate cortex). They indicate the strengths and limitations of the fMRI. Perhaps the most profound implication of the Shaywitzses' work is the biology behind a learning disability. They demonstrate a persistent nature of a functional disruption in the left-hemispheric neural systems and indicate that the disorder is lifelong.

The final chapter (Chapter 32) by MacArthur provides a comprehensive analysis of what we have learned about LD from qualitative research. Although a definition of qualitative research is hard to pinpoint, some characteristics noted by MacArthur indicate a focus on understanding people, events, and constructs in their full context. An essential characteristic of qualitative research is commitment to understanding social issues in their natural context with all its complexity. There is an open nature to the investigation that focuses on the meaning of events, ensuring the trustworthiness of the data, and checking the validity of the interpretations. In his review, several studies have relied primarily on a qualitative analysis of interviews to understand the views of individuals with LD. Usually interview transcripts are analyzed inductively and the responses are guided by general questions. MacArthur outlines the limitations in this approach but indicates that unique perspectives of individuals with LD are not often heard in quantitative models of analysis.

In summary, the authors of these chapters review significant advances in knowledge made in the field of LD. Although the chapters are diverse in terms of research programs reviewed, some clear themes emerge. For example, there is a clear biology to LD, the correlates of which are reflected in a number of psychological processes. There appears to be a reliance on operational definitions of LD that do not rely on discrepancy criteria. Furthermore, several instructional programs with critical commonalities have been effective across a broad array of academic areas. A number of legal and political influences have provided distraction to developments within the field, yet strong, theoretically based research is emerging in multiple areas. In addition, a number of methodological approaches have converged in showing that students with LD have qualitatively and quantitatively distinctive characteristics that vary from those of their normally achieving peers. There remain, of course, many unresolved areas within the field. Some of these continue to relate to consensus on definition, whereas others relate to isolating those components of instruction necessary for effective outcomes. Though each chapter fleshes out the details of various research programs, the reader discovers numerous and important directions for future research.

2

A Brief History of the Field of Learning Disabilities

Daniel P. Hallahan
Devery R. Mock

Without a historical perspective, the uniqueness of present-day contributions and "discoveries" tends to be overemphasized. But in fact these contributions represent extensions, modifications, verifications, or duplications of previously observed phenomena or stated positions. Unless we use the past as points of reference and guides, investigators of [learning disabilites] may either recommit past follies or "rediscover" the contributions of their professional progenitors when they should instead extend and correct the works of those who pioneered before them.

—WEIDERHOLT (1974, p. 1)

It is not easy to separate the wheat from the chaff, the sheep from the goat, or the contribution from the folly. In the field of learning disabilities (LD), professionals are asked to make this distinction almost daily. Some contributions in the field extend previous research and shed new light on old problems, for example, the relationship between phonological awareness and reading ability (Adams, 1990). However other "discoveries" are not so fruitful, for example, neurological patterning (Delacato, 1966).

Weiderholt (1974) suggested that the ultimate value of a "contribution" depends not on the persuasive power of its supporters but on the "contribution's" relative place in history. Thus, to distinguish the proverbial wheat from chaff, Weiderholt argued for the "contribution" in its historical context. In so doing we look to the past, well beyond even the 1975 passage of the Education for All Handicapped Children Act (EAHCA), to a history that spans centuries and conti-

nents. This history includes research investigating behaviors as disparate as aphasia and social competence and interventions ranging from Direct Instruction to forced laterality. It is a history that begins with the observed relationship between brain injury and behavior and progresses to and beyond the systematic identification of students with specific disability. In keeping with others who have chronicled these events (Hallahan & Mercer, 2001; Lerner, 2000; Mercer, 1997; Wiederholt, 1974), we have approached this subject chronologically and divided the history of LD into several periods. We have chosen to use the periods suggested by Hallahan and Mercer (2001): European Foundation Period (c. 1800–1920); U.S. Foundation Period (c. 1920–1960); Emergent Period (c. 1960–1975); Solidification Period (c. 1975–1985); Turbulent Period (c. 1985–2000). Individually these periods illustrate the interests, theories, and tools of the field at various points in time. Collectively, these periods evidence progress and serve as guides for distinguishing the contribution from the folly.

European Foundation Period (c. 1800–1920)

During this period, some European physicians and researchers explored the relationship between brain injury and behaviors, primarily disorders of spoken language. Later, in the second half of this period, this research gave way to investigations concerning presumed brain abnormalities and disorders of reading. Many of the achievements of this period, although limited by 19th-century technology, remain seminal achievements in the field of LD. The work of individuals such as Gall (Gall & Spurzheim, 1809), Broca (1861), and Hinshelwood (1895, 1917), however flawed and limited by the technology of their time, serve as the very "points of reference and guides" that Wiederholt (1974) extolled.

One of the first individuals to explore the relationship between brain injury and mental impairment was a physician named Franz Joseph Gall. Prior to Gall, the brain was viewed as "a single organ from which flowed vital energy under the influence of the will into all parts of the body" (Head, 1926, p. 3). Based on his observations of patients with brain injury, Gall asserted that separate areas of the brain controlled specific functions. Sir Henry Head, in his classic two-volume work on aphasia, paraphrased a letter published in 1802 describing Gall's assertions:

> The apparently uniform mass of the brain is made up of organs which subserve the manifestations of our vital and moral faculties; these consist of three groups: (1) those which concern purely the exercise of vital force; (2) the inclinations and affections of the soul; and (3) the intellectual qualities of the mind. Each of these is localised in a different portion of the brain. The organ of the vital force resides in the brain stem. . . . The inclinations and affections of the soul belong to the basal ganglia, whilst the intellectual qualities of the mind are situated in various parts of the cerebral hemispheres. Hence the moral and intellectual characteristics can be deduced from measurements of the skull, which is modified by the underlying brain. (1926, pp. 4–5)

As Head noted, the letter summarizing Gall's discoveries contained two themes—one related to the revolutionary idea of localization of function in the brain, the other to what was to become the basis for what was called "craniology" or "phrenology." Unfortunately for Gall, his name became more associated with phrenology than with his discovery of localization of brain function. By the middle of the 19th century, he was considered a charlatan within the medical community.

According to Head, Gall also missed the mark with respect to his conceptualization of what later would come to be known as Broca's aphasia. He was the first to describe cases of speech loss based on injury to the left frontal lobe. However,

> although many instances came before him, he appears to have looked upon them as confirmatory of a localization of faculties determined on other grounds. For him normal speech was due to the perfect exercise of certain aspects of memory, each of which was situated in some particular part of the anterior lobes of the brain. . . .
>
> Gall . . . appears to have looked upon speech as the direct mechanical expression of the concepts, inclinations, feelings and talents of man, each of which he localized in a particular part of the brain. (1926, p. 11)

Beginning in the 1820s, John Baptiste Bouillaud, dean of the Medical School of the College of France, performed autopsies of patients with known brain injury. This work confirmed Gall's notion of localization of brain functioning. Bouillaud posited that movement and sensory perception were controlled in the cortex of the brain and speech in the frontal anterior lobes.

Later, Pierre Paul Broca used autopsies to further Bouillaud's work and concluded that speech functions actually reside in the inferior left frontal lobe, an area that would later be named Broca's area. His name also became linked to a particular type of slow, laborious, dysfluent speech—Broca's aphasia.

In 1874, Carl Wernicke published a book containing 10 case studies of brain-injured patients with language disorders. These patients had fluent speech, but often it was devoid of meaning. In addition, these individuals manifested difficulty in recognizing and comprehending words. Wernicke labeled this disorder "sensory aphasia." With time, this particular type of aphasia as well as the area of the left temporal lobe responsible for the disorder would bear Wernicke's name.

As research in language disorders progressed, interest developed in disorders related to reading. In 1872, Sir William Broadbent published an account of six cases of persons whose histories supported the idea that speech and language is controlled by the left frontal lobe. One of these cases was that of an otherwise intelligent adult who lost the ability to read and name familiar objects while retaining the ability to write and converse. Later in 1877, Adolph Kussmaul reported on observations made by van den Abeele, which left "little room to doubt that a complete text-blindness may exist, although the power of sight, the intellect, and the power of speech are intact": "A woman, forty-five years of age, was struck with apoplexy while in the enjoyment of the most blooming health. . . . Two months after the attack she discovered that she could no longer read printing and writing. She saw the text, distinguished the forms of the letters, and could even copy the text, but was incapable of translating words into spoken words and thoughts" (1877, p. 776). Kussmaul attached the label "word-blindness" to this specific brand of reading disability.

In 1884, Berlin, a German ophthalmologist, introduced the term, "dyslexia." He believed "dyslexia" was preferable to "word blindness" for a condition of neurological origin (Anderson & Meier-Hedde, 2001). In a later book, Berlin presented six cases of adults with dyslexia, each of whom had lost the ability to read even though each had normal language ability (Berlin, 1887, cited in Anderson & Meier-Hedde, 2001).

In 1896, W. Pringle Morgan, an English physician, published the first case study of a child with congenital word-blindness. A French physician, John Hinshelwood, inspired by the work of Morgan and others, studied a particular patient from 1894 to his death in 1903. Upon performing the autopsy, Hinshelwood located the cause of the reading disability in the left angular gyrus. In 1917, Hinshelwood published *Congenital Word-Blindness*, a volume in which he noted the disproportionate number of males with this disorder and posited the potential heritability of congenital word-blindness. In addition, Hinshelwood asserted that the primary area of disability was faulty visual memory for words and letters. For this reason, he recommended one-to-one training designed to increase visual memory for words.

U.S. Foundation Period (c. 1920–1960)

By 1918, all states had passed laws requiring compulsory education for children. Thus, this period, one relatively comparable to Weiderholt's (1974) "transition phase," begins as teachers across the United States attempted to affect widespread literacy. Consequently, researchers in this period moved beyond observing and explaining abnormal behavior. Instead, many found themselves working with children in educational settings where remediation, not etiology, became the focus. Out of necessity, these researchers built on the work of their European predecessors and developed diagnostic categories, assessment tools, and remedial interventions that would influence future practice. Not surprisingly, much of this work was focused on reading disability.

In 1921, Grace Fernald coauthored an article describing remedial reading practices that had been used with students at the UCLA Clinic School (Fernald & Keller, 1921). In this article Fernald advocated for an emphasis on teaching the reading and writing of words as wholes using a technique that integrated several sensory modalities including visual, auditory, kinesthetic, and tactile (VAKT). As rationale for this procedure, Fernald (1943) provided historic examples of the teaching of reading via the kinesthetic modality. These references included Plato, Horace, Quintilian, Charlemagne, and Locke. To her credit, Fernald kept extensive records of student progress, and although she did not conduct research with the methodological rigor expected today, she was able to report notable performance gains in the areas of reading, spelling, penmanship, foreign language, and arithmetic.

Samuel Torrey Orton, the father of the International Dyslexia Society (formerly Orton Dyslexia Society), worked as a neuropathologist at the State Pychopathic Hospital in Iowa City, Iowa. In this capacity, Orton participated in a 2-week mobile clinic for students with learning problems where he made observations regarding students with low academic achievement, many of whom had low reading achievement. Of the 14 students in the clinic referred for reading problems, most demonstrated IQs in the near-average to above-average range, which led Orton to hypothesize that IQ was not always reflective of true intellectual capacity, especially in students with reading deficits—a view shared by many present-day reading researchers (Siegel, 1989). Orton summarized and published this work in *Reading, Writing, and Spelling Problems in Children* (Orton, 1937).

Although Orton built on much of Hinshelwood's work, he came to disagree with his predecessor on numerous points. Orton believed that the prevalence of reading disability was much higher than Hinshelwood's 1 per 1,000, perhaps even as high as 10% of the total school population (Orton, 1939). In addition, Orton (1939) maintained that the skill of reading involved more areas of the brain than the angular gyrus. He put forth the theory of mixed dominance, wherein the brain stored mirror images of visual representations. Students with reading disabilities lacked cerebral dominance and were therefore unable to suppress these stored, mirrored representations. Mixed dominance therefore resulted in reversals of letters and words in both reading and writing. He labeled this phenomenon "strephosymbolia," explaining that students with reading disabilities were not blind to words; instead, they "twisted" the symbols comprising words. Although Orton's work would later perpetuate the myth that individuals with dyslexia "see things backward," he left an enduring legacy in remediation practices. He stressed the need for explicit phonics and blending instruction using a multisensory approach. This practice is explained in *Remedial Work for Reading, Spelling, and Penmanship* (Gillingham & Stillman, 1936), a reference guide that has recently been published in its eighth edition.

Orton's research associate in the mobile clinic was Marion Monroe. After taking a position at a facility for delinquent boys with mental retardation, the Institute for Juvenile Research, Monroe developed a synthetic phonetic approach to the teaching of reading. She published her experiments in the book *Children Who Cannot Read* (Monroe, 1932) and later went on to train teachers in several field-based projects in areas around Chicago. Like Fernald, Monroe published studies lacking methodological rigor by today's standards; however, she did report impressive achievement gains in reading.

Monroe, like Orton, bequeathed to the field of LD educational practices that affected progress in years to come. For example, Monroe pioneered the practice of calculating a reading index, the discrepancy between actual and expected level of reading achievement for a student. Using this index, she could identify students who needed specific assistance. Perhaps Monroe's greatest gift to the field of LD came about through her meticulous reporting of case studies of children with reading disabilities. In particular, Monroe advocated finding patterns of errors in order to decide on remedial prescriptions: "Reading errors are of many kinds and may be classified into various types. Two children, reading the same paragraph, may make the same number of errors, receive the same reading grade, and yet their mistakes may be wholly different in nature. Their reading performances may be quantitatively the same but qualitatively unlike" (1932, p. 34).

At the Institute of Juvenile Research, Marion Monroe had a colleague named Samuel Kirk who was working at the institute as part of his graduate training in psychology. Monroe tutored Kirk in the diagnosis and remediation of severe reading disability. Although Monroe's influence is not immediately apparent in Kirk's master's thesis comparing the Fernald kinesthetic method to the look–say method, it is impossible to ignore her influence, as well as that of Orton, in Kirk's doctoral dissertation. In completing the requirements of the doctoral program at the University of Michigan, Kirk studied brain–behavior relationships by surgically creating brain lesions in rats and testing them for handedness and strephosymbolia (Kirk, 1935, 1936). After completing his doctorate, Kirk took a position at the University of Illinois and established the first experimental preschool for children with mental retardation. In taking on the task of educating these children, Kirk found a need for assessments that could isolate and identify abilities and disabilities. The result was the Illinois Test of Psycholinguistic Abilities (ITPA; Kirk, McCarthy, & Kirk, 1961). Although the ITPA would later be widely criticized (Engelmann, 1967; Hallahan & Cruickshank, 1973; Hammill & Larsen, 1974; Mann, 1971; Ysseldyk & Salvia, 1974), it enjoyed widespread use through the 1970s. Kirk's work, flowing directly out of Monroe's tutelage, produced the historically important ideas that (1) children with disabilities (later specified as LD) have intraindividual differences, and (2) assessment is a critical tool for guiding instruction.

In addition to reading, researchers practicing during the U.S. Foundation Period began to investigate disabilities in perception, perception–motor, and attention. Much of the early research in this area focused on adults with brain injury. Kurt Goldstein was a physician and director of a hospital for soldiers who had incurred head wounds in World War I. In this role, Goldstein observed and documented a constellation of behaviors seeming to accompany brain injury. These behaviors included hyperactivity, forced responsiveness to stimuli (i.e., indiscriminant reaction to stimuli), figure-background confusion, concrete thinking, perseveration, meticulosity, and catastrophic reaction (Goldstein, 1936, 1939). In keeping with the popular Gestalt school of thought, Goldstein argued that these phenomena were best understood not by looking for a specific physiological cause but by viewing the individual and his or her related manifestations as a whole. He was concerned with the functioning of the entire individual in all aspects of behavior.

The work of Goldstein served as an impetus for other researchers who were interested in applying his findings to children. Much of this work took place at one institution—Wayne County Training School in Northville, Michigan, about 20 miles from the University of Michigan. (In fact, several key figures in the field of special education during this period worked at Wayne County, e.g., Alfred Strauss, Heinz Werner, Edgar Doll, William Cruickshank, Newell Kephart, Laura Lehtinen, and Samuel Kirk.) Two German émigrés—Alfred Strauss, a neuropsychiatrist, and Heinz Werner, a developmental psychologist—were key in translating Goldstein's findings to those of children with mental retardation.

Strauss and Werner divided the children into two groups: those with exogenous mental retardation and those with endogenous mental retardation. The former were presumably brain injured; the latter presumably had familial mental retardation. In a series of laboratory studies, they found that the exogenous group of children exhibited more forced responsiveness to auditory and visual stimuli (Werner & Strauss, 1939b, 1940, 1941). In addition, Strauss and Kephart (1939) found children with exogenous retardation to be more disinhibited, impulsive, erratic, and socially unaccepted than children with endogenous retardation.

The work of Werner and Strauss did not go without criticism. In particular, Sarason (1949) pointed out that there were serious flaws in the way they distinguished their exogenous from endogenous groups. Nevertheless, they had found reliable differences between the two groups, suggesting that mental retardation was not a homogenous state. Further reinforcing this idea was a study of what happened to the two groups after admission to Wayne County. They found that after 4 to 5 years in the institution, the IQ of students with exogenous retardation decreased while the IQ of the endogenous group increased an average of 4 points (Strauss & Kephart, 1939). Based on this information, the researchers began designing learning environments to better fit the needs of students with exogenous retardation. In such environments, inessential stimuli were attenuated and essential accentuated. This line of research produced two classic volumes: *Psychopathology and Education of the Brain-Injured Child* (Strauss & Lehtinen, 1947) and *Psychopathology and Education of the Brain-Injured Child: Progress in Theory and Clinic* (Vol. 2) (Strauss & Kephart, 1955).

Werner and Strauss also espoused approaching standardized test scores with caution. Similar to Monroe, they advocated that clinicians dig deeper to find out the reasons why a particular error was made.

Werner (1937) contended that to understand normal child psychology, as well as mental deficiency, one must go beyond mere standardized achievement test scores. Werner and Strauss (1939a) argued for what they termed "functional analysis," "the examination of an individual in critical situations which elicit the impaired functions" (p. 61). Furthermore, they stated, "It is clear that the results of functional analysis, rather than the data from achievement tests, should serve as the guide for remedial work. The methods, techniques and materials for training must be chosen for their adequacy in relation to the functional impairment" (p. 62).

And so it was that:

> the conceptual posture of Werner and Strauss, coupled with their research into the differentiation between exogenous and endogenous mental retardation, did much to destroy the then-popular notion that mental retardation was a homogenous state. Concern for the diagnosis of particular disabilities and educational procedures based upon the Werner and Strauss recommendations became an intrinsic element of the basic principles upon which the field of LD was constructed. (Hallahan & Cruickshank, 1973, p. 65)

William Cruickshank was the person to carry forward Werner and Strauss's ideas as he helped pioneer the emerging field of LD. After completing his doctorate, Cruickshank began working with children with cerebral palsy and found that these children performed similarly to those with exogenous mental retardation studied by Werner and Strauss. In fact, the children with cerebral palsy displayed more forced responsiveness to background in figure-background studies than did children without cerebral palsy. Cruickshank therefore recommended that the education of students with cerebral palsy take place in distraction-free environments. Upon making such recommendations, Cruickshank organized a demonstration pilot study in Montgomery County, Maryland, titled the Montgomery County Project. The results of the study were published in *A Teaching Method for Brain-Injured and Hyperactive Children* (Cruickshank, Bentzen, Ratzeburg, & Tannhauser, 1961). The case histories of the students in this study suggest that according to present-day criteria, many would be considered learning disabled or learning disabled with comorbid attention-deficit/hyperactivity disorder (ADHD).

Like that of Werner and Strauss, Cruickshank's educational program reduced irrelevant stimuli, enhanced relevant stimuli, and provided highly structured assignments. The academic instruction took the form of readiness training involving perceptual and perceptual–motor exercises, homework, and arithmetic. Little attention was given to the development of reading skills. This program increased perceptual–motor abilities and decreased levels of distractibility but unfortunately had no effects on academic achievement or IQ. In addition, the increases in perceptual–motor abilities and attention disappeared in the 1-year follow-up. Despite the questionable efficacy of his educational program, Cruickshank is singularly important to the history of LD. He was responsible for building a bridge between the research previously conducted with students with mental retardation to children who would now be considered learning disabled.

Emergent Period (c. 1960–1975)

At the close of the Foundation Period, researchers had discovered tools for identifying and educating students with disabilities. They had sufficient knowledge to claim existence of a specific construct, a construct not yet referred to as LD. Thus, the time was ripe for the emergence of LD into the public domain. During the period spanning 1960 to 1975, parents and teachers became acquainted with the notion of LD and founded organizations to advocate for children with this disability, federal officials began to take notice of the rising tide of public concern for students with this disability, and researchers created interventions that would later set standards for practice. As a result, this period is characterized by the efforts of numerous individuals and groups to put forward comprehensive definitions and effective educational programming.

The term "learning disability" first appeared in print in *Educating Exceptional Children* (Kirk, 1962). Kirk (1962) defined LD as a retardation, disorder, or delayed development in one or more of the processes of speech, language, reading, writing, arithmetic, or other school subject resulting from a psychological handicap caused by a possible cerebral dysfunction and/or emotional or behavioral disturbances. It is not the result of mental retardation, sensory deprivation, or cultural and instructional factors. (p. 263)

Later in 1963, Kirk used this term in addressing a group of parents at the Conference on the Exploration into Problems of Perceptually Handicapped Children. The parents were searching for a name for a proposed national organization. After listening to Kirk, they named their new organization the Association for Children with LD (ACLD), now known as the LD Association of America.

Two years later, Kirk's former student, Barbara Bateman, put forth a definition that reintroduced Monroe's concept of reading index. This definition proposed the following:

Children who have learning disorders are those who manifest an educationally significant discrepancy between their estimated potential and actual level of performance related to basic disorders in the learning process, which may or may not be accompanied by demonstrable central nervous system dysfunction, and which are not secondary to generalized mental retardation, educational or cultural deprivation, severe emotional disturbance, or sensory loss. (1965, p. 220)

From this definition, LD became inextricably tied to the notion of achievement–aptitude discrepancy.

The federal government soon became interested in the field of LD and sponsored a project titled "Minimal Brain Dysfunction: National Project on LD in Children." The project was staffed by three task forces, two of which focused primarily on defining LD. Interestingly, the two task forces were of markedly different constitution and thus produced remarkably different definitions. Task Force I was composed of medical professionals who elected to define the term "minimal brain dysfunction." This disorder affected

children of near average, average, or above average general intelligence with certain learning

or behavior disabilities ranging from mild to severe, which are associated with deviations of function of the central nervous system. These deviations may manifest themselves by various combinations of impairment in perception, conceptualization, language, memory, and control of attention or motor function . . .

These aberrations may arise from genetic variations, biochemical irregularities, perinatal brain insults or other illnesses or injuries sustained during the years which are critical for the development and maturation of the central nervous system, or from unknown causes. (Clements, 1966, pp. 9–10)

Task Force II was composed of educators who sought to create an alternative definition to that proposed by Task Force I. Unable to reach consensus on a single definition, they put forth two. The first stressed Kirk's earlier notion of intraindividual differences. Children with LD were thus

those (1) who have educationally significant discrepancies among their sensory-motor, perceptual, cognitive, academic, or related developmental levels which interfere with the performance of educational tasks; (2) who may or may not show demonstrable deviation in central nervous system functioning; and (3) whose disabilities are not secondary to general mental retardation, sensory deprivation, or serious emotional disturbance. (Haring & Bateman, 1969, pp. 2–3)

The second definition brought forward Monroe and Bateman's concept of discrepancy. It stated:

Children with LD are those (1) who manifest an educationally significant discrepancy between estimated academic potential and actual level of academic functioning as related to dysfunctioning (sic) in the learning process; (2) may or may not show demonstrable deviation in central nervous system functioning; and (3) whose disabilities are not secondary to general mental retardation, cultural, sensory, and/or educational deprivation or environmentally produced serious emotional disturbance. (Haring & Bateman, 1969, p. 3)

As these two task forces were attempting to name and define the construct that is LD, the Education of the Handicapped Act was signed into law. Contrary to the wishes of many parents and despite the progress of the field, the 1966 Education of the Handicapped Act did not extend federal assistance and protection to students with LD. Although many parent groups advocated for their children and exerted pressure on federal policymakers, parents of children with more traditional disabilities held more political sway (E. Martin, personal communication, January 2001). These parents were concerned that the reallocation of limited resources would mean fewer services for their children. They argued that children with LD were already served through programs such as Title I. Interestingly, similar arguments were also heard in 2001 as policymakers attempted to revamp the field of LD (Fletcher, 2001).

In 1968, *The First Annual Report of the National Advisory Committee on Handicapped Children* was published. The U.S. Office of Education formed and charged this committee with writing a report and definition of LD that could be used to set policy and secure funding. This committee was chaired by Kirk and hence offered a definition similar to the definition Kirk published in his 1962 textbook. The definition read:

Children with special (specific) LD exhibit a disorder in one or more of the basic psychological processes involved in understanding or in using spoken and written language. These may be manifested in disorders of listening, thinking, talking, reading, writing, spelling, or arithmetic. They include conditions which have been referred to as perceptual handicaps, brain injury, minimal brain dysfunction, dyslexia, developmental aphasia, etc. They do not include learning problems that are due primarily to visual, hearing or motor handicaps, to mental retardation, emotional disturbance, or to environmental disadvantage. (U.S. Office of Education, 1968, p. 34)

Following this report and the formation of the first major professional organization—the Division for Children with LD (DCLD) of the Council for Exceptional Children—Congress passed the Children with Specific LD Act. Neither this act nor Public Law (PL) 91-230 made LD a formal category; however, Part G of the law permitted the U.S. Office of Education to award discretionary grants to support teacher education, research, and model service delivery programs in LD (Martin, 1987).

Like many of his predecessors, Newell Kephart worked at the Wayne County Training School. Kephart (1960, 1971) proposed the idea of a "perceptual–motor match." This theory held that motor development preceded visual development and kinesthetic sensations resulting from motor movement provide feedback; therefore, motor training should precede visual perceptual training. Beyond this, Kephart also asserted that laterality, the ability to discriminate left from right on one's body, precedes the ability to discriminate left from right in space. He therefore recommended remediating the reversal errors of poor readers through training in laterality.

Like Kephart, several other researchers focused their attentions on visual and visual–motor disabilities. Gerald Getman, an optometrist, published a manual of training activities that focused on general coordination, balance, eye–hand coordination, eye movements, form perception and visual memory (Getman, Kane, Halgren, & McKee, 1964). Also during this period, Marianne Frostig developed a pencil-and-paper test, *The Marianne Frostig Developmental Test of Visual Perception*, assessing eye–motor coordination, figure–ground visual perception, form constancy, position in space, and spatial relations (Frostig, Lefever, & Whittlesey, 1964). Raymond Barsch created the "Movigenic Curriculum" (Barsch, 1967) in which he attempted to train students for efficient movement in the environment, and Glen Doman and Carl Delacato attempted to program "neurological organization" in children with brain injury (Delacato, 1959, 1963, 1966). Among other things, Doman and Delacato advocated limiting children's use of one side of their body in order to promote unilaterality. They believed that mixed dominance was a sign of brain injury and a cause of reading disabilities. Although these programs enjoyed brief periods of popularity, they were eventually criticized and dismissed. The Doman–Delacato program, in particular, came under heavy fire from critics (Hallahan & Cruickshank, 1973; Robbins & Glass, 1969). Hence, the Emergent Period produced many real contributions to the field of LD, but it also yielded quite a few follies (Weiderholt, 1974).

Before moving to the next period, we briefly discuss another important figure from the Emergent Period: Helmer Mykle-bust. Whereas many during this period were pursuing lines of research focused on visual and visual–motor development, Myklebust focused on language development. In work-ing with deaf children, Helmer Myklebust encountered children with normal hearing acuity and poor auditory comprehension. In attempting to explain this phenomenon, Myklebust proposed that these students and others with LD had difficulty in interneu-rosensory learning. Doris Johnson was criti-cal in helping Mykelbust translate his ideas to classroom practices. Together, they advo-cated instructional programming in which (1) training in comprehension preceded training in expression, (2) whole words and sentences were trained to the exclusion of nonsense words and individual sounds, and (3) training in phonetically dissimilar words preceded training in words that are similar (Johnson & Myklebust, 1967).

Like Monroe and Bateman, Myklebust found it useful to consider a student's ability compared with his or her achievement level. He introduced the idea of a "learning quo-tient," consisting of expected potential com-pared with realized potential. Expected po-tential was the average of mental age (the higher of verbal and nonverbal mental age), life age, and grade age (included to reflect opportunity for school learning). Realized potential was taken from scores on stan-dardized achievement tests.

Solidification Period (c. 1975–1985)

According to Hallahan and Mercer (2001), from 1975 to 1985 the field of LD entered a period of calm that foreshadowed a later pe-riod of turbulence. In these years the field so-lidified both the definition and federal regu-lations for identifying students with LD. In addition, researchers, for the most part, abandoned the follies of the past and focused on empirically validated applied research. Although there was some turmoil related to professional organizations, this upheaval was brief and limited in scope and effect.

Definition and Federal Regulations

In 1975, Gerald Ford signed EAHCA into law. This law required school districts to

provide free and appropriate educations to all of their students, including students with LD. As EAHCA reached full implementa-tion in 1977, the U.S. Office of Education put forth a definition of LD. This definition was essentially the same one proposed by National Advisory Committee on Handi-capping Conditions (NACHC) in 1968 and remains, with minor changes, the same defi-nition used today. It read:

> The term "specific learning disability" means a disorder in one or more of the psychological processes involved in understanding or in us-ing language, spoken or written, which may manifest itself in an imperfect ability to listen, speak, read, write, spell, or to do mathemati-cal calculations. The term does not include children who have LD which are primarily the result of visual, hearing, or motor handicaps, or mental retardation, or emotional distur-bance, or of environmental, cultural, or eco-nomic disadvantage. (U.S. Office of Educa-tion, 1977, p. 65083)

In addition to this definition, the U.S. Of-fice of Education also proposed a formula that could be used by individual states to identify students with LD, but because of negative public response, this discrepancy formula was not included. However, the U.S. Office of Education's regulations did retain the general idea of the need for a se-vere discrepancy between achievement and intellectual ability for identification as learning disabled.

In opposition to the definition used in EAHCA, the National Joint Committee on LD (NJCLD), a body consisting of several professional organizations and the ACLD, proposed a definition that did not include a psychological process clause. By intentional-ly excluding this clause, the NJCLD dis-tanced itself from the perceptual and per-ceptual–motor training programs of its not so distant past. This definition stated:

> LD is a generic term that refers to a heteroge-neous group of disorders manifested by signif-icant difficulties in the acquisition and use of listening, speaking, reading, writing, reason-ing or mathematical abilities. These disorders are intrinsic to the individual and presumed to be due to central nervous system dysfunction. Even though a LD may occur concomitantly with other handicapping conditions (e.g., sen-sory impairment, mental retardation, social

and emotional disturbance) or environmental influences (e.g., cultural differences, insufficient-inappropriate instruction, psychogenic factors), it is not the direct result of those conditions or influences. (Hammill, Leigh, McNutt, & Larsen, 1981, p. 336)

Shortly after EAHCA had reached full implementation, the U.S. Office of Education funded five centers for applied research in LD. Dale Bryant directed the Columbia University center and his colleagues carried out research in memory and study skills, arithmetic, basic reading and spelling, the interaction of readers and texts, and reading comprehension. At the University of Illinois at Chicago, Tanis Bryan led research in social competence and attributions regarding success and failure, and at the University of Kansas, Donald Deshler directed research in educational interventions for adolescents with LD. James Ysseldyke directed the institute at the University of Minnesota. These researchers addressed the decision-making process used to identify students with LD. At the University of Virginia, Dan Hallahan directed research on children with LD who have attention problems, and John Lloyd led research on metacognitive strategies directly used in completing academic tasks.

Turbulent Period (c. 1985–2000)

In his 1974 historical review of the field of LD, Weiderholt wrote: "Despite [the] rapid growth during the 1960s and '70s, or perhaps because of it, the LD field is currently confronted with several major problems. These include problems of definition, territorial rights, and an adequate data base" (p. 43). These problems that Weiderholt identified continued and intensified in the following years. If the Solidification Period represented the calm before the storm, the Turbulent Period was the storm. Between the publication of Weiderholt's history and the 1998–1999 school year, the number of students identified as having LD doubled. Currently more than 2.8 million students are identified as having LD (U.S. Department of Education, 2000). This rapid increase in the size of the population with LD escalated the level of intensity regarding issues that were once noncontroversial or unrecognizable in the Solidification Period.

Throughout this period, professional and government organizations continued to put forward definitions of LD with the intent at arriving at some form of consensus within the field. In 1986, the ACLD (now the LD Association of America) proposed a definition of LD in which the authors stressed the chronic and lifelong nature of the condition as well as the potential effects disabilities may have on "self-esteem, education, vocation, socialization, and/or daily living activities" (Association for Children with LD, 1986, p. 15). This definition was unique in that it lacked an exclusion clause. A year later, the Interagency Committee on LD (ICLD; 1987) proposed a definition similar to that of the NJCLD, except for two points. The committee included social skills deficits as a type of LD and listed attention-deficit disorder as a potential comorbid disorder with LD. In 1988, the NJCLD revised its definition. This revision yielded a definition consistent with the lifelong nature of LD found in the Learning Disabilities Association of America (LDA) definition and discordant with the social skills deficit as LD found in the LDA and ICLD definitions. The definition read:

> LD is a general term that refers to a heterogeneous group of disorders manifested by significant difficulties in the acquisition and use of listening, speaking, reading, writing, reasoning, or mathematical abilities. These disorders are intrinsic to the individual, presumed to be due to central nervous system dysfunction, and may occur across the life span. Problems of self regulatory behaviors, social perception, and social interaction may exist with LD but do not by themselves constitute a LD. Although LD may occur concomitantly with other handicapping conditions (for example, sensory impairment, mental retardation, serious emotional disturbance) or with extrinsic influences (such as cultural differences, insufficient or inappropriate instruction), they are not the result of those conditions or influences. (National Joint Committee on LD, 1988, p. 1)

Despite the varied definitions that were put forth between 1975 and 1997, the reauthorization of the Individuals with Disabilities Education Act (IDEA) included essentially the same definition found in the 1975 EAHCA. Thus, despite all the progress the field had made in those 22 years, the federal regulations authorizing special education for students with LD clung to an understanding that had in fact been proposed by Kirk as early as 1962.

The pursuit of applied research that began in the Solidification Period continued through the Turbulent Period. Much of this effort grew out of the research begun at the five institutes (Hallahan & Mercer, 2001). Investigations focused on deficits in cognition, metacognition, social skills, and attributions in students with LD. In addition, training regimens for the remediation of these deficits, as well as curriculum-based assessment, all emanated from the earlier research programs of the institutes.

In addition to the research carried out by the institutes established in the Solidification Period, research in phonological processing became a focus in the Turbulent Period. Researchers found that phonological awareness, the ability to identify and manipulate the units of sound in our spoken language, to be one of the most powerful predictors of later reading skill (National Reading Panel, 2000). Moreover, reading researchers have come to view phonological awareness as a component part of effective reading remediation. Lyon (1998) stated: "We have learned that for 90% to 95% of poor readers, prevention and early intervention programs that combine instruction in phoneme awareness, phonics, fluency development, and reading comprehension strategies, provided by well trained teachers, can increase reading skills to average reading levels" (p. 9). The recognized importance of phonological awareness has even led to change in the way researchers define dyslexia. Dyslexia is now believed to be a disability "reflecting insufficient phonological processing abilities" (Lyon, 1995, p. 9).

The research of the Turbulent Period has also produced evidence supporting a biological basis for LD. Albert Galaburda and Norman Geschwind conducted postmortem studies in which they found differences in the size of the planum temporale between dyslexics and nondyslexics (Galaburda, Menard, & Rosen, 1994; Galaburda, Sherman, Rosen, Aboitiz, & Geshwind, 1985; Geschwind & Levitsky, 1968; Humphreys, Kaufman, & Galaburda, 1990). Neuroimaging studies have revealed that the left hemisphere of the brain seems to show ab-

normal functioning in individuals with dyslexia (Joseph, Noble, & Eden, 2001). In addition, researchers have found a high degree of heritability for reading disability and speech and language disorders (Wood & Grigorenko, 2001).

Although the research conducted in the Turbulent Period has answered many questions, this research has also highlighted some pressing problems within the field. Foremost among these problems seems to be the utility of the discrepancy formula in identifying students with LD. The notion of using a discrepancy between ability and achievement, first proposed by Monroe and later advocated by Bateman and Myklebust, was adopted by most states as part of their identification process (Frankenberger & Fronzaglio, 1991). Critics have argued that this formula does not reliably identify students with LD (Fletcher et al., 2001; Vellutino, Scanlon, & Lyon, 2000). Furthermore, students with and without discrepancies do not significantly differ on measures of phonological awareness, orthographic coding, short-term memory, and word retrieval (Fletcher et al., 2001). Researchers are therefore pursuing alternatives to the discrepancy based identification procedure. These alternatives include phonological assessments (Torgesen, 2001; Torgesen & Wagner, 1998) and treatment validity approaches (Fuchs & Fuchs, 1998; Gresham, 2001).

Another issue of urgency is the disproportionate representation of some ethnic groups in the LD category. Although the degree of disproportion is not as great as for some other categories, such as mental retardation or behavior disorders, African Americans are slightly overrepresented in the LD category—18.3 percent of students ages 6 to 21 in the LD category are African American whereas 14.8 percent of the resident population ages 6 to 21 are African American. And American Indians are even more disproportionately represented in the LD category—1.3% of students ages 6 to 21 in the LD category are American Indians whereas 1.0% of the resident population 6 to 21 are American Indians (U.S. Department of Education, 2000).

The fact that disproportionate representation in the LD category is not a major issue for the aggregated data from across the

United States should not blind us to the fact that both African American and Hispanic students are disproportionately identified as LD in some states: "The nationally aggregated data have been interpreted to suggest no overrepresentation of either black or Hispanic students in LD. But state-level data tell a more complex story. . . . Clearly there is overrepresentation for these two minorities in the LD category *in some states*" (National Research Council, 2002, p. 67).

In addition, professionals inside and outside the field are wrestling with the issue of placement options for students in special education. Sparked by the regular education initiative (REI) proposed by Madeleine C. Will (1986), the former Assistant Secretary of Education, the controversial debate pitting full inclusion against a continuum of placement options continues to divide and define the field of LD.

Finally, the field is also wrestling with the debate between modernism and postmodernism. Proponents of postmodernism view disability as a social construction based on incorrect, immoral assumptions regarding difference. They seek to create a caring society that values and accepts differences of any kind. Eschewing the need to pursue objective validation of teaching methods, postmodernism's "main effect has been to reassure aspiring cultural critics that they can play a significant role in the treatment of disabilities without having to do anything so tiresome as, for instance, work directly with children to obtain the relevant data necessary to help them become more *functionally* independent" (Sasso, 2001, p. 190). Modernists, however, subscribe to a medical model that places the locus of disability within the individual. Furthermore, they look to empirical research to validate teaching practices. Teachers, therefore, use research-based instructional techniques to enhance learner functioning and reduce differences.

The questions facing the field of LD are many and varied. Some of the answers to these questions may prove to be true "contributions" to the field. Others may only be the follies against which Weiderholt warned. The future of the field of LD seems to hinge on this very issue: Will we choose contributions, or will we choose follies? Fortunately, we need not make this choice blindly. Although it is difficult to predict what the future will bring, we do have our past, our rich and varied history. This history will direct our future. It is our point of reference and our guide (Weiderholt, 1974), and this history has shown us, time and again, that that which endures is based on solid, empirical underpinnings.

References

Adams, M. J. (1990). *Beginning to read: Thinking and learning about print.* Cambridge, MA: MIT Press.

Anderson, P. L., & Meier-Hedde, R. (2001). Early case reports of dyslexia in the United States and Europe. *Journal of Learning Disabilities, 34,* 9–21.

Association for Children with LD. (1986). ACLD definition: Specific learning disabilities. *ACLD Newsbriefs,* 15–16.

Barsch, R. H. (1967). *Achieving perceptual–motor efficiency: A space-oriented approach to learning.* Seattle, WA: Special Child Publications.

Bateman, B. (1965). An educational view of a diagnostic approach to learning disorders. In J. Hellmuth (Ed.), *Learning disorders* (Vol. 1, pp. 219–239). Seattle, WA: Special Child Publications.

Berlin, R. (1884). Uber dyslexie [About dyslexia]. *Archiv fur Psychiatrie, 15,* 276–278.

Berlin, R. (1887). *Eine besondere art der wortblindheit [A specific kind of word blindness].* Wiesbaden, Germany: J. F. Bergman.

Broadbent, W. H. (1872). On the cerebral mechanism of speech and thought. *Proceedings of the Royal Medical and Chirurgical Society of London, 4,* 24–29.

Broca, P. P. (1861). Remarques sur le siège de la faculté du langage articulé, suivies d'une observation d'amphemie (perte de la parole) [Remarks on the seat of the faculty of articulate language, followed by an observation of aphemia]. *Bulletin de la Société Anatomique, 36,* 330–357.

Clements, S. D. (1966). Minimal brain dysfunction in children: Terminology and identification: Phase one of a three-phase project. *NINDS Monographs, 9* (Public Health Service Bulletin No. 1415). Washington, DC: U.S. Department of Health, Education and Welfare.

Cruickshank, W. M., Bentzen, F. A., Ratzeburg, F. H., & Tannhauser, M. T. (1961). *A teaching method of brain-injured and hyperactive children.* Syracuse, NY: Syracuse University Press.

Delacato, C. H. (1959). *The treatment and prevention of reading problems: The neurological approach.* Springfield, IL: Charles C Thomas.

Delacato, C. H. (1963). *The diagnosis and treatment of speech and reading problems.* Springfield, IL: Charles C Thomas.

Delacato, C. H. (1966). *Neurological organization and reading.* Springfield, IL: Charles C Thomas.

Engelmann, S. (1967). Relationship between psychological theories and the act of teaching. *Journal of School Psychology, 5,* 92–100.

Fernald, G. M. (1943). *Remedial techniques in basic school subjects.* New York: McGraw-Hill.

Fernald, G. M., & Keller, H. (1921). The effect of kinaesthetic factors in the development of word recognition in the case of non-readers. *Journal of Educational Research, 4,* 355–377.

Fletcher, J. M., Lyon, G. R., Barnes, M., Stuebing, K. K., Francis, D. J., Olson, R. K., Shaywitz, S. E., & Shaywitz, B. A. (2001, August). *Classification of LD: An evidence-based evaluation.* Paper presented at the LD Summit, U.S. Department of Education, Washington, DC.

Fletcher, M. A. (2001, October 5). Overhaul planned for special education: Administration decries U.S. law. *The Washington Post,* p. A3.

Frankenberger, W., & Franzaglio, K. (1991). A review of states' criteria for identifying children with LD. *Journal of Learning Disabilities, 24,* 495–500.

Frostig, M., Lefever, D. W., & Whittlesey, J. R. B. (1964). *The Marianne Frostig Developmental Test of Visual Perception.* Palo Alto, CA: Consulting Psychology Press.

Fuchs, L. S., & Fuchs, D. (1998). Treatment validity: A unifying concept for reconceptualizing the identification of LD. *Learning Disabilities Research and Practice, 13,* 204–219.

Galaburda, A. M., Menard, M. T., & Rosen, G. D. (1994). Evidence for aberrant auditory anatomy in developmental dyslexia. *Proceedings of the National Academy of Science USA, 91,* 8010–8013.

Galaburda, A. M., Sherman, G. F., Rosen, G. D., Aboitiz, F., & Geschwind, N. (1985). Developmental dyslexia: Four consecutive patients with cortical anomalies. *Annals of Neurology, 18,* 222–233.

Gall, F. J., & Spurzheim, J. C. (1809). *Reserches sur le système nerveux en général, et sur celui du cerveau en particulier [Studies on the nervous system, with particular attention to the brain].* Paris: Schoell.

Geschwind, N., & Levitsky, W. (1968). Human brain: Left–right asymmetries in temporal speech. *Science, 161,* 186–187.

Getman, G. N., Kane, E. R., Halgren, M. R., & McKee, G. W. (1964). *The physiology of readiness, an action program for the development of perception for children.* Minneapolis, MN: Programs to Accelerate School Success.

Gillingham, A., & Stillman, B. W. (1936). *Remedial work for reading, spelling, and penmanship.* New York: Sachett & Wilhelms.

Goldstein, K. (1936). The modification of behavior consequent to cerebral lesions. *Psychiatric Quarterly, 10,* 586–610.

Goldstein, K. (1939). *The organism.* New York: American Book.

Gresham, F. (2001, August). *Reponsiveness to intervention: An alternative approach to the identification of LD.* Paper presented at the LD Summit, U.S. Department of Education, Washington, DC.

Hallahan, D. P., & Cruickshank, W. M. (1973). *Psychoeducational foundations of learning disabilities.* Englewood Cliffs, NJ: Prentice-Hall.

Hallahan, D. P., & Mercer, C. D. (2001, August). *LD: Historical perspectives.* Paper presented at the LD Summit, U.S. Department of Education, Washington, DC.

Hammill, D. D., & Larsen, S. C. (1974). The effectiveness of psycholinguistic training. *Exceptional Children, 41,* 514.

Hammill, D. D., Leigh, J. E., McNutt, G., & Larsen, S. C. (1981). A new definition of learning disabilities. *Learning Disability Quarterly, 4,* 336–342.

Haring, N. G., & Bateman, B. (1969). Introduction. In N. G. Haring (Ed.), *Minimal brain dysfunction in children: Educational, medical, and health related services* (pp. 1–4). Washington, DC: U.S. Department of Health, Education, and Welfare.

Head, H. (1926). *Aphasia and kindred disorders of speech.* London: Cambridge University Press.

Hinshelwood, J. (1895). Word-blindness and visual memory. *Lancet, 2,* 1564–1570.

Hinshelwood, J. (1917). *Congenital word-blindness.* London: H. K. Lewis.

Humphreys, P., Kaufmann, W. E., & Galaburda, A. M. (1990). Developmental dyslexia in women: Neuropathological findings in three patients. *Annals of Neurology, 28,* 727–738.

Interagency Committee on LD. (1987). *LD: A report to Congress.* Bethesda, MD: National Institutes of Health.

Johnson, D. J., & Myklebust, H. R. (1967). *LD: Educational principles and practices.* New York: Grune & Stratton.

Joseph, J., Noble, K., & Eden, G. (2001). The neurobiological basis of reading. *Journal of Learning Disabilities, 34,* 566–579.

Kephart, N. C. (1960). *Slow learner in the classroom.* Columbus, OH: Merrill.

Kephart, N. C. (1971). *Slow learner in the classroom* (2nd ed.). Columbus, OH: Merrill.

Kirk, S. A. (1935). Hemispheric cerebral dominance and hemispheric equipotentiality. In Anonymous, *Comparative Psychology Monographs.* Baltimore: Johns Hopkins Press.

Kirk, S. A. (1936). Extrastriate functions in the discrimination of complex visual patterns. *Journal of Comparative Psychology, 21,* 145–159.

Kirk, S. A. (1962). *Educating exceptional children.* Boston: Houghton Mifflin.

Kirk, S. A., McCarthy, J. J., & Kirk, W. D. (1961). *Illinois Test of Psycholinguistic Abilities* (Experimental ed.). Urbana: University of Illinois Press.

Kussmaul, A. (1877). Word deafness and word blindness. In H. von Ziemssen & J. A. T. McCreery (Eds.), *Cyclopedia of the practice of medicine* (pp. 770–778). New York: William Wood.

Lerner, J. W. (2000). *LD: Theories, diagnosis, and teaching strategies* (8th ed.). Boston: Houghton Mifflin.

Lyon, G. R. (1995). Toward a definition of dyslexia. *Annals of Dyslexia, 45,* 3–27.

Lyon, G. R. (1998). *Overview of reading and litera-*

cy initiatives (Report to Committee on Labor and Human Resources, U.S. Senate). Bethesda, MD: National Institute of Child Health and Human Development, National Institutes of Health.

Mann, L. (1971). Psychometric phrenology and the new faculty psychology. *Journal of Special Education, 5*, 3–14.

Martin, E. W. (1987). Developmental variation and dysfunction: Observations on labeling, public policy, and individualization of instruction. In M. D. Levine & P. Satz (Eds.), *Middle childhood: Development and dysfunction* (pp. 435–445). Baltimore: University Park Press.

Mercer, C. D. (1997). *Students with LD* (5th ed.). Upper Saddle River, NJ: Merrill.

Monroe, M. (1932). *Children who cannot read.* Chicago: University of Chicago Press.

Morgan, W. P. (1896). A case of congenital word blindness. *British Medical Journal, 2*, 1378.

National Joint Committee on LD. (1988). *Letter to NJCLD Member Organizations.* Washington, DC: Author.

National Reading Panel. (2000, April). *Report of the National Reading Panel: Teaching children to read* (NIH Publication No. 00–4654). Bethesda, MD: National Institute of Child Health and Human Development, National Institutes of Health.

National Research Council. (2002). *Minority students in special and gifted education.* (M. S. Donovan & C. T. Cross, Eds.). Washington, DC: National Academy Press.

Orton, S. T. (1937). *Reading, writing, and speech problems in children.* New York: W. W. Norton.

Orton, S. T. (1939). A neurological explanation of the reading disability. *The Educational Record, 20*(Suppl. 12), 58–68.

Robbins, M., & Glass, G. V. (1969). The Doman–Delacato rationale: A critical analysis. In J. Hellmuth (Ed.), *Educational therapy* (Vol. II, pp. 321–377). Seattle, WA: Special Child Publications.

Sarason, S. B. (1949). *Psychological problems in mental deficiency.* New York: Harper.

Sasso, G. M. (2001). The retreat from inquiry and knowledge in special education. *Journal of Special Education, 34*, 178–193.

Siegel, L. S. (1989). IQ is irrelevant to the definition of LD. *Journal of Learning Disabilities, 22*, 469–486.

Strauss, A. A., & Kephart, N. C. (1939). *Rate of mental growth in a constant environment among higher grade moron and borderline children.* Paper presented at American Association of Mental Deficiencies.

Strauss, A. A., & Kephart, N. C. (1955). *Psychopathology and education of the brain-injured child, Vol. II: Progress in theory and clinic.* New York: Grune & Stratton.

Strauss, A. A., & Lehtinen, L. E. (1947). *Psychopathology and education of the brain-injured child.* New York: Grune and Stratton.

Torgesen, J. K. (2001, August). *Empirical and theoretical support for direct diagnosis of LD by as-sessment of intrinsic processing weaknesses.* Paper presented at the LD Summit, U.S. Department of Education, Washington, DC.

Torgesen, J. K., & Wagner, R. K. (1998). Alternative diagnostic approaches for specific developmental reading disabilities. *Learning Disabilities Research and Practice, 13*, 220–232.

U.S. Department of Education. (2000). *Twenty-second annual report to Congress on the implementation of the Individuals with Disabilities Education Act.* Washington, DC: Author.

U.S. Office of Education. (1968). *The first annual report of National Advisory Committee on Handicapped Children.* Washington, DC: U.S. Department of Health, Education and Welfare.

U.S. Office of Education. (1977). Assistance to states for education of handicapped children: Procedures for evaluating specific LD. *Federal Register, 42*(250), 65082- 65085.

Vellutino, F. R., Scanlon, D. M., & Lyon, G. R. (2000). Differentiating between difficult-to-remediate and readily remediated poor readers: More evidence against the IQ-achievement discrepancy definition of reading disability. *Journal of Learning Disabilities, 33*, 223–238.

Werner, H. (1937, May). Process and achievement: A basic problem of education and developmental psychology. *Harvard Educational Review,* pp. 353–368.

Werner, H., & Strauss, A. A. (1939a). Problems and methods of functional analysis in mentally deficient children. *Journal of Abnormal and Social Psychology, 34*, 37–62.

Werner, H., & Strauss, A. A. (1939b). Types of visuo-motor activity in their relation to low and high performance ages. *Proceedings of the American Association on Mental Deficiency, 44*, 163–168.

Werner, H., & Strauss, A. A. (1940). Causal factors in low performance. *American Journal of Mental Deficiency, 45*, 213–218.

Werner, H., & Strauss, A. A. (1941). Pathology of figure-background relation in the child. *Journal of Abnormal and Social Psychology, 36*, 236–248.

Wernicke, C. (1874). *Der aphasische symptomenkomplex.* Breslau, Poland: Cohn & Weigert.

Wiederholt, J. L. (1974). Historical perspectives on the education of the learning disabled. In L. Mann & D. Sabatino (Eds.), *The second review of special education* (pp. 103–152). Philadelphia: JSE Press.

Will, M. C. (1986). Educating children with learning problems: A shared responsibility. *Exceptional Children, 52*, 411–415.

Wood, F. B., & Grigorenko, E. L. (2001). Emerging issues in the genetics of dyslexia: A methodological review. *Journal of Learning Disabilities, 34*, 503–511.

Ysseldyke, J. E., & Salvia, J. A. (1974). Diagnostic prescriptive teaching: Two models. *Exceptional Children, 41*, 181–186.

3

Classification and Definition of Learning Disabilities: An Integrative Perspective

Jack M. Fletcher
Robin D. Morris
G. Reid Lyon

This chapter addresses research on the classification, definition, and identification of learning disabilities (LD), and implications for public policy. For the past 20 years, we have been addressing issues related to the classification and definition of LD (Fletcher, Lyon, et al., 2002; Fletcher & Morris, 1986; Lyon et al., 2001; Morris, 1988; Morris, Satz, & Blashfield, 1981). We have attempted to identify classification as a central issue in LD research, showing that the results of any given study depend greatly on the underlying classification of LD. The classification model chosen leads to definitions of LD and related disorders that, in turn, influence the methods used for its identification. How children are identified as having LD has significant influence on the results of any study.

Historically, LD has existed as a disorder that was difficult to define. Implicit classifications viewed LD as "unexpected" underachievement. The primary approach to identification involved a search for intraindividual variability as a marker for the "unexpectedness" of LD, along with an emphasis on the exclusion of other causes of underachievement that would be "expected" to produce underachievement (Lyon et

al., 2001). In 1977, recommendations for operationalizing the federal definition of LD were provide to states after passage of Public Law (PL) 94-142 to help identify children in this category of special education (U.S. Office of Education, 1977). In these regulations, LD was defined as a heterogeneous group of disorders with a common marker of intraindividual variability, (i.e., "unexpectedness"), representing a discrepancy between IQ and achievement. Unexpectedness was also indicated by exclusionary criteria, such as sensory disorders, socioeconomic disadvantage, inadequate instruction, and emotional-behavioral disorders that presumably lead to "expected" underachievement.

Implementation of this model and its focus on intraindividual differences in public policy have led to an industry that dominates identification procedures in schools. This industry develops IQ and achievement tests, produces research on the best way to measure discrepancy, and trains a large cadre of personnel who give these tests and help ensure compliance with procedural guidelines adopted by states. As states vary considerably in how the federal definition is operationalized, and schools in how identification methods are implemented and interpreted, there is substantial variability in which students are served in special education as learning disabled across schools, districts, and states (MacMillan & Siperstein, 2002; Mercer, Jordan, Allsop, & Mercer, 1996).

Classification research over the past 10 to 15 years has provided little evidence that IQ discrepancy demarcates a specific type of LD that differs from other forms of underachievement (Fletcher, Lyon, et al., 2002). This research has also questioned the classification validity of most proposed exclusionary criteria, noting little evidence that children with "expected" forms of achievement differ from those with "unexpected" underachievement beyond the identification criteria (Lyon et al., 2001). Although the case against IQ discrepancy and exclusion is strongest for word-level reading disabilities, enough research has been completed on the underlying psychometric model to cast doubt on applications to other forms of LD in reading, math, and written expression (Stuebing et al., 2002).

Other research, especially in reading, has shown that LD appears dimensional, not categorical, and has not been able to produce markers that qualitatively distinguish different forms of LD from other forms of underachievement (Shaywitz, Escobar, Shaywitz, Fletcher, & Makuch, 1992). In word-level reading disabilities, for example, a major determinant of reading ability is clearly phonological processing, which distinguishes word-level reading disability (RD) from other forms of LD and from typically achieving readers, but only on a quantitative basis (Liberman, Shankweiler, & Liberman, 1989; Share & Stanovich, 1995; Vellutino, Scanlon, & Fletcher, 2002). Greater severity of phonological processing deficits produces more severe reading difficulties, but strengths in phonological processing also produce better reading. Normal variability on a continuum is also consistent with genetic research on word-level RD, where RD is strongly heritable (Grigorenko, 2001; Olson, Forsberg, Gayan, & DeFries, 1999). However, the same genetic susceptibilities that lead to poor reading also account for proficiency in reading (Gilger, 2002). Given the accumulation of knowledge about word-level RD, the most common form of LD, how can it be described as "unexpected?"

Intraindividual Differences versus Problem-Solving Models

In response to these findings, two models have emerged, both of which are represented as competing policy recommendations for LD and other high-incidence disorders identified in the Individuals with Disabilities Education Act (IDEA). The first involves individual differences and focuses on within child ability discrepancies as the basis for LD (Kavale & Forness, 2000). The second, commonly referred to as the problem-solving model (Reschly, Tilly, & Grimes, 1999), is an outcomes-oriented approach in which the child's response to instruction is paramount. The former is a child attribute model focused toward organismic hypotheses regarding the nature of LD, whereas the latter is more oriented toward the context in which the child learns, focused as it is on instruction. However, from a classification perspective, the two models are more similar than different, as we describe herein. Both models are best conceptualized as dimensional, retain the concept of "unexpectedness," are based on the notion of discrepancy, do not rely on policy-based special education categories, focus on specific academic behaviors, and have as a goal the development of effective interventions. Moreover, although the models identify children as LD based on different attributes, the measurement issues are virtually identical. Both involve ability–expectancy discrepancies and rely on individual differences for treatment implementation. The next section describes each model in turn. We then highlight the similarities and differences from a classification perspective and provide three examples derived largely from the intraindividual differences model (IQ discrepancy, subtypes, aptitude by treatment interventions), to illustrate the convergence of the two models.

Intraindividual Differences Model

The essence of this model was clearly specified in a recent consensus paper from 10 major groups interested in LD organized by the National Center for Learning Disabilities (NCLD) and the Office of Special Education Programs (2002). This paper notes that "while IQ tests do not measure or predict a student's response to instruction, measures of neuropsychological functioning and information processing could be included in evaluation protocols in ways that document the areas of strength and vulnerability needed to make informed decisions about eligibility for services, or more importantly, what services are needed. An essential characteristic of SLD is failure to achieve at a level of expected performance based upon the student's other abilities" (p. 18).

This statement clearly highlights the role of intraindividual differences as a marker for discrepancy and unexpected underachievement. It also highlights the limitations of IQ–achievement discrepancy as a marker for LD, largely on the basis of lack of relationships with intervention outcomes. As opposed to a single marker such as IQ discrepancy, unexpectedness is operationalized as unevenness in development. The child with LD has strengths in many areas but weaknesses in some core attributes that lead to underachievement. The LD is unexpected as the weaknesses lead to difficulties with achievement and adaptive functions, but not all areas of adaptation. Building on reading research, proponents of this view call for better classifications that more clearly delineate the different profiles associated with LD, help delineate different types of LD, and also differentiate LD from other childhood disorders, such as mental retardation and behavioral disorders such as attention-deficit/hyperactivity disorder (ADHD). This approach leads to definitions based on *inclusionary* criteria and systematic attempts to identify children as having LD based on characteristics that relate to intraindividual differences (Lyon et al., 2001). It relies heavily on norm-referenced assessment.

A major assumption of this model is that better classifications will lead to enhanced treatment of children with LD. The weakness of the model, especially from the perspective of the problem-solving model, is the focus on test scores in isolation of the child's classroom performance (Reschly & Tilley, 1999). The result is more testing of children, reinforcing the model currently in place with new and presumably improved norm-referenced measures. In addition, this trend leaves unanswered the questions of what to do with children who do not achieve adequately who have relatively flat test profiles and, more important, how such approaches lead to better outcomes for children with LD. Of particular concern is the tendency of the intraindividual differences model to focus on behaviors that are not directly related to intervention, such as processing skills (Torgesen, 2002). Both issues are often addressed by attempts to define subtypes of LD based on the hypothesis that more homogeneous groupings lead to improved outcomes through more targeted interventions. But even here, interactions beyond the primary area of difficulty (reading, math) are hard to identify.

Problem-Solving Model

The second model is put forth as a marked departure from historical conceptions of LD and an alternative to the intraindividual differences model. Referred to as a problem-solving model, it is based on the view that what is paramount for LD is how to treat it. Classifications, intraindividual differences, and subtypes are all notions that have not proved beneficial for intervention and are therefore not useful (Rechsly & Tilly, 1999). These notions are viewed as outgrowths of organismic, "medical" models that require knowledge of the cause in order to affect a treatment. Thus, in its extreme version, the problem-solving model is purportedly devoid of theoretical assumptions and classifications. It reflects an empirical approach to the discovery of "what works" and is focused largely on improvements in the behaviors leading to identification.

In implementation, the model is noncategorical, at least regarding special education categories in IDEA. It relies on functional analyses of learning and behavior that are ipsative, not normative. The referent population is typically locally defined. For LD, methods that involve progress monitoring, such as curriculum-based assessment (Fuchs & Fuchs, 1998; Speece & Case, 2001), are major tools for identification.

The problem-solving model implicitly retains the concepts of unexpectedness and discrepancy but bases them on assessments of learning and progress over time. For example, the initial decision regarding whether a child is discrepant from school and/or parent expectations, essential to this model, is a discrepancy classification (Ysseldyke & Marston, 1999). The decision is wrought with the same difficult issues that the more traditional normative classification systems possess. If a child is from a low-performing school, does that mean they are not poor readers if their performance is in line with school expectations? Similarly, if a child is from a high-functioning school, should parental expectations that their child be an outstanding reader represent the basis for such decisions? Even if one uses curriculum-based measurements as an alternative to more traditional norm-referenced psychometric measures, there is always the decision to be made as to whether a child has met, or not met, the specified academic skill or ability level for their group. This is clearly a classification problem because of the need to define the comparison group, the academic skills/abilities to be evaluated, and the criteria for progress.

In the problem-solving model, the progress of children is constantly monitored, and those who do not show adequate development of reading or math receive targeted interventions (Reschley et al., 1999). Identification of the student as having LD is based on failure to respond to intervention, another classification decision that involves explicit criteria for sorting kids into those who respond and do not respond. Such a decision is based on a model of change. Any determination of change requires a baseline postintervention attribute comparison, which is another type of discrepancy model. Thus, in the problem-solving model, decisions are made about who needs interventions and the types of interventions they need. These are clearly decisions that reflect implicit classifications of students, interventions, intervention effectiveness, and how they should be matched. Otherwise all children would receive the same interventions. Anything in between reflects classification, which leads to definitions, and, in turn, identification. The task is always to make explicit the implicit nature of these classifications. When this is done, the models are more similar than different but focus on different characteristics of the same process.

Thus, although it is common to cast these models as opposing views, we take the position that for LD, the two perspectives are actually quite compatible. Whereas the intraindividual difference perspective may lead to excessive testing and a focus on classification that does not consistently optimize identification of children with LD, the problem-solving model is not independent of classification issues, or even the concept of intraindividual differences. This model simply uses a different type of classification approach that produces issues for identification that are not terribly different from those characteristic of the intraindividual-differences model. Moreover, although the problem-solving model assumes null results for subtype by treatment (or aptitude by treatment) interventions, there is clear evidence for such interactions, and these interventions are at the heart of the problem-solving model. If not, why should schools attempt to provide different treatments for children with reading, math, and behavioral difficulties? In an extreme application, why provide any differences in instruction to any child? The key, from our perspective, is that the components of the intraindividual model that are especially viable focus on academic skills and rely less on dimensions involving processing or special education diagnostic categories. But much of the research that shows viability has focused on models relating processes to outcomes and classifications that form groups using explicit, multidimensional criteria based on the relevant dimensions. The groupings facilitate communication but are not necessary for the intraindividual-differences model and do not necessarily require significant normative assessment frameworks.

Differences in Models

In these examples, we are not ignoring the differences in these models and the assumptions they make. A model based intraindividual differences focuses on ability–ability discrepancies, whereas the problem-solving model is based on changes in the same ability over time. The former can be either normative based, or ipsative based, as all decisions are based on individual children, an inherently ipsative process. The latter is typically relative to a behavioral baseline and based on ipsative change, but there are always questions concerning the normative basis for evaluating changes across different education contexts. However, the presumption that ability–ability discrepancies are related to intervention outcomes at the level of processing, a secondary level of analysis, or even neurobiological correlates is at best weakly established and largely reflects relationships with initial status. But that does not mean that such outcomes are not possible, just that past models, particularly those focused on policy-based special education groups, have not been found to be valid. These types of differentiations are also found in the problem-solving model, where expectancy–ability discrepancy is used to identify children who need intervention (Tilly, Reschly, & Grimes, 1999). As Tilly and colleagues (1999) state when defining a discrepancy, "Data collection provides appropriate quantitative and qualitative descriptions of a target behavior and of relevant setting expectations, yielding a quantitative discrepancy between the two" (p. 311). Similarly, they state that "the magnitude of the discrepancy is quantified, based on a comparison between learner performance and local educational demands" (p. 311). The reliance on local norms is a major issue for large-scale implementation and begs the question of why these models eschew norm-referenced achievement tests. Such tests have excellent reliability and validity, providing quick "snapshots" of level of performance.

Another difference may be more historical in nature than reflective of current thinking, which involves Cronbach's (1957) disillusionment with his early statement that "there is some best group of treatments to use and some best allocation of persons to treatment" (p. 680). Tilley and colleagues (1999) suggest that this disillusionment came because the research could not identify interactions between interventions and information-processing modality, neuropsychological profiles, or learning styles and orientations. They do suggest that there was evidence of "prior knowledge" affecting later learning and academic outcomes but do not consider this to be evidence of the type of aptitude by treatment interaction proposed by Cronbach. From the intraindividual-differences model, such findings are

clear markers of the interaction of past biological propensies and environmental experiences and represent a strong case for aptitude by treatment interactions, particularly from an individual-differences orientation.

The perceived incompatibility of these two models ultimately reflects confusion about different levels of classification, the relation of classification and identification, and a failure to recognize that no single classification is suitable for all purposes. In the remainder of this chapter, we briefly review that nature of classification, highlighting differences in classification and identification. We discuss the past 20 years of classification research in the context of models of intraindividual differences, highlighting levels at which subtype by treatment interventions has emerged. We also discuss classification and identification issues from the perspective of problem-solving models, outlining the classification hypotheses implicit in this approach as well as how such models do indeed make use of the concept of intraindividual differences. In the end, we hope to make a case for broader understanding of both perspectives as part of a more integrated understanding of LD with significant implications for public policy.

Nature of Classifications

Classifications are heuristics that facilitate the partitioning of a larger set of entities into smaller, more homogeneous subgroups based on similarities and dissimilarities on a set of defining attributes. When entities are assigned to the subgroups making up the classification, the process is appropriately called identification, representing operationalization of the definitions that emerge from the classification. Diagnosis is the process of applying these operational definitions to these children to decide membership in one or more partitions. Even deciding that a child needs academic interventions is a diagnostic decision and does not imply the necessity of an organismic or medical model. Although we use terminology that describes groupings, the groupings are essentially decisions made about the placement of individuals on a set of correlated dimensions. The decisions are somewhat arbitrary, reflecting measurement error and the fact that the dimensions are correlated. The critical issues are the validity and reliability of the partitions. Valid classifications do not exist solely because partitions can be made. Rather, the partitions making up a valid classification can be differentiated according to attributes (external variables) not used to establish the subgroups. In addition to these validity considerations, good classifications are also reliable (i.e., are not dependent on the method of classification and replicate in other samples) and have adequate coverage (i.e., permit identification of the majority of entities of interest). They also facilitate communication, prediction, and other activities, though different classifications may be better for some than other purposes (Blashfield & Draguns, 1976).

Most endeavors in the social and behavioral sciences, as well as the natural sciences, involve classification. In the behavioral sciences, the underlying classification is often implicit and not recognized. In classification research, classifications are made explicit and treated as hypotheses about the reliability, validity, coverage, and utility of a hypothetical subgrouping of interest. In essence, classification research is concerned with the independent variables present even in single-subject designs that serve to isolate a child, group, or other subdivision for study. Any research study is an evaluation of a set of dependent variables as well as the independent variables that led to the specification of the entities under investigation (Blashfield, 1993; Fletcher, Francis, Rourke, Shaywitz, & Shaywitz, 1993; Morris & Fletcher, 1988; Skinner, 1981).

In research and practice on LD, classification occurs in identifying children as needing intervention, as having LD or typically achieving; as having LD versus being mentally retarded or with ADHD; within LD, as reading versus math impaired. When exclusionary criteria are applied, LD represents a subgroup of "unexpected" underachievement. It is differentiated from expected underachievement due to emotional disturbance, economic disadvantage, cultural and linguistic diversity, and inadequate instruction (Kavale & Forness, 2000). From a classification perspective, these levels of classification represent hypotheses that should be evaluated. Such hypotheses are present in both the intraindividual-differences model and the problem-solving model and can only be evaluated by using variables that are different from those used to establish the classification.

Classification, Definition, and Identification

Many of the issues involving different models for identifying children with LD reflect confusion about the relationship of classification, definition, and identification. The relationship is inherently hierarchical in that the definitions derived from classifications yield criteria for identifying members into the subcomponents making up the classification. Thus, definitions of LD typically derive from an overarching classification of childhood disorders that differentiate LD from mental retardation and various behavior disorders, such as ADHD. This classification yields definitions and criteria based on attributes that distinguish LD from mental retardation and ADHD. These criteria can be used to identify children into different parts of the classification model.

It is pretentious and inaccurate to maintain that any form of identification is independent of an overarching classification. Moreover, when the classification is not explicitly articulated, identification will become fuzzy and lead to unnecessarily heterogeneous groupings. Thus, a major step in the development of identification methods for LD was the dropping of even broader concepts such as minimal brain dysfunction (MBD) and the recognition that MBD consisted of at least two groups of children: those with difficulties primarily in the academic domain (LD) and those with difficulties primarily in the behavioral domain (ADHD) (Satz & Fletcher, 1980). Although there is overlap in which children may be identified into these categories, one hypothesis is that this overlap reflects comorbidity, or the presence of two disorders in the same child (Fletcher, Shaywitz, & Shaywitz, 1999). Another hypothesis is that this overlap represents one disorder with dual attributes. Although some propose that differentiating these disorders is not essential, as in the recent advancement of the notion of atypical brain development as an overarching classification of children with various developmental difficulties (Gilger & Kaplan, 2002), this concept is not very different from the use of MBD as a syndrome encapsulating children with LD and/or ADHD. Knowing that a child is identified with MBD (or with atypical brain development) says little about intervention or prognosis. However, identification with LD or ADHD (or both LD and ADHD) has clear implications for intervention (academic remediation, medication, behavior modification) and prognosis (Fletcher et al., 1999). At this level of classification, there are well-established interactions of subgroup membership, interventions, and outcomes. Would we proceed by putting all children with LD on stimulant medication regardless of the ADHD component or, conversely, using scarce resources to put a child with ADHD and no RD into an intensive phonologically based intervention program?

Classification in Intraindividual Differences and Problem-Solving Models

Regardless of the model, classifications are implicit in any attempt to identify a child as needing academic or behavioral attention, as having LD, or as needing help with reading and/or math. In the intraindividual-difference model, the classification is often made explicit as norm-referenced assessment batteries are completed that presumably measure attributes derived from theoretical links to the achievement problem that, in turn, are derived from the classification that lead to identification into defined subgroups. But the problem-solving model also uses implicit classifications. First, the act of identifying a child as needing attention or as not responding to intervention is an application of a classification model. Similarly, different outcomes are assessed in measuring progress in reading versus math. Assessment of response to intervention for academic and behavioral difficulties is not equivalent. Why would one assess response to a behavioral intervention with a reading outcome? Although different attributes are measured for identification purposes in the intraindividual versus problem-solving models, the underlying methods (and the difficulties implementing them) are identical. The major difference is that the intraindividual model involves discrepancies in *different* abilities typically assessed at the *same* time point, whereas the problem-solving model typically involves the assessment of the *same* abilities at *different* time points. But the measurement issues in determining significant differences between, for example, two abilities are identical to those involved in the assessment of significant changes in the same ability at two time points (Morris, Fletcher, & Francis, 1993). These issues can be understood with a brief discussion of the concept of an ability profile as a representation of similarities and dissimilarities—the essence of classifications.

Ability Profiles: Similarities and Dissimilarities

Both the intraindividual differences model and the problem-solving model involve the assessment of unevenness (similarities and dissimilarities) in ability development. This is clearly apparent in the intraindividual model, where different tests are given to determine achievement and cognitive processing strengths and weaknesses. Thus, differences in IQ and achievement, reading and math, or language and spatial skills can be represented as a profile that displays the strengths and weaknesses of a child (in a clinical evaluation) or group of children (in research), reflecting dimensions on which the child or groups of children are similar and dissimilar.

Profiles vary on multiple dimensions commonly represented as shape (or pattern), elevation (or level), and scatter (or variability). A correlation coefficient, for example, is an index of profile similarity/dissimilarity that is based solely on shape and scatter with no consideration of whether the profiles differ in elevation. Differences in elevation are commonly represented along a severity dimension. An index of similarity such as Cattell's rp or squared Euclidean distance takes into account both shape and elevation when evaluating profiles for similarity and dissimilarity. Two profiles with the same shape could be highly correlated but might be represented at different levels of severity, so that incorporating both dimension of shape and elevation is usually important (Morris & Fletcher, 1988).

In the intraindividual-differences model, variations in attribute profiles are implicitly at the heart of most conceptual models for classifying childhood disorders and the basis for identification. If children were identical, all ability–ability profiles would be flat, consistent with a normative score at the mean of the population, and classification would be irrelevant (Morris et al., 1993). Measurement error introduces variability (scatter) around the mean and will make profiles uneven in shape and different in elevation. These measurement issues also limit the validity of hard and fast cut points for diagnostic cut points as well as whether significant change has occurred with an intervention. For example, a child with a 14-point discrepancy between two correlated abilities is not very different from one with a 7-point difference. Similarly, a child who reads 14 words per minute below expectation (note how expectation must be introduced into the discussion) is not very different from one who reads 7 words per minute below expectation. Determining the discrepancy in outcomes and expectations depends on the reliability of the measure of reading, the number of time points, and the age of the child. We presume that the joint effects of experience and biology combine to increase the variability of ability–ability and ability–time profiles and to an extent that is greater than that induced by measurement error. Much of what happens in research on dependent variables is the determination of the extent to which these variations can be accounted for by introduction of a classification (e.g., comparison of LD and typically achieving groups), with further inferences concerning the basis by which the classification accounts for this variability (instruction, home environment, brain function). A paradox for the intraindividual-differences model is the fact that profiles that reflect reduced elevation but that are relatively flat are produced by the same processes (environment, biology) that produce unevenness. Don't children who are comparably impaired in reading and math have LD? They have essentially greater impairments in language and working memory than children with difficulties only in reading and math. But not calling them learning disabled (unless they fit better in another part of the classification) is a true hall of mirrors.

These children are essentially either more severe or have two disorders. The intraindividual-differences model does not account well for variations in elevation.

In LD (and other dimensional disorders), we emphasize the importance of a multivariate approach (Doehring, 1978; Satz & Fletcher, 1980) at the level of both the dependent and independent variables. At this point in the evolution of scientific research on LD, studies of single variables are not terribly meaningful beyond the pilot phase. For example, research on word-level RD that involves a dependent variable without considering its relationships with phonological awareness or word reading cannot provide a strong explanation of a group difference or correlation of the dependent variable with reading. Similarly, comparing groups of children defined as having LD without specifying the area of academic impairment (e.g., accuracy vs. fluency of single-word reading, math vs. reading vs. both reading and math) or relationships with other disorders (e.g., ADHD) is less meaningful. It will be difficult to establish whether any differences are specific to the basis for grouping or to some other correlated, but not measured, attribute. If we have learned anything from research on LD over the past century, it is that the results of any study depend greatly on how the sample is defined, which ultimately reflects the nature and explicitness of the classification underlying the independent variable in the study. This is true even in single-subject designs as a decision had to be made that the child needed to be the single subject (i.e., required intervention). That this issue has not permeated practice and the day-to-day identification and provision of services to children with LD in schools—or that researchers still use school-identified samples—should be of concern to everyone involved with these children.

Whereas these issues clearly apply to the intraindividual-differences model, we stipulate that they also apply to the problem-solving model, and in areas beyond the assessment of change. As we stated earlier, there is an implicit classification of LD as children with reading, math, and behavior difficulties are assessed with outcomes appropriate to the academic domain. Another type of classification occurs when children are subdivided into those who need intervention and those who do not. Children are often further classified into those who respond and those who do not respond to initial intervention and then those who respond to, or do not respond to, increasingly intense forms of interventions. The bases for both decisions are essentially profiles that vary in shape, elevation, and scatter. However, these profiles usually represent changes in ability development over time and may be represented as a learning curve. Such curves vary in level (intercept) and shape (slope) and also are associated with measurement error that is ideally lower than that attributed to intercept and slope (Fuchs & Fuchs, 1998). Even in a single-subject-design framework, the graphs of functional assessment results tied to changes in the intervention have identical level and shape characteristics. The psychometric issues underlying the evaluation of these ipsative profiles are similar to those involved in normative profiles in the intraindividual-differences model (Morris et al., 1993). The profiles represent multiple time points and the results of such assessments also depend on how the sample is defined. The learning profiles of children with both RD and ADHD on a reading fluency probe likely differ from those associated with RD or ADHD as single disorders, although this type of question apparently has not been asked. One of the critical questions in all these models is the decision made regarding which attributes should be the focus of intervention and how one decides when the wrong attribute has been selected.

In the next section, we consider research on the intraindividual-differences model, examining areas in which the concept of discrepancy has been useful and not useful. That section addresses the issue of individual differences and their relevance to LD, as well as the related issue of aptitude by treatment interventions. We then address the treatment of this research by the problem-solving model, largely showing how the strengths of this model are compatible with the results of research from the intraindividual-differences model.

IQ–Achievement Discrepancy

The issue of IQ discrepancy is an example of how the intraindividual-differences mod-

el has not been useful. From the perspective of the problem-solving model, this classification is based on attributes that are not related to outcomes and detract from a focus on intervention. For the intraindividual-differences model, this classification exemplifies the importance of a hypotheses-testing approach. It is important to recognize that the IQ-discrepancy model is typically in fact a two-group classification of RD. It illustrates clearly that a classification can lack validity but with no impact on identification. As Lyon, Fletcher, and Barnes (in press) recently summarized (see also Fletcher, Lyon, et al., 2002; Lyon et al., 2001), studies of IQ–achievement discrepancy have taken place largely in the domain of RD. The studies include two recent meta-analyses of studies comparing cognitive and achievement correlates in children in RD groups based on IQ-discrepancy and low achievement definitions. There are also studies that examine prognosis, response to intervention, and heritibility in IQ-discrepant and low-achievement groups of children with RD. As the two meta-analyses show, the available studies are extensive, covering the age range into adults. Measures of reading outcomes predominantly involve word recognition but extend to reading comprehension and fluency measures, as well as school-identified samples where the specific identification measures are loosely specified. These studies involve both genders and a range of socioeconomic status (SES) levels. Finally, other forms of LD are addressed (e.g., math disability), along with speech and language disorders (Tomblin & Zhang, 1999). The psychometric issues are well understood and singularly explain why an IQ-discrepancy model is not likely viable (Stuebing et al., 2002).

The two meta-analyses of cognitive correlates of RD are most instructive, representing about 25 years of accumulated research. Hoskyn and Swanson (2000) identified 69 studies conducted from 1975 to 1996, coding 19 that met stringent IQ and achievement criteria. Effect sizes were computed to compare groups of students with higher IQ and poor reading achievement (IQ discrepant) and students with both lower IQ and poor reading achievement (low achievement, or LA). They reported negligible to small differences on several measures of reading and phonological processing (range = –0.02 to 0.29), but larger differences on measures of vocabulary (0.55) and syntax (0.87). They concluded, "children with RD share a common phonological core deficit with LA achievers. However, the results indicated that the deficits shared by the two groups are much broader than a phonological core" (p. 102).

Stuebing and colleagues (2002) identified 46 studies from a sample of over 300 from 1973 to 1998. These studies included measures of behavior, academic achievement, and cognitive abilities. From these studies, effect sizes were computed for behavior, achievement, and cognitive domains. The effect-sizes estimates were negligible for behavior (–0.05; 95% confidence interval = –0.14, 0.05) and achievement (–0.12; 95% confidence interval = –0.16, –0.07). A small effect size was found for cognitive ability (0.30; 95% confidence interval = 0.27, 0.34).

As the effect sizes were heterogeneous in the achievement and cognitive ability areas, specific tasks within the each domain were examined. Achievement outcomes involving word recognition, oral reading, and spelling showed small effect sizes indicating poorer performance by the IQ-discrepant groups. However, outcomes on reading comprehension, math, and writing yielded negligible effect sizes. The small effect sizes for word recognition, oral language, and spelling may reflect the use of word recognition tasks to define poor readers in many of the studies and the correlation of these definitional measures with similar measures not used to form groups.

For tasks involving cognitive ability, results were similar to those of Hoskyn and Swanson (2000). Those cognitive abilities closely related to reading disability yielded negligible effect sizes: phonological awareness (–0.13; 95% confidence interval = –0.23, –0.02), rapid naming (–0.12; 95% confidence interval = –0.30, 0.07), memory (0.10; 95% confidence interval = –0.01, 0.19), and vocabulary (0.10; 95% confidence interval = –0.02, 0.22). Outside the domain of tasks closely related to reading, measures of IQ not used to define the group yielded large effect-size differences favoring, as expected, the IQ-discrepant group. Cognitive skills such as those measured by IQ

subtests (spatial cognition, concept formation) yielded small to medium effect sizes, also indicating higher scores by the IQ-discrepant group. Many measures outside the phonological domain shared negligible to small effect size differences despite the large differences (about standard deviation) in IQ between the aggregated IQ-discrepant and LA groups. Altogether the difference across the 46 studies in cognitive ability was about three-tenths of a standard deviation, demonstrating substantial overlap between the groups on phonological, language, and nonphonological tasks.

In examining psychometric issues, Stuebing and colleagues (2002) found that variation in effect sizes across studies could be modeled simply by the scores on the IQ and reading tasks used to define the groups (i.e., sampling variation across studies) and the correlation of these definitional variables with the tasks used to compare the two groups. Thus, variation in effect sizes largely reflected differences in how groups are formed, clearly showing the importance of classification issues, not true differences between the groups as so defined.

The results of these two meta-analyses are consistent despite differences in the criteria for selecting studies and do not provide strong support for the validity of classifications based on IQ discrepancy. Other studies have examined the IQ-discrepant model in relation to intervention outcomes and prognosis. As Aaron (1997) reported in a review of earlier studies, there is little evidence of relationships of IQ scores or groupings based on discrepancy and reading outcomes. Fletcher, Lyon, and colleagues (2002) reviewed six recent studies that examined the outcomes of remedial and prevention studies in relation to IQ or IQ discrepancy (Foorman et al., 1997; Foorman, Francis, Fletcher, Schatschneider, & Mehta, 1998; Hatcher & Hulme, 1999; Torgesen et al., 1999; Vellutino, Scanlon, & Lyon, 2000; Wise, Ring, & Olson, 1999). Five of the six studies found no relationships. The only study to identify a relationship (Wise et al., 1999) found that Full Scale IQ predicted 5% of the variance in word reading outcomes on one measure of word reading. However, this effect was not apparent on two other measures of word reading or assessments of phonological processing ability. As Vellutino and colleagues (2000) stated, "the IQ-achievement discrepancy does not reliably distinguish between disabled and non-disabled readers.... Neither does it distinguish between children who were found to be difficult to remediate and those who are readily remediated, prior to initiation of remediation, and it does not predict response to remediation" (p. 235).

Similar results are apparent for studies of prognosis in naturally occurring (nonremediated) samples, where longitudinal outcomes do not differentiate IQ-discrepant and low achieving children identified with RD or relate strongly (Flowers, Meyer, Lovato, Felton, & Woods, 2001; Francis, Shaywitz, Stuebing, Shaywitz, & Fletcher, 1996; Share, McGee, & Silva, 1989; Shaywitz et al., 1999; Vellutino, Scanlon, & Lyon, 2000). Similarly, O'Malley, Francis, Foorman, Fletcher, and Swank (2002) reported that children identified into IQ-discrepant and LA groups in grade 2 were similar on kindergarten assessments of different precursor skills.

Altogether, the results of these studies do not provide evidence for the validity of models of intraindividual differences based on the two-group classification of children into IQ-discrepant and LA groups. These findings involve multiple outcomes, approaches to defining IQ discrepancy and LA, and extend to different types of LD. Especially critical are the largely null results for relations of IQ or IQ discrepancy with intervention outcomes and long- term development. Consistent with the NCLD (2002) position paper and other consensus documents (Donavon & Cross, 2002), neither IQ scores nor IQ discrepancy appear relevant for treatment planning. Thus, this model for intraindividual differences lacks support and should be abandoned.

Subtypes of Learning Disability

A second approach to intraindividual differences involves the search for subtypes of LD. In introducing this extensive area of research, it is important to recognize that any attempt to differentiate subgroups of LD is a subtyping study. Thus, attempts to compare children who vary in academic strengths and weakness are just as important as the studies that attempt subtyping

based on neuropsychological or cognitive measures. The latter are more commonly recognized as subtypes, but the former are vital, as they not only clearly demonstrate subgroup by outcome interactions in several domains but also help establish the viability of the concept of LD. As such, it is easier to support the use of norm-referenced achievement tests in the assessment of children with LD than the use of neuropsychological and cognitive tests as a demonstration of intraindividual differences.

ACHIEVEMENT SUBTYPES

The division of children with LD into groups based on the level and pattern of academic underachievement has a long history (Dool, Stelmack, & Rourke, 1993; Fletcher, 1985; Rourke & Finlayson, 1978). These studies, which most commonly compare children with disabilities in reading, math, and both reading and math, show that all forms of LD are not the same in a wide range of external attributes. As such, they support the heterogeneity of LD and the need to tie LD to specific domains of academic functioning. These subdivisions extend to variations in reading disability, where children can be differentiated by patterns of strengths and weaknesses in word recognition, fluency, and comprehension. Thus, there is a significant literature comparing children with adequate word recognition and poor reading comprehension with those who have both word recognition and reading comprehension deficits (Cornoldi & Oakhill, 1996, reviewed in Lyon et al., in press). There is an emerging literature on children with deficits only in word recognition or fluency with those who have deficits in both domains. Finally, there is extensive literature on interactions of RD and ADHD (Fletcher et al., 1999).

This literature permits some interesting conclusions. These subgroups, typically defined by patterns on achievement tests, are clearly differentiated on cognitive attributes not used to define the groups, as well as from children who are typically achieving and those with ADHD and lower IQ scores (Dool et al., 1993; Fletcher, 1985). They also differ in heritability and neurobiological correlates (Grigorenko, 2001). The cognitive differences are clearly indicated in

Figure 3.1, which compares children defined on the basis of achievement, IQ, and behavioral assessments (rating scales) into those with only RD (word recognition), only math disability (computations), only ADHD, typically achieving, and those with IQ test scores below 80, representing an operationalization of a mental deficiency criterion. In fact, this cut point is too high and most likely should be set lower to capture children with mental retardation. Children were defined as having LD based on either a low achievement (less than 25th percentile) or a 1.5 standard error discrepancy definition. The dependent measures were selected from a set of cognitive and neuropsychological tests expected to differentiate children with LD from those who are typically achieving, as well as those with RD (phonological awareness, rapid naming, vocabulary, paired associate learning), math disability (concept formation, procedural learning, visual–motor integration), and ADHD (sustained attention, concept forma-

tion, procedural learning). Figure 3.1 clearly shows profile differences in the groups on the shape and level of performance on these variables. In particular, the group with RD shows strengths in procedural learning and weaknesses in phonological awareness. The groups with ADHD and math disability show differences from one another on the measures of concept formation and procedural learning, which also differentiate them from the typically achieving children. The low-average IQ group has a flatter profile and is distinguished primarily on the basis of elevation differences. Finally, some variables distinguish the RD and MD groups from those that are typically achieving, but not from one another (rapid naming, paired associate learning, visual–motor integration). These results, which are apparent across multiple studies of subsets of these variables (see Lyon et al., in press), help establish the external validity of this classification of mental deficiency, different types of LD, and ADHD. It should be noted

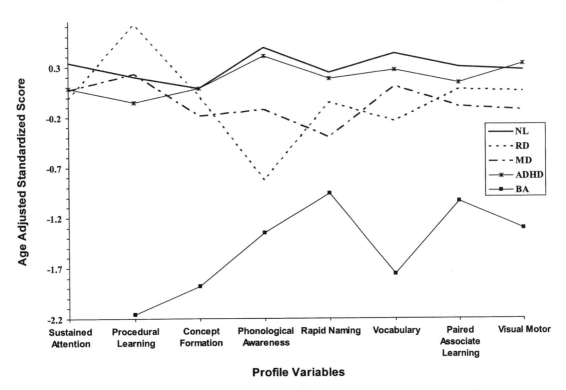

FIGURE 3.1. Comparisons of cognitive profiles for children with only reading disability (RD), only math disability (ND), and typical achievement (NL).

that although we discuss this classification as a set of subgroups, a categorical classification is not implied. In fact, this is a subdivision based on cut points on dimensional assessments of reading, math, IQ, and behavioral assessments of inattention and hyperactivity. There are many different classification models, which require the use of multiple dimensions, academic vectors, or prototypes that do not require dichotomous diagnostic decisions.

In Figure 3.2, we compare children with RD, MD, and both RD and MD with the low-IQ group on the same variables. Note that the group with both RD and MD differs in elevation from the single-deficit groups and the low-IQ group. There are also configuration differences that essentially parallel the patterns seen in the single-deficit group. The severe and parallel patterns around the phonological awareness dimension stand out, but statistical tests

show that the patterns on variables related to MD also suggest similarities (Klorman et al., 2002). Thus, children with RD and MD have essentially both disorders with more pervasive impairment of working memory and language. Imagine how results of different studies of LD will vary depending on whether the study evaluates either, or both, math and reading.

In Figure 3.3, we compare children with RD, ADHD, and both RD and ADHD with typically achieving children. Note that the group with RD and ADHD differs in elevation from the single-dimension groups but shows patterns that parallel their profiles. In addition, the group with ADHD shows relatively little cognitive morbidity on these measures. Studies of children with ADHD that do not evaluate reading and math may exaggerate the extent of impairment on cognitive tests. This suggestion is clearly supported by Figure 3.4, which shows profiles

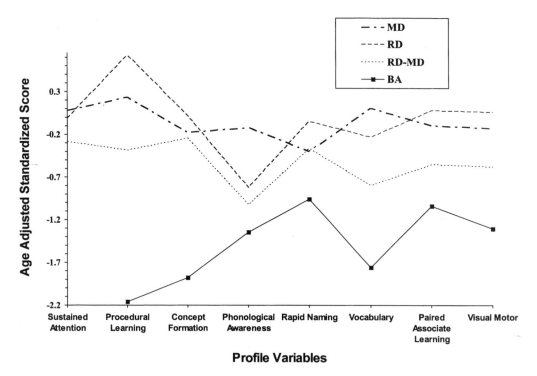

FIGURE 3.2. Comparisons of cognitive profiles for children with math disability (MD), reading disability (RD), both reading and math disability (RD-MD), and attention-deficit/hyperactivity disorder and no learning disability (ADHD).

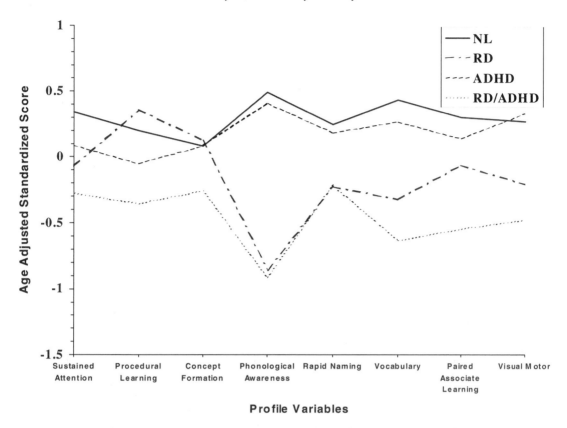

FIGURE 3.3. Comparisons of cognitive profiles for children with reading disability and no ADHD (with or without math disability) (RD), reading disability and ADHD (with or without math disability) (RD/ADHD), only attention-deficit/hyperactivity disorder (ADHD), and typical achievement (NL).

for children with MD, ADHD, MD and ADHD, and typically achieving children. Again, children with both MD and ADHD differ largely on elevation, while patterns differentiate ADHD and MD from typically achieving children.

Other research shows distinctions among children with RD based on patterns of word recognition, fluency, and comprehension. For example, children with impairments on fluency but not word recognition show difficulties with rapid naming and other measures that index speed of processing (Wolf & Bowers, 1999), but not phonological awareness. Children with poor reading comprehension and adequate decoding show problems with language comprehension and metacognitive variables involving inferencing ability, integration of textual information, and abstraction (Cornoldi & Oakhill, 1996; Lyon et al., in press). In ad-

dition, there are subgroup-by-treatment interactions on variables related to treatment and prognosis. In terms of treatment, empirical demonstrations show that children with word-level RD do not respond to metacognitive strategy instruction, or to math interventions, but respond well to interventions that incorporate explicit intervention in phonics and the alphabetic principle (Lovett & Barron, 2002). In addition, children show differential responsiveness to various interventions based on patterns involving accuracy of word recognition versus fluency of text reading (Lovett & Barron, 2002). In terms of prognosis, long-term outcomes are demonstrably poorer for children with LD that also involves ADHD, or for ADHD that involves academic difficulties (Satz, Buka, Lipsitt, & Seidman, 1998; Spreen, 1989). It is likely that any LD that involves more than one academic area, or that oc-

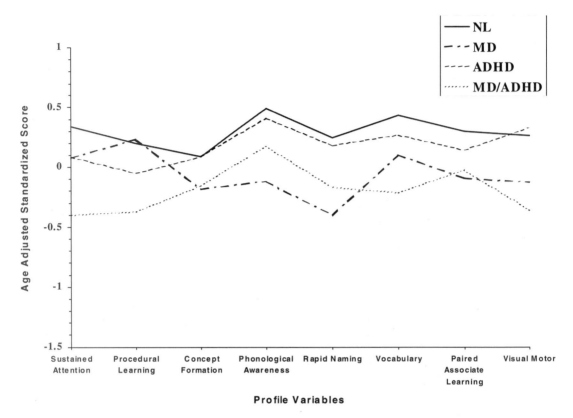

FIGURE 3.4. Comparisons of cognitive profiles for children with only math disability (MD), math disability and ADHD (MD/ADHD), only attention-deficit/hyperactivity disorder (ADHD), and typical achievement (NL).

curs in conjunction with an oral language disorder, shows poorer outcomes.

These examples of external validity may seem trivial or obvious. But they are important in the face of blanket assertions that there is no evidence for subgroup by treatment or aptitude by treatment interactions (Tilley et al., 1999). These findings are the strongest support for the intraindividual-difference model, with further support in neuroimaging studies and genetic studies showing difference in the neurobiological correlates of different subgroups of LD (Grigorenko, 2001; Lyon et al., in press). This classification does not imply a categorical model, especially as the distinctions are on correlated dimensions. The underlying classification model is not monothetic, which means that all attributes must be present for classification, or even the type of polythetic classifications used in psychiatric classification. Here there is a set of attributes, defined by theoretical links between cog-

nitive models of learning and achievement outcomes, none of which are necessary or sufficient. Rather, the model is most akin to prototype models where there are ideal types and variation around the ideal type, or vector models that link academic domains in multidimensional space.

Where the issues emerge is with attempts to use the variables that we have shown validate classifications of children as having LD as subclassifications based on cognitive or neuropsychological profiles. Thus, the LD subtyping literature seeks more homogeneous subgroups in the belief that this approach is related to intervention, prognosis, or neurobiological correlates. There is a vast literature on aptitude by treatment interactions in education that also posits relations of cognitive attributes, learning styles, and putative neurological functions. As we see in the next two sections, there are justifiable concerns about what this extensive body of research has produced.

COGNITIVE/NEUROPSYCHOLOGICAL
SUBTYPES OF LD

Children with LD are heterogeneous. Even within well-defined samples of readers with LD, there is large within-sample variance on some skills. This observation may explain, in part, why readers with LD have been reported to differ from controls on so many variables (Doehring, 1978). The literature on subtyping of LD is voluminous (Hooper & Willis, 1989; Lyon et al., in press; Newby & Lyon, 1991; Rourke, 1985). It has largely not been linked to theoretical models of the development of academic skills, brain function, or other relevant bodies of work. Much of the research consists of dumping archival data sets into a statistical algorithm, so that results vary considerably across studies. There is little demonstration that the patterns that emerge have implications for intervention or prognosis. These concerns fit into a larger literature that questions whether there is value in assessing processing skills in children with LD, thus questioning the assumptions underlying the intraindividual-differences model. Some possible exceptions are the focus of the remainder of this section. One focuses on rational grouping of readers with LD into subtypes on the basis of clinical observations and/or theories related to reading disability (Lovett & Barron, 2002; Lovett, Ransby, & Barron, 1988; Wolf & Bowers, 1999; Wolf, Bowers, & Biddle, 2001). A second approach exemplifies the use of empirical multivariate statistical methods to identify homogeneous subtypes of readers with LD (Lyon, 1985a; Morris et al., 1998).

RATIONAL SUBTYPING

As an example of a rational (clinical) approach to subtypes, Lovett (1984, 1987; Lovett, Steinbach, & Frijters, 2000) proposed two subtypes of reading disability based on the hypothesis that word recognition develops in three successive phases. The three phases are related to (1) accuracy in identifying printed words, (2) automatic recognition, and (3) automatization followed by as components of the reading process become consolidated in memory. Children who fail at the first phase are termed "accuracy disabled," whereas those who achieve age-appropriate word recognition but are deficient in the second or third phase are termed "rate disabled."

The strength of the Lovett subtype research program is its extensive external validation (Lovett & Barron, 2002; Newby & Lyon, 1991). In a study of the two subtypes (rate-disabled vs. accuracy-disabled subtype) and a typically achieving sample matched on word recognition ability to the rate-disabled group, accuracy-disabled readers were deficient in a wide array of oral and written language areas different from the reading behaviors used to identify subtype members. The deficiencies of the rate-disabled group were more apparent in deficient connected text reading and spelling (Lovett, 1987). Reading comprehension was impaired on all measures for the accuracy-disabled group and was highly correlated with word recognition skill, but the rate-disabled group was impaired on only some comprehension measures. These additional subtype-treatment interaction studies (Lovett et al., 1988; Lovett, Lacerenza, et al., 2000; Lovett, Ransby, Hardwick, & Johns, 1989) found some differences between accuracy- and rate-disabled groups on contextual reading outcomes, whereas word recognition improved for both groups.

Lovett's program is founded on explicit developmental reading theory, which has been translated into a developmental model of subtypes of reading, illustrates methodological robustness, and offers detailed, thoughtful alternative explanations for the complex external validation findings (Newby & Lyon, 1991). Important treatment-outcome findings are muted somewhat by reading gains on standardized measures that do not move many children into the average in spite of statistically significant results. Unfortunately, the classic question of how one defines average (or expected) is an unanswered classification question that may be complicated due to contextual differences among school, classrooms, and so on. Another problem is that if all children have effective instruction that moves them into the average range, then the "expected" or "average" changes and new children are again identified as discrepant. Thus, there is little evidence for significant subtype by treatment interactions (Lyon & Flynn, 1989), but this program is continuing.

More recent research continues to emphasize the importance of this basic distinction between accuracy and rate but tends to rely on cognitive measures of processing. In the double-deficit model developed by Wolf and associates (Wolf & Bowers, 1999; Wolf, Bowers, & Biddle, 2001), the authors propose that while phonological processing contributes considerably to word recognition deficits, reading involves the ability to read both accurately and fluently. This view receives especially strong support from studies of RD in languages other than English, where the relationship of phonology and orthography is more transparent. Thus, children with RD in German and Italian are still characterized by difficulties that are more apparent in how rapidly they read words and text, not by accuracy (Paulescu et al., 2001; Wimmer & Mayringer, 2002). In these studies, a phonological defect is apparent in poor spelling, but a subgroup also emerges that reads and spells adequately but has fluency deficits that are independent of problems with phonological processing. When isolated deficits in fluency occur, the most reliable correlate occurs on tasks that require rapid naming of letters and digits. Thus, Wolf and associates have postulated the *double-deficit model* of subtypes.

This model specifies three subtypes, one characterized by deficits in both phonological processing and rapid naming, another with impairments only phonological processing, and a third with impairments only in rapid automatized naming. Wolf and associates have summarized evidence, largely rational, but with some evidence of validity, based on comparisons on other cognitive skills, that supports this subtyping scheme. Although it has been suggested that the two deficits are additive in children with double deficits, and that the double-deficit group is more severe, there are inherent measurement and methodological problems identified by Schatschneider, Carlson, Francis, Foorman, and Fletcher (2002) and Compton, DeFries, and Olson (2001) with this assertion. When both phonological processing and rapid naming are impaired, the child is more severely impaired in both dimensions, which makes it difficult to match single- and double-deficit-impaired children. Thus, children with double deficits tend to have more severe problems on either phonology

or rapid naming, as well as in reading, compared to children with single deficits. An alternative is to use an empirical approach to subtyping to determine whether these subtypes emerge, which we address in the next section.

Prior to discussing empirical subtyping, note that Wolf and colleagues (2001) base subtyping at the level of processing, whereas Lovett, Lacerenza and colleagues (2000) base their schemas on patterns of reading deficits. Other subtyping schemes also base the classification on patterns of reading subskills. For example, Castles and Coltheart (1993) found evidence for two subtypes or children with RD based on patterns of errors in reading pseudowords and exception (irregular) words. Relating these findings to a body of research on acquired disorders of reading (alexia), they distinguished children with phonological dyslexia from those with surface dyslexia. However, there has been virtually no external validation of these subtypes. Stanovich, Siegel, and Gottardo (1997) suggested that whereas phonological dyslexia could be validated, surface dyslexia appeared unstable and transitory.

EMPIRICAL SUBTYPING METHODS

There are numerous examples of empirical subtyping studies derived from achievement, neurocognitive, neurolinguistic, and combined classification models. Multiple models of LD in reading have emerged through the application of multivariate statistical approaches. An integrated analysis of several prominent reading-disability subtype systems that have been intensively investigated suggests some areas of convergence in the literature (Hooper & Willis, 1989). In particular, memory-span, phonological, and orthographic processing in reading appear to be central in defining subtypes. Although a dichotomy of auditory–linguistic versus visuospatial reading disability subtypes have been commonly proposed, this division has not been effectively validated (Newby & Lyon, 1991), nor is the evidence strong for any nonlinguistic variable as an explanation for the reading difficulties experienced by children with dyslexia. Because of these findings, we would not expect subgroup by treatment interactions when auditory versus visual processing subtypes, or other older neuropsychological and information processing subtype models, are used for classification purposes. The theoretical model behind the choice of attributes for a classification model is critical to its ultimate validity and success.

In a series of studies employing multivariate cluster-analytic methods, Lyon (1985a, 1985b) identified six subtypes of older readers with LD (11- to 12-year-old children) and five subtypes of younger readers with LD (6- to 9-year-old children) on measures assessing linguistic skills, visual–perceptual skills, and memory-span abilities. The theoretical viewpoint guiding this subtype research was based on Luria's (1966, 1973) observations that reading ability is a complex behavior effected by means of a complex functional system of cooperating zones of the cerebral cortex and related subcortical structures. Within the context of this theoretical framework, it could be hypothesized that a deficit in any one or several zones of the functional system could impede the acquisition of fluent reading behavior. The identification of multiple subtypes within both age cohorts suggested the possibility that several different types of LD readers exist, each characterized by different patterns of neuropsychological subskills relevant to reading acquisition.

We emphasize this example as it explicated attempts to identify subtype by treatment interventions, a research priority that is still infrequently addressed. Follow-up subtype-by-treatment interaction studies using both age samples (Lyon, 1985a, 1985b) only partially supported the independence of the subtypes with respect to response to treatment. It was found, however, that subtypes characterized at both age levels by significant deficits in blending sounds, rapid naming, and memory span did not respond to intervention methods employing synthetic phonics procedures. Rather, members of this linguistic-deficit subtype first had to learn phonetically regular words by sight and then learn the internal phonological structure using the whole word as a meaningful semantic context. Again, this was true for both younger and older disabled readers within the linguistic-deficit subtype.

In the past 10 years, the frequency of empirical subtyping studies has diminished. It is clear that many of these approaches to subtyping are largely atheoretical and simply involved the application of multivariate statistical algorithms to cognitive and academic variables. The resultant solutions were highly variable, and often unreliable. Although there was some general replication across groups in terms of the types of clusters that are identified, the subtypes themselves were often difficult to relate to what is known about domain-specific reading or other learning disabilities.

One recent empirical subtyping study provided support not only for the double-deficit model, but also for models that separate "specific" forms of reading disability from garden-variety forms of reading disability (Morris et al., 1998). This study differed from previous empirical approaches to subtyping in that it was based on a theoretical model emphasizing the role of phonological processing in reading disability (Liberman et al., 1989; Stanovich, 1988). It also used other theories to select potential variables. Thus, measures of rapid naming, short-term memory, vocabulary, and perceptual skills were included. From a methodological perspective, the sample was large and was selected on an *a priori* basis for a subtyping study (i.e., it was not just a sample of convenience). Multiple definitions were used to identify children. In addition to children defined with dyslexia, children with dyslexia and math disability as well as isolated math disabilities, permutations involving ADHD, and typically achieving children were included. The application of the clustering algorithms was rigorous and followed guidelines ensuring both internal and external validity (Morris & Fletcher, 1988).

Figure 3.5 portrays the nine resultant subtypes. All profiles are depicted as *z*-scores relative to the sample mean. Here it is apparent that there are five subtypes with specific reading disability, two subtypes representing more pervasive impairments in language and reading, and two representing typically achieving groups of children. Six of the seven reading disability subtypes share, however, an impairment in phonological awareness skills. The five specific subtypes largely vary in rapid automatized naming and verbal short-term memory. Here we can see a large subtype in Figure

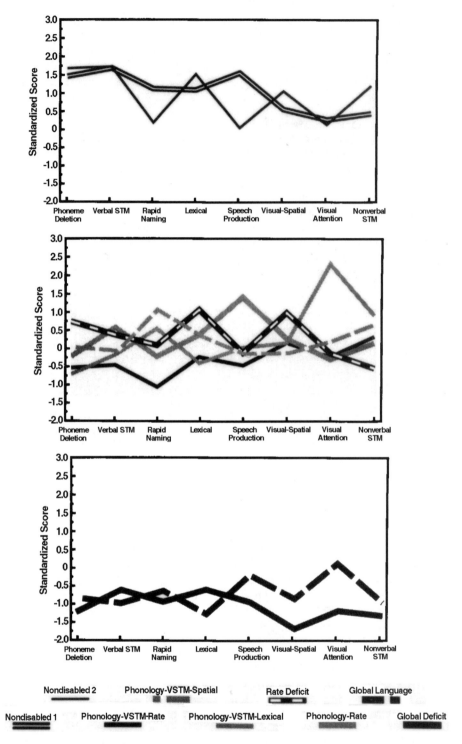

FIGURE 3.5. Cognitive profiles for nine subtypes of reading produced by cluster analysis. The two subtypes in the upper panel are typically achieving children and are largely differentiated from other subtypes by level of performance. The subtypes in the lower panel are lower in overall level of function, representing pervasive impairments of language, and are differentiated by level and shape. The five subtypes in the middle panel show specific patterns of strengths and weaknesses distinguishable largely by shape (Morris et al., 1998). V = verbal; STM = short-term memory.

3.5 that has impairments in phonological awareness, rapid naming, and verbal short-term memory. There are two subtypes with impairments in phonological awareness and verbal short-term memory, varying in lexical and spatial skills, a subtype with phonological awareness and rapid naming difficulties, and a subtype that is not impaired in phonological awareness but has deficits on any measure that required rapid processing, including rapid naming. This latter subtype is not impaired in word recognition but has difficulties on measures of reading fluency and comprehension, consistent with double-deficit model (Wolf & Bower, 1999). The five specific subtypes can be differentiated from the garden-variety subtypes on the basis of their vocabulary development. Those children with specific subtypes of reading disability have vocabulary levels that are in the average range; children with more pervasive disturbances of reading and language have vocabulary levels that are in the low-average range.

Altogether, these results are consistent with the central role of phonological processing in word-level RD, as well as Wolf and Bower's double-deficit model. The results are also consistent with Stanovich's (1988) phonological core-variable-differences model. This model postulates that phonological processing is at the core of all word-level RD. But RD is often more than just phonological processing problems. Children may have problems outside the phonological domain that do not contribute to the word recognition difficulties. These problems could be represented by impairments in vocabulary that would interfere with comprehension, more pervasive disturbances of language that would lead to a garden-variety form of RD, or even fine motor and visual perceptual problems that are demonstrably unrelated to the reading component of RD. The value of these distinctions in relation to treatment, however, is largely unexplored.

Summary: Subtyping Studies

Studies of subtypes based on processing skills do not suggest much evidence for subtype by treatment interactions. Such subtypes can be evaluated on other external variables. There is some evidence for differences in cognitive correlates, heritability, and prognosis, but it pales in relationship to classifications based on academic and behavior subtypes. For academic subtypes, the interactions with outcomes are obvious.

Where these studies have been helpful is the identification of components of intervention that are essential for promoting enhanced achievement in children with LD. At least for RD, progress in the development of interventions proceeded directly from research on the cognitive development of language and reading and on intraindividual differences among poor readers. The notion in the problem-solving model that one simply intervenes until effective treatments are identified has not been actualized and would not be expected to help develop interventions for LD. Indeed, research that focus largely on "what works" in the absence of a cumulative, integrated body of knowledge does not yield effective interventions. Thus, as Cummins (1999) suggested, we lack methods for the effective instruction of English-language learners precisely because the field has been focused on program evaluation outcomes and not on a cumulative body of knowledge that includes mechanism. At the same time, focusing on intraindividual differences does not necessarily lead to classifications that facilitate intervention, as in a problem-solving model.

Aptitude by Treatment Interactions

Whereas the intraindividual-differences model focuses on different subtype hypotheses and derives from cognitive psychology and neuropsychology, the problem-solving model focuses on the failure of aptitude by treatment interactions research as outlined in the special education literature. In the aptitude by treatment interaction literature, the focus is not so much on subgroups as it is on within-child traits. These traits represent natural characteristics of the child—either strengths or weaknesses—that should be matched to characteristics of different interventions. Thus, children might be classified as "auditory" or "visual" learners, or "left-brained" or "right-brained." The intervention would attempt to either strengthen a deficit or bypass the deficit by focusing on a strength. The left-brained child, for example, would be taught to verbally mediate math problems to compensate for "right brain" weaknesses.

Years of investigation of these hypotheses have led to largely null results. Interactions involving modality, learning styles, or putative neurological factors have not interacted with treatment characteristics. Similarly, evidence that children in different categories of special education (e.g., LD vs. mental retardation) need or respond differently to various interventions is not apparent. As Reschly and colleagues (1999) point out, the effect of the search for aptitude by treatment interactions leads in directions that do not result in better outcomes for children in special education and may be iatrogenic, as the model does not result in a focus on direct treatment of the target behaviors, such as reading and math.

We do not dispute the null results for aptitude by treatment interactions. However, it is important to recognize that this is an older literature where cognitive models of the development of reading and math skills were seriously underdeveloped. Moreover, rejection of interactions of special education categories in policy does not negate the relevance of the underlying dimensions themselves, just the classification in federal regulations. Here the criteria are demonstrably short on validity and reflect purposes other than a scientifically based classification. Nonetheless, it is not apparent that children with LD benefit from interventions that do not focus on the actual area of deficiency—reading, math, and so on. In addition, identification for special education services must hinge on more than a score on a norm-referenced test, given the measurement issues that are involved. Here the value of the problem-solving model in focusing identification on the results of an intervention with convergence from other sources of data is apparent. Concern, however, that the rejection of aptitude by treatment models invalidates classifications and automatically involves a noncategorical model is misleading. To reiterate, the problem-solving model does involve the notion of discrepancy. It is dimensional and does use information about differences among children. When the effects of initial status or severity are considered, there is evidence of "aptitude" by treatment interactions.

Foorman and colleagues (1998) demonstrated that children who were weakest in phonological awareness showed the best response to basal curriculums that taught the alphabetic principal explicitly. Lovett and Barron (2002) predict treatment outcomes based on assessments of phonological awareness and rapid naming. This information was captured by interactions of initial status and curriculum. Initial status as related to outcomes is vital for both the intraindividual-differences and problem-solving models.

An Integrated Model

Throughout this chapter, we have argued that the intraindividual-differences model and the problem-solving model have evolved to a point where they implicitly reflect common themes and assumptions about LD. In this respect, research on the intraindividual-differences model shows that the underlying classifications are dimensional, representing a set of correlated vectors regarding child attributes. The model is strongest when focused on the primary manifestations of LD, which involve reading, math, and writing. It is weakest in looking for ability–ability discrepancies as a marker for LD, especially in relation to intervention issues. Processing strengths and weaknesses do not have strong relationships with treatment outcome, although they may have relationships with etiology.

At the same time, there are relationships with discrepancies in academic behaviors, treatment outcomes, and prognosis that support the viability of a version of the intraindividual-differences model. The normative basis is especially useful for making decisions about level of performance and comparability of treatments. But normative test scores or variations in them are not strong markers of intervention outcomes, especially if the goal is to monitor progress as an indicator of outcome. These tests are usually designed to be highly stable and are not sensitive to small units of change (Francis, Shaywitz, Stuebing, Shaywitz, & Fletcher, 1994). These models lead to paradoxes where more severely impaired children are not viewed as having LD because their profiles are flatter. In fact, flatness occurs because of variations in severity and the correlation among the attributes. It is very difficult to argue that children with garden-variety LD versus specific LD are qualitatively different as opposed to representing more severe impairment in key component skills that in turn suppress other correlated abilities.

The problem-solving model is less focused on within-child variation but retains the concept of discrepancy with environmental (i.e., class and school) or social expectations. The discrepancy is usually relative to expectations that apply to the local context. This model also relies on dimensional classifications, even though these classifications are rarely articulated. It is strongly focused on outcomes and purports to be atheoretical and disinterested in within-child characteristics, though exactly how such a model would decide for whom a reading (vs. math) intervention was warranted or establish a need for more or less intervention absent classification considerations is difficult to conceptualize. The measurement issues underlying how children are identified under the problem-solving model are identical to those in the intraindividual-differences model despite the focus on different attributes of the child. The intraindividual-differences model is misleading in the belief that ability–ability discrepancies in themselves are markers of biological variability as test scores are a product on biology and environment (Fletcher & Taylor, 1984). In addition, the rejection of the problem-solving model of norm-referenced testing is also inadequate, leading to excessive reliance on local norms that could be wasteful in terms of resources. Indeed, methods based on curriculum-based assessment and progress monitoring—critical for problem-solving models—typically attempt to establish a broader normative base than just a local educational context.

Integrating these models requires that we reorganize the inherently multilevel nature of children in schools. These multiple levels are depicted in Figure 3.6, which shows that the child is nested within the classroom, which is nested within the school, which in turn is nested in the community. The child attributes are measured over time. Any modeling of differences in child attributes, or changes over time, must take into account these different levels of analysis. In particular, response to intervention will involve interactions of the children with char-

Nested Analysis of Growth in Reading

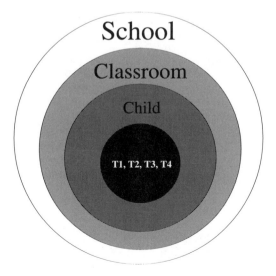

FIGURE 3.6. Multilevel model of growth in reading skills. Time is nested within the child, which is nested within the classroom, which is nested within the school. Not depicted is the nesting of the school within the community.

acteristics of the curriculum, classroom, or teacher level of the model. These two levels must always be considered.

The type of classification will always depend on its purpose. If the goal is to identify children for special education services, test scores and ability discrepancies are not sufficient. Children should not be placed in special education without evidence of failure to respond to quality instruction. At the same time, there are different models of response to instruction, and it is not correct that norm-referenced tests are completely insensitive to change (Reschly & Tilley, 1999). It depends on the model of change. As Torgesen (2002) has demonstrated, the child who responds should change his or her rank in the population, moving into the average range. This begs the question of "average" in that its definition will change as interventions affect many children. But the key is to measure children in multiple ways over time and look at the strengths and weaknesses of these different assessments. Thus, while progress monitoring using curriculum-based measures is vital for identification (Fuchs & Fuchs, 1998), the snapshots of behavior provided by norm-referenced achievement tests can complement this approach. Both types of measures complement identification for special education services and help remove the inherently relative orientation of curriculum-based measures. Such approaches also provide broader pictures of the child, particularly if the assessment includes domains of achievement and behavior. But even here we are not suggesting that, in practice, children need significant batteries of tests. Rather, the goal should be to identify intervention needs and monitor a child's progress, which can be complemented by methods derived from both models. Children do learn in social contexts, so that specifications of the learning environment are essential to establishing response to intervention. This extends to the school and community level of analysis in Figure 3.6. Schools that are dysfunctional, or communities that do not interact with the school, can be expected to produce large numbers of children with learning difficulties.

In policy, the strengths of these two models must be put in place in a revision of the intraindividual-differences model that has dominated special education eligibility determinations in IDEA. Ability discrepancies that only involve child attributes are clearly not adequate. But children should not be eligible for services solely based on deviations from local expectations or an absence of normative low achievement. The notion of discrepancy and unexpectedness is maintained in both models. All children are capable of learning, and there are no true nonresponders—just slow responders (Denton & Mathes, in press). It is absurd not to call children with profiles that are relatively flat learning disabled, or to avoid the weaknesses of distinctions with mild mental retardation in the absence of some intervention need that emerges in the child's response to instruction. Thus, for identification and eligibility purposes, LD should be conceptualized as "unexpected" largely in the absence of response to adequate instruction, and the "discrepancy" a matter of not learning to expectations. Regardless, any policy-based decisions should be evaluated on the basis of whether children benefit from the revisions in the underlying classification model, which are implicitly represented in any such policy.

References

Aaron, P. G. (1997). The impending demise of the discrepancy formula. *Review of Educational Research, 67,* 461–502.

Blashfield, R. K. (1993). Models of classification as related to a taxonomy of learning disabilities. In G. R. Lyon, D. B. Gray, J. F. Kavanagh, & N. A. Krasnegor (Eds.), *Better understanding learning disabilities: New views from research and their implications for education and public policies* (pp. 17–26). Baltimore: Brookes.

Blashfield, R. K., & Draguns, J. G. (1976). Towards a taxonomy of psychopathology. The purposes of psychiatric classification. *British Journal of Psychiatry, 129,* 574–583.

Castles, A., & Coltheart, M. (1993). Varieties of developmental dyslexia. *Cognition, 47,* 149–180.

Chronbach, L. J. (1957). The two disciplines of scientific psychology. *American Psychologist, 12,* 671–684.

Compton, D. L., DeFries, J. C., & Olson, R. K. (2001). Are RAN- and phonological awareness deficits additive in children with reading disabilities? *Dyslexia, 7,* 125–149.

Cornoldi, C., & Oakhill, J. (Eds.). (1996). *Reading comprehension difficulties: Processes and intervention.* Mahwah, NJ: Erlbaum.

Cummins, J. (1999). Alternative paradigms in bilingual education research: Does theory have a place? *Educational Researcher, 29,* 26–32.

Doehring, D. G. (1978). The tangled web of behavioral research on developmental dyslexia. In A. L. Benton & D. Pearl (Eds.), *Dyslexia* (pp. 123–137). New York: Oxford University Press.

Donovan, M. S., & Cross, C. T. (2002). *Minority students in special and gifted education.* Washington, DC: National Academy Press.

Dool, C. B., Stelmack, R. M., & Rourke, B. P. (1993). Event-related potentials in children with learning disabilities. *Journal of Clinical Child Psychology, 22,* 387–398.

Fletcher, J. M. (1985). Memory for verbal and nonverbal stimuli in learning disability subgroups: Analysis by selective reminding. *Journal of Experimental Child Psychology, 40,* 244–259.

Fletcher, J. M., Foorman, B. R., Boudousquie, A. B., Barnes, M. A., Schatschneider, C., & Francis, D. J. (2002). Assessment of reading and learning disabilities: A research-based, intervention-oriented approach. *Journal of School Psychology, 40,* 27–63.

Fletcher, J. M., Francis, D. J., Rourke, B. P., Shaywitz, S. E., & Shaywitz, B. A. (1993). Classification of learning disabilities: Relationships with other childhood disorders. In G. R. Lyon, D. B. Gray, J. F. Kavanagh, & N. A. Krasnegor (Eds.), *Better understanding learning disabilities: New views from research and their implications for education and public policies* (pp. 27–56). Baltimore: Brookes.

Fletcher, J. M., Lyon, G. R., Barnes, M., Stuebing, K. K., Francis, D. J., Olson, R. K., Shaywitz, S. E., & Shaywitz, B. A. (2002). Classification of learning disabilities: An evidenced-based evaluation. In R. Bradley, L. Danielson, & D. P. Hallahan (Eds.), *Identification of learning disabilities: Research to policy* (pp. 185–250). Mahwah, NJ: Erlbaum.

Fletcher, J. M., & Morris, R. (1986). Classification of disabled learners: Beyond exclusionary definitions. In S. J. Cici (Ed.), *Handbook of cognitive, social, and neuropsychological aspects of learning disabilities* (pp. 55–80). Hillsdale, NJ: Erlbaum.

Fletcher, J. M., Shaywitz, S. E., & Shaywitz, B. A. (1999). Comorbidity of learning and attention disorders: Separate but equal. *Pediatric Clinics of North America, 46,* 885–897.

Fletcher, J. M., & Taylor, H. G. (1984). Neuropsychological approaches to children: Towards a developmental neuropsychology. *Journal of Clinical Neuropsychology, 6,* 39–56.

Flowers, L., Meyer, M., Lovato, J., Wood, F., & Felton, R. (2001). Does third grade discrepancy status predict the course of reading development? *Annals of Dyslexia, 51,* 49–71.

Foorman, B. R., Francis, D. J., Winikates, D., Mehta, P., Schatschneider, C., & Fletcher, J. (1997). Early interventions for children with reading disabilities. *Scientific Studies of Reading, 1,* 255–276.

Foorman, B. R., Francis, D. J., Fletcher, J. M.,

Schatschneider, C., & Mehta, P. (1998). The role of instruction in learning to read: Preventing reading failure in at-risk-children. *Journal of Educational Psychology, 90,* 37–55.

Francis, D. J., Shaywitz, S. E., Stuebing, K. K., Shaywitz, B. A., & Fletcher, J. M. (1994). The measurement of change: Assessing behavior over time and within a developmental context. In G. R. Lyon (Ed.), *Frames of reference for assessment of learning disabilities* (pp. 29–58). Baltimore: Brookes.

Francis, D. J., Shaywitz, S. E., Stuebing, K. K., Shaywitz, B. A., & Fletcher, J. M. (1996). Developmental lag versus deficit models of reading disability: A longitudinal, individual growth curves analysis. *Journal of Educational Psychology, 88,* 3–17.

Fuchs, L. S., & Fuchs, D. (1998). Treatment validity: A unifying concept for reconceptualizing identification of learning disabilities. *Learning Disabilities Research and Practice, 13,* 204–219.

Gilger, J. W. (2002). Current issues in the neurology and genetics of learning-related traits and disorders: Introduction to the special issue. *Journal of Learning Disabilities, 34,* 490–491.

Gilger, J. W., & Kaplan, B. J. (2002). Atypical brain development: A conceptual framework for understanding developmental learning disabilities. *Developmental Neuropsychology, 20,* 465–482.

Grigorenko, E. L. (2001). Developmental dyslexia: An update on genes, brains, and environments. *Journal of Child Psychology and Psychiatry, 42,* 91–125.

Hatcher, P., & Hulme, C. (1999). Phonemes, rhymes, and intelligence as predictors of children's responsiveness to remedial reading instruction. *Journal of Experimental Child Psychology, 72,* 130–153.

Hooper, S. R., & Willis, W. G. (1989). *Learning disability subtyping: Neuropsychological foundations, conceptual models, and issues in clinical differentiation.* New York: Springer-Verlag.

Hoskyn, M., & Swanson, H. L (2000). Cognitive processing of low achievers and children with reading disabilities: A selective meta-analytic review of the published literature. *School Psychology Review, 29,* 102–119.

Kavale, K. A., & Forness, S. R. (2000). What definitions of learning disability say and don't say: A critical analysis. *Journal of Learning Disabilities, 33,* 239–256.

Klorman, R., Thatcher, J. E., Shaywitz, S. E., Fletcher, J. M., Marchione, K. E., Holahan, J. M., Stuebing, K. K., & Shaywitz, B. A. (2002). Effects of event probability and sequence on children with attention deficit/hyperactivity, reading, and math disorder. *Biological Psychiatry, 52,* 773–846.

Liberman, I. Y., Shankweiler, D., & Liberman, A. (1989). The alphabetic principle and learning to read. In D. Shankweiler & I. Y. Liberman (Eds.), *Phonology and reading disability: Solving the reading puzzle* (pp. 1–34). Ann Arbor: University of Michigan Press.

Lovett, M. W. (1984). A developmental perspective

on reading dysfunction: Accuracy and rate criteria in the subtyping of dyslexic children. *Brain and Language, 22,* 67–91.

Lovett, M. W. (1987). A developmental approach to reading disability: Accuracy and speed criteria of normal and deficient reading skill. *Child Development, 58,* 234–260.

Lovett, M. W., & Barron, R. W. (2002). The search for individual and subtype differences in reading disabled children's response to remediation. In D. L. Molfese & V. J. Molfese (Eds.), *Developmental variations in learning* (pp. 309–338). Mahwah, NJ: Erlbaum.

Lovett, M. W., Lacerenza, L., Borden, S. L., Frijters, J. C., Steinbach, K. A., & DePalma, M. (2000). Components of effective remediation for developmental reading disabilities: Combining phonological and strategy-based instruction to improve outcomes. *Journal of Educational Psychology, 92,* 263–283.

Lovett, M. W., Ransby, M. J., & Barron, R. W. (1988). Treatment, subtype, and word type effects in dyslexic children's response to remediation. *Brain and Language, 34,* 328–349.

Lovett, M. W., Ransby, M. J., Hardwick, N., & Johns, M. S. (1989). Can dyslexia be treated? Treatment-specific and generalized treatment effects in dyslexic children's response to remediation. *Brain and Language, 37,* 90–121.

Lovett, M. W., Steinbach, K. A., & Frijters, J. C. (2000). Remediating the core deficits of reading disability: A double-deficit perspective. *Journal of Learning Disabilities, 33,* 334–358.

Luria, A. R. (1966). *Higher cortical functions in man.* New York: Basic Books.

Luria, A. R. (1973). *The working brain.* New York: Basic Books.

Lyon, G. R. (1985a). Educational validation studies of learning disability subtypes. In B. P. Rourke (Ed.), *Neuropsychology of learning disabilities: Essentials of subtype analysis* (pp. 228–256). New York: Guilford Press.

Lyon, G. R. (1985b). Identification and remediation of learning disability subtypes: Preliminary findings. *Learning Disability Focus, 1,* 21–35.

Lyon, G. R., Fletcher, J. M., & Barnes, M. C. (in press). Learning disabilities. In E. J. Mash & R. A. Barkley (Eds.), *Child psychopathology* (2nd ed.). New York: Guilford Press.

Lyon, G. R., Fletcher, J. M., Shaywitz, S. E., Shaywitz, B. A., Torgesen, J. K., Wood, F. B., Schulte, A., & Olson, R. (2001). Rethinking learning disabilities. In C. E. Finn, Jr., A. J. Rotherham, & C. R. Hokanson, Jr. (Eds.) *Rethinking special education for a new century* (pp. 259–287). Washington, DC: Thomas B. Fordham Foundation and Progressive Policy Institute.

Lyon, G. R., & Flynn, J. M. (1989). Educational validation studies with subtypes of learning disabled readers. In B. P. Rourke (Ed.), *Neuropsychological validation of learning disability subtypes* (pp. 243–242). New York: Guilford Press.

MacMillan, D. L., & Siperstein, G. N. (2002).

Learning disabilities as operationally defined by schools. In R. Bradley, L. Danielson, & D. P. Hallahan (Eds.), *Identification of learning disabilities: Research to policy* (pp. 287–333). Mahwah, NJ: Erlbaum.

Mercer, C. D., Jordan, L., Allsop, D. H., & Mercer, A. R. (1996). Learning disabilities definitions and criteria used by state education departments. *Learning Disability Quarterly, 19,* 217–232.

Morris, R. (1988). Classification of learning disabilities: Old problems and new approaches. *Journal of Consulting and Clinical Psychology, 56,* 789–794.

Morris, R., & Fletcher, J. M. (1988). Classification in neuropsychology: A theoretical framework and research paradigm. *Journal of Clinical and Experimental Neuropsychology, 10,* 640–658.

Morris, R. D., Fletcher, J. M., & Francis, D. J. (1993). Conceptual and psychometric issues in the neuropsychological assessment of children: Measurement of ability discrepancy and change. In I. Rapin & S. Segalovitz (Eds.), *Handbook of neuropsychology* (Vol. 7, pp. 341–352). Amsterdam: Elsevier.

Morris, R., Satz, P., & Blashfield, R. (1981). Neuropsychology and cluster analysis: Potential and problems. *Journal of Clinical Neuropsychology, 3,* 79–99.

Morris, R. D., Stuebing, K. K., Fletcher, J. M., Shaywitz, S. E., Lyon, G. R., Shankweiler, D. P., Katz, L., Francis, D. J., & Shaywitz, B. A. (1998). Subtypes of reading disability: Variability around a phonological core. *Journal of Educational Psychology, 90,* 347–373.

National Center for Learning Disabilities & the Office of Special Education Programs. (2002). *Specific learning disabilities: Finding common ground.* New York: Author.

Newby, R. F., & Lyon, G. R. (1991). Neuropsychological subtypes of learning disabilities. In J. E. Obrzut & G. W. Hynd (Eds.), *Neuropsychological foundations of learning disabilities: A handbook of issues, methods, and practice* (pp. 355–385). New York: Academic Press.

Olson, R. K., Forsberg, H., Gayan, J., & DeFries, J. C. (1999). A behavioral-genetic analysis of reading disabilities and component processes. In R. M. Klein & P. A. McMullen (Eds.), *Converging methods for understanding reading and dyslexia* (pp. 133–153). Cambridge, MA: MIT Press.

O'Malley, K. J., Francis, D. J., Foorman, B. R., Fletcher, J. M., & Swank, P. R. (2002). Growth in precursor reading skills: Do low-achieving and IQ-discrepant readers develop differently? *Learning Disability Research and Practice, 17,* 19–34.

Paulescu, E., Demonet, J. F., Fazio, F, McCrory, E., Chanoine, V., Brunswick, N., Cappa, S. F., Cossu, G., Habib, M., Frith, C. D., & Frith, U. (2001). Dyslexia: Cultural diversity and biological unity. *Science, 291,* 2165–2064.

Reschly, D. J., & Tilly, W. D. (1999). Reform trends and system design alternatives. In D. J. Reschly,

W. D. Tilly, & J. P. Grimes (Eds.), *Special education in transition: Functional assessment and noncategorical programming* (pp. 19–48). Longmont, CO: Sopris West.

Reschly, D. J., Tilly, W. D., & Grimes, J. P. (Eds.). (1999). *Special education in transition Functional Assessment and Noncategorical Programming.* Longmont, CO: Sopris West.

Rourke, B. P. (Ed.). (1985). *Neuropsychology of learning disabilities: Essentials of subtype analysis.* New York: Guilford Press.

Rourke, B. P., & Finlayson, M. A. J. (1978). Neuropsychological significance of variations in patterns of academic performance: Verbal and visual-spatial abilities. *Journal of Pediatric Psychology, 3,* 62–66.

Satz, P., Buka, S., Lipsitt, L., & Seidman, L. (1998). The long-term prognosis of learning disabled children. In B. K. Shapiro, P. J. Accardo, & A. J. Capute (Eds.), *Specific reading disability: A view of the spectrum* (pp. 223–249). Timonium, MD: York Press.

Satz, P., & Fletcher, J. M. (1980). Minimal brain dysfunctions: An appraisal of research concepts and methods. In H. E. Rie & E. D. Rie (Eds.), *Handbook of minimal brain dysfunctions: A critical view* (pp. 669–715). New York: Wiley.

Schatschneider, C., Carlson, C. D., Francis, D. J., Foorman, B. R., & Fletcher, J. M. (2002). Relationships of rapid automatized naming and phonological awareness in early reading development: Implications for the double deficit hypothesis. *Journal of Learning Disabilities, 35,* 245–256.

Share, D. L., McGee, R., & Silva, P. A. (1989). IQ and reading progress: A test of the capacity notion of IQ. *Journal of American Academy of Child and Adolescent Psychiatry, 28,* 97–100.

Share, D. L., & Stanovich, K. E. (1995). Cognitive processes in early reading development: Accommodating individual differences into a model of acquisition. *Issues in Education: Contributions From Educational Psychology, 1,* 1–57.

Shaywitz, S. E., Escobar, M. D., Shaywitz, B. A., Fletcher, J. M., & Makuch, R. (1992). Evidence that dyslexia may represent the lower tail of a normal distribution of reading ability. *New England Journal of Medicine, 326,* 145– 150.

Shaywitz, S. E., Fletcher, J. M., Holahan, J. M., Shneider, A. E., Marchione, K. E., Stuebing, K. K., Francis, D. J., & Shaywitz, B. A. (1999). Persistence of dyslexia: The Connecticut longitudinal study at adolescence. *Pediatrics, 104,* 1351–1359.

Skinner, H. (1981). Toward the integration of classification theory and methods. *Journal of Abnormal Psychology, 90,* 68–87.

Speece, D. L., & Case, L. P. (2001). Classification in context: An alternative approach to identifying early reading disability. *Journal of Educational Psychology, 93,* 735–749.

Spreen, O. (1989). Learning disability, neurology, and long-term outcome: Some implications for the individual and for society. *Journal of Clinical & Experimental Neuropsychology, 11,* 389–408.

Stanovich, K. E. (1988). Explaining the differences between the dyslexic and the garden-variety poor reader: The phonological-core variable difference model. *Journal of Learning Disabilities, 21,* 590–604.

Stanovich, K. E., Siegel, L. S., & Gottardo, A. (1997). Converging evidence for phonological and surface subtypes of reading disability. *Journal of Educational Psychology, 89,* 114–128.

Stuebing, K. K., Fletcher, J. M., LeDoux, J. M., Lyon, G. R., Shaywitz, S. E., & Shaywitz, B. A. (2002). Validity of IQ-discrepancy classifications of reading disabilities: A meta-analysis. *American Educational Research Journal, 39,* 469–518.

Tilly, W. D., Reschly, D. J., & Grimes, J. (1999). Disability determination in problem-solving systems: Conceptual foundations and critical components. In D. J. Reschly, W. D. Tilly, & J. P. Grimes (Eds.), *Special education in transition: Functional assessment and noncategorical programming* (pp. 285–321). Longmont, CO: Sopris West.

Tomblin, J. B., & Zhang, X. (1999). Language patterns and etiology in children with specific language impairment. In H. Tager-Flusberg (Ed.), *Neurodevelopmental disorders* (pp. 361–382). Cambridge, MA: MIT Press.

Torgesen, J. K. (2002). Empirical and theoretical support for direct diagnosis of learning disabilities by assessment of intrinsic processing weaknesses. In R. Bradley, L. Danielson, & D. P. Hallahan (Eds.), *Identification of learning disabilities: Research to policy* (pp. 563–613) Mahwah, NJ: Erlbaum.

Torgesen, J. K., Wagner, R. K., Rashotte, C. A., Rose, E., Lindamood, P., Conway, J., & Garvan, C. (1999). Preventing reading failure in young children with phonological processing disabilities: Group and individual responses to instruction. *Journal of Educational Psychology, 91,* 579–594.

U.S. Office of Education. (1977). Assistance to states for education for handicapped children: Procedures for evaluating specific learning disabilities. *Federal Register, 42,* G1082–G1085.

Vellutino, F. R., Scanlon, D. M., & Fletcher, J. M. (2002). *Research in the study of reading disability (dyslexia): What have we learned in the past four decades?* Unpublished manuscript.

Vellutino, F. R., Scanlon, D. M., & Lyon, G. R. (2000). Differentiating between difficult to remediate and readily remediated poor readers: More evidence against the IQ Achievement discrepancy definition of reading disability. *Journal of Learning Disabilities, 33,* 223–238.

Wimmer, H., & Mayringer, H. (2002). Dysfluent reading in the absence of spelling difficulties: A specific disability in regular orthographies. *Journal of Educational Psychology, 94,* 272–277.

Wise, B. W., Ring, J., & Olson, R. K. (1999). Training phonological awareness with and without explicit attention to articulation. *Journal of Experimental Child Psychology, 72,* 271–304.

Wolf, M., & Bowers, P. G. (1999). The double deficit hypothesis for the developmental dyslexias. *Journal of Educational Psychology, 91,* 415–438.

Wolf, M., Bowers, P. G., & Biddle, K. (2001). Naming-speed processes, timing, and reading: A conceptual review. *Journal of Learning Disabilities, 33,* 387–407.

Ysseldyke, J., & Marston, D. (1999). Origins of categorical special education services in schools and a rationale for changing them. In D. J. Reschly, W. D. Tilly, & J. P. Grimes (Eds.), *Special education in transition: Functional assessment and noncategorical programming* (pp. 1–18). Longmont, CO: Sopris West.

4

Learning Disabilities and the Law

Cynthia M. Herr
Barbara D. Bateman

If a special educator of the 1950s or 1960s had been asked how likely it was that by the late 1970s every aspect of the daily practice of special education would be governed by detailed federal law, the answer probably would have been, "Not likely." However, it has come to pass, and now few special educators remember what special education looked like before it was subject to legal mandate at every turn.

The focus of this chapter is how the law, both legislation and litigation, affects the field of learning disabilities (LD). We examine the impact of law on (1) evaluation and eligibility for services determinations, (2) the development of individualized education programs (IEPs) and the provision of a free appropriate public education, and (3) the provision of education in the least restrictive environment. For example, the Individuals with Disabilities Education Act requires IEPs for all eligible students. These IEPs (at least in law) control the special education and related services to be delivered to students. If an eligible student's behavior interferes with learning, IDEA requires that the IEP contain a behavior intervention plan which must, of course, be implemented. Prior to IDEA, there was no such requirement

and, rarely, such a practice. Clearly, law has an impact on special education practice.

We also discuss the possibility that LD research and practice can or should affect the law. We examine, for example, what influence, if any, our ever-increasing knowledge of the effectiveness of specific methodologies for students with LD has had on the law. We focus primarily on court decisions in major cases involving students with LD. The cases presented are representative, not exhaustive. State hearing decisions have not been presented because they are too numerous, often inconsistent, and do not constitute legal precedent.

Before looking specifically at LD cases, it is important to look briefly at the law behind the cases.

Litigation and Legislation

Litigation (i.e., case law) can prompt legislation, which, in turn, produces more litigation, which then interprets and applies the legislation. That litigation can then result in new or amended legislation. And the cycle goes on. An early example of the effect of special education litigation on legislation was the influence that two cases in the early 1970s had on legislation passed in 1975. The *Pennsylvania Association for Retarded Children (PARC) v. Pennsylvania* (1972) and *Mills v. D. C. Board of Education* (1972) cases arose out of grassroots movements by parents of children with disabilities to force public schools to provide education for their children, many of whom had been excluded from public schools or segregated in separate schools for children with disabilities. From these cases came the impetus for passage of the Education of All Handicapped Children Act (EAHCA) of 1975. Originally called Public Law (PL) 94-142, it is now called the Individuals with Disabilities Education Act, or IDEA. The major provisions of IDEA, which relate to zero-reject, free appropriate public education (FAPE), discipline, child find, due process hearings, and other procedural protections, were patterned closely after the court orders of *PARC* and *Mills*.

The IDEA legislation then resulted in new litigation. The landmark special education case of *Hendrick Hudson Central School District Board of Education v. Rowley* (1982) illustrates how case law (litigation) clarifies and interprets legislation. Even though the purpose of IDEA is to provide FAPE to every child with a disability, the statute itself fails to fully define the critical word "appropriate." The U.S. Supreme Court, therefore, defined "appropriate education" in *Rowley*: "[T]he education to which access is provided [must] be sufficient to confer some educational benefit upon the handicapped child" (pp. 200–201). The Court further concluded that "the 'basic floor of opportunity' provided by the Act consists of access to specialized instruction and related services which are individually designed to provide educational benefit to the handicapped child" (p. 202).

Later cases such as *Honig v. Doe* (1988), which dealt with the discipline of students with disabilities, and *Delaware County Intermediate Unit No. 25 v. Martin K.* (1993), dealing with methodology for a student with autism, led to IDEA amendments in 1990 and 1997. The cycle of litigation–legislation–litigation–legislation will continue in the field of special education. Following the 1997 amendments to IDEA, we are now in a cycle of litigation which will interpret and clarify those changes, as well as continue to resolve other disputes.

Three major pieces of federal legislation affect the education of individuals with disabilities, including those with LD: (1) IDEA, (2) Section 504 of the Vocational Rehabilitation Act of 1973, and (3) the Americans with Disabilities Act (ADA) of 1990. There is some overlap across these three acts. Because the great majority of cases in the field of LD have been filed under IDEA, we deal only with this legislation in this chapter. IDEA, first enacted in 1975, governs the provision of special education and related services to all children with disabilities ages 3–21 who qualify under IDEA.

Because IDEA coverage extends only through secondary school graduation or age 21, cases of alleged discrimination against college students and employees with LD are brought under Section 504 and/or the ADA. In most of these cases, individuals are seeking accommodations in admissions, assessment, or the workplace or working conditions. A review of these cases is beyond this discussion. With a few notable exceptions (e.g., *Guckenberger v. Boston University* [1997]), most plaintiffs with LD have not prevailed. The common issues are whether the plaintiff with LD is actually a "disabled" person as defined by Section 504 and ADA (i.e., whether she or he has a "substantial limitation" in a major life activity) and/or whether the disputed accommodation would involve a fundamental alteration in the program or job. The remainder of this chapter presents cases brought under IDEA.

Evaluation and Eligibility

The processes of evaluating individuals for LD and determining their eligibility for services and protection from discrimination raise two main issues which various courts have addressed: (1) whether an individual has a learning disability and (2) whether a student's academic problems are the result of a learning disability or some other factor. Embedded in the first issue is the highly controversial issue of what standard should be used to determine whether an individual has a learning disability.

Does an Individual Have a
Learning Disability?

IDEA defines a learning disability both by what it is and what it is not:

> The term means a disorder in one or more basic psychological processes involved in understanding or in using language, spoken or written, that may manifest itself in an imperfect ability to listen, think, speak, read, write, spell, or to do mathematical calculations, including conditions such as perceptual disabilities, brain injury, minimal brain dysfunction, dyslexia, and developmental aphasia. . . .
>
> The term does not include learning problems that are primarily the result of visual, hearing, or motor disabilities, of mental retardation, of emotional disturbance, or of environmental, cultural, or economic disadvantage. (34 C.F.R. § 300.7(b)(10))

Of all the categories of disability defined in IDEA, the category of specific learning disability is the only category for which specific evaluation procedures and criteria are provided:

> A team may determine that a child has a specific learning disability if—
>
> (1) The child does not achieve commensurate with his or her age and ability levels in one or more of the areas listed . . . if provided with learning experiences appropriate for the child's age and ability levels; and
>
> (2) The team finds that a child has a severe discrepancy between achievement and intellectual ability in one or more of the following areas:
>
>   (i) Oral expression.
>   (ii) Listening comprehension.
>   (iii) Written expression.
>   (iv) Basic reading skill.
>   (v) Reading comprehension.
>   (vi) Mathematics calculation.
>   (vii) Mathematics reasoning.
>   (34 C.F.R. § 300.541(a))

The majority of litigation which relates to LD evaluation and eligibility involves disagreements between parents and districts about whether a student has a learning disability. In both *Hiller v. Board of Education of the Brunswick Central School District* (1990) and *Norton v. Orinda Union School District* (1999), the courts agreed with the districts that the students did not have LD because there was no significant discrepancy between the students' achievement and their intellectual abilities. In *Welton v. Liberty 53 School District* (2001), the court also agreed with the district that Eric Welton did not have a learning disability in reading and math, as the parents insisted, because Eric's academic performance in these areas met state criteria. The district and the court agreed, however, that Eric did have a learning disability in the area of written language because his performance fell below the state's criterion in this area.

Generally, courts have tended to look at three factors when deciding whether a student has a learning disability: (1) the presence of a severe discrepancy between achievement and ability, (2) the student's need for special education, and (3) state criteria for a learning disability. For example, in *Ridgewood Board of Education v. N.E.* (1999), the court found that a student had a learning disability because both an independent consultant and the district's child study team found that the student demonstrated a severe discrepancy between his ability and his achievement even though the district claimed that the student did not meet New Jersey's requirement that he have a "perceptual impairment."

Rarely does a court look beyond the above factors to determine whether a student has a learning disability. The court in *Corchado v. Board of Education of Rochester City School District* (2000) is a notable and refreshing exception to this practice. Despite the fact that the evidence indicated that the student had average academic performance, the *Corchado* court said:

> The IHO's [independent hearing officer] reasoning, in effect, precludes a child whose academic achievement can be described as "satisfactory" from being able to demonstrate that documented disabilities adversely affected the student's academic performance. This should not and cannot be the litmus test for eligibility under IDEA.
>
> Each child is different, each impairment is different, and the effect of the particular impairment on the particular child's educational achievement is different. (p. 375)

The *Corchado* court decision illustrates perfectly one of the major controversies that exists today concerning the determination of whether an individual has a learning disability. The controversy centers on the use of discrepancy formulas to determine whether a "severe discrepancy" between achievement and ability exists. Nowhere in the regulations for IDEA is the term "severe discrepancy" defined. A discrepancy formula was proposed for IDEA in 1976 but was soundly rejected by the field. Nevertheless, almost all schools rely on a state- or district-level discrepancy formula, even though these are usually intended only as guidelines. New York, for example, demands a "discrepancy of 50% or more between suggested achievement and actual achievement" (8 N.Y.C.R.R. § 200.1(mm)(6)). Reliance on discrepancy formulas has flourished and is now nearly universal. The thrust of IDEA in identifying children who have LD is reliance on professional judgment, based on a full and thorough individual and individualized evaluation. However, practice has moved increasingly toward reliance on a formula and on a predetermined, one-size-fits-all, limited selection of standardized tests. Factors other than law have weighed heavily in shaping these practices. One factor, ironically, is a fear of legal actions. Many psychologists and educators mistakenly believe that reliance on a quantitative formula and the one-size-fits-all testing procedure can be more easily defended in a hearing or court than can professional judgment in selecting and interpreting assessment procedures. Other factors limiting the law's influence include the system being overwhelmed by increasing numbers of students needing special education and inadequate resources, including insufficient numbers of personnel trained and experienced in evaluating and recognizing LD.

This is clearly an area where neither the law nor LD practice has positively influenced the other. Instead both the law and LD practice seem stuck 30 years in the past when the use of discrepancy models was considered appropriate (Stanovich, 1999).

In an acknowledgment of the controversies that surround the field of LD, including issues of evaluation and eligibility, the Office of Special Education Programs (OSEP) of the federal Department of Education held a Learning Disabilities Summit in Washington, DC, in August 2001. One of the purposes of that summit was to begin discussions and examination of research findings,

as promised by OSEP in the final regulations for IDEA 1997 (64 Fed. Reg. 12637), to determine whether changes should be proposed to the procedures for evaluating children suspected of having a learning disability.

Are Academic Difficulties Caused by a Learning Disability or Other Factor?

Although the issue of whether an individual has a learning disability is the most frequently litigated issue in the area of evaluation and eligibility, it is not the only issue that reaches the courts. Several cases have addressed the issue of whether a student's academic difficulties were really the result of a learning disability or whether they were the result of other factors such as speech or behavior problems. *Kelby v. Morgan Hill Unified School District* (1992) illustrates the difficulties districts, hearing officers, and courts can have in trying to sort out whether a student's academic problems are the result of a learning disability or behavior problems. Parents often argue that the behavior problems are the result of a student's frustration because of academic failure, while districts may argue that the behavior problems cause the student to have academic problems. In *Kelby,* the district, the hearing officer, the district court, and the circuit court all agreed that Richard Kelby's academic problems were due to behavioral issues even though two independent evaluators stated that Richard had a learning disability due to processing deficits. In *Capistrano Unified School District v. Wartenberg* (1995), the Court of Appeals for the Ninth Circuit disagreed with the district's decision that Jeremy Wartenberg's academic failure was due to his misbehavior. In reaching its decision, the court held that "Jeremy's social maladjustment could not be separated out from his organic disorder, and that his misconduct was primarily caused by his organic disorder rather than a non-covered problem" (p. 810).

Though some may argue that a student's disability label does not matter as long as the student receives appropriate services, the court in *Friedman v. Vance, Montgomery County Board of Education* (1996) disagreed. Here the issue was whether Alexander should receive services under a speech/language label or under an LD label. The district court concluded "by a preponderance of evidence, that Alexander ha[d] a learning disability" (p. 657). The court went on to point out that the disability designation was not irrelevant: "By missing the learning disability problems, over and above the speech and language problems, the IEP lacks a full set of goals and objectives, and those that are present consist of mere sketches of the full range of services needed" (p. 657).

Although the issues of evaluation and eligibility are not insignificant, legislation and litigation have had a far greater effect on learning disability practice in the area of IEPs and the provision of FAPE.

IEPs and FAPE

The law has clearly had a significant impact on LD practice in the areas of the development of IEPs and the provision of FAPE to students with LD. Before 1975 and the earliest versions of IDEA, there was no legal requirement for IEPs and school districts were not required to provide children with disabilities with FAPE. Whether or not one believes that IEPs serve a useful purpose in the provision of special education to students with learning or other disabilities, they are mandated by law as a means to ensure that students served under IDEA receive FAPE. Many cases have been filed by parents claiming that their children with LD have been denied FAPE because of either procedural or substantive errors in the development of the IEP or in the document itself. The U.S. Supreme Court in *Rowley* (1982) made it clear that states must comply with both the procedural and substantive requirements of IDEA: "Therefore, a court's inquiry in suits brought under §1415(e)(2) is twofold. First, has the State complied with the procedures set forth in the Act? And second, is the individualized educational program developed through the Act's procedures reasonably calculated to enable the child to receive educational benefit" (p. 206)?

Procedural Issues

The extensive and detailed procedural requirements of IDEA relate to parents' rights

to access records, participate in decision making, obtain an independent educational evaluation, receive prior written notice of district proposals and refusals, consent to initial evaluation and special education placements, present complaints, initiate a hearing and appeal, have the student's placement maintained while disputes are pending, and more. The *Rowley* court particularly emphasized the importance of the procedural aspects of IEP development: "Congress placed every bit as much emphasis upon compliance with procedures . . . as it did upon the measurement of the resulting IEP against a substantive standard" (pp. 205–206).

Lake (2000) has summarized about 150 hearings and cases involving IEP procedural errors related to timeliness, notice, team members and participation, IEP form and development, IEP content, and implementation. Some procedural errors are deemed "harmless" and do not result in a denial of FAPE. Those serious violations which do constitute a denial of FAPE are those that result in an actual loss to the student of educational opportunity or benefit or that deny parents the opportunity for full and meaningful participation in the IEP process.

Courts have ruled that LD students were denied FAPE by (1) districts' failure to give parents adequate notice of their procedural protections (*Hall v. Vance County Board of Education*, 1985; *Briere v. Fair Haven Grade School District*, 1996), (2) districts' failure to follow IEP procedures such as timelines and essential content of IEPs (*Hall v. Vance*, 1985; *Briere v. Fair Haven Grade School District*, 1996; *Evans v. Board of Education of the Rhinebeck Central School District*, 1996; *Susquenita School District v. Raelee*, 1996; *Flowers v. Martinez Unified School District*, 1993; *Egg Harbor Township Board of Education v. S.O.*, 1992; *Lascari v. Ramapo Indian Hills Regional High School District*, 1989), (3) a district's unilateral decision to graduate a student (*Kevin T. v. Elmhurst Community School District*, 2001), and (4) a district's failure to follow IDEA's guidelines for evaluating students with specific learning disability (*Evans v. Board of Education of the Rhinebeck Central School District*, 1996).

Other courts have determined that similar procedural violations did not reach the level of denying FAPE to students (*Salley v. St. Tammany Parish School Board*, 1996; *Welton v. Liberty 53 School District*, 2001; *Judith S. v. Board of Education of Community Unit School District No. 200*, 1998; *Livingston v. Desoto County School District*, 1992; *Doe v. Defendant I.*, 1990; *Hiller v. Board of Education of the Brunswick Central School District*, 1990).

The major way that these cases have affected LD practice is in the heightened awareness among professionals of the many procedural requirements regarding the development of IEPs and the provision of services to students with LD. However, as the following section demonstrates, a heightened awareness among professionals does not always mean that students receive appropriate services.

Substantive Issues

In this section we discuss the most significant issue courts have dealt with since IDEA was enacted, which is: To how much benefit is a student with a disability entitled in the provision of FAPE? We also discuss a second issue, that of methodology, which is gaining increasing importance in special education, especially in the provision of an appropriate education to students with LD.

THE BENEFIT STANDARD

When *Rowley* was decided in 1982, it was necessary for the Supreme Court to determine the type of standard (maximize potential, provide equal opportunity, etc.) to be used to judge program "appropriateness." The Supreme Court chose the "reasonably calculated to enable the child to receive *educational benefit* [italics added] standard," now widely called the "ed benefit" or the *Rowley* standard. In each individual case, a second inquiry is required, namely, to *how much benefit* is this child entitled? Benefit is often measured by progress. In this context, an appropriate program for an intellectually gifted 15-year-old would potentially allow her to progress or benefit more than an appropriate program would benefit a 4-year-old who had severe mental retardation.

Thus, the question of whether FAPE (including sufficient benefit) has been provided must always be a fact-specific, individual-

ized inquiry. The *Rowley* court, therefore, declined to establish any one test for the adequacy of the benefit, beyond making it clear that IDEA does not require the school to provide the best program possible or to maximize each child's potential. Within those limits, several federal circuit courts of appeal have weighed in.

The Fourth Circuit examined the "how much benefit" issue in *Hall v. Vance County Board of Education* (1985). The district contended that the student with LD's social promotions plus minimal improvement on standardized reading tests over a 4-year period showed sufficient benefit to constitute FAPE. The court considered the student's progress in light of the student's own intellectual capabilities and observed:

> *Rowley* recognized that a FAPE must be tailored to the individual child's capabilities and that while one might demand only minimal results in the case of the most severely handicapped children, such results would be insufficient in the case of other children. Clearly, Congress did not intend that a school system could discharge its duty under the EAHCA [predecessor to the IDEA] by providing a program that produces some minimal academic advancement, no matter how trivial. (p. 636)

The Third Circuit, in the case of a dyslexic student, said that IDEA "calls for more than a trivial educational benefit" (*Ridgewood*, 1999, p. 247). In *Capistrano* (1995), the Ninth Circuit was explicit in detailing an appropriate program to meet Jeremy's educational needs and then concluding that Jeremy's IEP did not meet those needs but that the private LD school did. Among Jeremy's named needs were frequent feedback, clear commands, structured school environment, small class size, consistent behavior management, and individualized attention. The court also found that Jeremy's public school IEP moved him too much between classes; assigned him too many teachers; and failed to provide the structure, consistency, and attention that Jeremy needed.

In contrast to the Ninth Circuit's *Capistrano* decision, the Eighth Circuit in *Fort Zumwalt v. Clynes* (1997) concluded that Nicholas Clynes had received sufficient educational benefit even though, after 5 years of school, Nicholas's word attack skills were at a first-grade level and he did not know the alphabet. The court was impressed that Nicholas earned passing marks in the third grade and that he had been promoted to fourth grade just before his parents removed him from the public school. The dissenting judge had a different view:

> [T]he IEP for 1991–1992 was not designed to provide "personalized instruction with sufficient support services to permit [Nicholas] to benefit educationally from that instruction." By submitting an IEP substantially similar to others that had previously produced so few positive results, and by exhibiting an unwillingness to explore any different approaches, Fort Zumwalt did not extend to Nicholas the free and appropriate education mandated by IDEA. . . . Nicholas's achievements, particularly in the area of reading skills, can at best be described as trivial. This cannot be the sort of education Congress had in mind when it enacted IDEA. (p. 617)

When appellate judges disagree so sharply on whether a student received FAPE, it should not be surprising that we are sometimes confused. Many district courts have also wrestled with the issue of how much benefit a child with a learning disability should expect under IDEA. In *Pascoe v. Washingtonville Central School District* (1998), the court ruled that a 17-year-old student with severe dyslexia had received enough benefit because the student earned credits toward a high school diploma and had passed the New York Regent's Competency Tests even though the student's reading and writing skills were at about a second-grade level. The court also noted that although several experts expressed the opinion that the student could have made substantial progress in reading and writing in the right environment, "such potential does not establish that the IEP in issue was inappropriate" (p. 35).

Even before IDEA's 1997 amendments significantly increased the focus on level of benefit and on objective evidence of progress, some district courts held that limited educational progress was not sufficient to prove educational benefit. In *Egg Harbor Township Board of Education* (1992), the court stated that "while the benefits or lack of them actually realized by a child are not dispositive of the question of whether the program was sufficient to satisfy *Rowley's*

'floor of benefit', [citation deleted] they are certainly one indicator" (p. 7). *Evans v. Board of Education of the Rhinebeck Central School District* (1996) held that the district's program could not provide educational benefit to the student because the proposed teacher "was not qualified to teach adolescents or to instruct, train or otherwise consult with teachers as to how to work with Frank [the student] using the approach he requires" (p. 348). Since the 1997 IDEA amendments, several courts have increased the bar of what constitutes enough educational benefit to provide a FAPE.

A federal district court in Indiana recently dealt in detail with LD and FAPE issues *(Nein v. Greater Clark County School Corp.,* 2000). From kindergarten through fourth grade, Lucas attended an elementary school in the Greater Clark District (Indiana). He was identified in first grade as having a severe learning disability. In first grade, Lucas's Wechsler Intelligence Scale for Children (WISC; Wechsler, 1991) Full Scale IQ was 95. Nevertheless, in January of fourth grade, Lucas was reading below second-grade level and was spelling at first-grade level. In November of Lucas's fifth-grade year, a hearing officer (as quoted by the district court) found the district had denied Lucas FAPE: "The ability to read is a fundamental ingredient in a free appropriate education that can be diminished only by a finding that the disabled child is clearly incapable of achieving reading skills transferable to life settings. The failure to use an approach that will provide Student with the tools to become an independent reader is alone an important reason why the LEA did not provide an appropriate education" (p. 970).

The district court went on to explain, "If an IEP must be designed to take into account a child's individual educational needs, it logically follows that the child's capacity to learn should also be considered in evaluating the IEP" (p. 974).

After noting that district personnel did not demonstrate any expertise or significant training in teaching students with dyslexia, the court reviewed and refuted the school district's claims that they had provided sufficient benefit to Lucas (i.e., a Chevrolet education) while the parents were demanding a Cadillac:

At the risk of carrying these metaphors too far, for a student like Lucas, the ability to read is truly the key that opens the door to all other aspects of an education. In terms of the automotive metaphor, Greater Clark was providing the Neins with a Chevrolet without a transmission—even if the engine might run, no power ever reached the wheels. Because the Milestones program produced no *transferable* progress in three years, as both the initial hearing officer and the Board of Appeals found, the program was plainly failing to provide even a minimally *adequate* educational benefit. (p. 977)

The court also saw through the district's claim that adequate benefit was shown by Lucas's grades (in fact, they were modified) and his promotions (retention was against district policy) as did the court in *R.R. v. Wallingford Board of Education* (2001), which held:

Despite the student's attainment of passing grades and his regular advancement from grade to grade, we are not persuaded by the Board's argument that the student was making satisfactory progress. The record is replete with test results indicating that, despite having been placed in a mainstream ninth grade class, the student had not progressed in reading ability beyond a third or fourth grade level. (p. 123)

Indisputably, the benefit standard has been newly highlighted and emphasized, and most of us agree the standard has been raised. Congress's insistence on improving special education outcomes requires, among other changes, greater utilization of effective teaching practices (i.e., effective methodology).

METHODOLOGY AS A SUBSTANTIVE ISSUE
OF FAPE

This section examines recent changes in the law and the effects of those changes. However, we must begin with an important non-change.

From 1975 to the present time, IDEA has defined *special education* as "specially designed instruction, at no cost to parents, to meet the unique needs of a chid with a disability . . ." (34 C.F.R. § 300.26(a)). There is no change here. But, in the 1999 regulations, the U.S. Office of Education defined

specially designed instruction as "adapting, as appropriate to the needs of an eligible child under this part, the content, *methodology* (emphasis added) or delivery of instruction . . ." (34 C.F.R § 300.26(b)(3)).

As significantly, Attachment 1 (titled *Analysis of Comments and Changes*) to the 1999 IDEA regulations (64 Fed. Reg. 12552) discusses the foregoing change to the definition of specially designed instruction:

Case law recognizes that instructional methodology can be an important consideration in the context of what constitutes an appropriate education for a child with a disability. At the same time, these courts have indicated that they will not substitute a parentally-preferred methodology for sound educational programs developed by school personnel in accordance with the procedural requirements of the IDEA to meet the educational needs of an individual child with a disability.

In light of the legislative history and case law, it is clear that in developing an individualized education there are circumstances in which the particular methodology that will be used is an integral part of what is "individualized" about a student's education and, in those circumstances will need to be discussed at the IEP meeting and *incorporated into the student's IEP* (emphasis added). For example, for a child with a learning disability who has not learned to read using traditional instructional methods, an appropriate education may require some other instructional strategy.

In all cases, whether methodology would be addressed in an IEP would be an IEP team decision. (64 Fed. Reg. 12552)

If we recall that every IEP must contain "a statement of the special education . . . to be provided" (20 U.S.C. § 1414(d)(1)(A)(iii)), that special education is specially designed instruction and that methodology is included therein, we can only conclude, as has the U.S. Office of Education, that there are times at which methodology is an essential ingredient in FAPE and must, therefore, be included in the IEP.

Though some degree of deference may still be due the school's choice of methodology under the 1997 IDEA, it seems clear that any presumption of appropriateness of that school choice now is properly seen as rebuttable. Under IDEA, the parents have the right to dispute any matter related to the provision of FAPE (34 C.F.R. § 300.507(a)(1)). Methodology is, in many cases, the key element in FAPE and must be subject to dispute resolution.

If any further evidence is required that methodology may be and sometimes must be on the IEP, one has only to look at the new mandates for the IEP team to address Braille for students with visual impairments, to consider positive behavior interventions for students with behavior issues, and to conduct functional behavior assessments as necessary. These are all squarely methodologies. When any techniques and/or methodologies are on an IEP, they, of course, may be disputed by the parent.

Hearing officers and courts are understandably reluctant to be involved in these disputes over methodology, and in spite of the emphasis on methodology found in the 1997 IDEA, some courts still refuse to entertain the issues of methodology. The court in *Kugler v. Vance* (1999), for example, declared, "The question of appropriate methodology for providing related services to Matthew is precisely the type of dispute that is inappropriate for judicial resolution" (p. 751). Even though many courts are reluctant to address issues of methodology, there are times at which courts must, as the provision of FAPE requires no less.

A federal district court has recently provided cogent guidance, well grounded in both law and special education, for decision makers faced with evaluating the appropriateness of a school district's IEP. In *Board of Education of the County of Kanawha v. Michael M.* (2000), "the entire dispute rests on the issue of whether the *methodology in the IEPs* [italics added] was reasonably tailored to accomplish the goals set forth in the IEPs" (p. 611). In approaching this dispute, the court laid out the following steps:

For a school district to sustain its burden of proving that its IEP was reasonably calculated at the time of creation to provide some educational benefit, the school district cannot simply provide conclusory statements that the IEP was adequate. The school district must show the following concrete information. First, the school district must show that it set forth the proper elements of the IEP. . . .

Second, the school district must show that the annual goals, benchmarks, and short-term objectives set forth in the IEP were reasonable. The goals must be realistic and attainable, yet more than trivial and de minimis. . . .

Third, the school district must show that the methodology that it employed was tailored to meet the annual goals, benchmarks, and short-term objectives set forth in the IEP. Stated differently, the special education and related services must be tailored to reasonably accomplish the goals in the IEP. (p. 610)

The court in *Nein* (2000) also dealt with methodology issues in determining whether Lucas had received an appropriate education. In the following excerpt from the case, Ms. Hoeppner is the school's special education teacher who had used a whole-language method with Lucas unsuccessfully. Ms. Dakin is one of the experts who testified about dyslexia.

[This testimony] does not show that Ms. Hoeppner either had actually implemented Ms. Dakin's recommendations or was planning to do so. Ms. Dakin made numerous recommendations, but the recommendation most at issue here was that Greater Clark implement a direct teaching reading program using multisensory, structured, sequential techniques. Ms. Hoeppner did not testify that Lucas' fifth grade IEP included the use of such a teaching program, or that she was planning to use such a teaching program. In fact, Lucas's IEP does not provide for the use of a direct teaching method or any other particular teaching technique to be used to improve his reading skills. As Ms. Hoeppner explained, because there are never any specific instructions in a student's IEP regarding teaching methodology or technique, Ms. Hoeppner would determine what teaching techniques to use with a particular student by looking at the broad goals contained in the student's IEP. There is simply no evidence in the record indicating that, if Ms. Hoeppner had had the opportunity to implement the fifth grade IEP, she was planning to use a teaching method or technique different from those she had used unsuccessfully with Lucas for the prior three years. (p. 979)

In fairness to the judicial system, it should be said that although many courts have flatly refused to examine methodology, a few, in addition to *Kanawha* and *Nein*, have braved the waters. Among these is the *Evans* (1996) court. Frank Evans was a 15-year-old with severe dyslexia. The Rhinebeck School District proposed a program for Frank that consisted of one-on-one multisensory instruction in reading and writing for 60 minutes 4 days a week along with enrollment in a special education class for English; support services in math and science; and modifications in testing, classwork, and homework. Dyslexia experts agreed that due to the severity of Frank's LD, he needed an intensive program of individualized, integrated, multisensory, sequential training in order to receive academic benefit. The court found that "despite her [Frank's special education teacher] intensive individual instruction eight times per week, and homework and classwork modifications, Frank's performance declined" (p. 348). As a result of such evidence and the testimony of dyslexia experts, the court found that the Rhinebeck School District had not used a methodology designed to ensure an appropriate education for Frank.

We can expect to see more cases come before the courts which require decisions about methodology for students with LD, especially those who have severe reading disabilities. It may be that in a field in which the controversy about how best to teach reading has long raged, law and litigation will actually have as much effect on changing LD practice as has the abundance of research on reading from the last 50 years!

ACCOMMODATIONS FOR STUDENTS WITH LD

The issue of providing accommodations for students with LD is one that has only infrequently been raised in the courts. In *Doe v. Withers* (1993), the parents of a student with LD claimed that their son's teachers and school officials had refused to provide the accommodations required by his IEP. Douglas's IEP allowed him to take tests orally for his mainstream classes. This accommodation had been provided when Douglas was in elementary and middle school. When Douglas entered high school, all his teachers but one agreed to comply with the oral-testing accommodation. Because his history teacher refused to allow him to take tests orally, Douglas failed his history class. As a result, he was barred from participating in extracurricular activities. The court ordered the district to provide all necessary tutoring and reteaching to prepare Douglas to take an

oral test in American History. The court further awarded $15,000 damages, which the history teacher was required to pay to Douglas and his parents.

Recently, parents of students with LD settled a class action suit against the state of Oregon. The suit alleged that Oregon's statewide system of assessment (OSAS) discriminated against children with LD. In the settlement, *A.S.K. v. Oregon State Board of Education* (2001), Oregon agreed to adopt extensive recommendations of a panel of experts appointed to study Oregon's assessment system. In particular, the panel recommended:

> Accommodations should be considered allowable, valid, and scorable if they are used during instructional or on classroom assessments and are listed on a student's IEP until research evidence invalidates the score interpretation. Rather than consider all accommodations first invalid until proven to be valid, ODE should consider all accommodations valid unless and until research provides evidence that an accommodation alters the construct or level of the OSAS measure. (Disability Rights Advocates, 2001, p. 30)

As more and more states adopt statewide assessment systems that require students to pass tests in order to receive a high school diploma or qualify for college entrance or scholarships, this issue of appropriate accommodations is likely to be raised more frequently. We can expect to see more of these cases in the future.

Placement and Least Restrictive Environment

The IDEA legal requirements related to placement are remarkably simple. Every eligible student is entitled to an individualized placement decision based on his or her IEP and selected from a full continuum of alternative placements. When the student's education cannot be "achieved satisfactorily" in a regular classroom, another setting is allowed. According to the federal Office of Special Education Programs (Letter to Trahan, 1998):

> The overriding rule in any placement under Part B is that the child's placement must be in-

dividually determined based on his or her unique abilities and needs. Recognizing that regular class placement may not be appropriate for every disabled child, the Part B regulations require that school districts make available a range of placement options, known as the continuum of alternative placements, to meet the unique educational needs of students with disabilities. 34 C.F.R. § 300.551(a). This requirement for the continuum reinforces the importance of the individualized inquiry, not a "one size fits all" approach, in determining what placement is least restrictive for each student with a disability. (p. 403)

What Is a "Placement"?

In 1977, when IDEA first went into effect, most special educators thought "placement" meant *where* a program (curriculum, instruction, and related activities) was delivered. The program was the "what" of the child's education; the placement was the "where." However, it was soon evident that the courts did not necessarily see it the same way.

In *Concerned Parents v. New York City Board of Education* (1980), the Second Circuit court held that "the term 'educational placement' refers only to the general type of educational program in which the child is placed" (p. 753). This, of course, makes it difficult to interpret the many references in IDEA to identification, evaluation, program, and placement. Ordinarily in law, different words have different referents. The end result is some confusion over when and where, if at all, a line can be drawn between program and placement.

Over time, the prevailing issue in placement has become one of balancing IDEA's requirement for an appropriate education with the philosophy of including all students in regular classes. There have been many cases filed by parents of students with LD which dispute a district's choice of placement for a student.

Least Restrictive Environment

The concept of least restrictive environment (LRE) in IDEA apparently has its historical roots in the legal principle that when the government abridges or restricts life, liberty, or property, it must do so in the least intrusive, least drastic, or least harmful man-

ner that satisfies the government's purpose. In the 1960s, institutionalized patients with mental illness began to sue successfully for the right to move into the most "ordinary" programs and facilities (unlocked wards, weekend passes into the community, etc.) in which they were capable of responsibly participating, rather than being kept in unduly restrictive and often horribly inhumane conditions. This LRE principle would also apply, for example, if a prison or government hospital has to choose between a lobotomy or medication to control a prisoner's otherwise uncontrollable violent behavior.

The applicability of this least drastic, intrusive, or harmful doctrine to public school special and general education classrooms seems forced, at best. Similarly, the proposition that chronological age (rather than mental age, social age, needs, interests, abilities or performance level) is the only appropriate basis for grouping students in school is a stretch for many.

The term "LRE" is used in at least two fundamentally different ways in special education—either as one *particular place* on the continuum of placements (i.e., a regular classroom) or as *whatever placement* maximizes options, functioning levels, or possibilities for a given student and allows his or her education to be "achieved satisfactorily." Some courts have used the first notion, reflexively and without analysis, to mean placement in the mainstream of public education. More thoughtful courts have used the second and have sometimes acknowledged that the mainstream is not the LRE for a particular student.

LRE AS MANDATED MAINSTREAMING

In *Amann v. Stow School System* (1992), the court denied the parents' choice of a private school placement for a 14-year-old with LD because the private school provided no mainstreaming. The court quoted *Roland M.* in saying, "Mainstreaming may not be ignored, even to fulfill substantive educational criteria" (p. 621). The *Amann* court held this position in spite of the fact that the Massachusetts's educational benefit standard called for "maximum possible development." Likewise, the court in *Robert M. v. Hickok* (2000) rejected the parents' choice of a private school placement for their son Robert based on the erroneous premise that "federal law requires that children like Robert, whose intellectual abilities are only slightly less than those of his peers, be incorporated into regular classroom settings" (p. 531).

In a case in which parents and the school district had been unable to come to agreement on an IEP for the student in spite of numerous meetings, the Fourth Circuit found in favor of the district because the parents failed to demonstrate that their proposed placement would be the LRE for the student (*DeLullo v. Jefferson County Board of Education,* 1999). In a similar case, *Board of Education of the City School District of the City of New York* (1998), the court ruled that parents could not show that a private school placement was the LRE for the student. However, the court also ruled that the district's proposed program was not appropriate! The court left unanswered what placement *was* appropriate for the student. The issue of whether LRE properly applies to parents' placements is discussed later.

BALANCING LRE AND EDUCATIONAL BENEFIT

A number of courts have looked at the concept of LRE more broadly and have weighed educational benefit in balancing LRE with appropriate program. Courts have considered numerous factors when deciding what constitutes an appropriate placement. In *Egg Harbor* (1992), the court said, "Mainstreaming, however, is not the primary issue in this case. The question before us is the appropriateness of the educational program designed for S. by Egg Harbor" (p. 18). The court went on to quote the Burlington case: "The least restrictive environment guarantee . . . cannot be applied to cure an otherwise inappropriate placement" (*Burlington School Committee v. Massachusetts Department of Education,* 471 U.S. 359 [1985]) (p. 789). Following this reasoning, the *Egg Harbor* court ruled that Landmark School, a private school for students with LD, was an appropriate placement for S. and required the Egg Harbor district to pay for the placement.

In *Capistrano* (1995), the Ninth Circuit also ruled for a balance between mainstreaming and appropriateness of program. "Mainstreaming which results in total failure, where separate teaching would produce superior results, is not appropriate and satisfactory. Congress expressly limited its presumption in favor of mainstreaming to cases where mainstreaming is 'appropriate' and mainstream education can be provided 'satisfactorily'" (p. 812).

Even when private school placement is not at issue, courts must sometimes balance IDEA's preference for neighborhood school placement (34 C.F.R. § 300.552(c)) against other factors. The court in *Greenbush School Committee v. Mr. and Mrs. K.* (1996) said, "The default placement for a student under the Act is his or her local school, however, an IEP can override this default in situations where the student would not receive an educational benefit at the local school" (p. 203). In this case, the court found that the extreme animosity between the parents of a student with LD and the local school staff along with the student's "gripping" fear of attending the local school were sufficient to prevent the student from receiving educational benefit at the neighborhood school. The court, therefore, ordered the district to place the student at a different, nearby school in the same district.

The First Circuit, in *Milford School District v. William F.* (1997) reminds us that placement decisions must be made by a team of people who consider a number of factors. "The guidelines for a placement decision in New Hampshire law as in federal law provide for involving many interested persons and a wide variety of factors in the choice among alternative potential placements, and the law does not specify that any one factor or any one person's opinion must be given decisive weight" (p. 26).

Even the fact that a private school is religiously affiliated and not a special education school does not automatically preclude that school from being the LRE for a student. In *Matthew J. v. Massachusetts Department of Education* (1998), the court ruled that the Master's School, a private, non-special education, college-preparatory Christian school, appropriately addressed Matthew's need for no aggressive peers and a structured and supportive environment and was, therefore, the LRE.

Two recent cases delineate the critical importance of weighing educational benefit against mainstreaming in determining the LRE. In both cases, the district involved had failed to provide an appropriate education for a student with LD, and, as a result, the student had made negligible academic progress. In *Nein* (2000), the court stated: "Mainstreaming is not required in every case. . . . [I]t must be determined whether the child is benefitting educationally from mainstreaming. The evidence in the record here demonstrates that, for three years, Lucas did not benefit educationally from Greater Clark's educational plans. . . . Thus, there is a good reason in this case to discount Greater Clark's reliance on the IDEA's 'strong preference' for mainstreaming" (p. 981).

The court in *R.R.* (2001) ordered an out-of-district placement at a private LD school for an eighth-grade student who read at a third- or fourth-grade level in spite of the district's argument that the student would be deprived of elective courses and socialization with nondisabled peers. The court ruled, "On balance, we find the opportunities the student will miss in the Board's program pale beside his need for 'an intensive and unique program' in order to remedy his learning disability" (p. 124).

Issues of LRE continue to be raised in cases in which parents seek reimbursement for private school placements, even if those placements are residential, for their children with LD because the parents believe that district programs are inappropriate.

REIMBURSEMENT AS AN LRE ISSUE

Many LD placement cases arise when the parents believe the public school has failed to offer FAPE by not providing an appropriate instructional methodology and/or by not employing trained and experienced LD teachers. Typically, the parents remove the student to a private LD school and then seek reimbursement. Analytically, these cases pose two questions: Did the district provide FAPE, and if not, is the private placement proper under IDEA? However, a critical question is embedded in whether the private placement is proper, that is, whether IDEA's LRE preference applies to the parents' chosen placement. To date, the majority of courts have simply assumed that it

does and without any analysis have ruled against the parents. However, in *Florence County School District Four v. Carter* (1993), the U.S. Supreme Court ruled:

> There is no doubt that Congress has imposed a significant financial burden on States and school districts that participate in IDEA. Yet public educational authorities who want to avoid reimbursing parents for the private education of a disabled child can do one of two things: give the child a free appropriate public education in a public setting, or place the child in an appropriate private setting of the State's choice. This is IDEA's mandate, and school officials who conform to it need not worry about reimbursement claims. (p. 15)

The few courts that have looked at the question carefully since then have concluded that when the public sector fails to offer an appropriate program, LRE does *not* apply to bar reimbursement for a private placement, even if it is more restrictive. In *Cleveland Heights-University Heights City School District v. Boss* (1998), the Sixth Circuit pointed out the fallacy of expecting parents to pay for a private school education for their child when the district failed to provide an appropriate program.

> The District would have us read the IDEA to say, in effect: "If we fail to provide a disabled child with an appropriate education, the parents must pay for a private education, or let their child languish in our institution if the only placement more suitable to her needs and more closely approximating the ideal envisioned by the IDEA than what we offer is a specialized private school that admits only learning disabled students." Congress did not intend to place beneficiaries of the IDEA in the position of having to choose only among these unpalatable alternatives. (p. 400)

The parents of Raelee, a ninth-grader with LD, withdrew her from public school, placed her in a private school, and requested reimbursement from the school district. The court, in *Susquenita School District v. Raelee* (1996), ruled: "Although the Janus School did not provide Raelee the least restrictive setting possible, it was an appropriate placement in light of her educational needs and in view of the fact that Susquenita failed to offer an appropriate placement in a less restrictive setting" (p. 127).

Courts have used similar reasoning to order reimbursement to parents for residential placements when the residential placement provided the only appropriate program. In *Lascari* (1989), the court said:

We are sensitive to the possibility that parents may select a private school that affords their child an education that is more elaborate than is required. Conceivably, parents might select a boarding school even though a day program would furnish their child with an appropriate education. It would be anomalous, however, to recognize the parents' right to reimbursement, but to deny completely that right merely because they selected a school that furnished an education beyond that which the district is obliged to offer. It would also be anomalous to deny parents the right to reimbursement when the district failed to provide their child with an appropriate education and the only school that the parents could find was a boarding school. (p. 572)

In a case in which the parents of a student with a serious learning disability and a severe language disorder placed her in a private, residential school, the court found that "no non-residential alternatives to Maplebrook School were proposed by the District, nor were any such programs known to exist" (*Briere v. Fair Haven Grade School District*, 1996, p. 63).

However, a parent will not be entitled to reimbursement for a residential placement when a court finds that the district offered an appropriate program. In some courts, parents may also be denied reimbursement if the court finds that the child did not need a residential placement to benefit educationally. In *Lenn v. Portland School Committee* (1992), the parents of Daniel, a 17-year-old student with a learning disability, argued that their son needed a residential placement after being hospitalized for depression. The court ruled that the district's proposed program was reasonably calculated to be of significant educational benefit to Daniel. The court noted that the district program "would address Daniel's needs for specialized education . . . while enabling him to remain in his home community and interact daily with non-disabled peers" (p. 617).

In a similar case, *Salley v. St. Tammany Parish School Board* (1995), the parents of a fourth-grade student requested a residential placement for their daughter after she spent some time in a psychiatric hospital. The court found that "Many of the student's difficulties were related to her family relationships and were more adequately treated through counseling rather than removal to a residential facility" (p. 879). The court ruled that the district had offered an appropriate program that was less restrictive than the residential placement the parents requested.

In *Walczak v. Florida Union Free School District* (1998), the district proposed an IEP for a student with a learning disability which called for her placement in a self-contained class for developmentally disabled students. The Walczaks objected to this placement and argued that their daughter's needs could not be met in a day program and that she required a residential placement. The Walczaks also objected to the size (12 students) and composition (students with developmental disabilities) of the district's proposed class. The court found that "a clear preponderence of that evidence demonstrates that B.W. could make satisfactory academic and social progress in a twelve-student class in the BOCES day program" (p. 1143). The court, therefore, denied the parents' request for a residential placement.

As with most IDEA issues addressed by the courts, the question of what is the LRE for a particular student with a learning disability is complex and requires the balancing of many factors.

Conclusions and Further Thoughts

The statutory and case law that addresses services for students with LD is vast and sometimes conflicting. How has the field of LD been affected? Our response to this question is not based solely on the litigation and legislation we have reviewed in this chapter but also on our experiences as scholars and practitioners in the field of LD.

Arguably, legislation and litigation have had a detrimental affect on the practices of evaluating and determining the eligibility of students suspected of having a learning disability. Many students who are probably not learning disabled are receiving services under that label, and some students who should receive services are not. The IDEA definition of learning disability has lead to widespread misuse of standardized tests and discrepancy formulas. Even now that definition and the methods used to identify students with LD are being debated by nationally recognized researchers in the field of LD (Council for Exceptional Children, 2001). Regardless of whether the definition of LD is changed in the statute, a need will remain for district professionals who are truly knowledgeable about LD. School personnel must begin to used broader-based assessment procedures which go beyond simply comparing two scores from the WISC-III (Wechsler, 1991) and the Woodcock-Johnson III (Woodcock, McGrew, & Mather, 2001). There must be a move toward (or perhaps back to) greater reliance on teacher input, students' work products, observations, and other strategies to determine whether or not students are achieving at appropriate levels.

Special educators and administrators *must* be trained to recognize when methodology constitutes an integral part of a student's IEP. The new legal recognition that methodology may sometimes be required to be included on IEPs, especially for students with LD, is potentially important and positive. The inclusion of methodology on IEPs could be a major impetus for improved instructional practice for many students with LD. For this to happen, special educators and administrators must attend to the research on effective teaching methodology for students with LD, and they must be convinced that it is critical to implement such effective teaching procedures in special education programs and regular education classrooms which serve these students. Special educators must once again become teachers of "specialized" instruction. As Zigmond (1997) has said:

> Special education was once worth receiving; it could be again. In many schools, it is not now. Here is where practitioners, policymakers, advocates, and researchers in special education need to focus—on defining the nature of special education and the competencies of the teachers who will deliver it. Here is where the research-to-practice gulf must be bridged. Here is the issue we must resolve, or the hard-fought promise of IDEA will be empty, indeed. (p. 389)

In making decisions about placement for students with LD, districts have relied on the concept of "least restrictive environment" to eliminate many specialized classes for students with LD. In what sense, one might ask, is it "less restrictive" for a student to be with only nondisabled peers who do not and cannot share his or her perspectives and experiences?

Similarly, what is the underlying message when a student with LD is told that the only peers who are suitable are those who do not have LD? Is it really healthier for students with LD to be in regular classrooms where their disability puts them visibly and publicly on the bottom rung of dozens of daily ladders rather than being with other students with LD where they occupy all the rungs of the daily ladders, from top to bottom and in between? Little, if any, consideration is given by some districts to the self-esteem issues raised for students with LD placed all day in mainstream classes.

Some courts, at least, have recognized that program effectiveness as measured by student progress is at least as important as mainstreaming for students with LD. We firmly believe that it does students with LD little good to be mainstreamed and socialized in regular education classrooms for 12 years if the result is that those students leave high school reading at a second- or third-grade level and with serious self-esteem issues. Although the original intent of IDEA may have been to ensure access to public schools for students with disabilities, the current IDEA regulations make it clear that the appropriateness of a student's special education program must be judged, in large part, by the progress that student makes toward his or her educational goals.

We in the field of learning disabilities have learned much in the 40 years since Samuel Kirk (1962) coined the term "learning disability." We now know *how* best to teach students with LD so that they learn the skills and content that their nondisabled peers learn. The law provides an avenue for ensuring that students with LD benefit from this knowledge if we as practitioners follow the spirit of the law and provide truly individualized, *special* education to students with LD.

References

Amann v. Stow School System, 982 F.2d 644 (1st Cir. 1992).

Americans with Disability Act, 42 U.S.C. §§ 12101 et seq. (1994).

A.S.K. v. Oregon State Board of Education (Feb., 2001).

Board of Education of the City School District of the City of New York, 30 IDELR 64 (Review Officer Decision, 1998).

Board of Education of the County of Kanawha v. Michael M., 95 F. Supp. 2d 600 (S.D. W. Va. 2000).

Briere v. Fair Haven Grade School District, 948 F. Supp. 1242 (D. Vt. 1996).

Burlington School Committee v. Massachusetts Department of Education, 471 U.S. 359 (1985).

Capistrano Unified School District v. Wartenberg, 59 F.3d 884 (9th Cir. 1995).

Cleveland Heights-University Heights City School District v. Boss, 144 F.3d 391 (6th Cir. 1998).

Concerned Parents of New York City Board of Education, 629 F.2d 751 (2d Cir. 1980).

Corchado v. Board of Education of Rochester City School District, 86 F. Supp. 2d 168 (W.D.N.Y. 2000).

Council for Exceptional Children. (2001). The controversy over learning disabilities continues. *Today, 8*(4), 1, 5, 15.

Delaware County Intermediate Unit No. 25 v. Martin K., 831 F. Supp. 1206 (E.D. Pa. 1993).

DeLullo v. Jefferson County Board of Education, 194 F.3d 1304 (4th Cir. 1999).

Disability Rights Advocates. (2001). *Do no harm— High stakes testing and students with learning disabilities.* Oakland, CA: Author.

Doe v. Defendant I., 898 F.2d 1186 (6th Cir. 1990).

Doe v. Withers, 20 IDELR 422 (W. Va. Cir. Ct. 1993).

Education for All Handicapped Children Act, 20 U.S.C. § 1400 et seq. (1975).

Egg Harbor Township Board of Education v. S.O., 19 IDELR 15 (D.N.J. 1992).

Evans v. Board of Education of the Rhinebeck Central School District, 930 F. Supp. 83 (S.D.N.Y. 1996).

Florence County School District Four v. Carter, 510 U.S. 7 (1993).

Flowers v. Martinez Unified School District, 19 IDELR 898 (N.D. Cal. 1993).

Fort Zumwalt School District v. Clynes, 119 F.3d 607 (8th Cir. 1997).

Friedman v. Vance, Montgomery County Board of Education, 24 IDELR 654 (D. Md. 1996).

Greenbush School Committee v. Mr. and Mrs. K., 949 F. Supp. 934 (D. Me. 1996).

Guckenberger v. Boston University, 974 F. Supp. 106 (D. Mass. 1997).

Hall v. Vance County Board of Education, 774 F.2d 629 (4th Cir. 1985).

Hendrick Hudson Central School District Board of Education v. Rowley, 458 U.S. 176 (1982).

Hiller v. Board of Education of the Brunswick Central School District, 743 F. Supp. 958 (N.D.N.Y. 1990).

Honig v. Doe, 484 U.S. 305 (1988).

Individuals with Disabilities Education Act, Pub. L. 105–17, 111 Stat. 37 (1997) (codified at 20 U.S.C. §§ 1499–1487).

Judith S. v. Board of Education of Community. Unit School District No. 200, 28 IDELR 728 (N.D. Ill. 1998).

Kelby v. Morgan Hill Unified School District, 18 IDELR 831 (9th Cir. 1992).

Kevin T. v. Elmhurst Community School District No. 205, 34 IDELR 202 (N.D. Ill. 2001).

Kirk, S. A. (1962). *Educating exceptional children.* Boston: Houghton Mifflin.

Kugler v. Vance, 30 IDELR 749 (D. Md. 1999).

Lake, S. (2000). *IEP procedural errors: Lessons learned, mistakes to avoid.* Horsham, PA: LRP Publications.

Lascari v. Ramapo Indian Hills Regional High School District, 560 A.2d 1180 (N.J. 1989).

Lenn v. Portland School Committee, 19 IDELR 615 (D. Me. 1992).

Letter to Trahan, 30 IDELR 403 (Sept. 3, 1998).

Livingston v. Desoto County School District, 782 F. Supp. 1173 (N.D. Miss. 1992).

Matthew J. v. Massachusetts Department of Education, 989 F. Supp. 380 (D. Mass. 1998).

Milford School District v. William F., 129 F.3d 1252 (1st Cir. 1997).

Mills v. D.C. Board of Education, 348 F. Supp. 866 (D.D.C. 1972).

Nein v. Greater Clark County School Corp., 95 F. Supp. 2d 961 (S.D. Ind. 2000).

Norton v. Orinda Union School District, 168 F.3d 500 (9th Cir. 1999).

Pascoe v. Washingtonville Central School District, 29 IDELR 31 (S.D.N.Y. 1998).

Pennsylvania Association for Retarded Children (PARC) v. Pennsylvania, 343 F. Supp. 279 (E.D. Pa. 1972).

Ridgewood Board of Education v. N.E., 172 F.3d 238 (3rd Cir. 1999).

Robert M. v. Hickok, 32 IDELR 169 (E.D. Pa. 2000).

R.R. v. Wallingford Board of Education, 35 IDELR 32 (D. Conn. 2001).

Salley v. St. Tammany Parish School Board, 57 F.3d 458 (5th Cir. 1995).

Stanovich, K. E. (1999). The sociopsychometrics of learning disabilities. *Journal of Learning Disabilities, 32,* 350–361.

Susquenita School District v. Raelee, 96 F.3d 78 (3d Cir. 1996).

Vocational Rehabilitation Act of 1973, Pub. L. 93-112, 87 Stat. 394.

Walczak v. Florida Union Free School District, 142 F.3d 119 (2d Cir. 1998).

Wechsler, D. (1991). *Wechsler Intelligence Scale for Children—Third Edition*. San Antonio, TX: The Psychological Corporation.

Welton v. Liberty 53 School District, 35 IDELR 63 (W.D. Mo. 2001).

Woodcock, R. W., McGrew, K. S., & Mather, N. (2001). *Woodcock-Johnson III—Tests of Achievement*. Itasca, IL: Riverside.

Zigmond, N. (1997). Educating students with disabilities: The future of special education. In J. W. Lloyd, E. J. Kameenui, & D. Chard (Eds.), *Issues in education students with disabilities* (pp. 377–389). Mahwah, NJ: Erlbaum.

APPENDIX 4.1. Matrix of Referenced IDEA Cases and Issues

Case name[a]	IEPs/FAPE					LRE	
	Evaluation and eligibility	Procedural	How much benefit	Methodology	Accommodations	Placement	Reimbursement
Amann v. Stow School System (1992)						•	•
A.S.K. v. Or. State Board of Education (February 2001)					•		
Board of Education of the City School District of the City of New York (1998)						•	•
Board of Education of the County of Kanawha v. Michael M. (2000)				•			
Briere v. Fair Haven Grade School District (1996)		•				•	•
Capistrano Unified School District v. Wartenberg (1995)							
Cleveland Heights–University Heights City School District v. Boss (1998)			•			•	•
Concerned Parents of New York City Board of Education (1980)					•		
Corchado v. Board of Education Rochester City School District (2000)	•						
DeLullo v. Jefferson County Board of Education (1999)						•	•
Doe v. Defendant I. (1990)	•	•				•	•
Doe v. Withers (1993)					•		
Egg Harbor Township Board of Education v. S.O. (1992)		•	•			•	•
Evans v. Board of Education of the Rhinebeck Central School District (1996)		•	•	•		•	•
Flowers v. Martinez Unified School District (1993)		•					
Fort Zumwalt School District v. Clynes (1997)			•			•	•
Friedman v. Vance, Montgomery County Board of Education (1996)	•		•			•	•
Greenbush School Committee v. Mr. and Mrs. K. (1996)						•	•
Hall v. Vance County Board of Education (1985)		•	•			•	•

Case[a]						
Hendrick Hudson Central School District Board of Education v. Rowley (1982)			•			
Hiller v. Board of Education of the Brunswick Central School District (1990)	•	•				
Judith S. v. Board of Education of Community Unit School District No. 200 (1998)			•		•	•
Kathleen H. v. Massachusetts Board of Education (1998)						
Kelby v. Morgan Hill Unified School District (1992)						
Kevin T. v. Elmhurst Community School District No. 205 (2001)						
Kugler v. Vance (1999)	•					
Lascari v. Ramapo Indian Hills Regional High School District (1989)						
Lenn v. Portland School Committee (1992)			•	•	•	•
Livingston v. Desoto County School District (1992)		•	•		•	•
Matthew J. v. Massachusetts Department of Education (1998)					•	•
Milford School District v. William F. (1997)		•			•	•
Nein v. Greater Clark County School Corp. (2000)					•	•
Norton v. Orinda Union School District (1999)					•	•
Pascoe v. Washingtonville Central School District (1998)			•	•	•	•
Ridgewood Board of Education v. N.E. (1999)	•					
R.R. v. Wallingford Board of Education (2001)			•		•	•
Robert M. v. Hickok (2000)	•		•		•	•
Salley v. St. Tammany Parish School Board (1995)					•	•
Susquenita School District v. Raelee (1996)	•				•	•
Walczak v. Florida Union Free School District (1998)					•	•
Welton v. Liberty 53 School District (2001)	•				•	•

[a]For full citation, see reference list at the end of the chapter.

5

Learning Disability as a Discipline

Kenneth A. Kavale
Steven R. Forness

At a fundamental level, a discipline is defined as a branch of learning. All disciplines possess the primary goal of providing a comprehensive understanding of a particular phenomenon. Given the formal definition, learning disability (LD) would appear to qualify as a legitimate discipline but one far from achieving its primary goal. The reason is found in the fact that, at present, we appear to "know" far more than we "understand" about LD. The consequences of this limited understanding are found in the inability to answer a seemingly facile question: What is a learning disability? A discipline should be able to define itself without ambiguity.

A discipline should also demonstrate the quality of continually evolving into a more inclusive and structured domain. The LD discipline did not spring full grown from the brow of Kirk, Cruickshank, Kephart, and others. The LD discipline has evolved but not in any straight-line form making for easy progression. Because LD developed under the stress of practical exigencies, it shows gaps and bypaths as well as unfounded leaps of faith. Therefore, an essential

question remains: How far has the LD discipline progressed?

Historical Foundations

Origins

Wiederholt (1974) provided a useful history of LD that demonstrated its phased development from several types of disorders, most notably language, reading, and cognitive process problems. From the seminal study of exogenous mental retardation by Strauss and Werner (see Strauss & Lehtinen, 1947) to the rousing endorsement of Kirk's (1963) term "learning disabilities," LD was viewed as a neurologically based disorder manifested by unique processing disturbances that selectively interfered with acquiring and assimilating basic academic information.

The LD discipline also developed along social dimensions. Kavale and Forness (1995) showed how, within the structure of special education during the 1960s, there was a compelling need for a category such as LD. From misclassification of students in categorical special classes to lack of school-based services or educationally focused interventions for particular problems, a new category such as LD could resolve diagnostic predicaments and provide needed services.

The Problem of Definition

By the 1970s, the LD discipline was experiencing problems with the most enduring being the lack of consensus about definition (Doris, 1993). The origins of the LD definition are found in the National Advisory Committee on Handicapped Children (NACHC) (1968) report, but the present Individuals with Disabilities Education Act (IDEA) definition has not in fact changed substantially from the original NACHC definition. This definition, however, lacked precision then and now with its inherent ambiguity resulting in widely varying interpretation.

In a later survey, Tucker, Stevens, and Ysseldyke (1983) found consensus among "experts" about the viability of the LD category but considerable variability of opinion about almost all other issues. Critiques of the LD definition became so pervasive (e.g., Reger, 1979; Siegel, 1968) that the foundation was laid for discussions about whether LD really existed as a discrete entity. Kavale and Forness (2000) analyzed available LD definitions and concluded that, "LD has not been defined with much exactitude . . . [the definition] provides only a generalized picture of a portion of the school population experiencing academic difficulties . . . [but] accord about definition does not imply uniform interpretation, and any variation is likely to prevent precision in describing the nature of LD" (p. 245).

The fundamental "problem of definition" adversely affected the LD discipline. The LD definition belongs to the class of definition termed "stipulative," which possesses the quality of not needing to be true, only useful, and "as long as there is consensus and a perceived heuristic value, the definition is accepted and used" (Kavale & Forness, 2000, p. 247). A stipulative definition also need not be used for a common purpose, and varying interpretations may lead

to the development of essentially divergent disciplinary perspectives. On one side, there is LD as a scientific discipline whose goal was to predict and to explain LD. On the other side, there is LD as a political discipline whose goal is advocacy, policy directed at creating programs and services to meet the needs and interests of students with LD. Because these two disciplinary perspectives require different interpretations of the LD definition, there was little association between the goals and objectives of the scientific and the political LD disciplines.

The Scientific Discipline

The Strauss and Werner Paradigm

The scientific discipline of LD can be traced to investigations of brain function and dysfunction where Goldstein (1939) demonstrated that brain injury rarely caused specific disorders but rather usually included a variety of perceptual, cognitive, and behavioral disturbances that formed a syndrome. Werner and Strauss (1940) continued Goldstein's research program and their findings established the rudiments of the LD concept (see Strauss & Lehtinen, 1947). These ideas were reinforced by Clements's (1966) report on *minimal brain dysfunction* (MBD) where "specific learning disabilities" were one of the 10 most frequently agreed upon characteristics.

The MBD label did not receive general acceptance until Kirk's (1963) suggestion that the term "learning disability" might better focus on educational problems; might avoid medical implications; and might be better accepted by parents, teachers, and students. The LD concept was thus based primarily on the Strauss and Werner paradigm: (1) LD is associated with or caused by neurological dysfunction; (2) LD academic problems are related to process disturbance, most notably in perceptual–motor functioning; and (3) LD is associated with academic failure defined by discrepancy notions.

However, the evidence did not support the foundation of the Strauss and Werner paradigm because there were few useful group distinctions of a magnitude "that would unequivocally separate exogenous and endogenous functioning and that might provide a prototype for LD" (Kavale & Forness, 1984, p. 22). Kavale and Forness (1985) then demonstrated how the validity of the three primary ideas of the Strauss and Werner paradigm could also be challenged. In Kuhn's (1970) analysis of the history of science, such a situation should initiate a *paradigm shift*, but the LD discipline has never really abandoned these questionable suppositions. The reason is found in historical linkages (see Hallahan & Cruickshank, 1973) that demonstrate how the LD discipline was shaped by colleagues and students of Strauss and Werner who naturally incorporated their paradigm into conceptualizations about the nature of LD. This situation produced "a bias toward the Strauss and Werner 'paradigm' that is both profound and pervasive" (Kavale & Forness, 1985, p. 16).

Process Theories

In terms of theoretical structure, the emerging scientific LD discipline was dominated by process theories as conceptualized by Cruickshank, Ayres, Frostig, Kirk, Barsch, Getman, Kephart, Cratty, Myklebust, Delacato, and others. The process approach was based on the idea that the mind contained a variety of processes whose efficient functioning was prerequisite for learning.

The dominant-process theories began to witness vigorous philosophical attacks (e.g., Mann, 1971) as well as questions about the "true" relation between processes and academic learning (e.g., Kavale, 1981b, 1982). Soon following were empirical findings discounting the benefits of perceptual–motor training (Hammill, 1972; Kavale & Mattson, 1983), psycholinguistic training, (Hammill & Larsen, 1974; Kavale, 1981a), and modality-matched instruction (Arter & Jenkins, 1979; Kavale & Forness, 1987c). The negative evidence led Vellutino, Steger, Moyer, Harding, and Niles (1977) to ask, "Has the perceptual deficit hypothesis led us astray?" (p. 375). The often contentious academic debate about the process orientation of LD soon spread to professional organizations where "the controversy polarized the field, and most professionals more of less identified with the process orienta-

tion or with direct instruction. The political center of the learning disability movement practically dissolved in the mid 1970s . . . the professional climate a the time was acrimonious and often vituperative" (Hammill, 1993, p. 303). The scientific LD discipline thus had many competing voices which meant that their "messages had limited impact and influence on the way the field behaved. In many respects, there was a political vacuum in the LD field that was filled at various times by various organizations for various reasons" (Kavale & Forness, 1998, p. 262).

Theoretical Development

Although process theories were initially predominant in the scientific LD discipline, they were generally found invalid, and alternative theoretical ideas began to appear. Wong (1979a, 1979b) discussed the problems associated with LD theory at the time in terms of its unidimensional nature and isolated context and then critically reviewed seven theories about LD. In a later analysis, Torgesen (1986) suggested that LD theory was best described in terms of three broad paradigms including the neuropsychological (understanding cognitive abilities in terms of the specific brain systems that support them), information processing (cognitive ability as symbol manipulation analogous to a computer), and applied behavior analysis (behavior explained in terms of observable relationships between stimuli and responses).

Applied behavior analysis theory was combined with information processing theory to form cognitive behavior modification theory (Meichenbaum, 1977) whose cognitive elements were derived from Flavell's (1978) construct of metacognition (self-awareness and self-regulation). This new theory described the possibility that students with LD may have performance deficits rather than ability problems that were manifested by passive responses to the learning environment (Torgesen, 1977). By emphasizing *how* a student learns as opposed to *what* a student learns, Wong (1987) suggested that metacognitive theory moved the scientific LD discipline away from deficit-based conceptualizations.

Although paradigmatic pluralism moved

the scientific LD discipline away from narrow and unidimensional conceptualizations, LD theory had not yet advanced to support a true scientific LD discipline (Kavale, 1987c). Much research was produced that could not be rationally connected to any theoretical perspective and thus was not generalizable. To remedy the situation, the Bureau of Education for the Handicapped funded five research institutes in 1977 where information processing, social competence, LD in adolescents, identification of students with LD, and attention and metacognitive difficulties were investigated (see Deshler, 1978). The institutes were generally judged favorably (see Keogh, 1983) but some criticism was directed at the University of Minnesota institute investigating identification and decision making about LD (see McKinney, 1983).

Research

The volume of inquiry about the nature of LD began to increase significantly (Hallahan & Cruickshank, 1973). The empirical base continued to outpace theoretical development, however, with an increasing unwieldyness and inconsistency associated with research findings. The difficulties stemmed from two factors: (1) the heterogeneity of the LD population and (2) the incomplete descriptions of the characteristics of research subjects. Surveys of the research literature (e.g., Kavale & Nye, 1981) found that many studies failed to report essential sample characteristics, and even if reported, the studies were done in a manner that did not permit precise comparison between samples.

The problem of heterogeneity remained a significant barrier to enhanced understanding of LD (Gallagher, 1986). One solution offered was empirical subtyping techniques that used methods from numerical taxonomy to see how large data sets describing LD characteristics clustered to form discrete and independent groupings (Feagans, Short, & Meltzer, 1991). A major goal was to find not only diagnostic entities but also remedial groupings that might be the basis of subtype-by-treatment interactions (e.g., Lyon, 1985; McKinney & Speece, 1986). The subtype approach was not without problems, most notably the lack of a formalized description of LD that made its parallel to numerical taxonomy in botany and zoology less than exact (Kavale & Forness, 1987a).

Although LD research was generally deemed satisfactory (Swanson & Trahan, 1986), critiques of LD research were common from the beginning. Cohen (1976) discussed the "fuzziness" and the "flab" where LD research was "suffocating in correlation coefficients between fuzzies. These findings contribute little to man's basic knowledge or to his theoretical models" (p. 135). Nevertheless, the scientific LD discipline continued to explore its research base with attempts to clearly define issues and to provide suggestions for future directions (see Vaughn & Bos, 1987).

Basic vs. Applied Research

Over time, research emphasis became controversial with differing opinions about the merits of basic versus applied research. Some lamented the lack of basic research in LD while others argued that the field was better served by applied research efforts that teachers could immediately put to use in their classrooms. Swanson (1988) presented a compelling case for the critical role of basic research in developing a metatheory of LD: "Theory in turn, allows for the development of a genuine service, prevents the practice of data collection that does not contribute to an understanding of events, organizes existing studies, and reveals the complexity of simple events" (p. 206). But this view was challenged by those with an applied research bias where treatment was considered primary; theory was "nice" but not critical (e.g., Gavalek & Palincsar, 1988).

Philosophical Disputes

The scientific LD discipline also experienced philosophical disputes. During the late 1980s, LD was accused of possessing an enduring reductionist philosophy that resulted in the belief "a) that learning disabilities can be reduced so as to allow definition of a single verifiable entity (or set of entities), b) that the teaching/learning process is most effective when most reduced (e.g., controlled, focused, and segmented)" (Poplin, 1988b, p. 398).

Heshusius (1989b) argued against the scientific LD discipline's predominant "Newtonian mechanistic paradigm [where] all complexity is to be broken down into components" (p. 404). Iano (1986) offered a similar critique of the "natural science–technical" model where the focus was on analyzing a totality into parts. Generally, it was suggested that the scientific LD discipline needed to move from its positivist roots and would be better served by a holistic paradigm that attempted to *understand* complexity rather than trying to reduce it to simplicity (Poplin, 1988a). These ideas were not readily endorsed (e.g., Forness, 1988; Forness & Kavale, 1987) but were staunchly defended (e.g., Heshusius, 1989a; Iano, 1987).

The scientific LD discipline continued to hear claims about the holistic/nonmechanistic paradigm being "good" and "better" but little evidence to that effect. Once the scientific basis of LD was assailed with philosophical arguments, ideology became an increasingly important consideration in shaping the LD discipline. Although LD had its roots in medicine, the real-world of schools provided the possibility of social influence and political beliefs directing actions.

Learning Disability and Marxist Ideology

The late 1970s saw the rise of such an ideology in Marxist views where schooling was assumed to serve only the interests of elites, to reinforce inequalities, and to foster attitudes that maintained the status quo (Sharp, 1980). For example, Carrier (1986) indicated that, "Marxist models suggest that learning disability theory might be explicable as a set of beliefs which legitimate capitalist inequality and social relations" (p. 124) where LD was assumed to be associated with "sociogenic brain damage." Sleeter (1986) reinterpreted the history of LD from a conflict perspective that suggested LD was a special education category created to explain the school failure of white, middle-class students. Kavale and Forness (1987b) suggested that Sleeter's arguments were fallacious and based on assumptions that were "unremittingly racist, exclusive, and undemocratic" (p. 7). Consequently, "There is a permeating unreality to these analyses that

bears little resemblance to any LD that was known then or is known now" (Kavale & Forness, 1998, p. 257).

This genre of LD analysis reached its zenith with *The Learning Mystique: A Critical Look at "Learning Disabilites"* (Coles, 1987), which described a social "interactivity" theory of LD and viewed any biophysical formulation of LD as "'blaming the victim' [because] systemic, economic, social, and cultural conditions are the principle influences contributing to learning failure" (p. 209). In reality, "Marxist analyses fail to enhance our understanding LD in any meaningful fashion" (Kavale & Forness, 1998, p. 258), and the scientific LD discipline could not advance if Coles's (1987) views were accepted. First, it was a unidimensional view stressing sociopolitical influences while rejecting biophysical influences. Second, there was a resistance to accept even validated scientific evidence about the nature of LD. Yet, apologists continued to uncritically accept Coles's view that "the real reason that children function poorly usually is not that anything is wrong with the children, but, rather because of injustices in the school system and in society" (Miller, 1990, p. 87). What all these Marxist analyses really meant was moot because "the proposed solutions are solely political in character and usually require nothing less than a revolutionary restructuring of present society. The proposed solutions are simplistic because they fail to recognize the reality (and complexity) of phenomena and are dangerous because they emphasize egalitarian fantasies that serve only to exacerbate existing relations" (Kavale & Forness, 1998, p. 260).

Some solutions discussed the necessity for "looking through other lenses and listening to other voices" (see special series in the *Journal of Learning Disabilities*) which combined Marxist ideology with New Age wisdom to describe "the problems we face as accomplices in creating and maintaining bureaucracies and other structures that contribute to the current injustices of 'ableism', racism, and classism" (Poplin, 1995, p. 393). The difficulty was that the resultant *sociocultural constructionism* placed any scientific LD in a secondary position, resulting in a loss of rationality and increasing difficulty in resolving important questions such as, "What is LD?"

The Consequences of Ideology

The increasingly ideological bent of LD had significant negative consequences for the scientific LD discipline. Was LD myth or reality? For example, the myth idea was expressed thusly: "it should by now be clear that there is no such thing as learning disability" (McKnight, 1982, p. 352). Finlan (1994) called LD an "imaginary" disease "that was an "ill-conceived movement that has run amok and is placing millions of youngsters in a disabling trajectory toward failure and low self-esteem from which there is little hope of escape" (p. 8). These critical analyses only described the LD concept in terms of what it had become. These descriptions of LD ignored the associated "specific" adjective and attempted to fabricate an expansive LD including students who may require special education but who may not meet the parameters defining specific LD. Thus, "LD moved from a specific condition ('all LD include learning problems') to a general condition ('all learning problems include LD')" (Kavale & Forness, 1998, p. 265).

Theoretical Advances

Despite the corrosive effects of social constructions of LD, the scientific LD discipline continued to produce major research contributions directed at understanding LD (Vaughn & Bos, 1994). For example, the linguistic development and behavior of students with LD was comprehensively described (Wiig, 1990). The mathematics area was also investigated (e.g., Cawley, Fitzmaurice, Shaw, Kahn, & Bates, 1979; Ginsburg, 1997) with particular attention to *dyscalculia* (Kosc, 1974).

Reading (*dyslexia*), the most common academic deficit among students with LD, became a major focus. Rather than primarily a visual–perceptual problem, reading difficulties began to be viewed as basic linguistic deficits (Vellutino, 1977). Among the most important advances was the recognition of the importance of phonology (Liberman & Shankweiler, 1985), especially phonemic awareness as a fundamental reading skill (e.g., Stanovich, 1988; Wagner & Torgesen, 1987). Reading difficulties were further described with respect to the greater amount of processing needed to read (Snowling, 1981), the inability to group words based on rhyme (Bradley & Bryant, 1985), the significantly longer time required to process auditory stimuli (McCroskey & Kidder, 1980), and short-term auditory memory or encoding limitations (Kamhi, Catts, & Mauer, 1990). The areas of written language deficits (e.g., Graham, 1990; Montague, Maddux, & Dereshiwsky, 1990), spelling problems (e.g., Bruck, 1988; Carpenter, 1983), and handwriting (*dysgraphia*) (e.g., Deuel, 1995; Gerard & Junkala, 1980) were also investigated.

From the early 1980s, it became apparent that the scientific LD discipline was primarily oriented toward a metacognitive foundation for explaining performance differences (e.g., Bauer, 1987; Wong, 1985). This foundation also included enhanced understanding about attention (e.g., Riccio, Gonzalez, & Hynd, 1994), memory (Swanson & Cooney, 1991), especially working memory (Swanson, 1993), and attributions (Borkowski, Johnston, & Reid, 1986), especially the notion of "learned helplessness" (Pearl, Bryan, & Donahue, 1980). The elements of metacognition were explored with respect to metacomprehension (Bos & Filip, 1984), self-monitoring (Reid, 1996), metamemory (Lucangeli, Galderisi, & Cornoldi, 1995), mnemonics (Mastropieri & Scruggs, 1989), and scaffolding (Stone, 1998). Clearly, the earlier emphasis on perceptual-motor variables for explaining LD were replaced by a more cognitive information processing view (Lyon & Krasnegor, 1996).

A New Research Agenda

Although the rate of LD publication increased significantly (see Gerber, 1999–2000; Summers, 1986), the theoretical development of the field still appeared to lag behind (Kavale, 1993). A number of theories were proposed (see Torgesen, 1993), but none could fully explain the deficits experienced by an increasingly heterogenous LD population: "The difficulty is that not all students with learning disabilities demonstrate all these component deficits all the time. Consequently, any single variable can explain only learning disabilities in particular and not learning disabilities in general" (Kavale & Nye, 1991, p. 152).

Moats and Lyon (1993) discussed factors

that may have hampered the development of the scientific LD discipline. What they called for was a new LD research agenda that was initiated by the National Institute of Child Health and Human Development (NICHD) (see Lyon, 1995b). The NICHD then funded research centers that would (1) identify critical learning and behavioral diagnostic characteristics, (2) develop valid early predictors of achievement, (3) map the course of different types of LD, (4) identify comorbid conditions that develop in response to school failure, and (5) assess the efficacy of different treatment methods for different types of LD (Lyon, 1995a).

The NICHD learning disability research centers have pursued a curious means to study LD, however. A number of findings have been reported but one has to search for findings related to LD because the samples studied typically included students with dyslexia or attention-deficit/hyperactivity disorder (ADHD). The concepts of LD, dyslexia, and ADHD are not equivalent, and it should not be believed that either dyslexia or ADHD is better defined than LD. As suggested by Kavale and Forness (1998), "It could be argued that dyslexia (reading problems) and ADHD (attention problems) are symptoms of LD and not LD itself. What are we to make of a student with LD who possesses neither a reading nor an attention problem? What are we to do with the many students with LD who possess both a reading and a math problem?" (p. 269).

Evaluating the Scientific Discipline

The significant theoretical and empirical contributions over the past 25 years indicate that the scientific LD discipline has become well established but continues to face a curious dilemma: Far more is known than understood about LD. There is little pessimism, however, and although there has been sometimes quarrelous debate, Gerber (1999–2000) indicated the following:

> My position is that the debate itself has been an incalcuable benefit. It has unleashed 40 years of scholarly interest and effort. That effort, in turn, has debunked bromides, generated valuable new methods and techniques, re-

search capacities, and several promising insights. It has called into question our entire understanding of intelligence, learning, and disability. It has shaken a simplistic, received taxonomy of human learning differences to its root and readied us for more complex theory, measurement, and research. These are not small or inconsequential intellectual achievement and, despite impatience to improve the practical lives of real children, continuing on this path is likely to yield still greater rewards. (pp. 40–41)

The Political Discipline

Advocacy

The political discipline of LD stands in contrast to the scientific discipline. In place of the goal of understanding, the political LD discipline possesses the primary goal of advocacy, social action directed at creating programs and services to meet the needs and interests of students with LD. Although a legitimate and necessary activity, advocacy for LD should not exceed the understanding of LD. For example, Biklen and Zollers (1986) outlined a focus for advocacy in the LD field that included increasing public awareness of the LD experience and minimizing negative consequences associated with LD. There was no mention of enhancing the LD construct, however, and little discomfort surrounding the fact that LD was neither defined nor understood in any precise sense.

The political LD discipline appeared to possess an advocacy focus from its start. In 1992, the *Journal of Learning Disabilities* republished one of its inaugural articles, written by Ray Barsch in 1968. The article addressed the issue about whether the emerging LD should be viewed as a disability category or a concept where LD "is a term to be applied to any learner who fails to benefit from an existing curriculum into which he has been placed" (p. 12). Barsch further suggested that "learning disabilities are to be found wherever there are learners. Narrow definition of a precise set of symptoms will inevitably lead to massive exclusion" (p.12). Such exclusion has not occurred and ever greater numbers of students are being served under the LD rubric.

Pseudoscience

Although increased numbers are positive for the political LD discipline, the scientific LD discipline suffers because of the continued movement away from attempts to more clearly delineate the basic structure of LD. For example, in the place of real scientific advancement, there is pseudoscientific discussion about the presence or absence of LD in historical figures (e.g., Aaron, Phillips, & Larsen, 1988; Thompson, 1971). There is often little compelling medical or psychological data to support such posthumous diagnoses (Adelman & Adelman, 1987). Why engage in such discussion? The answer is found in advocacy as demonstrated by Miner and Siegel (1992) in their case study of W. B. Yeats, "We hope that children, parents, and teachers working with their problem will be inspired by the brilliant accomplishments of someone who may have had dyslexia" (p. 375). Thomas (2000) debunked the LD of Albert Einstein and suggested that such discussion may have positive inspirational effects "but the consequence is of claiming that Einstein had a learning disability without sufficient historical evidence are deleterious. It distorts the historical record and calls into question the credibility of other claims regarding the learning disabilities of prominent persons" (p. 157). The emphasis on advocacy trivializes the scientific discipline because a situation is created in which "a simple axiom captures the state of LD: the more you don't know what you are talking about, the greater the number of students likely to be served under the label about which you don't know what you are talking about" (Kavale & Forness, 1998, p. 266).

Numbers

Advocacy for LD has been enormously successful and the LD category now accounts for about 52% of all students with disabilities served in special education with an actual count exceeding 2.5 million. An increase of this magnitude is unprecedented and unparalleled. Could any rational speculation in 1970 ever anticipate that more than one-half of all students identified for special education might be subsumed under a single category?

Should LD be the size that it is? The question is difficult to answer primarily because the scientific LD discipline has not provided a "true" prevalence estimate. In place of epidemiological studies, LD prevalence is often established through policy statements issued by national organizations, but "this process is inherently political. The decisions about prevalence are not based on scientific grounds—but political considerations—primarily, the call to serve more students under the LD rubric. Under such circumstances, LD prevalence estimates become unidirectional with a strong bias towards increasing prevalence" (Kavale & Forness, 1998, p. 248).

The extraordinary number of students with LD has resulted in a loss of integrity for the field. There is less and less confidence about whether or not a student is "truly" LD, but this really does not seem to matter because more students are being served. The political LD discipline assumes that as long as students experiencing any sort of school difficulty receive special education, the field is doing well. The situation led Senf (1987) to describe LD as a sponge wiping up the spills of general education: "The LD sponge grew so fast because it was able to absorb a diversity of educational/behavioral/socioemotional problems irrespective of their cause, their stabilization, their remediation, or their progress" (p. 91).

Discrepancy, Underachievement, and Learning Disability

The success of the political LD discipline may be viewed as a consequence of the lack of a comprehensive understanding of LD. The current definition of LD has been problematic primarily because of difficulties in operationalizing it (Kavale & Forness, 2000). Although there has been some agreement about basic concepts (e.g., central nervous system dysfunction and process deficits), these elements have been difficult to measure and, consequently, validate. The difficulties in using the LD definition in practice led to rules and regulations stipulating discrepancy as the primary criterion to be used for LD identification (U.S. Office of Education, 1977). The discrepancy concept was introduced in a definition offered by Bateman (1965) and was considered a proxy for the idea that LD was associated with unexpected school failure (under-achievement). The discrepancy concept was quickly embraced and soon became the pri-mary (and often sole) criterion used for LD identification (Mercer, Jordan, Allsop, & Mercer, 1996).

The discrepancy concept precipitated much debate about statistical and psychome-tric issues (e.g., Cone & Wilson, 1981; Reynolds, 1984–1985; Shepard, 1980) but the real problem, from the scientific LD dis-cipline viewpoint, was that discrepancy rep-resented the operational definition of under-achievement (Kavale, 1987b). Consequently, discrepancy was really not a proxy for LD it-self, but when it was used as the sole identifi-cation criterion, discrepancy by definition becomes the equivalent of LD. Under-achievement and LD are not equivalent con-cepts, which suggests that discrepancy might be better viewed as a necessary but not suffi-cient criterion for LD identification (Kavale, 1987b). When placed in such a context, dis-crepancy remains an important foundation concept for LD and makes any discussion about its "demise" untenable (see Aaron, 1997).

The reliance on the single criterion of dis-crepancy for LD identification resulted in increasing vagueness about the LD concept: "LD is not some scientifically proven, hard-to-identify disease but a made-up category in which to place children" (Finlan, 1994, p. 7). Although the discrepancy criterion was efficient, its use soon undermined the system. First, it was not applied rigorously, leading to the finding that sometimes up to 50% of LD samples did not demonstrate the required level of discrepancy (e.g., Kavale & Reese, 1992; Kirk & Elkins, 1975; Shepard, Smith, & Vojir, 1983). Sec-ond, many students identified as LD were simply judged to be "clinical cases" who were provided special education for reasons other than being LD (Gelzheiser, 1987).

Learning Disability and Low Achievement

The vagaries in the LD identification process were demonstrated in studies con-ducted by the University of Minnesota Insti-tute for Research on Learning Disabilities (IRLD) (see Ysseldyke, Algozzine, Shinn, &

McGue, 1982). The findings appeared to show a large degree of overlap between test scores of LD and low achievement (LA) groups to the point where it was not possi-ble to differentiate group membership un-equivocally. These findings were taken to mean that efforts at differentiating LD and LA were futile, and that LD had become an "over-sophisticated concept" (see Algozzine & Ysseldyke, 1983) that was best replaced by a more general category encompassing primarily LA. A "reprieve" for the LD con-cept was offered (see Wilson, 1985), along with caution about concluding that LD and LA could not be distinguished: "The fact that many diagnosticians . . . do not distin-guish learning disabilities from generic low performance does not mean it cannot be done" (Bateman, 1992, p. 32).

Kavale, Fuchs, and Scruggs (1994) reex-amined the study by Ysseldyke and col-leagues (1982) using quantitative synthesis methods (meta-analysis). On average, it was found that it was possible to reliably differ-entiate 63% of the LD group from the LA group. Conversely, 37% could not be differ-entiated, and this figure represented the de-gree of overlap which stands in sharp con-trast to the 95% LD–LA overlap reported in the IRLD study. There was modest group differentiation in the ability area (ES = 0.304) but large group differentiation (ES = 0.763) in the achievement area with the LD group representing the lowest of the low achievers; the LD group was thus discrepant while the LA group was not.

Algozzine, Ysseldyke, and McGue (1995) countered with the suggestion that although students with LD may be the lowest of the low achievers, they did not represent a *qual-itatively* different population in the same sense as described for severe mental retarda-tion (MR) (Dingman & Tarjan, 1960) and specific reading disability (Rutter & Yule, 1975). When an identified LD group com-pared to an LA group demonstrates small differences in ability and large differences in achievement, the LD group demonstrates a "severe discrepancy" which is the basis for defining "two distinct populations. Because the LD group was lower on achievement di-mensions but not on ability, they are, in ad-dition to being the lowest of the low achiev-ers, a different population defined by an ability–achievement distinction represented in a different achievement distribution but not in a different ability distribution" (Kavale, 1995, p. 146).

Gresham, MacMillan, and Bocian (1996) also found an average 61% (ES = 0.28) LD–LA differentiation and concluded that "LD children performed more poorly in academic achievement than LA children" (p. 579). In terms of ability (IQ) levels, there was less group differentiation, suggesting that the LD group "could be reliably differentiated using measures of cognitive ability and tested academic achievement" (p. 580). With reference to reading achievement, Fuchs, Fuchs, Mathes, and Lipsey (2000) found that 72% of an LA group performed better in reading than the LD group (ES = 0.61) and concluded that "school personnel in fact do identify as LD those children who have appreciably more severe reading problems compared to other low-performing students who go unidentified" (p. 95).

Learning Disability and Intelligence

The discrepancy notion continued to be assailed with arguments about whether or not IQ was necessary in defining LD (Siegel, 1989; Stanovich, 1991). The arguments surrounded questions about what IQ tests measure and possible confounding about cause-and-effect relations between IQ and reading disability. Meyen (1989) objected to these arguments because they "question the efficacy of the category of learning disabilities itself as a means to identify students who warrant special education services" (p. 482) and would create a situation where "we would largely serve low achievers and have no basis for determining whether or not a student is achieving at a reasonable level given his or her ability" (p. 482). The discrepancy criterion is necessary for LD identification because of the long-standing assumption that IQ levels for students with LD need to be at near average or above levels in order to "discriminate between poor achievement that is expected (that is, on the basis of intellectual ability or sensory handicaps) and poor achievement that is not expected (that is, the probable presence of LD)" (Scruggs, 1987, p. 22).

The possible elimination of IQ in defining LD also led to the suggestion that LD might really be associated with any IQ level (e.g.,

Ames, 1968; Belmont & Belmont, 1980). Historically, students with IQ levels between 70 (or perhaps 75) to 85 (or perhaps 90) have been the most problematic portion of the school population. These "slow learners" (SL) (see Ingram, 1935) were not routinely eligible for special education because they neither met the 2 standard deviations (SDs) below the mean IQ criterion for MR or the severe discrepancy criterion for LD (i.e., no unexpected low achievement). The political LD discipline appears to have decided to subsume the SL group (about 14% of the school population) under the LD rubric. One consequence of incorporating the SL group is an increase in the proportion of students with LD who have IQ levels in the low average range (IQ = 70–84) (e.g., Gottlieb, Alter, Gottlieb, & Wishner, 1994; Shepard et al., 1983). The parameters of LD have thus changed to include a new class of students who possess learning difficulties *and* low average intelligence "but in doing so has contorted its basic character and undermined its scientific integrity" (Kavale & Forness, 1998, p. 251).

Learning Disability and Mental Retardation

The primary problem with the acceptance of a below average IQ criterion for LD was the confounding created with MR (MacMillan, Gresham, Bocian, & Lambros, 1998). Gresham et al. (1996) demonstrated how the percentage of students classified as mentally retarded was inversely related to the percentage of students classified as learning disabled (*r* = –.24) with the result being large increases in LD and significant decreases in MR to the point where the MR prevalence rate was at an illogical 0.6% (see Forness, 1985). The potential confounding between LD and MR created a situation where students with similar cognitive abilities and disabilities were served in one state as LD and in another as MR (MacMillan, Siperstein, & Gresham, 1996). For example, MacMillan and colleagues (1996) found, in a school referred sample of 150 students, 43 with IQ ≤ 75 but only 6 classified as mentally retarded while 18 classified as learning disabled. Similarly, Gottlieb and colleagues (1994) found the mean IQ level of an urban LD group to be 1.5 SDs lower than a comparison suburban LD group and

suggested that the real operational definition of LD was as follows: "Low-achieving,
low ability children who do not exhibit aggressive or bizarre behavior and whom
teachers cannot accommodate in their general education classrooms" (pp. 458–459).

The potential confounding between LD
and MR means that the basic LD concept of
specificity might be lost. As IQ level becomes lower, learning failure becomes less
unexpected and is likely to be exhibited
across *all* achievement domains. In contrast,
specific LD was assumed associated with intraindividual differences where achievement
deficits were found in one or more (but not
all) domains (Stanovich, 1986). Without the
specific adjective, LD becomes a more generalized concept that is closer conceptually
to MR, particularly at the borderline levels.
"When combined with the perception that
LD is a 'better,' less stigmatizing, and more
acceptable classification, the desire for LD,
rather than MR designation becomes irre-
sistible and the [political LD discipline] appears quite willing to accommodate this desire" (Kavale & Forness, 1998, p. 250).

"Losing" Learning Disability

When clear differentiation among categories
is lacking, it is the LD category that acts like
an "educational sponge," not MR or emotional or behavior disorder (E/BD). The scientific advancement of MR and E/BD have
not been impeded by an increasingly heterogeneous population like that "absorbed" by
LD (Kavale, 1987a). Although the "LD
sponge" is seemingly successful, MacMillan, Gresham, Siperstein, and Bocian
(1996), in commenting on the magnitude of
the increased LD numbers, indicated that
"were these epidemic-like figures interpreted by the Center for Disease Control, one
might reasonably expect to find a quaran-
tine imposed in the public schools of America" (p. 169).

When identified by schools, an essentially
"new" LD group is generated that does not
resemble LD groups identified for research
purposes who were probably selected with
criteria more closely paralleling those found
in federal regulations or state education
codes (e.g., MacMillan, Gresham, & Bocian, 1998; MacMillan & Speece, 1999).
The "system-identified" students with LD

(Morrison, MacMillan, & Kavale, 1985)
produced "problem learners with markedly
different characteristics than those proposed
by formal models" (Gerber, 1999–2000, p.
40), primarily because the reason for identification was "planning for services" rather
than determining "eligibility" (see Keogh,
1994). Thus, schools view eligibility and
classification as secondary concerns (Bocian, Beebe, MacMillan, & Gresham,
1999), which is probably the reason why
only half the population with LD actually
meets the discrepancy criterion. Gottlieb
and colleagues (1994) suggested that "the
discrepancy that should be studied most intensively is between the definition of learning disability mandated by regulation and
the definition employed on a day-to-day basis in urban schools" (p. 455).

The trend toward school-identified LD
undermines the scientific LD discipline because the original construct becomes essentially "lost." In schools, the primary eligibility criterion becomes the need for special
education services rather than a decision
about LD or not LD (Coutinho, 1995). All
the high-incidence mild disabilities (LD,
MR, E/BD) are, to some degree, essentially
"judgmental categories," and because LD is
often judged to be the best choice, LD becomes the "catch-all" classification where
the student in question may possibly require
special education services but whether or
not he or she is "truly" learning disabled remains moot. "Thus, LD covers not only students experiencing specific academic difficulties but also those who possess learning
problems with an overlay of lowered intellectual ability or mild behavior problems"
(Kavale & Forness, 1998, p. 250). Such an
LD is a far cry from the originally conceived
scientific construct and raises the important
question about whether or not this is what
LD should now be.

Conclusion

The LD discipline is presently a major play-
er in special education as exemplified by the
significant increase in publications addressing LD (Durrant, 1994). But caution is necessary because "It would be wrong to interpret this increased rate of publication as any
kind of evidence of scientific progress.

Clearly, the topic, LD, instigated many scholars to spend a good deal of time thinking and writing about the phenomenon. However, it is reasonable to ask if the time was well spent" (Gerber, 1999–2000, p. 33).

It would be a mistake to believe that the time studying LD has not been well spent, but this is not to suggest that it has been solely a "good" time. The "bad" time has created a disciplinary split where a scientific LD discipline and a political LD discipline operate with different goals and objectives. The scientific LD discipline seeks to understand LD and provide a clear and unencumbered view of the nature of LD. The political LD discipline possesses the goal of identifying ever-increasing numbers of students to provide the special education they presumably require. The difficulty is that the students identified by the political LD discipline often bear little resemblance to the description of LD offered by the scientific LD discipline. Thus, a new and different population with LD is created that significantly complicates the goal of understanding desired by the scientific LD discipline.

For the scientific LD discipline, the problems are not entirely conceptual. There appears to be an implicit understanding about the characteristics of LD (see Swanson & Christie, 1994), which suggests that problems with identifying LD surround the way the definition has been operationalized (Kavale & Forness, 2000). Presently, the formal LD definition does not explicitly include the concept of discrepancy (within the context of underachievement), and yet discrepancy is often the only criterion articulated in the operational definitions used in practice. This is not good science, and the scientific LD discipline should seek to provide a new formal definition that explicitly states what LD represents based on several decades of accumulated understanding about the nature of LD.

For the political LD discipline, the advocacy focus needs to shift from the goal of increasing numbers to providing the best instruction possible. The scientific LD discipline has provided powerful, research-based interventions (e.g., Gersten, 1998; Swanson & Hoskyn, 1998) but the enduring research-to-practice gap has limited implementation in the real world of schools (Gersten & Dimino, 2001; Malouf & Schiller, 1995). Implementing best practice with integrity and fidelity should be the primary focus of the political LD discipline.

The real goal should be a reduction in the tensions existing between the scientific and political LD disciplines. "The LD field must strive to attain a better balance between politics and science. Science must not be viewed as some esoteric activity" (Kavale & Forness, 1998, p. 270) and there needs to be increased belief in the axiom that "there is nothing so practical as a good theory" (see Polansky, 1986). Nevertheless, "Politics is a necessary component of any phenomenon . . . [and] . . . although politics is the mechanism for structuring LD in the real world . . . it does engender much bickering that is counterproductive in producing greater understanding of LD" (Kavale, Forness, MacMillan, & Gresham, 1998, p. 316). With reduced tensions between scientific and political LD, a more unified discipline may be created that possesses greater potential for resolving basic issues.

Even a more unified LD discipline may likely face new vexing issues (see Swanson, 2000). Nevertheless, a more unified LD discipline will be in a better position to resolve issues without a predominant politicized character that is not often informed by scientific understanding. The likely outcome would be more rational solutions and the elimination of discussions about whether or not the LD discipline might be in danger of extinction (see Mather & Roberts, 1994). Doing away with the perceived problem (i.e., LD) offers no resolution because of the continuing "moral and legal obligation to provide individuals with LDs with appropriate service" (p. 56). Instead of being on the defensive (see Keogh, 1987), the LD discipline should take the offensive in proclaiming that "active debate over concepts, policies, and practices of LD produces benefits by creating, attracting, and focusing intellectual (as well as material) resources in a universe of problems that although complex, tangled, ambiguous, even poorly defined are nonetheless real and important to those who engage over them" (Gerber, 1999–2000, p. 30). Thus, LD should be celebrated and, with a more unified perspective, perhaps move beyond its depiction for some 20 years as a "battered discipline" (Haight, 1980).

References

Aaron, P. G. (1997). The impending demise of the discrepancy formula. *Review of Educational Research, 67,* 461–502.

Aaron, P. G., Phillips, S., & Larsen, S. (1988). Specific reading disability in historically famous persons. *Journal of Learning Disabilities, 21,* 523–538.

Adelman, K. A., & Adelman, H. S. (1987). Rodin, Patton, Edison, Wilson, Einstein: Were they really learning disabled? *Journal of Learning Disabilities, 20,* 270–279.

Algozzine, B., & Ysseldyke, J. (1983). Learning disabilities as a subset of school failure: The over-sophistication of a concept. *Exceptional Children, 50,* 242–246.

Algozzine, B., Ysseldyke, J. E., & McGue, M. (1995). Differentiating low-achieving students: Thoughts on setting the record straight. *Learning Disabilities Research and Practice, 10,* 140–144.

Ames, L. B. (1968). A low intelligence quotient often not recognized as the chief cause of many learning difficulties. *Journal of Learning Disabilities, 1,* 735–738.

Arter, J. A., & Jenkins, J. R. (1979). Differential diagnostic-prescriptive teaching: A critical appraisal. *Review of Educational Research, 49,* 517–555.

Barsch, R. H. (1992). Prospectives on learning disabilities: The vectors of new convergence. *Journal of Learning Disabilities, 25,* 6–16.

Bateman, B. (1992). Learning disabilities: The changing landscape. *Journal of Learning Disabilities, 25,* 29–36.

Bateman, B. D. (1965). An educational view of a diagnostic approach to learning disabilities. In J. Hellmuth (Ed.), *Learning disorders* (Vol. 1, pp. 219–239). Seattle, WA: Special Child Publications.

Bauer, R. H. (1987). Control processes as a way of understanding, diagnosing, and remediating learning disabilities. In H. L. Swanson (Ed.), *Advances in learning and behavioral disabilities: Memory and learning disabilities* (Vol. 2, pp. 41–79). Greenwich, CT: JAI Press.

Belmont, I., & Belmont, L. (1980). Is the slow learner in the classroom learning disabled? *Journal of Learning Disabilities, 13,* 496–499.

Biklen, D., & Zollers, N. (1986). The focus of advocacy in the LD field. *Journal of Learning Disabilities, 19,* 579–586.

Bocian, K. M., Beebe, M. E., MacMillan, D. L., & Gresham, F. M. (1999). Competing paradigms in learning disabilities classification by schools and the variations in meaning of discrepant achievement. *Learning Disabilities Research and Practice, 14,* 1–14.

Bos, C. S., & Filip, D. (1984). Comprehension monitoring in learning disabled and average students. *Journal of Learning Disabilities, 17,* 229–233.

Borkowski, J. G., Johnston, M. B., & Reid, M. K. (1986). Metacognition, motivation, and the transfer of control processes. In S. J. Ceci (Ed.), *Handbook of cognition, social, and neuropsychological aspects of learning disabilities* (Vol. 2, pp. 147–174). Hillsdale, NJ: Erlbaum.

Bradley, L., & Bryant, P. (1985). *Rhyme and reason in reading and spelling.* Ann Arbor: University of Michigan Press.

Bruck, M. (1988). The word recognition and spelling of dyslexic children. *Reading Research Quarterly, 23,* 51–69.

Carpenter, D. (1983). Spelling error profile of able and disabled readers. *Journal of Learning Disabilities, 16,* 102–104.

Carrier, J. G. (1986). *Learning disability: Social class and the construction of inequality in American education.* New York: Greenwood Press.

Cawley, J. F., Fitzmaurice, A. M., Shaw, R., Kahn, H., & Bates, H. (1979). LD youth and mathematics: A review of characteristics. *Learning Disability Quarterly, 2,* 29–44.

Clements, S. D. (1966). *Minimal brain dysfunction in children: Terminology and identification.* Washington, DC: U.S. Department of Health, Education and Welfare.

Cohen, S. A. (1976). The fuzziness and the flab: Some solutions to research problems in learning disabilities. *Journal of Special Education, 10,* 129–136.

Coles, G. S. (1987). *The learning mystique: A critical look at "learning disabilities."* New York: Fawcett Columbine.

Cone, T. E., & Wilson, L. R. (1981). Quantifying a severe discrepancy: A critical analysis. *Learning Disability Quarterly, 4,* 359–371.

Coutinho, M. (1995). Who will be learning disabled after the revolution of IDEA? Two very distinct perspectives. *Journal of Learning Disabilities, 28,* 664–668.

Deshler, D. D. (1978). New research institutes for the study of learning disabilities. *Learning Disability Quarterly, 1,* 68–78.

Deuel, R. K. (1995). Developmental dysgraphia and motor skills disorders. *Journal of Child Neurology, 10,* 56–68.

Doris, J. (1993). Defining learning disabilities: A history of the search for consensus. In G. R. Lyon, D. B. Gray, J. F. Kavanagh, & N. A. Krasnegor (Eds.), *Better understanding learning disabilities* (pp. 97–116). Baltimore: Brookes.

Durrant, J. E. (1994). A decade of research on learning disabilities: A report card on the state of the literature. *Journal of Learning Disabilities, 27,* 25–33.

Feagans, L. V., Short, E. J., & Meltzer, L. J. (Eds.). (1991). *Subtypes of learning disabilities: Theoretical perspectives and research.* Hillsdale, NJ: Erlbaum.

Finlan, T. G. (1994). *Learning disability: The imaginary disease.* Westport, CT: Bergin & Garvey.

Flavell, J. H. (1978). Metacognitive aspects of problem solving. In L. B. Resnick (Ed.), *The nature of intelligence* (pp. 231–235). Hillsdale, NJ: Erlbaum.

Forness, S. R. (1985). Effects of public policy at the state level: California's impact on MR, LD, and ED categories. *Remedial and Special Education, 6,* 36–43.

Forness, S. R. (1988). Reductionism, paradigm shifts, and learning disabilities. *Journal of Learning Disabilities, 21,* 421–424.

Forness, S. R., & Kavale, K. A. (1987). Holistic inquiry and the scientific challenge in special education: A reply to Iano. *Remedial and Special Education, 8,* 47–51.

Fuchs, D., Fuchs, L. S., Mathes, P. G., & Lipsey, M. W. (2000). Reading differences between low-achieving students with and without learning disabilities: A meta-analysis. In R. Gersten, E. P. Schiller, & S. Vaughn (Eds.), *Contemporary special education research: Syntheses of the knowledge base on critical instructional issues* (pp. 81–104). Mahwah, NJ: Erlbaum.

Gallagher, J. J. (1986). Learning disabilities and special education: A critique. *Journal of Learning Disabilities, 19,* 595–601.

Gavelek, J. R., & Palincsar, A. S. (1988). Contextualism as an alternative worldview of learning disabilities: A response to Swanson's "Toward a metatheory of learning disabilities." *Journal of Learning Disabilities, 21,* 278–281.

Gelzheiser, L. M. (1987). Reducing the number of students identified as learning disabled: A question of practice, philosophy, or policy? *Exceptional Children, 54,* 145–150.

Gerard, J. A., & Junkala, J. (1980). Task analysis, handwriting, and process based instruction. *Journal of Learning Disabilities, 13,* 49–58.

Gerber, M. M. (1999–2000). An appreciation of learning disabilities: The value of blue–green algae. *Exceptionality, 8,* 29–42.

Gersten, R. (1998). Recent advances in instructional research for students with learning disabilities: An overview. *Learning Disabilities Research and Practice, 13,* 162–170.

Gersten, R., & Dimino, J. (2001). The realities of translating research into classroom practice. *Learning Disabilities Research and Practice, 16,* 120–130.

Ginsburg, H. P. (1997). Mathematics learning disabilities: A view from developmental psychology. *Journal of Learning Disabilities, 30,* 20–33.

Goldstein, K. (1939). *The organism, a holistic approach to biology derived from pathological data in man.* New York: American Book.

Gottlieb, J., Alter, M., Gottlieb, B. M., & Wishner, J. (1994). Special education in urban America: It's not justifiable for many. *Journal of Special Education, 27,* 453–465.

Graham, S. (1990). The role of production factors in learning disabled students' composition. *Journal of Educational Psychology, 82,* 781–791.

Gresham, F. M., MacMillan, D. L., & Bocian, K. M. (1996). Learning disabilities, low achievement, and mild mental retardation: More alike than different? *Journal of Learning Disabilities, 29,* 570–581.

Haight, S. L. (1980). Learning disabilities—The battered discipline. *Journal of Learning Disabilities, 13,* 452–455.

Hallahan, D. P., & Cruickshank, W. M. (1973). *Psychoeducational foundations of learning disabilities.* Englewood Cliffs, NJ: Prentice-Hall.

Hammill, D. D. (1972). Training visual perceptual processes. *Journal of Learning Disabilities, 5,* 552–559.

Hammill, D. D. (1993). A brief look at the learning disabilities movement in the United States. *Journal of Learning Disabilities, 26,* 295–310.

Hammill, D. D., & Larsen, S. C. (1974). The effectiveness of psycholinguistic training. *Exceptional Children, 41,* 5–14.

Heshusius, L. (1989a). Holistic principles: Not enhancing the old but seeing A-new. A rejoinder. *Journal of Learning Disabilities, 22,* 595–602.

Heshusius, L. (1989b). The Newtonian mechanistic paradigm, special education, and contours of alternatives: An overview. *Journal of Learning Disabilities, 22,* 403–415.

Iano, R. P. (1986). The study and development of teaching. With implications for the advancement of special education. *Remedial and Special Education, 1,* 50–61.

Iano, R. P. (1987). Rebuttal: Neither the absolute certainty of prescriptive law nor a surrender to mysticism. *Remedial and Special Education, 8,* 52–61.

Ingram, C. P. (1935). *The education of the slow-learning child.* New York: Ronald Press.

Kamhi, A. G., Catts, H. W., & Maurer, D. (1990). Explaining speech production deficits in poor readers. *Journal of Learning Disabilities, 23,* 632–636.

Kavale, K. A. (1981a). Functions of the Illinois Test of Psycholinguistic Abilities (ITPA): Are they trainable? *Exceptional Children, 47,* 496–510.

Kavale, K. A. (1981b). The relationship between auditory perceptual skills and reading ability: A meta-analysis. *Journal of Learning Disabilities, 14,* 539–546.

Kavale, K. A. (1982). Meta-analysis of the relationship between visual perceptual skills and reading achievement. *Journal of Learning Disabilities, 15,* 42–51.

Kavale, K. A. (1987a). On regaining integrity in the LD field. *Learning Disabilities Research, 2,* 60–61.

Kavale, K. A. (1987b). Theoretical issues surrounding severe discrepancy. *Learning Disabilities Research, 3,* 12–20.

Kavale, K. A. (1987c). Theoretical quandaries in learning disabilities. In S. Vaughn & C. S. Bos (Eds.), *Research in learning disabilities: Issues and future directions* (pp. 19–29). Boston: College-Hill/Little, Brown.

Kavale, K. A. (1993). A science and theory of learning disabilities. In G. R. Lyon, D. B. Gray, J. F. Kavanagh, & N. A. Krasnegor (Eds.), *Better un-*

derstanding learning disabilities (pp. 171–195). Baltimore: Brookes.

Kavale, K. A. (1995). Setting the record straight on learning disability and low achievement: The tortuous path of ideology. *Learning Disabilities Research and Practice, 10,* 145–152.

Kavale, K. A., & Forness, S. R. (1984). The historical foundation of learning disabilities: A quantitative synthesis assessing the validity of Strauss and Werner's exogenous versus endogenous distinction of mental retardation. *Remedial and Special Education, 6,* 18–24.

Kavale, K. A., & Forness, S. R. (1985). Learning disability and the history of science: Paradigm or paradox? *Remedial and Special Education, 6,* 12–23.

Kavale, K. A. & Forness, S. R. (1987a). The far side of heterogeneity: A critical analysis of empirical subtyping research in learning disabilities. *Journal of Learning Disabilities, 20,* 374–382.

Kavale, K. A. & Forness, S. R. (1987b). History, politics, and the general education initiative: Sleeter's reinterpretation of learning disabilities as a case study. *Remedial and Special Education, 8,* 6–12.

Kavale, K. A., & Forness, S. R. (1987c). Substance over style: A quantitative synthesis assessing the efficacy of modality testing and teaching. *Exceptional Children, 54,* 228–234.

Kavale, K. A., & Forness, S. R. (1995). *The nature of learning disabilities: Critical elements of diagnosis and classification.* Mahwah, NJ: Erlbaum.

Kavale, K. A., & Forness, S. R. (1998). The politics of learning disabilities. *Learning Disability Quarterly, 21,* 245–273.

Kavale, K. A., & Forness, S. R. (2000). What definitions of learning disability say and don't say: A critical analysis. *Journal of Learning Disabilities, 33,* 239–256.

Kavale, K. A., Forness, S. R., MacMillan, D. L., & Gresham, F. M. (1998). The politics of learning disabilities: A rejoinder. *Learning Disability Quarterly, 21,* 306–317.

Kavale, K. A., Fuchs, D., & Scruggs, T. E. (1994). Setting the record straight on learning disability and low achievement: Implications for policymaking. *Learning Disabilities Research and Practice, 9,* 70–77.

Kavale, K. A., & Mattson, P. D. (1983). "One jumped off the balance beam": Meta-analysis of perceptual-motor training. *Journal of Learning Disabilities, 16,* 165–173.

Kavale, K. A., & Nye, C. (1981). Identification criteria for learning disabilities: A survey of the research literature. *Learning Disability Quarterly, 4,* 383–388.

Kavale, K. A., & Nye, C. (1991). The structure of learning disabilities. *Exceptionality, 2,* 141–156.

Kavale, K. A., & Reese, J. H. (1992). The character of learning disabilities: An Iowa profile. *Learning Disability Quarterly, 15,* 74–94.

Keogh, B. K. (1983). A lesson from Gestalt psychology. *Exceptional Education Quarterly, 4,* 115–127.

Keogh, B. K. (1987). Learning disabilities: In defense of a construct. *Learning Disabilities Research and Practice, 3,* 4–9.

Keogh, B. K. (1994). A matrix of decision points in the measurement of learning disabilities. In G. R. Lyon (Ed.), *Frames of reference for the assessment of learning disabilities* (pp. 15–26). Baltimore: Brookes.

Kirk, S. A. (1963, April). Behavioral diagnosis and remediation of learning disabilities. In *Proceedings of the First Annual Meeting of the ACLD Conference on Exploration into the Problems of the Perceptually Handicapped Child* (pp. 1–7). Chicago: Author.

Kirk, S. A., & Elkins, J. (1975). Characteristics of children enrolled in the child service demonstration centers. *Journal of Learning Disabilities, 8,* 630–637.

Kosc, L. (1974). Developmental dyscalculia. *Journal of Learning Disabilities, 7,* 164–177.

Kuhn, T. S. (1970). *The structure of scientific revolutions* (2nd ed.). Chicago: University of Chicago Press.

Liberman, I. Y., & Shankweiler, D. (1985). Phonology and the problem of learning to read and write. *Remedial and Special Education, 6,* 8–17.

Lucangeli, D., Galderisi, D., & Cornoldi, C. (1995). Specific and general transfer effects following metamemory training. *Learning Disabilities Research and Practice, 10,* 11–21.

Lyon, G. R. (1985). Educational validation of learning disability subtypes. In B. P. Rourke (Ed.), *Neuropsychology of learning disabilities: Essentials of subtype analysis* (pp. 228–253). New York: Guilford Press.

Lyon, G. R. (1995a). Critical research needs in learning disabilities: A programmatic response from the NICHD. *Thalmus, 15,* 10–11.

Lyon, G. R. (1995b). Research initiatives in learning disabilities: Contributions from scientists supported by the National Institute of Child Health and Human Development. *Journal of Child Neurology, 10,* 120–126.

Lyon, G. R., & Krasnegor, N. A. (Eds.). (1996). *Attention, memory, and executive function.* Baltimore: Brookes.

MacMillan, D. L., Gresham, F. M., & Bocian, K. M. (1998). Discrepancy between definitions of learning disabilities and school practices: An empirical investigation. *Journal of Learning Disabilities, 31,* 314–326.

MacMillan, D. L., Gresham, F. M., Bocian, K. M., & Lambros, K. M. (1998). Current plight of borderline students: Where do they belong? *Education and Training in Mental Retardation and Developmental Disabilities, 33,* 83–94.

MacMillan, D. L., Gresham, F. M., Siperstein, G. N., & Bocian, K. M. (1996). The labyrinth of IDEA: School decisions on referred students with subaverage general intelligence. *American Journal on Mental Retardation, 101,* 161–174.

MacMillan, D. L., Siperstein, G., & Gresham, F. (1996). A challenge to the viability of mild mental retardation as a diagnostic category. *Exceptional Children, 62,* 356–371.

MacMillan, D. L., & Speece, D. L. (1999). Utility of current diagnostic categories for research and practice. In R. Gallimore, L. P. Bernheimer, D. L. MacMillan, D. L. Speece, & S. Vaughn (Eds.), *Developmental perspectives on children with high-incidence disabilities* (pp. 111–133). Mahwah, NJ: Erlbaum.

Malouf, D. B., & Schiller, E. P. (1995). Practice and research in special education. *Exceptional Children, 61,* 414–424.

Mann, L. (1971). Psychometric phrenology and the new faculty psychology: The case against ability assessment and training. *Journal of Special Education, 5,* 3–14.

Mastropieri, M. A., & Scruggs, T. E. (1989). Constructing more meaningful relationships: Mnemonic instruction for special populations. *Educational Psychology Review, 1,* 83–111.

Mather, N., & Roberts, R. (1994). Learning disabilities: A field in danger of extinction? *Learning Disabilities Research and Practice, 9,* 49–58.

McCroskey, R. L., & Kidder, H. C. (1980). Auditory fusion among learning disabled, reading disabled, and normal children. *Journal of Learning Disabilities, 13,* 69–76.

McKinney, J. D. (1983). Contributions of the institutes for research on learning disabilities. *Exceptional Education Quarterly, 4,* 129–144.

McKinney, J. D., & Speece, D. L. (1986). Academic consequences and longitudinal stability of behavioral subtypes of learning disabled children. *Journal of Educational Psychology, 78,* 365–372.

McKnight, R. T. (1982). The learning disability myth in American education. *Journal of Education, 164,* 351–359.

Meichenbaum, D. (1977). *Cognitive behavior modification: An integrative approach.* New York: Plenum Press.

Mercer, C. D., Jordan, L., Allsop, D. H., & Mercer, A. R. (1996). Learning disabilities definitions and criteria used by state education departments. *Learning Disability Quarterly, 19,* 217–232.

Meyen, E. (1989). Let's not confuse test scores with the substance of the discrepancy model. *Journal of Learning Disabilities, 22,* 482–483.

Miller, J. L. (1990). Apolcalypse or renaissance or something in between? Toward a realistic appraisal of "The learning mystique." *Journal of Learning Disabilities, 23,* 86–91.

Miner, M., & Siegel, L. S. (1992). William Butler Yeats: Dyslexic? *Journal of Learning Disabilities, 25,* 372–375.

Moats, L. C., & Lyon, G. R. (1993). Learning disabilities in the United States: Advocacy, science, and the future of the field. *Journal of Learning Disabilities, 26,* 282–294.

Montague, M., Maddux, C. D., & Dereshiwsky, M. I. (1990). Story grammar and comprehension and production of narrative prose by students with learning disabilities. *Journal of Learning Disabilities, 23,* 190–197.

Morrison, G. M., MacMillan, D. L., & Kavale, K. A. (1985). System identification of learning disabled children: Implications for research sampling. *Learning Disability Quarterly, 8,* 2–10.

National Advisory Committee on Handicapped Children. (1968). *First annual report, special education for handicapped children.* Washington, DC: Department of Health, Education, and Welfare.

Pearl, R., Bryan, T., & Donahue, M. (1980). Learning disabled children's attributions for success and failure. *Learning Disability Quarterly, 3,* 3–9.

Polansky, N. A. (1986). "There is nothing so practical as a good theory." *Child Wefare, 65,* 3–15.

Poplin, M. S. (1988a). Holistic/constructivistic principles of the teaching/learning process: Implications for the field of learning disabilities. *Journal of Learning Disabilities, 21,* 401–416.

Poplin, M. S. (1988b). The reductionist fallacy in learning disabilities: Replicating the past by reducing the present. *Journal of Learning Disabilities, 21,* 389–400.

Poplin, M. S. (1995). Looking through other lenses and listening to other voices: Stretching the boundaries of learning disabilities. *Journal of Learning Disabilities, 28,* 392–398.

Reger, R. (1979). Learning disabilities: Futile attempts at a simplistic definition. *Journal of Learning Disabilities, 12,* 529–532.

Reid, R. (1996). Research in self-monitoring with students with learning disabilities: The present, the prospects, the pitfalls. *Journal of Learning Disabilities, 29,* 317–331.

Reynolds, C. R. (1984–1985). Critical measurement issues in learning disabilities. *Journal of Special Education, 18,* 451–476.

Riccio, C. A., Gonzalez, J. J., & Hynd, G. W. (1994). Attention-deficit hyperactivity disorder (ADHD) and learning disabilities. *Learning Disability Quarterly, 17,* 311–322.

Rutter, M., & Yule, W. (1975). The concept of specific reading retardation. *Journal of Child Psychology and Psychiatry, 16,* 181–197.

Scruggs, T. E. (1987). Theoretical issues surrounding severe discrepancy: A discussion. *Learning Disabilities Research, 3,* 21–23.

Senf, G. M. (1987). Learning disabilities as sociologic sponge: Wiping up life's spills. In S. Vaughn & C. Bos (Eds.), *Research in learning disabilities: Issues and future directions* (pp. 87–101). Boston: Little, Brown/College Hill.

Sharp, R. (1980). *Knowledge, ideology, and the politics of schooling: Towards a Marxist analysis of education.* London: Routledge & Kegan Paul.

Shepard, L. (1980). An evaluation of the regression discrepancy method for identifying children with learning disabilities. *Journal of Special Education, 14,* 79–91.

Shepard, L. A., Smith, M. L., & Vojir, C. P. (1983). Characteristics of pupils identified as learning disabled. *American Educational Research Journal, 20,* 309–331.

Siegel, E. (1968). Learning disabilities: Substance or shadow? *Exceptional Children, 35*, 433–437.

Siegel, L. S. (1989). I. Q. is irrelevant to the definition of learning disabilities. *Journal of Learning Disabilities, 22*, 469–478, 486.

Sleeter, C. E. (1986). Learning disabilities: The social construction of a special education category. *Exceptional Children, 53*, 46–54.

Snowling, M. J. (1981). Phonemic deficits in developmental dyslexia. *Psychological Research, 43*, 219–234.

Stanovich, K. E. (1986). Cognitive processes and the reading problems of learning disabled children: Evaluating the assumption of specificity. In J. K. Torgesen & B. Y. L. Wong (Eds.), *Psychological and educational perspectives on learning disabilities* (pp. 87–131). Orlando, FL: Academic Press.

Stanovich, K. E. (1988). Explaining the differences between the dyslexic and the garden-variety poor reader: The phonological-core variable-difference model. *Journal of Learning Disabilities, 21*, 590–604.

Stanovich, K. E. (1991). Discrepancy definitions of reading disability: Has intelligence led us astray? *Reading Research Quarterly, 26*, 7–29.

Stone, C. A. (1998). The metaphor of scaffolding: Its utility for the field of learning disabilities. *Journal of Learning Disabilities, 31*, 344–364.

Strauss, A. A., & Lehtinen, L. E. (1947). *Psychopathology and education of the brain-injured child*. New York: Grune & Stratton.

Summers, E. G. (1986). The information flood in learning disabilities: A bibliometric analysis of the journal literature. *Remedial and Special Education, 7*, 49–60.

Swanson, H. L. (1988). Toward a metatheory of learning disabilities. *Journal of Learning Disabilities, 21*, 196–209.

Swanson, H. L. (1993). Working memory in learning disability subgroups. *Journal of Experimental Child Psychology, 56*, 87–114.

Swanson, H. L. (2000). Issues facing the field of learning disabilities. *Learning Disability Quarterly, 23*, 37–50.

Swanson, H. L., & Christie, L. (1994). Implicit notions about learning disabilities: Some directions for definitions. *Learning Disabilities Research and Practice, 9*, 244–254.

Swanson, H. L., & Cooney, J. B. (1991). Learning disabilities and memory. In B. Y. L. Wong (Ed.), *Learning about learning disabilities* (pp. 103–127). New York: Academic Press.

Swanson, H. L., & Hoskyn, M. (1998). Experimental intervention research on students with learning disabilities: A meta-analysis of treatment outcomes. *Review of Educational Research, 68*, 277–321.

Swanson, H. L., & Trahan, M. (1986). Characteristics of frequently cited articles in learning disabilities. *Journal of Special Education, 20*, 167–182.

Thomas, M. (2000). Albert Einstein and LD: An evaluation of the evidence. *Journal of Learning Disabilities, 33*, 149–157.

Thompson, L. J. (1971). Language disabilities in men of eminence. *Journal of Learning Disabilities, 4*, 39–50.

Torgesen, J. K. (1977). The role of non-specific factors in the task performance of learning disabled children: A theoretical assessment. *Journal of Learning Disabilities, 10*, 27–35.

Torgesen, J. K. (1986). Learning disabilities theory: Its current state and future prospects. *Journal of Learning Disabilities, 19*, 399–407.

Torgesen, J. K. (1993). Variations on theory in learning disabilities. In G. R. Lyon, D. B. Gray, J. F. Kavanagh, & N. A. Krasnegor (Eds.), *Better understanding learning disabilities* (pp. 153–170). Baltimore: Brookes.

Tucker, J., Stevens, L. J., & Ysseldyke, J. E. (1983). Learning disabilities: The experts speak out. *Journal of Learning Disabilities, 16*, 6–14.

U.S. Office of Education. (1977, December 29). Assistance to states for education of handicapped children: Procedures for evaluating specific learning disabilities. *Federal Register, 41*(230), 52404–52407.

Vaughn, S., & Bos, C. S. (Eds.). (1987). *Research in learning disabilities: Issues and future directions.* Boston: College-Hill/Little, Brown.

Vaughn, S., & Bos, C. (Eds.). (1994). *Research issues in learning disabilities: Theory, methodology, assessment, and ethics.* New York: Springer-Verlag.

Vellutino, F. R. (1977). Alternative conceptualizations of dyslexia: Evidence in support of a verbal-deficit hypothesis. *Harvard Educational Review, 47*, 334–354.

Vellutino, F. R., Steger, B. M., Moyer, S. C., Harding, C. J., & Niles, J. A. (1977). Has the perceptual deficit hypothesis led us astray? *Journal of Learning Disabilities, 10*, 375–385.

Wagner, R. K., & Torgesen, J. K. (1987). The nature of phonological processing and its causal role in the acquisition of reading skills. *Psychological Bulletin, 101*, 192–212.

Werner, H., & Strauss, A. A. (1940). Causal factors in low performance. *American Journal of Mental Deficiency, 45*, 213–218.

Wiederholt, J. L. (1974). Historical perspectives on the education of the learning disabled. In L. Mann & D. Sabatino (Eds.), *The second review of special education* (pp. 103–152). Philadelphia: JSE Press.

Wiig, E. H. (1990). Linguistic transitions and learning disabilities: A strategic learning perspective. *Learning Disability Quarterly, 13*, 128–140.

Wilson, L. R. (1985). Large-scale learning disability identification: The reprieve of a concept. *Exceptional Children, 52*, 44–51.

Wong, B. Y. L. (1979a). The role of theory in learning disabilities research: Part I. An analysis of problems. *Journal of Learning Disabilities, 12*, 585–595.

Wong, B. Y. L. (1979b). The role of theory in learning disabilities research: Part II. A selective review of current theories of learning and reading disabilities. *Journal of Learning Disabilities, 12*, 649–658.

Wong, B. Y. L. (1985). Metacognition and learning disabilities. In D. L. Forrest-Pressley, G. E. MacKinnon, & T. G. Waller (Eds.), *Metacognition, cognition, and human performance* (Vol. 2, pp. 137–180). New York: Academic Press.

Wong, B. Y. L. (1987). How do the results of metacognitive research impact on the learning disabled individual? *Learning Disability Quarterly, 10,* 189–195.

Ysseldyke, J. E., Algozzine, B., Shinn, M. R., & McGue, M. (1982). Similarities and differences between low achievers and students classified learning disabled. *Journal of Special Education, 16,* 73–85.

6

English-Language Learners with Learning Disabilities

Russell Gersten
Scott Baker

This chapter highlights key instructional issues related to English-language learners with learning disabilities (LD). It is divided into three sections. The first section discusses the issues of disproportionate representation of English-language learners in special education, and the LD category, in particular. The second section describes ongoing research by the authors on first-grade reading instruction for English-language learners. The goal of this research is to begin to articulate dimensions of teaching in general education settings that prevent reading failure for English-language learners who are grappling with the double demands of learning to read and learning a new language. The final section highlights key instructional issues involved in merging English-language development with academic instruction. It is based, in large part, on research we have conducted over the past decade and a research synthesis we conducted (Gersten & Baker, 2000c).

Disproportionate Representation of English-Language Learners in Special Education

It is telling that both the 1982 report by Heller, Holtzman, and Messick and the

2002 reports by the National Research Council (NRC) on the disproportionate representation of ethnic minority students in special education frame issues of disproportional representation in terms of the need to clearly specify the conditions under which disproportionate representation creates problems. The reports deemphasize the extensive focus on various quantitative estimates of minority student overrepresentation (or underrepresented) in different special education categories such as LD. Framing the issue this way has special relevance for English-language learners, especially those suspected of having a learning disability. The continuing relevance of some of the conditions specified in the 1982 report, in particular, have held up well over the 20-year period, not only in their contemporary importance but also in the unique ways they affect English-language learners.

Invalid Placement

Disproportionate representation may be a problem when certain groups of students are inappropriately identified as having a disability they do not, actually, possess. Underlying problems can often be the assessment measures and procedures used and/or subsequent interpretations used for the determination. As many chapters in this book indicate, the LD category, more than any other, presents the most controversial and problematic diagnostic challenge. And when the students under scrutiny are English-language learners, the challenge is particularly great.

In the Heller and colleagues (1982) report, the assessment controversy centered on what was then consistent overrepresentation of minority students in the mild mental retardation category, which at that time represented the largest group of students in special education. At issue was the use of intelligence tests with minority students (primarily African Americans) and related issues having to do with classic notions of test validity (Messick, 1980).

In the report, little was said specifically about assessment issues involving English-language learners. In a sense, this is curious in that a major stimulus for national attention turning toward the issue of overrepresentation of ethnic minority students in the mild mental retardation category was the classic research study by Jane Mercer (1970). Her sample included Hispanic as well as African American students. The key finding in Mercer's study was that many students from ethnic minority groups were diagnosed as educable mentally retarded but were not perceived as disabled, or to have problems functioning successfully, in their homes or communities. In other words, they were only perceived "disabled" when they were in school. Mercer questioned the legitimacy of labeling students as mentally retarded given this contradiction. This issue has great relevance for the LD category 30 years later. Mercer's sample included both Latino and African-American students.

However, major national attention was focused on overrepresentation of African Americans in special education at that time. The reader needs to recall that 1982 was at the beginning of what has become the largest wave of immigration in the history of the United States, a movement that has dramatically increased the number of English-language learners in the schools.

In the 2002 report, the entire assessment system for determining high-incidence disabilities (i.e., learning disabilities, behavior disorders, mild mental retardation) is under attack, especially in the case of learning disabilities. Traditional methods for determining the existence of a learning disability by measuring the discrepancy between ability and achievement has been criticized as conceptually flawed (Fuchs & Fuchs, 1998; Lyon et al., 2001), procedurally cumbersome (Shinn, 1989), and largely useless in being able to provide helpful information about potentially effective instructional options (Marston, 1989). These problems are exacerbated when the students being assessed are English-language learners because it is unclear whether low scores on either intelligence or achievement tests are due to actual problems, language difficulties, or unfamiliarity with cultural conventions.

Increasingly, the claim is made that a better way of determining the existence of a learning disability is to document that learning problems are pervasive over time and occur despite the presence of instructional approaches that enable the majority of the referred student's peers to learn successfully. One way this conceptual definition of a learning disability has been operationalized is low rates of learning growth measured by consistent academic measures administered regularly over time (Lyon, 1994).

Reconceptualizations of LD are beginning to have an impact on the field, albeit a relatively small one so far. A 2002 report from the National Research Council indicates that alternative models of disability identification that include low rates of academic growth as a key identification variable are producing positive benefits for students (Ikeda et al., 2002).

Another focus in the 2002 NRC report is the importance of special interventions in the regular classroom to address learning problems, particularly in reading, as early as possible. Both of these issues—determining rates of academic growth over time as a key criterion of a disability and intervening as early as possible with students experiencing learning problems—have significant implications for English-language learners.

For native English speakers, these new proposals have an intuitive appeal and there is substantial evidence of student benefit. Essentially, students who enter school with low literacy skills, or who make low rates of literacy growth over time, are considered to be at risk for school failure. As part of the pre-referral intervention process, these students are provided with instructional opportunities—typically more intensity or just more instruction—which their peers who are not at risk do not receive. By intervening early, the expectation is that many students who would normally not receive help until they experienced sufficient failure to qualify for special education are provided with early assistance that will help them improve their rate of learning and enable them to keep pace with their peers. In this way, a formal referral to special education can be avoided.

But for a large percentage of English-language learners, lower levels of initial English literacy skills can be expected on average because they have not learned English at home the way monolingual English-speaking students have. More important, the very concept of adequate rates of academic growth (at least in English) is largely unknown unless a great deal is known about the proficiency these students have in their native language and in English. In addition, it is important to know about the details of the instructional environment these students experience, which may be very different than that of their native English-speaking peers.

Optimal instructional programs for English-language learners, especially when pre-referral assessments and interventions are at their most intense for native English speakers, are complex and controversial. Only in the past 2 years have researchers started to study them, and none of the research is yet complete. Many continue to advocate that native language programs are necessary until a student reaches an adequate level of English-language proficiency. For example, this was the position taken by the National Academy of Sciences report on beginning reading (Snow, Burns, & Griffin, 1998), although the panel did agree there was absolutely no empirical support for such a position. Others (Anderson & Roit, 1998) have reasoned that learning to read in English as early as possible is important in that reading and writing are excellent venues for the development of English-language proficiency.

When English-language learners are taught predominantly in their native language and gradually introduced to English, a number of conceptual problems present themselves in trying to determine what aca-demic learning problems exist and what to do about them (Gersten, 1996b).

It is unclear what rates of growth in languages other than English are important for English-language learners, and to what extent growth in a student's native language will serve as a sufficient safeguard against eventual problems with English acquisition, especially the acquisition of the formal, abstract language of academic disciplines. Ultimately, when English is introduced in third, fourth, or fifth grades, it is unclear when and how to separate normal problems in learning a new language (i.e., English) from problems that constitute a legitimate learning disability that require the need for special education services. All students grapple with the issue that English has a terribly complex and often irregular system for converting letters or letter combinations into sounds compared to a language such as Spanish or Arabic. For these reasons, many have identified disproportionately low rates of English-language learners in certain districts in the category of LD (e.g., Gersten & Woodward, 1994; Harry, 1992).

For English-language learners who are taught to read in English very early in school, it is similarly unclear the extent to which the challenges they face learning a new language and acquiring academic content simultaneously (Gersten, 1996a) change from becoming normal challenges faced by English-language learners into learning problems indicating the presence of a learning disability.

In summary, the idea of early, preventive interventions advocated in the 2002 report makes a great deal of sense for native English speakers. We have solid evidence regarding what constitutes a strong program in beginning reading (Snow et al., 1998), how reading progress can be monitored frequently over time (Fuchs, 1986), and how to intervene successfully to increase students' learning trajectories. For English-language learners, however, it is unclear how well this model fits.

Poor Quality Instruction in General Education and Its Impact on Special Education Referrals for English-Language Learners

Disproportionate representation is a problem when students from certain ethnic groups are more likely to be referred and placed in special education than are their peers. One of the causes cited in the Heller and colleagues (1982) report was that the quality of instruction provided to students in low-income schools with high ethnic minority populations may often be problematic. The 1982 report recognized the inherent complexity of trying to determine what constitutes quality instruction for students in general education. For the most part, the report offered rather instructional guidelines for determining quality.

A major difference between the Heller and colleagues (1982) report and the 2002 NRC report is that the initial report primarily had at its disposal research on which particular instructional settings or placements seemed to produce better outcomes— regular classes or separate special education classes—"rather than on the characteristics of effective instruction" (Heller et al., 1982, p. 21). In contrast, the 2002 report devotes a good deal of attention to which types of instructional approaches appear to be most effective or promising for students regardless of setting.

It is interesting to consider the parallel between lack of research on effective instructional approaches for students with learning disabilities identified in the Heller and colleagues (1982) report and the current void in the knowledge base on the best ways to teach English-language learners. Since 1982, there have been significant advances in what we know about components of effective instruction for students with learning disabilities (Gersten, Baker, Pugach, Scanlon, & Chard, 2001; Swanson & Hoskyn, 1998). That knowledge base is evident in the 2002 report.

For example, the 2002 NRC report clearly lays out important components of programs in beginning reading. Specific recommendations are also provided for high-quality first- and second-tier interventions when students do not respond successfully to initial instruction.

It is important to note that this level of instructional specificity is *not* part of the knowledge base for English-language learners. This void will change, however, if the report by the National Research Council (August & Hakuta, 1997) on effective education for English-language learners is fol-

lowed. This report clearly states that large program evaluation studies, which have characterized much of the federally supported research on English-language learners, have not produced particularly useful results. This research has tried, essentially, to determine whether it is better to teach students in English or their native language (usually Spanish) in the primary grades. In noting that the research suffers from methodological and conceptual problems, August and Hakuta (1997) conclude, "There is little value in conducting evaluations to determine which type of program is best" (p. 138).

This conclusion is analogous to the research of the 1970s and 1980s that attempted to determine which instructional setting or placement (self-contained class or general education classroom) was best for students with LD. For research with English-language learners, the solution is "not finding a program that works for all children and all localities, but rather finding a set of program components that works for the children in the community of interest, given that community's goals, demographics, and resources" (August & Hakuta, 1997, p. 138). Research carried out this way would have a significant impact on both of the conditions outlined previously that address when disproportionate representation of English-language learners in the LD category is a problem.

Despite the fact that little research has been conducted on components of effective instruction for English-language learners, the research that is available can provide an initial knowledge base to build on. In the next two sections we describe some of our research on this topic. We then address highlights of our attempt to synthesize the knowledge base on effective teaching of English-language learners using both meta-analytic and multivocal (qualitative) techniques for research synthesis (Gersten & Baker, 2000c).

The First-Grade Classroom Observational Study

We now have a reasonably sound research base on critical components for building literacy in the early grades and converging evidence of what approaches prevent reading failure and reduce inappropriate referral into special education (National Reading Panel, 2000; Snow et al., 1998). We have consistently argued that effective reading instruction principles are directly relevant for teaching reading to English-language learners, although significant modulation and adjustment are required (Gersten & Baker, 2000c; Gersten & Jiménez, 1994). Modulation, for example, would require much greater linkage of vocabulary instruction with word attack and analysis instruction for English-language learners than for native English speakers. Additional attention should also be paid to teaching phonemes and sounds that are prevalent in English but not existent in a student's native language (be it Korean or Tagalog, Spanish or Arabic). English-language learners would likely require many more opportunities to practice speaking and reading aloud, and more time on vocabulary development, including the teaching of meanings of words that will be quite familiar to virtually all native English speakers in first grade.

Two years ago, we began a study to begin to explore some of these hypotheses. We reasoned that given the limited knowledge base, it made the most sense to systematically observe beginning reading instruction in classrooms for evidence of how practicing teachers were addressing these issues. We collected and analyzed observation and reading outcome data for a set of 20 first-grade classrooms, in which English-language learners comprised the majority of students. Teachers in these classrooms were also implementing a research-based approach to early literacy based on the recently adopted California Reading and Language Arts Framework. Our goals for conducting observations were to analyze teaching practice by measuring what we referred to as quality of instruction on key instructional dimensions. We expected these goals would ultimately lead us to identifying key pedagogical factors critical to reading improvements for English-language learners learning to read in English.

Essentially, there are three general approaches for classroom observation instruments. First, there are low-inference measures such as the instruments used in the classic studies of beginning reading (Ander-

son, Evertson, & Brophy, 1979; Foorman, Francis, Fletcher, & Lynn, 1996; Stallings & Kaskowitz, 1974). Precise operational definitions are used to determine things such as the number of minutes of academic engaged time, the number of positive responses, and the latency of teacher feedback to students. Second, open-ended qualitative observations have been used to a considerable degree in classrooms of English-language learner, including much of our earlier work (e.g., Gersten, 1999; Jiménez & Gersten, 1999). In these studies, we immersed ourselves in approximately 15 classrooms serving English-language learners in grades 3 to 6, and took relatively open-ended field notes to describe patterns of instruction that appeared to be productive or ineffective in terms of teaching reading and language arts, and promoting English-language development. Although we employed a coding system to help us sort out and categorize eight major issues (Gersten, 1996b), observers' notes were open-ended, including verbatim excerpts, statements of working hypotheses with supporting evidence, and narrative descriptions of instruction. Finally, a moderate-level inference observational instrument, such as the one used in a recent study of teaching quality by Stanovich and Jordan (1998), includes aspects of both low-inference and open-ended instruments. Attempts are made to define key variables of interest in observable terms, but rather than observers attempting to quantify what they observe in real time, they use their professional judgment and knowledge of the observation setting to rate the quality of what they see many times on a Likert scale. For example, an observer might rate the quality of feedback a teacher provide students or the complexity of academic discourse between students.

We agreed on a moderate-level inference instrument for several reasons. We were still in the exploratory stages of investigating this issue; thus, a precise measure of rates of select classroom interactions would be premature. On the other hand, purely open-ended qualitative field notes did not seem the right fit for this type of study in that we had a definite sense of promising instructional variables, based on effective teaching research and effective reading instruction, and wanted some systematic database. Also, based on earlier qualitative research, we had reasonable hypotheses as to specific instructional techniques and modulations that could lead to enhancing the reading and language development of English-language learners and wished to see if these variables correlated with student growth in reading.

Items on the instrument were derived from four sources: (1) process–product studies on effective teaching of beginning reading (Anderson et al., 1979; Stallings & Kaskowitz, 1974); (2) reading instruction for students with significant reading problems (Leinhardt, Zigmond, & Cooley, 1981; Stanovich & Jordan, 1998); (3) descriptive studies of effective instructional environments for English-language learners (Tikunoff et al., 1991), and current thinking on best practice (Echevarria, Vogt, & Short, 2000); and (4) the knowledge base on teaching beginning reading.

Effective teaching research conducted over the past 25 years suggests numerous effective pedagogical strategies for the development of reading and early literacy skills. Variables such as the influence of time spent engaged in academic tasks—as well as the importance of preteaching, scaffolding, and quality of feedback—are recognized today as critical elements of classroom teaching. Many of these formed the framework for the study by Stanovich and Jordan (1998).

Description of the English-Language Learner Classroom Observation Instrument

The final instrument was composed of 29 items, which were rated on a 1–7 Likert scale, with 7 being most effective and 1 being least effective. The pilot version contained 50 items. Items were deleted, collapsed or revised due to (1) low base rate, (2) low interrater reliability, and (3) redundancy. Ratings were complemented by observers' qualitative notation of activities and responses observed during the observational period. To expand the scope of the data, observers continued to record low base-rate items on a separate sheet attached to the instrument.

The Observation Instrument was field tested in 1999 and 2000 in 25 California classrooms within three urban districts in California. In the final sample of 20 classrooms, 10 classrooms had some native English speakers while 10 consisted solely of English-language learners. Whereas 19 classrooms had Spanish-speaking, English-language learners, 30% of the classrooms also included other English-language learners (e.g., Vietnamese, Somali, and Cambodian). Each classroom selected for observation was made up of at least 75% English-language learners.

Growth in reading performance was assessed using the Dynamic Indicators of Basic Early Literacy Skills (DIBELS; Kaminski & Good, 1996), a series of 1-minute reading tasks representing phonemic awareness, alphabetic understanding, and oral reading fluency. An additional reading measure was adapted from the California Reading Results Reading Comprehension Assessment (California Reading and Literature Project, 1999).

Classrooms were observed during the entire instructional period for reading/language arts. California's reading standards mandate a minimum of 2.5 hours for reading/language arts instruction. Each classroom teacher was observed from two to four times toward the middle of the school year. To reduce the possibility of an interaction effect between observers and teachers, observers rotated through the various classrooms and consulted frequently to discuss the meaning of items and how to code different instructional events.

Interrater reliability was established through joint observations and frequent conferencing following independent completion of rating scales. The median interobserver agreement, with agreement defined as observers being within 1 point of each other, was 74% across the items with a range from 55% to 88%. For a moderate inference rating system, this was an acceptable level of agreement.

We developed six empirically derived subscales based on factor scores. These subscales and related items appear in Table 6.1. The internal consistency of the subscales was quite high. Cronbach's *alpha* for each subscale ranged from .80 to .95 with a median of .89.

Student Outcomes Related to Observed Instruction

In the 20 classrooms there were 229 English-language learners whose reading skills

TABLE 6.1. Empirical Subscales from the English-Language Learner Classroom Observation Instrument

1. *Explicit teaching/the art of teaching*
   - Models skills and strategies
   - Makes relationships overt
   - Emphasizes distinctive features of new concepts
   - Provides prompts
   - Length of literacy activities is appropriate
   - Adjusts own use of English during lesson

2. *Instruction geared toward low performers*
   - Achieves high level of response accuracy
   - Ensures quality of independent practice
   - Engages in ongoing monitoring of student understanding and performance
   - Elicits responses from all students
   - Modifies instruction for students as needed
   - Provides extra instruction, practice, and review
   - Asks questions to ensure comprehension

3. *Sheltered English techniques*
   - Uses visuals or manipulatives to teach content
   - Provides explicit instruction in English
   - Encourages students to give elaborate responses
   - Uses gestures and facial expressions in teaching vocabulary and clarifying meaning of content

4. *Interactive teaching*
   - Secures and maintains student attention during lesson
   - Extent to which students are "on task" during literacy activities
   - Selects and incorporates students' responses, ideas, examples, and experiences into lessons
   - Gives students wait time to respond to questions

5. *Vocabulary development*
   - Teaches difficult vocabulary prior to and during lesson
   - Structures opportunities to speak English
   - Provides systematic instruction to vocabulary development
   - Engages students in meaningful interactions about text

6. *Phonemic awareness and decoding*
   - Provides systematic instruction in phonemic awareness
   - Provides systematic instruction in letter–sound correspondence
   - Provides systematic instruction in decoding

were assessed in both winter and spring. Assessments at the beginning of the study would usually have occurred much closer to the start of the academic year, but this was not possible because preparations for the study were not completed until well into the fall term.

The range of performance on each outcome measure was considerable, indicating that some English-language learners appeared to be acquiring reading skills at an impressive rate while others were clearly struggling.

One potential explanation for different levels of reading performance is overall English-language proficiency. We used available school records for the most recent test data for English-language proficiency to divide the English-language learners into three groups. There were 208 English-language learners for whom language test data was available. Student scores indicated (1) very low levels of English-language proficiency, (2) moderate levels of proficiency (corresponding to limited English proficiency category on the Language Assessment Scales), or (3) those with strong levels of proficiency.

Table 6.2 presents these data. On two of the three reading measures, students at the lowest level of English language proficiency actually did slightly better than students who were moderately proficient. The difference is very small, however, and difficult to interpret. Not surprisingly, students at the highest level of English-language proficiency did much better than students in the two other groups, which supports the important role of English-language proficiency and English-language development.

Student Reading Outcomes by Instructional Ratings

It is informative to examine the range of reading scores of English-language learners in the 20 classrooms in relation to ratings of instruction effectiveness. Figure 6.1 presents the classroom mean for each of the 20 classrooms on our major reading outcome measure, oral reading fluency, adjusted for pretest performance on Letter Naming Fluency administered at the beginning of the study. The line around the mean represents the 95% confidence interval. The 20 classrooms are organized into quartiles on the

TABLE 6.2. Means for Reading Outcome Measures by English-Language Proficiency Status

Measure	Low (*n* = 84) Mean (*SD*)	Limited (*n* = 79) Mean (*SD*)	High (*n* = 45) Mean (*SD*)
Word Attack	43.4 (27.9)	47.5 (31.2)	69.1 (30.8)
Oral Reading Fluency	41.4 (34.2)	37.7 (27.5)	63.4 (34.4)
Reading Comprehension[a]	2.2 (2.9)	1.9 (2.8)	5.1 (3.1)

[a]Because of scheduling difficulties, not all students were administered the Reading Comprehension measure. The numbers of students tested on this measure were 83, 73, and 44, for the Low, Limited, and High groups, respectively.

basis of their overall rating of instructional quality. Within each quartile, the classrooms are ordered from low to high in terms of overall instructional rating.

Across quartiles, classrooms that were rated higher in terms of overall instructional quality had higher adjusted reading scores at the end of grade 1. In other words, the observations seemed to do a reasonable job demarcating broad groups of classrooms on the basis of instructional factors related to reading. Given the entire range, it does seem that factors associated with our ratings of instructional quality were moderately associated with improved reading outcomes.

Both authors of this chapter (RG and SB) were members of the observation team and spent a considerable amount of time in nearly all of the first-grade classrooms. Our observations were conducted during the entire reading and language arts block; thus we have considerable experience with these teachers from which we derive the following more qualitative impressions of instruction in these classrooms.

Perhaps our most dominant impression is the extensive variability in instructional effectiveness we observed. In a number of classrooms we saw instruction that was of extremely high quality—students were actively engaged throughout the reading lessons and the activities seemed interesting and challenging to students. Teachers targeted important reading skills.

In many classrooms, instruction was problematic. Students were rarely engaged

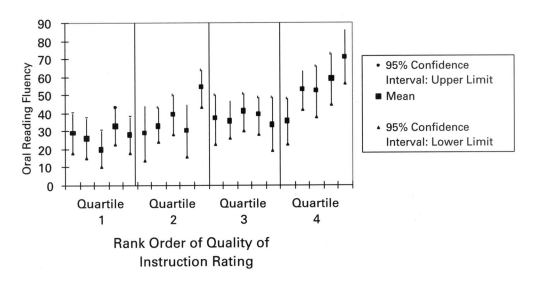

FIGURE 6.1. Quality of instruction ratings and student performance on oral reading fluency.

and teachers did not seem to have a real sense of what they wanted to accomplish or how to use the curriculum. Among the specific practices that seemed to distinguish teachers in the most effective classrooms from those in classrooms where instruction was most problematic, the following seemed particularly noteworthy: In the most effective classrooms there was a seamless quality to instruction that made the 2 hours much more productive and pass much more quickly. One activity blended naturally into the next and it was clear that teachers had planned carefully for these transitions. One of our observation items concerned the appropriateness of the length of literacy activities. In effective classrooms, activity length was more appropriate for 6-year-olds than in less effective classrooms. A 2-hour instructional block requires many different activities, especially with first-graders. In effective classrooms, activities rarely lasted more than 20 minutes or so. In problematic classrooms, activities might go on for 45 minutes or more; students got bored and started looking for more interesting things to do. Minor behavior problems increased in frequency and intensity as the length of the activity increased.

Although not captured as dramatically as we predicted, our field notes indicated that vocabulary instruction clearly distinguished the most effective classrooms from the least effective ones. In fact, as we had previously hypothesized (Gersten & Baker, 2000c), in some particularly effective classrooms, vocabulary served as a kind of anchor around which many other activities revolved. That is, vocabulary activities were incorporated throughout the reading lesson and were combined with other literacy activities.

During instruction to build phonemic awareness, for example, teachers would not only have students manipulate the sounds in target words, but they would also build vocabulary activities involving those words. Many of the target words were easy to visualize, which increased the relevance of the vocabulary segment of the lesson. Students and teachers would offer definitions and sentences involving target words and provide extended descriptions based on personal experience or knowledge. Teachers would provide pictures or offer line drawings on the board. Not only did infusing

vocabulary activities provide natural and structured breaks from the abstract phonemic awareness activities, but it fostered an exciting pace and rhythm to the lesson and provided a cognitively challenging task that students could participate in at many different levels.

Another factor that seemed to clearly separate successful from problematic classrooms was the incorporation of writing activities into the reading lesson in a highly integrated fashion. In most of the high-achieving classrooms, there was a strong emphasis on, or at least considerable time spent on, writing activities. In the most effective classrooms the connection between reading and writing activities was very clear.

In one effective classroom, for example, a connected set of reading and writing activities was extended over several days. With the teacher, students read a story about the jungle. As part of preparing to read the story they studied key vocabulary, a standard prereading task. In this classroom, students wrote these key words and others they encountered or thought about in a journal they would use to eventually write their own jungle story.

Over the course of 2 days, the teacher reviewed this story and target words a number of times, preparing students to write their own story. The teacher outlined a story structure that each student was expected to use and required that students include a certain number of words they had entered in their journals. When it was time for students to write their stories, they seemed prepared and eager for the task. There were a couple of key points in the lesson. First, there was a consistent and effective emphasis on vocabulary development. Second, the connection to reading and writing was explicit.

Merging English-Language Development and Reading/Language Arts Instruction: The Emerging Knowledge Base

In our final section, we respond to the recent challenge articulated by Rosalinda Barrera (cited in Jiménez, Moll, Rodríguez-Brown, & Barrera, 1999):

The real challenge for schools today is not the growing number of Latino/a children who speak Spanish (and must learn English) but the school's continuing need to do a far better job of delivering instruction to them in English. This would entail that schools and teachers acknowledge and understand these children as second-language learners and develop quality, content-rich ESL programs for them. . . . It also means that we must teach English reading and writing from a second-language. (p. 225)

In January 2002, in the Reauthorization of the Elementary and Secondary Education Act, Congress set a national goal of developing English-language proficiency within 3 years for all students who are English-language learners. This would include students with learning disabilities. Thus, it seems to be a particularly timely issue.

This section provides insights gained from our years of research in this area. A major emphasis of our research has been on codifying the knowledge base on how to teach English-language learners effectively in a second language, and how to merge English-language development with literacy instruction. The various studies have almost invariably included students with LD and we have tried to conceptualize implications for teaching this group of students.

Research we conducted began with a series of qualitative studies regarding the nature of instruction provided to English-language learners making the transition into all English-language instruction in grades 3–6 (Gersten, 1996a, 1996b, 1999; Gersten & Jiménez, 1994) describing both the strengths (Jiménez & Gersten, 1999) and problems in current practice (Gersten, 1999). Next we conducted a thorough review of both the qualitative and quantitative research on the topic and conducted a series of expert focus groups involving both researchers and professional educators with expertise in this topic (Gersten & Baker, 2000b, 2000c). Our major goal was to use these groups to articulate a vision of what most saw as critical issues and promising practices.

We use these sources as a means for articulating our sense of what we know about effective instructional practice, useful concepts in understanding components of best practice and critical issues that require further research. Our focus is in teaching students reading and other content areas in English in a sensitive, effective fashion while meeting the goal of promoting English-language proficiency.

Understanding the Components of a Comprehensive English-Language Development Program

In her study of an innovative approach for teaching reading comprehension of English-language learners with disabilities, Echevarria (1995) noted that "language is a primary vehicle for intellectual development" (p. 537). The connection between language development and acquisition of academic content and strategies for reading and problem solving is fundamental to virtually all instructional research for this population.

August and Hakuta (1997) note how all contemporary theories "share the important claim that academic language is different from language use in other contexts" (pp. 36–37). Despite widespread understanding of the distinction between these two types of language uses, it is still common for teachers to make the erroneous assumption that possessing command of conversational English means a child can follow abstract discussions of concepts such as antipathy, or specific gravity, or the causes of World War II.

Determining how to teach this language to students has been a challenge. Early attempts at English-language development (English as a second language [ESL]) instruction focused extensively on the formal structures of language (e.g., definitions, syntax, subject verb agreement, and placement of adjectives) using a mix of conversational English and more formal, literary language. This approach is now routinely criticized because it fails to capitalize on the central communicative function of language, it does not often generate student interest, and it results in limited generalization (Cummins, 1980; Tharp & Gallimore, 1988).

The 1980s saw the beginning of more "natural" conversational approaches to teaching English. These approaches were also criticized extensively on at least two grounds. First, they do not necessarily help students develop competence in the highly abstract, often decontextualized language of academic discourse. "Natural" conversations may help with development of conversational English (which many students seemed to be acquiring through everyday life in the United States anyway), but they rarely helped where help was needed most—with abstract, academic English, critical to understanding science, mathematics, history, and so forth.

A small but increasing number of researchers and scholars argued that English-language reading can serve as a powerful tool in building English-language proficiency and saw a reciprocal influence between learning to read in English and a child's English-language development. The stress on infusing English-language development into reading and language arts instruction and using literature and vocabulary in stories read as the core of an English-language development program is a major advance in our thinking.

Developing dialogue related to texts read by the student or by the teacher to the student seems a logical direction for English-language development instruction to proceed in. It would seem particularly critical for those involved in teaching students with LD, as there often is a strong language or language-related component to the disability. Literature seems an excellent venue for building the more formal language of school discourse in students.

Classes that merge English-language development activities with reading/language arts or other types of content area instruction are often called sheltered or content area ESL or immersion approaches. In the United States, these have largely been "homegrown" approaches to teaching, developed by districts, and sometimes individual teachers, to meet the needs of students.

With this approach, "teachers do not simplify—they amplify, they reiterate, reinstate, exemplify in diverse ways. . . . They construct support mechanisms (the reiterations, examples, diagrams) that . . . enable learners to access sophisticated concepts and relationships" (Walquis, 1998, cited in Gersten & Baker, 2000a). Use of English is modulated so that it is comprehensible to the student (Gersten, 1996a). In some cases, a student's native language may be used to help the student complete a task, clarify a point, or respond to a question.

The expert focus groups conducted by Gersten and Baker (2000c) noted some difficulties, in practice, with this approach.

Two problems that emerged were the following:

- Few districts have a curriculum program or approach that promotes students' proper use of the English language;
- Teachers often did not provide sufficient time for English-language development activities, and that content coverage tended to dominate time allocation.

In the words of one participant, this approach often fails, "to provide adequate time for English language learning" (Gersten & Baker, 2000b). In other words, participants felt that teachers often emphasize content acquisition over building English-language abilities. As one teacher noted, "It's important to use content as a basis for language development . . . [however] there is a risk during content instruction of neglecting language development."

Another major discussion item in the expert focus groups was the failure to systematically impart to students skills in speaking and writing standard English, even as late as middle school. Though many group members felt that the policy of never correcting students for grammatical or pronunciation problems during English-language instruction made sense during the early years of English-language development, there was general consensus that students need feedback on their formal English usage as they progress in school. Furthermore, teachers lack any kind of coherent system for providing it. One professional work group suggested that in the early phases of language learning, teachers should modulate the feedback they provide students and be sensitive to the problems inherent in correcting every grammar mistake students make. However, during later stages, one member reflected the feeling in the group by noting the "importance of identifying errors and providing specific feedback."

A recent research study by Fashola, Drum, Mayer, and Kang (1996) may provide some direction in this area. They noted how errors made by Latino students in English are usually predictable, and how these predictable errors could become the basis of *proactive curricula*: "Rather than simply marking a predicted error as incorrect, the teacher could explicitly point out that the phonological or orthographic rule in English is different from the one in "Spanish" (p. 840). Fashola and colleagues provide numerous examples of how teachers could proactively use knowledge of differences between Spanish and English to help their students avoid making these same predictable errors. Analogous strategies can be used for other languages, and especially to assist students whose home language is drastically different than English. This would appear to be a major focus for curriculum development in this area.

After reviewing these issues with expert focus groups and reading about problems with content area ESL in sources as diverse as virtually every newspaper in a large urban area and the *Harvard Educational Review* (Reyes, 1992), we concluded that an effective English-language development program should include a component devoted to helping students learn how to use the second language according to established conventions of grammar and syntax. On the other hand, providing some time each day when English-language learners have opportunities to work on all aspects of English-language development and providing academically challenging content instruction (be it in native language or English) are likely to be more easily achievable, especially if teachers take time to make goals clear.

A promising body of research suggests that peer-mediated approaches to instruction, such as peer-mediated instruction (Arreaga-Mayer, 1998) and collaborative strategic reading (Klingner & Vaughn, 1996, 2000), may be excellent venues for students not only to help build comprehension strategies and reading fluency but also to help in various aspects of English-language development.

These approaches involve heterogeneous small groups of students and provide clear guidelines for working together on various aspects of strategic reading, including summarizing, clarifying, using context clues to help understand word meanings, and generating questions for peers that help members focus on critical information. To date, there has been little specific inquiry on precisely which students benefit, the nature of discourse, and other fascinating and important issues that center on English-language de-

velopment, although both studies by Klingner and Vaughn (1996, 2000) begin to provide interesting insights.

To date, most of our knowledge base in this area remains more theoretical and experiential, as does virtually every topic in the education of English-language learners, than based on controlled research.

Guiding Principles for Best Practice

We conclude with a succinct overview of several additional instructional principles that seem to guide best practice. We limit this discussion to three critical instructional issues that seem to permeate many aspects of instruction.

BUILDING AND USING VOCABULARY AS A CURRICULAR ANCHOR

Vocabulary learning should play a major role in successful programs for English-language learners. The number of new vocabulary terms introduced at any one time should be limited. Criteria for selecting words should be considered carefully, so that words are selected that convey key concepts, are of high utility, are relevant to the bulk of the content being learned, and have meaning in the lives of students. The example cited earlier from a particularly effective first-grade classroom gives the reader a sense of how this goal can be accomplished. It is critical at all grade levels.

Restricting the number of words students are expected to learn per day will help them learn word meanings at a deep level of understanding. One expert teacher we have worked with previously provided insights into the methods she used to select and teach. She noted how she chose words for the class to analyze in depth that represented complex ideas—adjectives such as "anxious," "generous," and "suspicious," and nouns such as "memory"—words that English-language learners are likely to need help with and words that were linked to the story in meaningful and rich ways. Students had to read the story and look for evidence that certain events or descriptions that were connected to vocabulary instruction pertained to a particular character or incident. Intervention studies have also addressed vocabulary development directly supporting this approach (Rousseau, Tam, & Ramnarain, 1993).

USE OF VISUALS TO REINFORCE CONCEPTS AND VOCABULARY

The double demands of learning content and a second language are significant and the difficulty should not be underestimated. Because the spoken word is fleeting, visual aids such as graphic organizers, concept and story maps, and word banks give students a concrete system to process, reflect on, and integrate information.

The effective use of visuals during instruction with English-language learners has ranged from complex semantic visuals (Reyes & Bos, 1998) to visuals based on text structures, such as story maps and compare–contrast "think sheets."

Intervention studies and several observational studies have noted that the effective use of visuals during instruction can lead to increased learning. Rousseau and colleagues (1993) used visuals for teaching vocabulary (i.e., words written on the board and the use of pictures), and Saunders, O'Brien, Lennon, and McLean (1998) incorporated the systematic use of visuals for teaching reading and language arts. Visuals also play a large role in Cognitive Academic Language Learning Approach (CALLA), shown to be related to growth in language development (see Gersten & Baker, 2000b, for further discussion).

Implementation of even simple techniques such as writing key words on the board or a flip chart while discussing them verbally can support meaningful English-language development and comprehension. However, even the simple integration of visuals is drastically underused, and it seems that even when used, methods are typically inconsistent or superficial and do not support students' deep processing and thinking.

MODULATION OF COGNITIVE AND LANGUAGE DEMANDS

This last instructional strategy carries a different weight of importance, and we view it as the most speculative among those we have proposed. Yet, we think it is critical for successful English-language development. The proposition is that during English-language content instruction, effective teachers intentionally vary cognitive and language demands to achieve specific goals.

When cognitive demands are high, language expectations are simplified. In this case, for example, teachers may accept brief or truncated responses in English. In another part of the lesson, cognitive demands are intentionally reduced so that students can more comfortably experiment with extended English-language use.

This proposition was supported in each of the five expert focus groups conducted. It also appears consistent with contemporary theories of second-language acquisition (e.g., August & Hakuta, 1997). These examples from Gersten (1996a) convey a sense of how a teacher can adjust the language and cognitive demands within a lesson. The following is an example of a teacher using the constructs and principles of instructional conversations:

> "For example," the teacher, Mrs. Tapia asked, "What do you think the story will be about? Do you think this lady will be in the story?" She delicately elicited a wide range of predictions; each prediction was placed on the chart.

Student involvement was extremely high. Even the more passive students volunteered a prediction. The teacher provided prompts to students who seemed to be floundering, such as: "With a title like this and this picture on the cover, Fernando, what do you think this story will be about?' " Her style of feedback and mediation was interesting. She *never* judged a response incorrect or illogical. However, when a student predicted that the people in the story "will have a ranch," a statement that seemed to make no sense, she asked him why.

Even the more reticent students volunteer their predictions. All are recorded on the flip chart. At the conclusion of this brief story, a discussion of mood ensues. Mrs. Tapia asks, "What did you think about it?" One student answers, "It was kind of sad." Mrs. Tapia responds, "How do you know?" Miguel, one of the students she earlier described as a student with learning difficulties, says "Because old people." Mrs. Tapia praises Miguel for his insight. Because the idea is on the right track, even though the English grammar is incomplete, the response is evaluated for content rather than the extent to which it conformed to correct language use.

Responses are never labeled right or wrong, but sometimes students are asked to explain the rationale for their answers or opinions. Jorge, for example, explains that he "liked it because it was sad and it was happy," and he proceeds to provide several examples of sad and happy instances.

While discussing another story, the class had concluded that the leading character had transformed himself from a "bad man" (a thief) to a "good man" (one who helps people). Mrs. Tapia asked for examples. In my estimation, the story contained about 30. Even the most reticent students volunteered to provide evidence as to how we know the thief has become a good man. Every child who participated provided a reasonable piece of evidence. The momentum of the group propelled some otherwise reticent students to volunteer.

Summary and Conclusions

Both Heller and colleauges (1982) and NRC (2002) reports on disproportionate representation of minorities in special education highlight the fact that the quality of instruction provided to minority students in general education classrooms is deeply connected to any problems or issues that may lead to disproportionate representation. The erratic quality of instruction provided to many English-language learners has been frequently documented and would seem a pivotal area for major national efforts, and reform of special education for English-language learners with LD is impossible without significant improvements in the quality of instruction provided in general education. This chapter highlighted key issues in instruction for English-language learners and principles suggested to be effective in our own research and our previous review of the research base.

We stress that English-language development has been sorely neglected and provide examples and principles for how to merge English-language development with reading and language arts instruction to provide the beginnings of knowledge base for effective teaching of English-language learners in a second language and simultaneous growth in both oral and written English-language proficiency. We also note instructional factors that appear to explain, in part, growth in reading fluency and comprehension during first grade, arguably the most critical year for reading instruction.

An emerging body of research suggests that the use of approaches such as "sheltered English," whereby the linguistic demands placed on students are aligned with their knowledge of English, can lead to students' learning of complex, age-appropriate content, as well as English-language development. We have proposed that particularly effective teachers carefully modulate their use of English depending on their teaching goals. They decrease cognitive demands when English-language development is the primary goal and increase cognitive demands when content acquisition is the goal.

Increasingly, researchers argue that we need to think of components of instruction that lead to improved learning outcomes as opposed to broad instructional labels that, at best, crudely describe complex instructional interventions (August & Hakuta, 1997). We have attempted to highlight some of the principles of best practice that have begun to emerge. However, the empirical knowledge base remains slender on this critical topic.

Acknowledgments

Sections of this chapter are adapted from Gersten and Baker (2000a, 2000c).

References

Anderson, L., Evertson, C., & Brophy, J. (1979). An experimental study of effective teaching in first-grade reading groups. *Elementary School Journal, 79,* 193–223.

Anderson, V., & Roit, M. (1998). Reading as a gateway to language proficiency for language-minority students in the elementary grades. In R. M. Gersten & R. T. Jiménez (Eds.), *Promoting learning for culturally and linguistically diverse students: Classroom applications from contemporary research* (pp. 42–54). Belmont, CA: Wadsworth.

Arreaga-Mayer, C. (1998). Language sensitive peer mediated instruction for culturally and linguistically diverse learners in the intermediate elementary grades. In R. Gersten & R. Jiménez (Eds.),

Promoting learning for culturally and linguistically diverse students: Classroom applications from contemporary research (pp. 73–90). Belmont, CA: Wadsworth.

August, D., & Hakuta, K. (1997). *Improving schooling for language-minority children.* Washington, DC: National Academy Press.

California Reading and Literature Project. (1999). *Reading professional development institute focusing on results, K–3.* San Diego: California Reading and Literature Project.

Cummins, J. (1980). The cross-lingual dimensions of language proficiency: Implications for bilingual education and the optimal age issue. *TESOL Quarterly, 14*(2), 175–187.

Echevarria, J. (1995). Interactive reading instruction: A comparison of proximal and distal effects of Instructional Conversations. *Exceptional Children, 61,* 536–552.

Echevarria, J., Vogt, M., & Short, D. J. (2000). *Making content comprehensible for English-language learners: The SIOP model.* Boston: Allyn & Bacon.

Fashola, O. S., Drum, P. A., Mayer, R. E., & Kang, S. (1996). A cognitive theory of orthographic transitions: Predictable errors in how Spanish-speaking children spell English words. *American Educational Research Journal, 33*(4), 825–844.

Foorman, B. R., Francis, D. J., Fletcher, J. M., & Lynn, A. (1996). Relation of phonological and orthographic processing to early reading: Comparing two approaches to regression-based, reading-level-match designs. *Journal of Educational Psychology, 88,* 639–652.

Fuchs, L. (1986). Monitoring progress among mildly handicapped pupils: Review of current practice and research. *Remedial and Special Education, 7*(5), 5–12.

Fuchs, L. S., & Fuchs, D. (1998). Treatment validity: A unifying concept for reconceptualizing the identification of learning disabilities. *Learning Disabilities Research and Practice, 13,* 204–219.

Gersten, R. (1996a). The double demands of teaching English language learners. *Educational Leadership, 53*(5), 18–22.

Gersten, R. (1996b). Literacy instruction for language-minority students: The transition years. *Elementary School Journal, 96*(3), 227–244.

Gersten, R. (1999). Lost opportunities: Challenges confronting four teachers of English-language learners. *Elementary School Journal, 100*(1), 37–56.

Gersten, R., & Baker, S. (2000a). *Practices for English-language learners.* Topical Summary for the National Institute for Urban School Improvement.

Gersten, R., & Baker, S. (2000b). The professional knowledge base on instructional interventions that support cognitive growth for English-language learners. In R. Gersten, E. Schiller, & S. Vaughan, *Contemporary special education research: Syntheses of the knowledge base on critical instructional issues* (pp. 31–79). Mahwah, NJ: Erlbaum.

Gersten, R., & Baker, S. (2000c). What we know about effective instructional practices for English-language learners. *Exceptional Children, 66,* 454–470.

Gersten, R., Baker, S. K., Pugach, M., Scanlon, D., & Chard, D. (2001). Contemporary research on special education teaching. In V. Richardson (Ed.), *Handbook for research on teaching* (4th ed., pp. 695–722). Washington, DC: American Educational Research Association.

Gersten, R., & Jiménez, R. (1994). A delicate balance: Enhancing literacy instruction for students of English as a second language. *The Reading Teacher, 47*(6), 438–449.

Gersten, R., & Woodward, J. (1994). The language minority student and special education: Issues, themes and paradoxes. *Exceptional Children, 60*(4), 310–322.

Harry, B. (1992). *Cultural diversity, families, and the special education system: Communication and empowerment.* New York: Teachers College Press.

Heller, K. A., Holtzman, W. H., & Messick, S. (1982). *Placing children in special education: A strategy for equity.* Washington, DC: National Academy Press.

Ikeda, M. J., Grimes, J., Tilly, W. D., Allison, R., Kurns, S., & Stumme, J. (2002). Implementing an intervention-based approach to service delivery: A case example. In M. R. Shinn, H. M. Walker, & G. Stoner (Eds.), *Interventions for academic and behavior problems II: Preventive and remedial approaches* (pp. 53–70). Bethesda, MD: National Academy of Sciences Publications.

Jiménez, R., & Gersten, R. (1999). Lessons and dilemmas derived from the literacy instruction of two Latina/o teachers. *American Education Research Journal, 36*(2), 265–301.

Jiménez, R. T., Moll, L. C., Rodríguez-Brown, F. V., & Barrera, R. B. (1999). Latina and Latino researchers interact on issues related to literacy learning. *Reading Research Quarterly, 34*(2), 217–230.

Kaminski, R. A., & Good, R. H. (1996). Toward a technology for assessing basic early literacy skills. *School Psychology Review, 25,* 215–227.

Klingner, J. K., & Vaughn, S. (1996). Reciprocal teaching of reading comprehension strategies for students with learning disabilities who use English as a second language. *Elementary School Journal, 96,* 275–293.

Klingner, J. K., & Vaughn, S. (2000). The helping behaviors of fifth graders while using collaborative strategic reading during ESL content classes. *TESOL Quarterly, 34*(1), 69–98.

Leinhardt, G., Zigmond, N., & Cooley, W. (1981). Reading instruction and its effects. *American Educational Research Journal, 18,* 343–361.

Lyon, G. R. (1994). *Frames of reference for the assessment of learning disabilities: New views on measurement issues.* Baltimore: Brookes.

Lyon, G. R., Fletcher, J. M., Shaywitz, S. E., Shaywitz, B. A., Torgesen, J. K., Wood, F. B., Schulte, A., & Olson, R. (2001). Rethinking learning disabilities. In C. E. Finn, A. J. Rotherham, & C. R. Hokanson (Eds.), *Rethinking special education for a new century* (pp. 259–288). Washington, DC: Thomas B. Fordham Foundation and the Progressive Policy Institute.

Marston, D. (1989). Curriculum-based measurement: What is it and why do it? In M. R. Shinn (Ed.), *Curriculum-based measurement: Assessing special children* (pp. 18–78). New York: Guilford Press.

Mercer, J. R. (1970). Sociological perspectives on mild mental retardation. In H. C. Haywood (Ed.), *Social-cultural aspects of mental retardation.* New York: Appleton-Century-Crofts.

Messick, S. (1980). Test validity and the ethics of assessment. *American Psychologist, 35,* 1012–1027.

National Reading Panel. (2000). *Report of the National Reading Panel: Teaching children to read: An evidence-based assessment of the scientific research literature on reading and its implications for reading instruction.* Washington, DC: National Institute of Child Health and Human Development.

National Research Council. (2002). *Minority students in special and gifted education* (Committee on Minority Representation in Education, M. S. Donovan & C. T. Cross, Eds.). Washington, DC: National Academy Press.

Reyes, E., & Bos, C. (1998). Interactive semantic mapping and charting: Enhancing content area learning for language minority students. In R. Gersten & R. Jiménez (Eds.), *Promoting learning for culturally and linguistically diverse students: Classroom applications from contemporary research* (pp. 133–152). Belmont, CA: Wadsworth.

Reyes, M. (1992). Challenging venerable assumptions: Literacy instruction for linguistically different students. *Harvard Educational Review, 62*(4), 427–446.

Rousseau, M. K., Tam, B. K. Y., & Ramnarain, R. (1993). Increasing reading proficiency of language-minority students with speech and language impairments. *Education and Treatments of Children, 16,* 254–271.

Saunders, W., O'Brien, G., Lennon, D., & McLean, J. (1998). Making the transition to English literacy successful: Effective strategies for studying literature with transition students. In R. Gersten & R. Jiménez (Eds.), *Promoting learning for culturally and linguistically diverse students: Classroom applications from contemporary research* (pp. 99–132). Belmont, CA: Wadsworth.

Shinn, M. R. (Ed.). (1989). *Curriculum-based measurement: Assessing special children.* New York: Guilford Press.

Snow, C. S., Burns, S. M., & Griffin, P. (1998). *Preventing reading difficulties in young children.* Washington, DC: National Academy Press.

Stallings, J., & Kaskowitz, D. (1974). *Follow-through classroom observation evaluation 1972–1973* (SRI Project URU-7370). Stanford, CA: Stanford Research Institute.

Stanovich, P. J., & Jordan, A. (1998). Canadian teachers' and principals' beliefs about inclusive education as predictors of effective teaching in heterogeneous classrooms. *Elementary School Journal, 98,* 221–238.

Swanson, H. L., & Hoskyn, M. (1998). Experimental intervention research on students with learning disabilities: A meta-analysis of treatment outcomes. *Review of Educational Research, 68,* 277–321.

Tharp, R. G., & Gallimore, R. (1988). *Rousing minds to life.* Cambridge, UK: Cambridge University Press.

Tikunoff, W. J., Ward, B. A., van Broekhuizen, L. D., Romero, M., Castaneda, L. V., Lucas, T., & Katz, A. (1991). *Final report: A descriptive study of significant features of exemplary special alternative instructional programs.* Los Alamitos, CA: The Southwest Regional Educational Laboratory.

Walquis, A. (1998). *Legal declaration* (California case #C-98-2252 CAL).

7

Searching for the Most Effective Service Delivery Model for Students with Learning Disabilities

Naomi Zigmond

Learning disabilities (LD) as an *educational* phenomenon has a rather short history. Whereas public schools have recognized and provided services for students with physical, sensory, and intellectual handicaps since the beginning of the twentieth century, students with LD did not come to the attention of public schools until the 1960s, and large-scale provision of special education services for this population of students dates back only to 1975 and the passage by Congress of Public Law (PL) 94-142, the Education of All Handicapped Children Act.

From the very start, practitioners and school administrators assumed that there was no "one best way" to provide educational services for the LD population. As early as 1970, Kephart was advocating for a full continuum of services. For some students with LD, "the so-called hard-core case[s] whose interferences are so extensive that [they] will probably need major alterations of educational presentations for the length of [their] educational career[s]" (p. 208), Kephart recommended a segregated classroom. But for those with somewhat less severe problems, "whose interference with learning is such that much of the activities of the [general education] classroom become

meaningless . . . [and who] need more intensive assistance than the classroom teacher can be expected to provide" (p. 208), Kephart suggested what would later be known as a resource room model: "a clinical approach in which [the student with LD] is removed from the classroom for a short time, a half-hour or an hour a day. During this short period, individually or in small groups of two or three, intensive attack is made on his learning problems—not upon curriculum matters, but upon the learning problem itself and the methods by which he processes information" (p. 208). The child with minor learning problems, Kephart believed, had much more to gain from interactions with peers in the general education classroom than from intensive activities in a segregated program. This child could be helped by the regular classroom teacher and would be fully included in the mainstream.

In the first edition of Lerner's (1971) classic textbook on LD, she, too, called for a continuum of placements matched to the educational needs of the child with LD: special classes for students with severe problems, itinerant teaching services for children whose learning disability is not severe enough to warrant a special class, and resource rooms for most students with LD at both elementary and secondary school levels. By 1975, Hammill and Bartel were suggesting that special schools and special classes "should be used with considerable caution and viewed as a last resort" (p. 3). They, also, advocated for a resource room model that permitted "the pupil to receive instruction individually or in groups in a special room . . . [in which] the emphasis is on teaching specific skills that the pupil needs. At the end of his lesson, he returns to the regular classroom and continues his education there" (p. 4).

Data in the first annual report to Congress (U.S. Department of Health, Education and Welfare, 1979) confirmed that a continuum of service delivery models for students with LD was, indeed, in place: In the 1976–1977 school year, 81% of the students with LD were based in general education classes and received pullout special education services for less than half of the schoolday, 17% were served primarily in special classes, and 2% were in separate facilities. Twenty-one years later, the 22nd annual report to Congress (U.S. Department of Education, 2000) indicated that across the nation, the distribution of students with LD across service delivery models had shifted only slightly. In the 1997–1998 school year, 83% were based in general education classes, receiving pullout special services for less than half of the schoolday, 16% were served primarily in separate classes, and just under 1% were in separate facilities.

What these relatively stable numbers mask is the heated debate that has raged for at least 20 years and the flurry of research it generated on *which service delivery model is actually best* for serving students with LD in public schools. A similar question had first been asked by Lloyd Dunn in 1968 with reference to special education services for students with mild mental retardation, and response to his article spurred the adoption of resource room services in place of special day classes for these students in the 1970s. The question was raised again with the passage of PL 94–142, the Education of All Handicapped Children Act (1975), and answered ambiguously, with support for a continuum of services on the one hand and a preference for placement in the general education classroom on the other hand.

The question of which service delivery model is best for students with disabilities was hotly debated again in the mid-1980s, as essays on the failure of part-time and pullout special education began to proliferate. For students with LD, the focus of the debate was on the more than 80% of students who were already spending at least some of their time in general education classrooms. And the theme was consistent: Fundamental changes in the delivery model for special education were needed to increase the accomplishments of those students. Biklin and Zollers (1986) asserted that "students do not benefit from this [pull-out] special education" (p. 581). Hagarty and Abramson (1987) concluded that a "split scheduling approach for providing services . . . is neither administratively nor instructionally supportable" (p. 316). And Madeline Will (1986), then Assistant Secretary of Education and head of the Office of Special Education Programs, proclaimed, "Although well intentioned, the so-called 'pull out' approach to the educational difficulties of students with learning problems has failed in many instances to meet the educational needs of these students" (p. 413). Will and others (e.g., Gartner & Lipsky, 1987, 1989; National Association of State Boards of Education, 1992) called for completely integrated educational experiences for children with learning problems to achieve "improved educational outcomes" (Will, 1986, p. 413). Advocates for this new, fully inclusive service delivery model for special education pressed for elimination of all pullout programs in favor of full-time integration in general education classrooms.

In the 1997 reauthorization of the Individuals with Disabilities Education Act, the question of preferred service delivery model was raised again, and this time with a new urgency. With the additional requirement that students with disabilities participate in (and perform respectably on) statewide assessments and accountability procedures, pressures to favor one kind of placement (full inclusion in the general education classroom) over any other (providing some pullout services in some other place) mounted. In the public policy debates that ensued, little attention was paid to research evidence on the efficacy of the various service delivery models. Would a review of that body of work have helped to shape the debate about what is the most effective model and who should get what?

This chapter looks at research studies and research reviews that focus on the relative effectiveness of service delivery models for students with LD and other mild/moderate disabilities. In these studies, the students are generally school-identified using state and local guidelines. I argue, as many others have before me, that research evidence on the relative efficacy of one special education placement over another is scarce, methodologically flawed, and inconclusive, in large part because studies of the educational outcomes of students with disabilities in one place or another can rarely conform to the rigorous standards of experimental research. But I also argue that, in practical terms, "Which service delivery model is most effective?" is the wrong question to ask. This question assumes that each service delivery model (special class, resource room, itinerant, full inclusion) represents a clearly specified treatment and that each is implemented with fidelity. In other words, when a researcher says a group of children were getting "full inclusion" or "resource room" services, he or she and the readers know what educational experiences the students were receiving. This is simply not the case. I suggest that if the goal of research on service delivery models is to improve outcomes for students with LD, there are more important questions to ask, and a search for these more important questions should prompt a move away from outcomes-based experimental designs toward new ways of thinking about research on service delivery models and the educational processes they support.

Outcomes-Based Efficacy Studies of Service Delivery Models in Special Education

For more than three decades, special education researchers and scholars have researched, and synthesized research on, the relative usefulness of one place or another for serving students with disabilities. Dunn (1968) focused his review of the efficacy of special education placements on research conducted with students with mental retar-

dation or emotional handicaps, and on the usefulness of special class placements over placement in the regular class. He concluded, on the basis of a half dozen studies conducted in the 1960s, and a review of research published by Kirk in 1964, that there was no empirical support for educating students with mild disabilities in special classes. "Retarded pupils make as much or more progress in the regular grades as they do in special education [and] efficacy studies on special day classes for other mildly handicapped children, including the emotionally handicapped, reveal the same results" (Dunn, 1968, p. 8). Though Dunn called for the abandonment of special day classes for students with mild disabilities, he argued persuasively for part-time pullout special education services to meet their specialized educational needs.

Ten years later, Sindelar and Deno (1978) reported research results that supported that position. In a narrative review of 17 studies, Sindelar and Deno concluded that resource rooms were more effective than regular classrooms in improving academic achievement of students with LD. At about the same time, a meta-analysis of efficacy studies completed by Carlberg and Kavale (1980) reported more complex results. Carlberg and Kavale's calculations of effect sizes showed that students with mental retardation in special class placements performed as well, academically, as those placed in regular grades. But they also showed a modest academic advantage for students with learning or behavior disorders in special classes (both self-contained and resource programs) over those remaining in the regular class. Leinhardt and Palley (1982) also concluded from their research review that resource rooms were better than regular placements for students with LD. And 1 year later, Madden and Slavin (1983) reviewed seven studies on the efficacy of part-time resource placements compared to full-time special education classes and full-time placement in the mainstream and concluded that if increased academic achievement is the desired outcome, "the research favors placement in regular classes . . . *supplemented by well designed resource programs*" (italics added; p. 530).

Research support for supplemental resource room services was, however, overlooked in the national frenzy to reshape special education that swept the country in the mid-1980s. With the introduction of newer, *full-inclusion* service delivery models, particularly full-inclusion models for students with mild/moderate disabilities that used special education teachers in consulting or co-teaching roles, the early research comparing special pullout placements with regular class placements seemed dated and irrelevant. In those earlier studies, it was easy to draw stark contrasts between regular class placements where no special services were available to students with disabilities and pullout services staffed by trained teachers who provided special instruction. In the newer, more inclusive service delivery models, students with disabilities were supposed to be receiving specially designed instruction or supplemental aids and services right in the general education classroom without having to be pulled out. Research documenting student progress in these new full-inclusion models was needed, and it proliferated.

Some studies seemed to show positive trends when students were integrated into general education classrooms (see Affleck, Madge, Adams, & Lowenbraun, 1988; Baker, Wang, & Walberg, 1995; Deno, Maruyama, Espin, & Cohen, 1990; Schulte, Osborne, & McKinney, 1990; Walther-Thomas, 1997; Wang & Baker, 1985–1986). Some researchers found that full-time placement in a general education classroom resulted in student academic progress that was *just as good as* that achieved by students in separate settings in elementary schools (see Banerji & Dailey, 1995; Bear & Proctor, 1990). But others reported disappointing or unsatisfactory academic and social achievement gains from inclusion models (see Fox & Ysseldyke, 1997; Saint-Laurent et al., 1998; Sale & Carey, 1995; Vaughn, Elbaum, & Boardman, 2001; Zigmond & Baker, 1990; Zigmond et al., 1995). It should come as no surprise, then, that in a review of research on these newer special education service delivery models, Hocutt (1996) reported equivocal findings: "Various program models, implemented in both general and special education, can have moderately positive academic and social impacts for student with disabilities" (p. 77). She concluded that no model is effective for all students.

Manset and Semmel (1997) compared eight inclusion models for elementary students with mild disabilities, primarily LD, as reported in the research literature between 1984 and 1994. They reiterated Hocutt's conclusions: Inclusive programs can be effective for some, although not all, students with mild disabilities. Waldren and McKleskey (1998) appeared to agree. In their research, students with severe LD made comparable progress in reading and math in pullout and inclusion settings, although students with mild LD were more likely to make gains commensurate with those of peers without disabilities educated in inclusive environments versus receiving special education services in a resource room.

Holloway (2001) reviewed five studies conducted between 1986 and 1996 comparing traditional pullout services to fully inclusive service delivery models and models that combined in-class services with pullout instruction. Though his findings are limited to students with mild LD and to the outcome of reading, his conclusions did not give strong support for the practice of full inclusion. Reading progress in the combined model was significantly better than in either the inclusion-only model or the resource room-only model.

In recent research, Rea, Mclaughlin, and Walther-Thomas (2002) used qualitative and quantitative methods to describe two schools and their special education models: one that was fully inclusive and one with more traditional supplemental pullout services. They showed that students served in inclusive schools earned higher grades, achieved higher or comparable scores on standardized tests, committed no more behavioral infractions, and attended more schooldays than did students in the more traditional schools with pullout programs.

In a specific review of co-teaching as the inclusive service delivery model, Zigmond and Magiera (2002b) found only four studies that focused on academic achievement gains, three at the elementary level and one at the high school level. In the three elementary studies, co-teaching was just as effective in producing academic gains as resource room instruction or consultation with the general education teacher. In the high school study, students' quiz and exam grades actually worsened following the co-teaching experiment.

Murawski and Swanson (2002) in their meta-analysis of co-teaching research literature found six studies from which effect sizes could be calculated; dependent measures included grades, achievement scores, and social and attitudinal outcomes. Murawski and Swanson reported effect sizes for individual studies ranging from low to high with an average total effect size in the moderate range. Both literature reviews on co-teaching concluded that despite the current and growing popularity of co-teaching as a service delivery model, further research is needed to determine whether it is an effective service delivery option for students with disabilities, let alone a preferred one.

Limitations of Outcomes-Based Experimental Research

The more than three decades of efficacy research reviewed here provide no simple and straightforward answer to the question of which service delivery model is best for students with LD. Despite the fact that dozens and dozens of studies have been reported in refereed special education journals, Murawski and Swanson (2002) were right to ask, "Where are the data?" (p. 258). Studies worthy of consideration in a meta-analysis or narrative literature review, with appropriate controls and appropriate dependent measures, are few and far between. Of course, research on the efficacy of special education models is hard to conduct, let alone to conduct well. For example, definitions of service delivery models or settings vary from researcher to researcher, and descriptions of the treatments being implemented in those models or settings are woefully inadequate. Random assignment of students to treatments is seldom an option, and appropriately matched (sufficiently alike) samples of experimental and control students and teachers are rare. As a result, "place" or "service delivery model" are not phenomena that lend themselves to precise investigation.

Research designs used to explore the effectiveness of different service delivery models often employ pre–posttreatment group designs. The limitations of these research designs for studying the efficacy of special education have been reported in numerous research reviews, as far back as Kirk (1964) and Semmel, Gottlieb, and Robinson (1979). The criticisms are always the same. Some studies use control groups, often samples from among students experiencing "traditional" programs (sometimes referred to as business as usual) in nonexperimental schools. Most researchers use intact groups of students assigned to the teacher or the school building that volunteered to participate in the experimental treatment program, not random assignment of students to treatments. Often the experimental treatment is well described, although the degree of implementation is not. Descriptions of the control treatment and its degree of implementation (if indeed a control group is used) are rarely provided. Most often, neither treatment is described sufficiently, nor its implementation monitored sufficiently, to make replication possible. Thus, even if one study demonstrates reliable achievement changes, difficulty in identifying treatment variables makes replication impossible in virtually all cases. Achievement gains, or lack thereof, often cannot be related to replicable interventions and the fundamental question of whether *Model A* is better than *Model B* cannot actually be answered.

The accumulated experimental evidence to date produces only one unequivocal finding: Languishing in a regular education class where nothing changes and no one pays any attention to an individual is not as useful to students with learning and behavior disorders as getting some help (though it does not seem to matter for students with mild mental retardation). All other evidence on whether students with disabilities learn more, academically or socially, and are happier in one service delivery model or another is at best inconclusive. Resource programs are more effective for some students with disabilities than self-contained special education classes or self-contained general education classes, but they are less effective for other students with similar disabilities. Fully inclusive programs are superior for some students with disabilities on some measures of academic or social skill development and inferior for other students on other measures. The empirical research does not identify one most effective model; it also often finds equivalent progress being made by students with LD across models (i.e., the research reports nonsignificant differences in outcomes). Interpreting nonsignificant findings can be tricky. Do we conclude that the proverbial cup is half full or half empty? Do we acknowledge that it does not matter where students receive their special education services and allow parents or school personnel wide berth in making choices? Or, do we proclaim that one model is preferred over another for philosophical, social, or moral reasons, because the research shows that this model "doesn't hurt"?

Asking a Different Set of Questions

In trying to understand the relative usefulness of service delivery models of special education, the question "Which is more effective?" may be too simplistic and naïve. Not only is research to answer that question hard to do well, but the answer in the end is unsatisfying because it does not help explain *why* one model seems better than another or *how* to make the less effective model more effective. An alternative approach to the controlled experiment began to take shape for me out of a fortuitous introduction to William Cooley, Gaea Leinhardt, and the concept of explanatory observational studies (Cooley, 1978). By the late 1970s and early 1980s, classroom-based educational research had clearly established that *what students learn* from their classroom experiences is a function of *what they do* during class time (see Fisher & Berliner, 1979; Stallings, 1979). Research on classroom activities that contribute to student growth had begun to converge. However, there was still a need for more careful descriptions of student classroom experiences that significantly influenced the development of reading skills. Cooley, Leinhardt, and I set out on a study of reading instruction in self-contained classrooms for students with LD to explore the relative effectiveness of various classroom instructional practices for improving achievement. Two basic assumptions about effective reading instruction guided our data collection and analysis activities. First, we assumed that what students learn is a function of what they do in class, and that features of the curriculum and teacher behavior influence directly what students do and only

indirectly what they learn. Second, we did not define reading instruction as simply everything that went on during allocated reading time. Instead, we assumed that classroom activities fell into three broad categories: those *directly* related to reading (e.g., they involved students responding to print); those that *indirectly* supported some aspect of reading but were not reading (e.g., listening to the teacher or talking about a story); and those that were so tangential to the acquisition of reading as to be *nonreading* (working on mathematics skills, drawing, cutting, or pasting). We imposed this view of classroom instruction and reading behaviors on our observational system.

We designed a study that would provide accurate descriptive information on reading instruction in self-contained classrooms, and that would also permit exploration of the plausibility of specific causal relationships among specific process and outcome variables (see Figure 7.1). We assumed that how teachers structured the learning environment would make a difference in how students spent their time, and how students spent their time would influence the level of reading proficiency they attained at the end of the academic year. Figure 7.1 displays the causal model of how the variables were assumed to be influencing each other in the classroom. Solid black lines indicate significant relationships in which we assumed a causal directionality but in which both variables were measured at approximately the same time. Dotted lines indicate relationships that we predicted would be significant but were not. The main point of Figure 7.1 is to show that posttest was assumed to be dependent on student behaviors and instructional content; student behaviors were assumed to be influenced by prior test performance and teacher behaviors.

We spent more than 2 years studying 11 self-contained LD classrooms and more than 100 students with LD and their teachers. The data confirmed our expectations. What went on in classrooms and how each student experienced and responded to the instructional environment made a difference in terms of achievement growth. Students in these self-contained classrooms spent, on average, only 26 minutes of a 362-minute school day engaged in oral or silent reading; on average, they also made only a little progress in read-

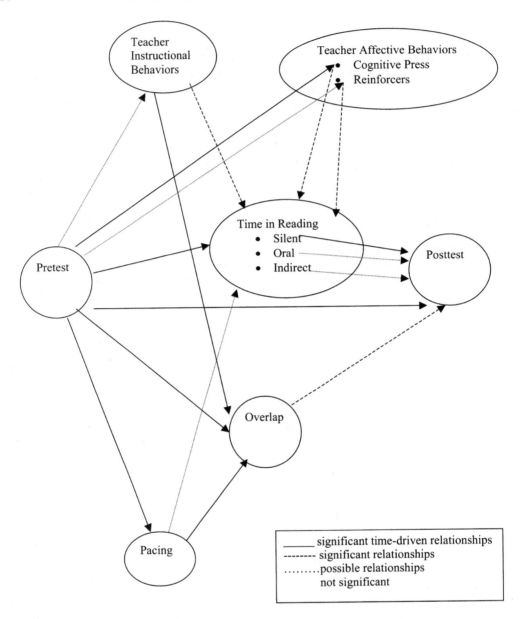

FIGURE 7.1. A model for explaining reading achievement. From Leinhardt, Zigmond, and Cooley (1981, p. 352). Copyright 1981 by the American Educational Research Association. Adapted by permission.

ing achievement. However, time spent on task by individual students with LD in direct and indirect reading activities was highly predictive of reading growth.

Looking "inside the Black Box"

This explanatory observational study convinced me that looking "inside the black box" at how students were spending their time and at what instructional and learning opportunities were being provided for them could not only help answer the questions of *why* one service delivery model might be better than another, but also *how* either could be improved. This conviction was strengthened in "The Case of Randy" (Zigmond & Baker, 1994). This article described the reading progress (or lack thereof) of one student with LD during a year in which special education services were provided in a part-time self-contained classroom, and 1 year later when they were provided in a fully inclusive, general education fifth-grade classroom. The data showed no significant differences in reading growth in the two service delivery models. The observational data helped to explain why.

> In the mainstream, Randy was "stretched." He was taught out of level, from a fifth grade book, when he was barely fluent in first grade level text. He was kept engaged on relevant tasks. His learning to read was directed and monitored by one of his two teachers almost all the time. The proportion of his allocated reading instruction time that he used to spend on independent seatwork he now spent in a whole group reading lesson, mostly listening or passively engaged. Though he was allocated less time for reading instruction in the mainstream, that time was spent more efficiently each day—with considerably less of Randy's reading time spent off task. But Randy also spent less time talking (about things reading-related) and writing than he had in the resource room. And despite all these differences in time allocation and time distribution, *minutes per week of time-on-task in oral and silent reading was virtually the same in the mainstream as the year before in the pull-out special education program.* (italics added; (Zigmond & Baker, 1994, pp. 115–116)

As we had previously established that students learn what they spend time doing (Leinhardt, Zigmond, & Cooley, 1981), and Randy had not spent any more time doing reading in one setting than in the other, his lack of differential reading progress was explainable. The observation data confirmed that it was not the setting but the teaching and learning opportunities made possible in the setting that would account for reading growth.

The observation data, or the look inside the service delivery model, however, revealed something more serious. In the mainstream fifth-grade class, Randy was not receiving a *special* education. He was not receiving individually tailored, remedial instruction on specific reading skills in which he was deficient. His fifth-grade education was no more special or uniquely suited to him than to anyone else in the class. This prompted us to shift our focus from the study of which service delivery model is more effective to what we came to think of as a more important question, "What kinds of instructional and learning opportunities are (or can be) made available to students with LD in different educational settings?" Sometimes using quantitative observation protocols and sometimes using qualitative ones, colleagues and I embarked on a series of studies to understand how general education classrooms worked, and the extent to which they were (or might be) appropriate venues for educating students with LD.

The first study was carried out in one urban elementary school (Baker & Zigmond, 1990). The students with LD in this school were school identified using state and district guidelines. Data on classroom ecologies were collected through informal and formal observations of reading, math, and special subject classes and interviews of school personnel. Across the entire school, our analyses revealed no evidence of differentiated instruction and no structures in the general education classrooms that could support it (Baker & Zigmond, 1990). Most classes operated with only one adult, the teacher. The primary mode of instruction in all classrooms was the single lesson taught to the whole group, or the same seatwork activity assigned to the whole class. The teachers in this school had uniform expectations for all students, and that mind-set was evident in the ways they organized and managed instruction. Teachers valued quiet and order. Instructional programs were routine. In fact, teachers seemed more committed to routine than to addressing individual differences, and they were more responsive to district mandates than to evidence from their students that the curriculum or pacing needed to be adapted. If this was what a student with LD in a fully inclusive service delivery model of special education could expect, we predicted that the model would not be efficacious (Baker & Zigmond, 1990).

Our experience in that urban elementary school was not unique. Again and again, we collected both qualitative and quantitative data to characterize general education classroom instruction. Again and again, we studied what *is* going on in general education classrooms, not what *could be* going on or what *should be* going on. And, again and again, we discovered how functional the current organization of classrooms was for the sets of learners that populated them, and how resourceful general education teachers could be in accommodating diversity without changing the basic organization and structure of their classroom. But we also noticed that whether left alone, or bombarded with intensive in-service training, general education teachers were more committed to accommodation than to learning, and more likely to emphasize order and quiet than individual differences and student needs.

We used these observations to counter the prevailing view that general education classrooms could be transformed into appropriate settings for the delivery of special education services to students with LD. We argued that, historically, students with LD assigned full time to a general education classroom were assumed to be capable of coping, on their own, with the ongoing mainstream curriculum. General education classrooms were not places where "special stuff" was (or could be) going on. Of course, despite our arguments, public policy and the social climate demanded a change toward a service delivery model for students with LD that eliminated virtually all pullout services. Now, students who had been diagnosed, and for whom an individualized education plan (IEP) had been written, were to be retained in the general education class full time, and special education resources were to be "pulled in," instead of the students being "pulled out." There were many variations on this theme (see Jenkins, Jewell, Leicester, Jenkins, & Troutner, 1990; Reynaud, Pfannenstiel, & Hudson, 1987; Stevens, Madden, Slavin, & Farnish, 1987; Wang, 1987; Zigmond & Baker, 1990), but in each of them, students who would otherwise have attended special education classrooms full or part time were returned full time to general education classes. Several authors (e.g., Lewis & Doorlag, 1991) described two components of instruction for mainstreamed students with LD. "In the **remediation** approach, the teacher instructs the student in skills that are areas of need. . . . Extra assistance might be provided to a fourth grader who spells at the second grade level. **Compensation**, on the other hand, attempts to bypass the student's weaknesses. For instance, to compensate for the reading and writing problems . . . the teacher might administer class tests orally" (Lewis & Doorlag, 1991, p. 240).

Wang (1989) described these same two components (but in the reverse order) as the *adaptive instruction* that should be available to students in full inclusion models.

Modifi[cation of] the learning environment to accommodate the unique learning characteristics and needs of individual students, and [provision of] direct or focused intervention to improve each student's capabilities to successfully acquire subject-matter knowledge and higher-order reasoning and problem-solving skills, to work independently and cooperatively with peers, and to meet the overall intellectual and social demands of schooling. (p. 183)

We believed it reasonable to investigate whether these practices were actually being implemented. My colleagues and I set out to explore, once more, the educational opportunities being provided for students with LD in full-inclusion models judged to be successful by teachers, administrators, parents, and professional colleagues—if students with LD were, in fact, experiencing *both* compensation (adapted learning environments) *and* remediation (direct or focused instruction in skills and strategies that would enable them to cope with the mainstream curriculum). If only compensation (adapted learning environments) was in place, students might be "managing the mainstream" but not learning fundamental skills and strategies that would allow them to become independent, self-directed learners. If only remediation (direct or focused instruction in skills and strategies that would enable them to cope with the mainstream curriculum) were going on, students might be spending a considerable portion of each day in failure experiences.

We studied five elementary school buildings that had, for several years, implemented fully inclusive service delivery models for students with LD. Observation and interview data in these buildings were searched for evidence of those two kinds of services for students with LD: (1) adaptations or accommodations that were designed to make the extant curriculum and instruction manageable for the student with LD by "bypassing" his or her deficits; and (2) focused, remedial instruction that would increase the capacity of the student with LD to cope with curriculum and materials, however they were presented. We found a lot of the former and, disappointingly, little of the latter.

> Conspicuously absent, as we watched special education teachers and general education teachers teach students with LD ... were activities focused on assessing individual students or monitoring progress through the curriculum. Concern for the individual was replaced by concern for a group—the smooth functioning of the mainstream class, the progress of the reading group, the organization and management of cooperative learning groups or peer tutoring. No one seemed concerned about individual achievement, individual progress, or individual learning. (Baker & Zigmond, 1995, p. 171)

The works just cited are but a few examples of research on service delivery models that have searched "inside the black box," and on the basis of our own studies, and those of many others (see Carr, 1995; Guetzloe, 1999; Harrington, 1997; Kauffman & Pullen, 1996; Klingner, Vaughn, Hughes, & Argulles, 1999; Shinn, Powell-Smith, & Good, 1996; Vaughn & Klingner, 1998) we have come to a conclusion that is not at all profound: Different settings offer different opportunities for teaching and learning. The general education classroom allows for access to students who do not have disabilities, access to curricula and textbooks to which most other students are exposed, access to instruction from a general education teacher whose training and expertise are quite different from those of a special education teacher, access to subject matter content taught by a subject matter specialist, and access to all the stresses and strains associated with the preparation for, taking of, and passing or failing of statewide assessments. If the goal is to have students learn content subject information, or learn how to interact with peers without disabilities, the general education setting is the place to do that.

Pullout settings allow for smaller teacher–student ratios and flexibility in the selection of texts, curricular objectives, and pacing of instruction; in the scheduling of examina-

tions; and in the assignment of grades. Special education pullout settings allow students to be learning different "stuff" in different ways and on a different schedule. If students need intensive instruction in basic academic skills well beyond the grade level at which peers without disabilities are learning how to read or do basic mathematics, if students need explicit instruction in controlling behavior or interacting with peers and adults, or if students need to learn anything that is not customarily taught to everyone else, a pullout special education setting may be more appropriate.

We continue to ask the more important question, "What kinds of instructional and learning opportunities are (or can be) made available to students with LD in different service delivery models?" in current ongoing research on co-teaching (e.g., Zigmond & Magiera, 2002a). In a co-teaching model, students with LD and their teacher are integrated into the general education classroom, and the two teachers share instructional responsibilities. But we have discovered that even that question does not dig deeply enough. Our search for "most effective" has failed to specify "most effective for whom?"

Looking at Individual Students

Special education has evolved as a means of providing specialized interventions to students with disabilities based on individual student progress on individualized objectives. The bedrock of special education is instruction focused on individual need. The very concept of "one best model" contradicts this commitment to individualization. Furthermore, results of research on how groups of students respond to treatment settings does not help the researcher or practitioner make an individualized decision for an individual student's plan. A better question to ask, if we dare, is, "For what kind of student with LD is one service delivery model more opportune than another?" That is, for which individual students with which individual profiles of characteristics and needs are the right opportunities likely to be provided through one service delivery model or another? We think that an answer to this much more complicated question would require new research designs and data analyses.

A first step in that direction might be to reanalyze group design data at the individual student level. For example, we collected achievement test data for 145 students with disabilities in three full inclusion programs as well as for many of their classmates without disabilities (Zigmond et al., 1995). Rather than reporting average growth of the students with LD, my colleagues and I reported the number and percentage of students with LD who made reliably significant gains (their gains exceeded the standard error of measurement of the reading test) during the experimental year. We also reported on the number and percentage of students with LD whose reading gains matched or exceeded the average gain of their grade level peers. And, finally, we reported on the number and percentage of students with LD whose achievement status (i.e., their relative standing in the grade-level peer group) had improved during the school year. These analytic techniques allowed for the exploration of setting effects individual by individual. Waldron and McLeskey (1998) followed this same tactic in their 1998 study. This approach seems more promising in terms of answering the question "most effective for whom?" than more traditional approaches used to date.

Final Comments

As early as 1979, federal monitoring of state programs was put into place not only to guard against too much segregation of students with disabilities but also to guard against "inappropriate mainstreaming" (U.S. Department of Health, Education and Welfare, 1979, p. 39). Although most would agree that students with mild disabilities should spend a large proportion of the schoolday with peers without disabilities, research does not support the superiority of any one service delivery model over another. Furthermore, effectiveness depends not only on the characteristics and needs of a particular student but also on the quality of the program's implementation. A poorly run model with limited resources will seldom be superior to a model in which there is a heavy investment of time, energy, and money. Good programs can be developed using any model; so can bad ones. Service delivery

model is less important than what is going on in the implementation of the program.

Thus, reflecting on the past 35 years of efficacy research, what do we know? We know that what goes on in a place is what makes the difference, not the location itself. We know that we learn what we spend time working on, and that students with disabilities will not learn to read or to write or to calculate if they do not spend more than the usual amount of time engaged in those tasks. We know that students with LD need explicit and intensive instruction. We know that some instructional practices are easier to implement and more likely to occur in some settings than in others. We know that we need more research that asks better and more focused questions about who learns what best where. And, we know that we need to explore new research designs and new data analysis techniques that will help us bridge the gap between efficacy findings and decision making on placements for individual students.

In response to the query, What is *special* about special education? We can say with some certainty that the model is not what makes special education "special" or effective. Effective teaching strategies and an individualized approach are the more critical ingredients in a special education, and neither of these are associated solely with one particular model of service delivery. That said, we must also remember that typical general education environments have been shown in research not to be supportive places in which to implement what we know to be effective teaching strategies for students with disabilities. Based on research evidence to date, placement decisions must continue to be made by determining whether a particular placement option will support those effective instructional practices that are required for a particular child to achieve his or her individual objectives and goals.

The search for the most effective model for delivery of special education services is a legitimate one, but it has tended to be fueled by passion and principle rather than by reason and rationality. Until we are ready to say that receiving special education services in a particular setting is good for some students with disabilities but not for others; that different educational environments are more conducive to different forms of teaching and learning; that different students need to learn different things in different ways; and that traditional group research designs may not capture these individual differences in useful ways, we may never get beyond the equivocal findings reported to date. We may even fail to realize that, in terms of the most effective of special education service delivery, we have probably been asking the wrong questions.

References

Affleck, J., Madge, S., Adams, A., & Lowenbraun, S. (1988). Integrated classroom versus resource model: Academic viability and effectiveness. *Exceptional Children, 54,* 339–348.

Baker, E. T., Wang, M., & Walberg, H. J. (1995, December/January). The effects of inclusion on learning. *Educational Leadership,* pp. 33–35.

Baker, J., & Zigmond, N. (1990). Snapshots of an elementary school: Are regular education classes equipped to accommodate learning disabled students? *Exceptional Children, 56*(6), 515–527.

Baker, J., & Zigmond, N. (1995). The meaning and practice of inclusion for students with learning disabilities: Themes and implications from the five cases. *Journal of Special Education, 29*(2), 163–180.

Banjerji, M., & Dailey, R. (1995). A study of the effects of an inclusion model on students with specific learning disabilities, *Journal of Learning Disabilities, 28,* 511–522.

Bear, G. G., & Proctor, W. A. (1990). Impact of a full-time integrated program on the achievement of non-handicapped and mildly handicapped children, *Journal of Exceptionality, 1,* 227–238

Biklin, D., & Zollers, N. (1986). The focus of advocacy in the LD field. *Journal of Learning Disabilities, 19,* 579–586

Carlberg, C., & Kavale, K. (1980). The efficacy of special versus regular class placement for exceptional children: A meta-analysis. *Journal of Special Education, 14,* 295–309.

Carr, M. (1995) A response to the responders. *Journal of Learning Disabilities, 28*(3) 136–138.

Cooley, W. W. (1978) Explanatory observational studies. *Educational Researcher, 7*(9), 9–15

Deno, S., Maruyama, G., Espin, C., & Cohen, C. (1990). Educating students with mild disabilities in general education classrooms: Minnesota alternatives, *Exceptional Children, 57,* 150–161.

Dunn, L. M. (1968). Special education for the mildly retarded—Is much of it justifiable? *Exceptional Children, 35,* 5–22.

Education of All Handicapped Children Act. (1975). Public Law 94-142, § 612 (5)(B).

Fisher, C. W., & Berliner, D. C. (1979). Clinical inquiry in research on classroom teaching and learning, *Journal of Teacher Education, 30*(6), 42–48.

Fox, N. E., & Ysseldyke, J. E. (1997). Implementing inclusion at the middle school level: Lessons from a negative example. *Exceptional Children, 64*(1), 81–98.

Gartner, A., & Lipsky, D. K. (1987). Beyond special education: Toward a quality system for all students. *Harvard Educational Review, 57,* 367–395.

Gartner, A., & Lipsky, D. K. (1989). *The yoke of special education: How to break it.* Washington, DC: National Center on Education and the Economy.

Guetzloe, E. (1999). Inclusion: The broken promise. *Preventing School Failure, 43*(3), 92–98.

Hagarty, G. J., & Abramson, M. (1987). Impediments to implementing national policy change for mildly handicapped students. *Exceptional Children, 53,* 315–323.

Hammill, D. D., & Bartel, N. R. (1975). *Teaching children with learning and behavior problems.* Boston: Allyn & Bacon.

Harrington, S. (1997). Full inclusion for students with learning disabilities. A review of the evidence. *School–Community Journal, 7*(1), 63–71.

Hocutt, A. M. (1996). Effectiveness of special education: Is placement the critical factor? *The Future of Children, 6*(1), 77–102.

Holloway, J. (2001, March). Inclusion and student with learning disabilities. *Educational Leadership,* pp. 86–88.

Individuals with Disabilities Education Act. (1997). Public Law 107-05, 20 U. S. C. §§ 1400 et seq.

Jenkins, J. R., Jewell, M., Leicester, N., Jenkins, L., & Troutner, N. (1990, April). *Development of a school building model for educating handicapped and at-risk students in general education classrooms.* Paper presented at the annual meeting of the American Educational Research Association, Boston.

Kauffman, J., & Pullen, P. (1996). Eight myths about special education. *Focus on Exceptional Children, 28*(5), 1–12.

Kephart, N. C. (1970). Reflection on learning disabilities: Its contribution to education. In J. I. Arena (Ed.), *Meeting total needs of learning disabled children: A forward look* (pp. 206–208). Pittsburgh, PA: Association for Children with Learning Disabilities.

Kirk, S. A. (1964). Research in education. In H. A. Stevens & R. Heber (Eds.), *Mental retardation: A review of* (pp. 57–99). Chicago: University of Chicago Press.

Klingner, J., Vaughn, S., Hughes, M. T., & Argulles, M. (1999). Sustaining research-based practices in reading: A 3-year follow-up. *Remedial and Special Education, 20*(5), 263–274.

Leinhardt, G., & Pallay, A. (1982). Restrictive educational settings? Exile or haven. *Review of Educational Research, 52,* 557–578.

Leinhardt, G., Zigmond, N., & Cooley, W. W. (1981). Reading instruction and its effects. *American Educational Research Journal, 18*(3), 343–361.

Lerner, J. W. (1971). *Children with learning disabil-*

ities: Theories, diagnosis, and teaching strategies. Boston: Houghton Mifflin.

Lewis, R. B., & Doorlag, D. H. (1991). Teaching special students in the mainstream (3rd ed.). New York: Merrill.

Madden, N. A., & Slavin, R. E. (1983). Mainstreaming students with mild handicaps: Academic and social outcomes. Review of Educational Research, 53, 519–569.

Manset, G., & Semmel, M. I. (1997). Are inclusive programs for students with mild disabilities effective? A comparative review of model programs. Journal of Special Education, 31, 155–180.

Murawski, W. W., & Swanson, H. L. (2002). A meta-analysis of co-teaching research: Where are the data? Remedial and Special Education, 22(5), 258–267

National Association of State Boards of Education. (1992). Winners all: A call for inclusive schools. Alexandria, VA: Author.

Rea, P. J., McLaughlin, V. L., & Walther-Thomas, C. (2002). Outcomes for students with learning disabilities in inclusive and pull-out programs, Exceptional Children, 68, 203–222

Reynaud, G., Pfannenstiel, T., & Hudson, F. (1987). Park Hill secondary learning disability program: An alternative service delivery model. Implementation manual. Kansas City: Missouri State Department of Elementary and Secondary Education. (ERIC Document Reproduction Services No. ED 28931)

Saint-Laurent, L., Dionne, J., Glasson, J., Royer, E., Simard, C., & Pierard, B. (1998). Academic achievement effects of an in-class service model on students with and without disabilities. Exceptional Children, 64, 239–253.

Sale, P., & Carey, D. M. (1995). The sociometric status of students with disabilities in a full-inclusion school. Exceptional Children, 62, 6–19.

Schulte, A. C., Osborne, S. S., & McKinney, J. D. (1990). Academic outcomes for students with learning disabilities in consultation and resource programs. Exceptional Children, 57, 162–172.

Semmel, M. I., Gotleib, J., & Robinson, N. (1979). Mainstreaming: Perspectives in educating handicapped children in the public schools. In D. Berliner (Ed.), Review of research in education (pp. 223–279). Itaska, IL: Peacock.

Shinn, M., Powell-Smith, K., & Good, R. (1996). Evaluating the effects of responsible reintegration into general education for students with mild disabilities on a case-by-case basis. School Psychology Review, 25(4), 519–539.

Sindelar, P. T., & Deno, S. L. (1978). The effectiveness of resource programming. Journal of Special Education, 12(1), 17–28.

Stallings, J. (1979). How to change the process of teaching reading in secondary schools, Educational Horizons, 57(4), 196–201.

Stevens, R., Madden, N., Slavin, R., & Farnish, A. (1987). Cooperative integrated reading and composition: Two field experiments. Reading Research Quarterly, 22, 433–454.

U.S. Department of Education. (2000). Twenty-second annual report to Congress on the implementation of the Individuals with Disabilities Education Act. Washington, DC: U.S. Government Printing Office.

U.S. Department of Health Education and Welfare. (1979). Progress toward a free appropriate public education: A report to congress on the implementation of Public Law 94-142, the Education of All Handicapped Children Act. Washington, DC: U.S. Government Printing Office.

Vaughn, S., Elbaum, B. E., & Boardman, A. G. (2001). The social functioning of students with learning disabilities: Implications for inclusion. Exceptionality, 9(1&2), 47–65.

Vaughn, S., & Klingner, J. (1998). Students' perceptions of inclusion and resource room settings. Journal of Special Education, 32(2), 79–88.

Waldren, N. L., & McCleskey, J. (1998). The effects of an inclusive school program on students with mild and severe learning disabilities, Exceptional Children, 64(3), 395–405.

Walther-Thomas, C. (1997). Co-teaching experiences: The benefits and problems that teachers and principals report over time. Journal of Learning Disabilities, 30(4), 395–407.

Wang, M. (1987). Toward achieving educational excellence for all students: Program design and student outcomes, Remedial and Special Education, 8(3), 25–34.

Wang, M. (1989). Accommodating student diversity through adaptive education. In S. Stainback, W. Stainback, & M. Forest (Eds.), Educating all students in the mainstream of education (pp. 183–197). Baltimore: Brookes.

Wang, M., & Baker, E. T. (1985–1986). Mainstreaming programs: Design features and effects. Journal of Special Education, 19(4), 503–521.

Will, M. C. (1986). Educating children with learning problems: A shared responsibility. Exceptional Children, 52(5), 411–415.

Zigmond, N., & Baker, J. (1990). Mainstreaming experiences for learning disabled students: A preliminary report. Exceptional Children, 57(2), 176–185.

Zigmond, N., & Baker, J. (1994). Is the mainstream a more appropriate educational setting for students with learning disabilities: The case of Randy. Learning Disabilities Research and Practice, 9(2), 108–117.

Zigmond, N., Jenkins, J., Fuchs, L., Deno, S., Fuchs, D., Baker, J. N., Jenkins, L., & Coutinho, M. (1995). Special education in restructured schools: Findings from three multi-year studies. Phi Delta Kappan, 76, 531–540.

Zigmond, N., & Magiera, K. (2002a). Co-teaching in secondary schools. Paper presented at the annual convention of the Council for Exceptional Children, New York.

Zigmond, N., & Magiera, K. (2002b). Current practice alerts: Co-teaching. Arlington, VA: Division for Learning Disabilities of the Council for Exceptional Children.

II
CAUSES AND BEHAVIORAL MANIFESTATIONS

8

Attention: Relationships between Attention-Deficit Hyperactivity Disorder and Learning Disabilities

Laurie E. Cutting
Martha Bridge Denckla

Learning disabilities (LD) represent a heterogeneous set of disorders that include difficulty (not predicted from measures of general cognitive aptitude) in a variety of academic and social domains. Over the years, researchers have studied the cognitive profiles and brain–behavior relationships associated with different types of LD. Of these, reading disabilities have been the most extensively researched (e.g., Adams, 1990; Lyon, 1995; Shaywitz & Shaywitz, 1999); other types of LD, such as math and written language disorders, have also been investigated, but to a lesser extent (e..g., Berninger, Abbott, Abott, Graham, & Richards, 2002; Berninger & Hart, 1992; Berninger & Rutberg, 1992; Berninger & Swanson, 1994; Geary, 1990, 1992, 1993; Hooper, Swartz, Wakely, de Kruif, & Montgomery, 2002; Mazzocco, 2001).

A variety of approaches have been taken to study LD. One approach has been to focus on the specific type of LD, such as reading disability, to try to determine from the "behavior" the brain and genetic underpinnings (e.g., Davis, Knopik, Olson, Wadsworth, & DeFries, 2001; DeFries & Alarcon, 1996; DeFries et al., 1997; Smith et al., 2001). Such research has yielded not only a

solid understanding of the cognitive characteristics of reading disability but also strong evidence for genetic and brain bases of reading disability, albeit that the precise genetic and brain mechanisms involved are still under exploration. Another approach to studying LD has been to study the phenotype of *known* genetic disorders that have a high prevalence of LD to understand more about brain–behavior relationships; study of genetically mediated LD allows for developing models of different subtypes of LD as well as understanding how different brain circuits may lead to similar behavior. The Learning Disabilities Research Center (LDRC) at the Kennedy Krieger Institute, under the direction of Dr. Martha Bridge Denckla, has taken this *gene-to-brain-to-behavior* approach in the study of LD, with a particular focus on the link between LD and attention-deficit hyperactivity disorder (ADHD).

Background, with Glossary

Before going into the specifics of this chapter, it seems prudent to provide readers with some background, including terminology, with which to appreciate the concepts and data.

First and foremost, we wish to explain why the chapter says much about ADHD but little about "attention," instead focusing on the cognitive domain of executive function as the relevant issue attached, as it were, to the diagnosis of ADHD. Much literature, culminating in Barkley's (1997a, 1997b) formulation of the concept of ADHD as a syndrome of deficient self-control, has redirected the research of the past decade in such a way that many authorities on the subject regret the nomenclature so prominently declaring "attention deficit." Many nonprofessional people still refer to a nonexistent term and even use as an adjective "ADD" (attention deficit disorder) even further spreading the misplaced emphasis on "attention." Briefly summarized, the evidence is overwhelming to the effect that in children and adults with ADHD, there is no "deficit" in "attention" (in the sense of resources in short supply); rather, there is a deficit in the deployment or allocation of attentional resources that characterizes both children and adults with the syndrome called ADHD. The allocation or deployment of attention is an "executive function," one of a group of functions collectively designated "executive." Evidence continues to accumulate in favor of a concept of ADHD that unifies the apparent "inattentiveness" with the other cluster, "hyperactivity/impulsivity" by virtue of the overarching executive function domain of self-control. Of course, allocation/deployment of attention exists within a subdomain of cognitive control, whereas the more glaring deficiencies of self-control manifest in "hyperactivity" or "impulsivity" belong to the subdomain of social–emotional control.

Cognitive neuroscience is more preoccupied with the attention/executive function distinction; the syndrome of ADHD, when discussed in relation to school problems and learning issues, resolves itself in this context into a broader executive impairment but a narrower attentional impairment than is implied by the name of the disorder, in the sense that more cognitive deficiencies than just attention are characteristic of the ADHD category. However, at the same time, only a particular subtype (not every component) of attention is substandard.

A term used by cognitive psychologists and cognitive neuroscientists, "executive function" refers to a set of control processes; so broad is the range of these control processes that the reader of any body of literature about "executive function" must "read the fine print" of operational definitions. Particularly important for educators is the inclusion within "executive function" of less lofty (and earlier developing) components such as inhibition and working memory; this *caveat* is stated because it is all too easy to elevate "executive function" to a synonym for "metacognition." When talking about young children in elementary school, the cognitive neuroscientists should be defining the term more as a set of infrastructural elements (inhibition and working memory) rather than organization/planning and other more future-oriented, higher-order components of executive function domain.

Neurology identifies executive function with the frontal lobe and its circuits, an aspect of brain architecture that is characterized by protracted, relatively slow maturation for over three postnatal decades. For the past 15 years, neurological research has emphasized the parallel circuits connecting different anatomic subdivisions of frontal lobe with separate, circuit-specific regions of basal ganglia and cerebellum. Magnetic resonance imaging (MRI) has, of course, facilitated study in living children of such parallel fronto–striato–cerebello–thalamo–frontal circuits. (Striatum refers to a portion of the basal ganglia.) These parallel circuits correspond to dedicated separate pathways for motor control, cognitive control, and social–emotional control; the segregation of circuits is "breached" at the level of the frontal cortex, such that only at the top (and last-to-reach-maturity) level is there "crosstalk" (integration) whereby the circuits influence each other.

Learning Disabilities Research at the Kennedy Krieger Institute

Over the past 12 years, the LDRC at the Kennedy Krieger Institute/Johns Hopkins School of Medicine has taken a behavioral neurogenetics approach to studying LD. The different disorders that have been the focus of this research are neurofibromatosis

Type 1 (NF-1), fragile X syndrome, and Tourette syndrome. The genetic etiology of both NF-1 and fragile X is known but has not been established as of yet for Tourette syndrome. In addition, because so many children with Tourette syndrome have ADHD, children with ADHD have served as a comparison group for this project.

The NF-1 project's original focus was to understand "nonverbal" LD; however, findings from this project, as well as other LDRC projects, have resulted in a shift in understanding; NF-1 is no longer regarded as accurately exemplifying "nonverbal" LD; furthermore, it has emerged that "nonverbal" LD in general (not just as associated with the NF-1 phenotype), in its purest sense, does not often occur. Instead, although individuals may have "nonverbal" deficits, they almost always also have other deficits, either in the verbal domain or in executive functioning. Another area of focus of the LDRC has been to examine the comorbidity of ADHD and investigate how that is related to the executive function deficits often seen in individuals with LD. Two disorders, NF-1 and Tourette syndrome, have been shown to be particularly applicable to understanding the overlap between the executive function that is the cog-

nitive component of ADHD and LD, often accompanied by executive dysfunction (see Figure 8.1). NF-1, in that its cognitive phenotype presents as a "classic" LD (particularly reading disability accompanied by ADHD), has yielded further understanding about these typically co-occuring disorders.

The Tourette syndrome project has yielded an understanding of the executive function-based influence of slow "processing speed"—another common characteristic of LD. Children with Tourette syndrome, 60% of whom also have ADHD, tend to exhibit slow "processing speed" with regard to cognitive tasks, whereas children with ADHD exhibit motoric slowing. Most important, findings with regard to ADHD have illustrated that the term "slow processing speed" would be more precisely expressed as "slow output speed," in that we have found deficiencies not of "processing," in the sense of intake functions, but of output or producing functions of the brain. This usage differs from the broader "processing" as an overarching term, in which case it subsumes "producing."

In the subsequent sections, we present selected findings from our research for NF-1 and Tourette syndrome, including our efforts to specify the neuropsychological pro-

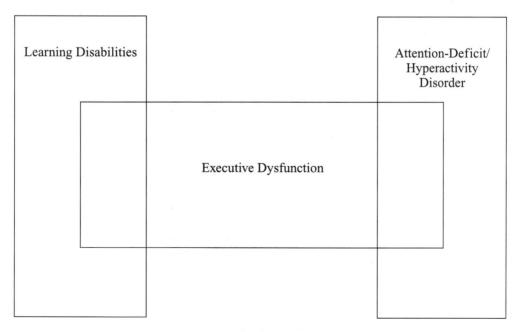

FIGURE 8.1. Overlap between LD and ADHD.

files as well as the underlying brain mechanisms of each. In addition, we discuss the implications of these findings with respect to idiopathic LD (i.e., that which as yet has no established genetic etiology).

Neurofibromatosis Type 1

Genetic and Physical Aspects of NF-1

NF-1 is one of the most common single-gene disorders, with an incidence of 2 to 3 cases per 10,000 in the population (Friedman, 1999) and equal prevalence rates across sex and race. Approximately 50% of all cases of NF-1 are familial, inherited in an autosomal dominant manner, with the remaining cases being spontaneous mutations (Crowe, Schull, & Neel, 1956). The locus of NF-1 abnormality has been found to be a rather large region on the long arm of chromosome 17 at 17q11.2 (Barker et al., 1987; Goldgar, Green Parry & Mulvihill, 1989; Gutman & Collins, 1993). Although there is a DNA test for NF-1, it is currently diagnosed based on physical symptoms from NIH consensus criteria (see Table 8.1). In addition, MRI findings have become more and more integral to the confirmation of NF-1.

NF-1 affects different aspects of the cutaneous, skeletal, and central nervous systems. Common manifestations of NF-1 include Lisch nodules, cutaneous and plexiform neurofibromas, axilary café au lait spots, nerve tumors, and optic gliomas (Stumpf, Alksne, & Annegers, 1988). In addition, T2 weighted hyperintensities, otherwise referred to as unidentified bright objects (UBOs), are seen on MRI scans,

typically in subcortical structures, and have been reported in 40 to 93% of children with NF-1 (Steen et al., 2001). While UBOs are commonly seen in individuals with NF-1, their biological and clinical significance is still not fully understood. Macrocephaly, or enlargement of the head, has long been observed in about 50% of individuals with NF-1; MRI studies are consistent with the interpretation that this is due to enlarged brains (megalencephaly; Cutting, Koth, Burnette, et al., 2000; Moore et al., 2000; Said et al., 1996; Steen et al., 2001). Recently, magnetic resonance spectroscopy imaging (MRSI) has revealed metabolic abnormalities in NF-1, with elevated N-acetylaspartate/Choline ratios in the thalamus (Wang et al., 2000).

Our Approach to Studying NF-1

There are several types of methodologies to use when studying genetic disorders; one approach is to study the impact of the genetic disorder on cognition by comparing performance of those affected to norms based on the general population (e.g., Dilts et al., 1996; Eliason, 1986; Moore, Slopis, Schomer, Jackson, & Levy, 1996; North et al., 1994). Another approach, one we also have taken, is to use a sibling-matched-pair (one NF-1-affected, one unaffected) design; this approach is exemplified in several of our published studies (e.g., Cutting, Huang, Zeger, Koth, & Denckla, 2002; Hofman, Harris, Bryan, & Denckla, 1994; Mazzocco et al., 1995). A sibling-matched-pair design, unlike that which involves an unrelated independent control group from the general population, takes into account familial and environmental factors (Mackintosh, 1998). Statistical "purists" have balked at the issue of nonindependence of the groups being compared. Both methodologies have advantages; however, within the context of trying to understand the direct gene-to-brain-to-behavior influences, the sibling-pair approach allows for a more focused understanding of the influence of the NF-1 gene on brain–behavior relationships.

TABLE 8.1. NIH Consensus Criteria for NF-1 Diagnosis

- Six or more café au lait macules
- Two or more neurofibromas or one plexiform neurofibroma
- Freckling in the axilla or inguinal region
- An optic glioma
- A distinct osseous lesion
- Two or more Lisch nodules
- A first-degree relative who meets the above criteria for NF-1

Note. Two or more must be present for diagnosis.

Cognitive Profile

Though there is virtually universal agreement that mental retardation is rare with

NF-1, the IQs of those affected are lower than the family of origin (indexed by siblings) would predict and are shifted into the lower portion of the normal range for the general population. In addition, LD is reported in approximately 25 to 61% of children with NF-1 (North et al., 1997; Riccardi, 1981; Stine & Adams, 1989), which is much higher than the estimates of 5 to 17.5% in the general population (Shaywitz and Shaywitz, 1999). Originally, it was thought that individuals with NF-1 had "nonverbal" LD (NVLD) because early studies documented significant impairments on Performance IQ and on a test called Judgment of Line Orientation, both considered to be tests of visuospatial ability (Benton, Hamsher, Varney, & Spreen, 1983, Weschler, 1974). Therefore, we embarked on studying NF-1 in the expectation of obtaining a clearer understanding of NVLD. However, since this time, a variety of studies, including many from our laboratory, have documented that NF-1 is strongly associated with deficits in the verbal domain (e.g., Cutting et al., 2000; Hofman, Harris, Bryan, & Denckla, 1994; Mazzocco et al., 1995; North et al., 1997); in fact, deficits in the verbal domain appear to be more widespread and academically debilitating than those in the "nonverbal" domain. An additional surprise in our research was that ADHD is associated with NF-1 to a much higher degree than expected from general familial prevalence of ADHD (Koth, Cutting, & Denckla, 2000). In particular, five studies, which we review herein, highlight different aspects of our findings about the cognitive profile of NF-1 and what they reveal about idiopathic LD (Cutting, Koth, & Denckla, 2000; Cutting et al., 2002; Hofman et al., 1994; Koth et al., 2000; Mazzocco et al., 1995).

In an initial study of 12 sibling pairs, Hofman and colleagues (1994) found that in addition to poor performance on tests of visuospatial ability (Judgment of Line Orientation; Block Design), children with NF-1 also had significantly lower-than-expected scores on measures of reading and writing ability; furthermore, even after controlling for IQ, a disproportionate representation of reading disabilities was characteristic of children with NF-1 as compared to their siblings. Mazzocco and colleagues (1995)

followed up the Hofman and colleagues study with a larger sample size (20 sibling pairs) and an expanded battery of visuospatial, language, reading, and attention abilities. Children with NF-1 were found to perform lower than expected (by reference to sibling) on a variety of language tests (Boston Naming Test, Phoneme Segmentation, Phonological Memory, Token Test, Letter–Word Identification, Passage Comprehension, and the Test of Written Language). Normal performance was observed on Rapid Automatized Naming, Word Fluency, and Grammaticality Judgment. Poorer-than-expected performance (by reference to sibling) was observed on only a few tests of visuospatial ability (Judgment of Line Orientation and Block Design), as well as two tests of controlled processing or executive function (a continuous performance test—number of omissions and the Wisconsin Card Sorting Test—categories). Discrepancy-based reading disability was again confirmed to be more prevalent in children with NF-1 as compared to their siblings; in addition, as is quite typically viewed as characteristic of reading disability, children with NF-1 showed deficits on phonological measures. Mazzocco and colleagues concluded from these findings that while children with NF-1 do have visuospatial deficits, deficits in the verbal domain were far more numerous and academically relevant, thus indicating that NF-1 is not a model for NVLD (and thereby resulting in the article's title proclaiming NF-1 the "not-so-nonverbal learning disability"). In terms of understanding reading disability, Mazzocco and colleagues commented that "children with NF-1 illustrate the conceptual difficulty underlying discrepancy-based reading disability, wherein language disorder influences both measures between which a discrepancy is calculated" (p. 519).

In an effort to understand similarities and differences between NF-1 and idiopathic reading disabilities, Cutting, Koth, and Denckla (2000) compared children with NF-1 to children with reading disabilities from the general population. Another goal of the study was to compare a discrepancy-based reading disabilities group with our NF-1 group to determine the impact of language deficits on ability to meet discrepancy-based definitions of reading disabilities.

As expected, children with NF-1 had deficits similar to those of children with reading disability; both groups had difficulty with reading and reading-related tests (Rapid Automatized Naming; Denckla & Rudel, 1976) and phoneme segmentation measures. Interestingly, the NF-1 group did not perform poorly on the Rapid Automatized Naming measure but did on both phonological measures, whereas the reading disability group performed poorly only on Rapid Automatized Naming, thus potentially providing some support for the dissociation between phonological and Rapid Automatized Naming measures (Wolf & Bowers, 1999). Other differences between the groups were that children with NF-1, unlike children with reading disability, showed deficits in visuospatial areas as well as a broader language deficit. Overall, this study showed that many children with NF-1 were not able to meet the discrepancy definition of reading disabilities because of their more "global" verbal impairments (i.e., lower Verbal IQ) but nonetheless showed the hallmark deficits (phonological) associated with reading disabilities.

One aspect of our study of NF-1 was to examine growth of certain cognitive functions. Based on the Hofman and colleagues (1994) and Mazzocco and colleagues (1995) studies, a pattern of "spared" and "impaired" tests (as compared to sibling's performance) emerged; those tests that were impaired were Vocabulary, Block Design, and Judgment of Line Orientation, whereas those tests that were "spared" were Picture Completion, Picture Arrangement, and Rapid Automatized Naming (letters and numbers). Ten sibling pairs were followed longitudinally and compared on the "spared" and "impaired" these tests (Cutting et al., 2002). Results showed that children with NF-1 did not "catch up" to their siblings on "impaired" measures; however, on the "spared" measures they continued to perform similarly to their siblings. On average, across the six cognitive measures, there was no significant difference between the groups in terms of growth rates. Interestingly, variation *among* families for level of performance was larger than variation among siblings (with and without NF-1) within a family on Vocabulary and Rapid Automatized Naming, thus providing evidence of significant familial effects on cognition, again confirming the need to consider investigating the NF-1-associated deficits within the familial context afforded by the sibling-pair design.

Because ADHD symptomology has been reported in children with NF-1, Koth and colleagues (2000) compared the prevalence of ADHD in children with NF-1 as compared to their unaffected siblings and parents. The goal of the study was to determine whether ADHD could be included in the phenotype of NF-1, or whether it was an unrelated disorder within families. Frequency of ADHD among children with NF-1, their siblings, and their parents was compared. Results indicated that a higher percentage of children with NF-1 (42%) had ADHD than either siblings (13%) or parents (5%), suggesting that ADHD is in part associated with the NF-1 cognitive phenotype. The origins of this association between ADHD and NF-1 are not entirely clear at this time. One of the features of NF-1 is UBOs, which are often seen the same brain structures implicated in ADHD (basal ganglia, thalamus, cerebellum, and brainstem). It may be that UBOs disrupt certain critical frontally related circuits, similar to those thought to be disrupted in idiopathic ADHD, thus giving rise to ADHD in children with NF-1. Future studies examining the relationship between presence of ADHD and presence and location of UBOs will be able to elucidate this issue.

In summary, findings regarding the cognitive phenotype of NF-1 indicate that children with NF-1 appear to have both visuospatial deficits and reading disabilities, the latter in the familiar context of many oral language deficiencies, a likely contribution to the lowering of their Verbal IQ (thus making fulfilling the criteria for a discrepancy-based LD more difficult). Findings from the Koth and colleagues (2000) study also indicate that NF-1 appears to be associated with ADHD. Thus, NF-1, while initially appearing to be a model of NVLD because of selective visuospatial deficits, has proven to be a model for what is typically seen in LD: difficulty with reading and language, with comorbid ADHD. In addition, ADHD/executive function may influence performance on certain tests; for example, it may be that the origin of poor performance on the Judgment of

Line Orientation stems from ADHD/executive function test-taking demands. Though the ADHD-related executive function deficits have not yet been fully explored in NF-1, further study, particularly in relation to lesions in the basal ganglia and cerebellum, may reveal critical circuits involved in ADHD in general and in its related executive function deficits. A challenge, not unique to the NF-1 studies, is to tease apart language contributions from the truly "central executive" issues when deficits on tests such as card sorting or word efficiency are employed in an "executive" battery.

Neuroimaging Findings

Neuroimaging findings with NF-1 have allowed for the study of areas of the brain that may affect specific aspects of cognition; in particular, examination of megalencephaly and UBOs in relation to cognition allows for exploration of disruption in specific brain regions and/or neural circuits that may contribute to selected cognitive deficits. To date, we have used two different imaging modalities, anatomical magnetic resonance imaging (aMRI) and MRSI in our study of NF-1.

It has been debated whether or not UBOs are related to cognitive impairment in NF-1; some studies have found a relationship while others have not (see Ozonoff, 1999). To address the ongoing controversy, Denckla and colleagues (1996) examined the number of locations of UBOs and volume of UBOs in relation to the relative "lowering" of IQ in children with NF-1 (as compared to their siblings). Findings showed that the number of locations (basal ganglia, cerebellum, brainstem, and other subcortical structures) occupied by UBOs accounted for 42% of the variance in the "lowering" of IQ in children with NF-1. It was concluded that "IQ [as a global measure of cognition] . . . might reasonably be more adversely affected by multiple interruptions in CNS [central nervous system] connections than by volume replacement in one or more specific locations" (p. 101).

In addition to the controversy as to whether UBOs are related to the cognitive deficits in NF-1, there has also been some suggestion from cross-sectional studies that UBOs decrease over time (DiMario &

Ramsby, 1998; Itoh et al., 1994). To address this issue further, we recently studied UBOs longitudinally in 12 children with NF-1 (Kraut et al., 2002); we examined a number of regions occupied by UBOs, number of UBOs per brain region, and UBO volume per brain region. Findings indicated that the number of regions occupied by UBOs, as well as UBO number and/or volume for all brain regions, diminished between the ages of 7 and 12; however, there was an increase during adolescence. The relationship of UBOs to changes in cognitive functioning over time was not examined in this study but will be a part of future studies in order to elucidate further the impact of UBOs and disruption of particular neuronal pathways on cognition, in particular with regard to the influence of disruption of neural circuits during critical time periods.

In an effort to better characterize UBOs, we used MRSI to examine the biochemical composition of the brain of males with NF-1 (Wang et al., 2000). Findings revealed that there was elevated Choline and normal N-acetylaspartate (NAA) in subjects who were less than 10 years old, but in subjects older than 10 years, there was reduced NAA and normal Choline. These changes (consistent in terms of NF-1-associated decreased NAA/Choline ratios) were found in UBOs in the basal ganglia and, surprisingly, most prominently (and independently of UBOs) in the thalamus. It was concluded from this study that the metabolic abnormities found using MRSI might indicate more widespread white matter abnormalies; specifically, elevated Choline in younger subjects may reflect increased myelin turnover, which might result in axonal injury (reflected by reduced NAA) in older subjects. This hypothesis has also been put forth by other investigators from other sources of information (e.g., neuropathological evidence; DiPaolo et al., 1995). Therefore, UBOs seen on aMRI scans may be indicators of larger, more global developmental white matter abnormalities in NF-1.

Other neuroimaging findings from our laboratory have focused on volumetric analyses. Cutting, Koth, Burnette, and colleagues. (2000) found that in a sample of 19 males with NF-1, approximately 50% were megalencephalic. Megalencephaly was not significantly associated with familial or sporadic origin of NF-1 or presence or absence of UBOs. However, megalencephaly was associated with verbal impairment (specifically, lower Vocabulary subtest scores). Further study of megalencephaly examining volume of lobar subdivisions and gray and white matter in relation to UBOs has revealed a more complex picture of megalencephaly in NF-1 (Cutting et al., in press), in particular with regard to presence of ADHD. Cutting and colleagues (in press) found a strong relationship between the presence of comorbid ADHD in males with NF-1 and megalencephaly. In this study, the brain volumes of 18 males with NF-1 were compared to those of 18 age-matched controls. Seven of the 18 males with NF-1 were diagnosed with ADHD. As compared to controls, males with NF-1 *without* ADHD were megalencephalic, whereas males with NF-1 *with* ADHD were *not* megalencephalic. However, all males with NF-1, regardless of ADHD status, showed increased volume of white matter in the frontal lobes; the NF-1 without ADHD group showed increased volume of white matter in the parietal lobes. Consistent with reports of decreased frontal lobe volumes in idiopathic ADHD, presence of ADHD in NF-1 was associated with a decrease in the volume of gray matter in the frontal lobe, namely, right prefrontal. Marked parietal white matter enlargement was seen if UBOs were present in the basal ganglia in NF-1 males who did not have ADHD. Findings from this study indicate that ADHD is an important comorbid diagnosis to consider and appears to be associated with a different neuroanatomical profile, specifically reduction in brain volume (as is also observed in idiopathic ADHD). In addition, strong evidence for the association of white matter abnormities with NF-1, regardless of comorbid ADHD, was found.

In summary, neuroimaging findings with NF-1 indicate a complex picture of a variety of anomalies: UBOs, megalencephaly, and metabolic evidence of neuronal and myelinic abnormalities. How these abnormalities in NF-1 are related to each other, as well as to cognition and presence of ADHD, is still under investigation. Understanding these relationships may further reveal our understanding of neural circuitry and brain regions that affect cognition in NF-1. This knowledge (at least at the level of systems and circuits, but not genes) may in turn be applicable to understanding brain-based origins of idiopathic ADHD and LD, as the systems and circuits involved, regardless of the reason such are abnormal, may be critically important.

Further Study of NF-1

We are currently undertaking study of NF-1 using multiple neuroimaging modalities (aMRI, MRSI, and functional MRI); this study involves sibling pairs as well as a control group and a reading disability group from the general population. One goal of the study is to understand how the chemical abnormalities that exist in the brains of children with NF-1 are related to the reading and language deficits associated with NF-1. Another goal is to determine how differences in brain activation when reading are linked to the cognitive and academic impairments associated with NF-1, and how these may be different/similar to those of children with idiopathic reading disabilities. Based on previous research findings, we are hypothesizing that chemical markers of neuronal abnormalities will exist in the thalamus (a "relay" station in the brain) and correlate with reading, language, and articulation deficits in NF-1, as defined by the "lowering" of the cognitive score of each child with NF-1 relative to that of his or her unaffected sibling. We also hypothesize that children with NF-1 will exhibit a pattern of activation in the language centers of the brain when performing reading-like tasks similarly to children with reading disabilities, but anomalously in comparison to normal readers. The goal of this study is to basic neurobiological factors and their affect on cognition, particularly reading and language (although ADHD will also be a factor) in NF-1 and reading disabilities, thus furthering our understanding of gene-to-brain-to-behavior relationships as related to reading and language disorders, as well as ADHD.

Tourette Syndrome

Tourette syndrome (TS) has been a focus of the LDRC over the last 12 years. TS is a neuropsychiatric disorder with a prevalence rate of approximately 1 per 1,000 males and 1 per 10,000 females and is characterized by a variety of waxing and waning and changing motor and vocal tics, and has an onset usually prior to 15 years of age (Leckman, King, & Cohen, 1999). Although the precise genetic mechanism for TS is not yet known, and is looking more polygenic than single-gene in mechanism, it has a strong genetic/familial component (Leckman & Cohen, 1999). Individuals with TS have a high rate of comorbidity with ADHD and obsessive–compulsive disorder (Golden, 1984; Singer, Schuerholz, & Denckla, 1995). It is estimated that approximately 50 to 60% of children with TS also have ADHD; moreover, it has been reported that approximately one-third of children with TS also have some type of LD (e.g., Burd, Kauffman, & Kerbeshian, 1992; Golden, 1984). The focus of study of TS in the LDRC was to understand the neuropsychological and neuroanatomical similarities and differences between children with TS, TS plus ADHD, and ADHD. In particular, the goal was to discern the role of ADHD, as mediated by its cognitive correlate, executive dysfunction, in producing LD; on the brain systems/circuits level, we focused on differences in prefrontal–subcortical systems that might differentiate these three groups. Our main findings were that LD and most aspects of executive dysfunction are not particularly characteristic of pure TS (when free of comorbid ADHD), with the sole exception of cognitive slowing. LD (written expression in particular) and an array of executive dysfunctions are more widespread in children with TS when ADHD is also present. Therefore, our most pertinent findings with regard to the TS project are actually in regard to what we have found about ADHD and its impact on manifestations of LD. Consequently, we provide some discussion of our findings with regard to TS; however, most of our discussion focuses on ADHD.

Cognitive Profile of TS and ADHD

Studies of several cohorts of children with TS from the LDRC have revealed that children with TS-only have relatively few impairments in executive functioning and do not have significant LD; instead, significant impairments in executive functioning and LD are present when there is comorbid ADHD

(Harris et al., 1995; Mahone, Koth, Cutting, Singer, & Denckla, 2001; Mahone et al., in press; Schuerholz et al., 1997; Schuerholz, Baumgardner, Singer, Reiss, & Denckla, 1996). For example, Harris and colleagues (1995) found that impairments in planning, cognitive flexibility, response inhibition, and self-monitoring were observed in the ADHD and TS+ADHD groups as reflected by poor performance on the Rey Osterreith Complex Figure, the Wisconsin Card Sorting Task (WCST; Categories Achieved and Set Breaks), and the Test of Variables of Attention (TOVA); however, the only impairments observed for the TS-only group were slow and variable reaction time on the TOVA, suggesting subcortical or basal ganglia involvement for this group. Other studies of groups of TS-only, TS+ADHD, and ADHD have further clarified differences between these groups (Schuerholz et al., 1996). Schuerholz and colleagues (1996) found that while 23% of the TS sample had an LD, this was because LD was present only in children who had TS *and* ADHD. Other findings from this study mirrored those of Harris and colleagues, with slow and variable reaction time observed in all groups; an unexpected finding in this study was poor performance on Letter–Word Fluency in the TS-only group. It was suggested from this finding that TS might be associated with a slowing in mental search ("bradyphrenia") resulting in poor linguistic productivity, different from motor slowing. This hypothesis was further clarified in a study of neuromotor functioning in children with TS-only, TS+ADHD, and ADHD-only (Schuerholz et al.). On timed motor movements, children with ADHD (with or without TS) were found to be slow relative to their age peers, while TS-only was associated with relatively unimpaired performance. Therefore, it was suggested that while both TS and ADHD are associated with slowing on choice reaction time tasks, this slowing is caused by different deficits. Children with TS show cognitive slowing, or "bradyphrenia," whereas children with ADHD show motoric slowing ("bradykinesia").

Mahone and colleagues (2001) recently examined two aspects of executive function, organization and response inhibition (thought to reflect dorsolateral and orbitofrontal circuitry), in a second cohort of children with TS-only, ADHD-only, and controls. It was hypothesized that children with TS-only would show deficits in organization, whereas children with ADHD would show deficits in both organization and response inhibition. In contrast to our previous studies, Mahone and colleagues examined not only total outcome scores but also process variables, or how the groups completed the task. In addition to overall performance, process variables examined included semantic clustering on a list-learning task (California Verbal Learning Test for Children; CVLT-C), clustering on semantic and letter–word fluency, intrusions on the CVLT-C, and errors on semantic and letter–word fluency. Findings were somewhat inconsistent with those of our previous studies: Differences were found only in the number of intrusions on the CVLT-C, which were abnormally elevated in *both* the TS and ADHD groups. No differences were observed between groups for total score on Letter Word Fluency or process variables from Letter Word Fluency. It was hypothesized that differences between these results and the Schuerholz and colleagues (1996) study may have been because of differences between samples; the more recent cohort had higher IQs and had been screened for a third comorbidity, obsessive–compulsive disorder (i.e., more stringently excluded). Mahone and colleagues speculated that "overgrowing," or compensation for subcortical deficiencies when afforded the maturation of the frontal cortex, might allow for normal performance on executive measures.

Other investigations stemming from the TS project have focused only on ADHD. For example, Reader, Harris, Schuerholz, and Denckla (1994) investigated executive function in 48 children with ADHD (no TS). Impairments were found on the WCST (number of categories achieved and set breaks) as well as the TOVA (errors of omission, slow and variable reaction time), but intact performance on Word Fluency as well as the Rey Complex Figure. The effect of comorbid reading disability (ADHD+RD) on executive function was also examined; findings indicated that there were no differences between the ADHD and ADHD+RD groups on any of the executive function measures with the exception of less variability on the TOVA for the ADHD+RD group.

Cutting, Koth, Mahone, and Denckla (in press), in an effort to further clarify how children with ADHD (who presumably have impairments in executive function) may show difficulty in the *process* of learning, recently examined the mechanisms underlying verbal learning in children with and without ADHD. Children with ADHD (none of whom had RD) were compared on both *process* and *product* scores from the CVLT-C. Findings indicated that while children with ADHD initially learned the same number of words as controls, they were weak in recalling the words after delays, suggesting that children with ADHD are less efficient learners. Sex-related findings revealed that regardless of ADHD diagnosis, boys and girls performed differently. Boys used semantic clustering less frequently and recalled fewer words from the middle region of the list than girls; girls also outperformed boys in terms of overall performance, *despite* lower verbal IQs. These findings showed that children with ADHD exhibit unexpected weaknesses in the *process* of learning.

In summary, neuropsychological findings from the TS project have yielded an understanding that most of the school-related difficulties reported in children with TS are most often associated with presence of ADHD-related deficits in executive function, although there is an issue with slowness (i.e., "processing speed") in this group, as well as with ADHD. (We have now seen this slowing phenomenon in our clinical experience with children referred for possible LD who also have TS.) Findings from various studies reveal that ADHD-related executive function deficits negatively influence not only in purely "academic" subjects but also the *process* of learning, in that children with ADHD do not apply effective learning strategies to material. More discussion of the implications of these findings is in the section "Future Directions," but nonetheless these findings do imply the need for further clarification of the role of ADHD and executive function in learning difficulties.

Neuroimaging Findings in TS and ADHD

Several volumetric neuroimaging studies that have been conducted through the LDRC lend support to the hypothesis that neurobiological mechanisms in TS and ADHD involve frontal/subcortical circuits. In ADHD, however, abnormalities have been found in cortical (frontal), subcortical (basal ganglia), and cerebellar structures. It may be that abnormalities in one or another, or even two or three of these structures, give rise to different types of severities of impairment in ADHD. Following we present a brief description of neuroanatomical findings from the LDRC.

In a study of the basal ganglia in children with TS, Singer and colleagues (1993) found in a group of predominantly male subjects that TS was associated with reversed asymmetry in the putamen and lenticular region. While control subjects showed left-greater-than-right asymmetry in the putamen and lenticular regions, TS subjects showed significantly less left predominance in these areas. Comorbid ADHD was associated with significantly smaller left globus pallidus volumes, and a separate subsequent follow-up study documented the same finding in boys with ADHD alone (Aylward et al., 1996). These studies support the hypothesis of subcortical abnormalities in both TS and ADHD, but considerably more subtle ones in "pure" TS cases (loss of normal L > R asymmetry).

Baumgardner and colleagues (1996) examined corpus callosum morphology in children (predominantly males) with TS-only, ADHD, and TS+ADHD. Results revealed dissociation between the anatomies of TS and ADHD. TS was associated with larger-than-normal volumes in four of five areas of the corpus callosum (splenium, isthmus/posterior body, midbody, and rostral body); conversely, ADHD was associated with smaller rostral body volumes. Paradoxically, the opposite direction of the two volumetric abnormalities led to apparently "normal" rostral body volumes of the comorbid TS+ADHD group, as though two pathologies, equal but opposite. These findings support the view that there are abnormalities in frontal/subcortical circuitry in both TS and ADHD, in that the anterior part of the corpus callosum provides interhemispheric connections for the frontal cortex; specifically, the rostral body has axons that link premotor and supplementary motor areas. Consistent with neuropsychological findings contrasting TS and ADHD

groups, neuroanatomical findings suggest that each disorder affects the nervous system somewhat differently (albeit in the same "neighborhood"). Our group's more recent work (Frederickson et al., 2002) elucidates the source of the fibers (white matter) that in pure TS enlarge the rostral corpus callosum. Interestingly, it should be noted that the abnormalities found in TS and ADHD in the corpus callosum are confined to boys, at least on the level of volumetric anatomy, according to another study from our group (Mostofsky et al., 1999).

Examination of gray and white matter cerebral volumes in TS and ADHD has revealed that whereas cortical abnormalities are present in both disorders, the cortical abnormality found in TS is much more subtle than that found in ADHD (Frederickson et al., 2002; Mostofsky et al., 2002). Frederickson and colleagues (2002) found right frontal lobe abnormalities in boys with TS, specifically an enlarged percentage of frontal lobe white matter as compared to overall frontal lobe tissue. Because of the known unidirectionality of the white matter involved (frontal lobe to basal ganglia), these findings, combined with those of the Singer and colleagues (1993) of loss of normal asymmetry in the basal ganglia, led Frederickson and colleagues to speculate that frontal lobe abnormalities may be primary and underlie the basal ganglia anomalies in TS. Mostofsky and colleagues (2002) recently examined gray and white matter frontal lobe and sublobar volumes of boys with ADHD. Results indicated, as many previous studies have also found, that boys with ADHD had smaller total cerebral volumes; this reduction was primarily due to smaller frontal lobe volumes. Within the frontal lobe, both gray and white matter volumes were reduced, suggesting that ADHD is associated with decreases in both the cell bodies and axons of the frontal lobe. Sublobar volumetric findings indicated reduction in prefrontal, premotor, and deep white matter volumes. These findings suggest that ADHD is associated not only with abnormalities in prefrontal cortex (which in this study included dorsolateral and orbitofrontal regions) but also with premotor cortex (which in this study included supplementary motor association areas, Broca's area, and the frontal eye fields). Abnormalities observed in cognitive ("executive functions"), social (disihibited or impulsive behavior), motor, and oculomotor tasks in ADHD, many from our laboratory (e.g., Barker et al., 2001; Denckla & Rudel, 1978; Mostofsky, Lasker, Singer, Denckla, & Zee, 2001; Reader et al., 1994; Shue & Douglas, 1992), lend support to Mostofsky and colleagues' findings of abnormalities in prefrontal and premotor cortex and suggest that rather than a single circuit being impaired in ADHD, a number of parallel fronto–striatal circuits, perhaps because of a common developmental abnormality, are impaired.

Cerebellar anomalies in ADHD suggest that this disorder also encompasses abnormalities in fronto–cerebellar circuits (Berquin et al., 1998; Mostofsky, Reisss, Lockhart, & Denckla, 1998). Mostofsky and colleagues (1998) found decreased size of the posterior vermis, specifically the inferior posterior lobe (lobules VIII-X), in boys with ADHD. Because there are connections between the cerebellum and prefrontal cortex, Mostofsky and colleagues speculated that these cerebellar abnormalities might contribute to the deficits observed in executive function thought to arise from prefrontal cortex.

In summary, neuroimaging findings regarding TS and ADHD reveal anomalies in frontal–subcortical structures. Both disorders show abnormal frontal lobe volumes, with additional abnormalities in subcortical structures. Nonetheless, the volumetric anomalies associated with each disorder are distinct in nature: TS appears to be associated with subtle cortical abnormalities. In contrast, there appear to be substantial findings with regard to ADHD in both widespread frontal–cortical and subcortical structures; the fact that reduction in frontal, basal ganglia, and cerebellar volumes have all been found reflect the multifaceted nature of this disorder and suggest that a variety of levels of anomalies in multiple pathways can result in ADHD.

It remains to be seen what would emerge from studying a large group of children with ADHD with aMRI, to discover who has one, two, or three levels of brain anomalies (including combinations of pairs) and what motor and cognitive profiles would correlate with each possible anatomic profile. Prognosis might well differ as functions of which and how many (one-, two-, or three-level) brain anomalies are present.

Future Directions

Though the findings of the LDRC at the Kennedy Krieger Institute over the past 12 years have resulted in further understanding of the relationships between LD and ADHD, with particular regard to the mediating influence of executive function overlapping these two, a lot remains to be understood. Although much of the research on LD has accumulated a body of knowledge about basic reading disabilities, the findings from the LDRC at the Kennedy Krieger Institute illustrate the complexities associated with elucidating deficits in higher-order functions. For example, the study of basic reading disability has resulted in knowledge about how to identify and remediate children with phonologically based basic reading disability; however, much remains to be understood about the complex interrelationships between executive function, language, and academic skills other than basic reading, such as reading comprehension, mathematics reasoning, and written expression. All these achievements require the ability to plan, organize, and self-monitor, several key components of executive function. In addition, deficits in the more "basic" level of executive function, response inhibition and working memory (associated with ADHD), in relation to all types of LD, including basic reading disabilities, are still not well understood. Systematic study of the interrelationships between the development of executive function, language, and skills in other academic areas besides basic reading is critical in terms of understanding how LD may manifest itself differently at each age and stage of development; for example, maturation of the frontal cortex may play a critical role in developing those skills for reading comprehension (beyond what is accounted for by basic reading) that require working memory and higher-order thinking.

Acknowledgments

This work was supported by the following National Institutes of Health grants: P50 NS 35359 (Learning Disabilities Research Center), ND 07414 (Post-doctoral Fellowship), and HD 24061 (Mental Retardation and Developmental Disabilities Research Center), as well as a grant from the Department of Defense (DAMD 17-00-1-0548).

References

Adams, M. J. (1990). *Beginning to read: Thinking and learning about print*. Cambridge, MA: MIT Press.

Aylward, E. H., Reiss, A. L., Reader, M. J., Singer, H. S., Brown, J. E., & Denckla, M. B. (1996). Basal ganglia volumes in children with attention deficit hyperactivity disorder. *Journal of Child Neurology, 11*, 112–115.

Barker, C. A., Garvey, M. A., Bartko, J. J., Denckla, M. B., Wasserman, E. M., Castellanos, F. X., & Ziemann, U. (2001). The ipsilateral silent period (iSP) in children with attention deficit hyperactivity disorder (ADHD). *Psychological Bulletin, 121*, 65–94.

Barker, D., Wright, E., Nguyen, K., Cannon, L., Fain, P., Goldgar, D., et al. (1987). Gene for von Recklinghausen neurofibromatosis is in the pericentrometic region of chromosome 17. *Science, 236*, 1100–1102.

Barkley, R. A. (1997a). *ADHD and the nature of self-control*. New York: Guilford Press.

Barkley, R. A. (1997b). Behavioral inhibition, sustained attention, and executive functions: Constructing a unifying theory of ADHD. *Psychological Bulletin, 121*, 65–94.

Baumgardner, T. L., Singer, H. S., Denckla, M. B., Rubin, M. A., Abrams, M. T., Colli, M. J., & Reiss, A. L. (1996). Corpus callosum morphology in children with Tourette syndrome and attention deficit hyperactivity disorder. *Neurology, 47*, 477–482.

Benton, A. L., Hamsher, K. D., Varney, N. R., & Spreen, O. (1983). Judgment of Line Orientation. In A. L. Benton et al. (Eds.), *Contributions to neuropsychological assessment: A clinical manual*. New York: Oxford University Press.

Berninger, V. W., Abbott, R. D., Abbott, S. P., Graham, S., & Richards, T. (2002). Writing and reading: Connections between language by hand and language by eye. *Journal of Learning Disabilities, 35*, 39–56.

Berninger, V. W., & Hart, T. (1992). A developmental neuropsychological perspective for reading and writing acquisition. *Educational Psychologist, 27*, 415–434.

Berninger, V. W., & Rutberg, J. (1992). Relationship of finger function to beginning writing: Application to diagnosis of writing disabilities. *Developmental Medicine and Child Neurology, 34*, 155–172.

Berninger, V. W., & Swanson, H. L. (1994). Modifying Hayes & Flower's model of skilled writing to explain beginning and developing writing. In E. Butterfield (Ed.), *Children's writing: Toward a process theory of development of skilled writing* (pp. 57–81). Greenwich, CT: JAI Press.

Berquin, P. C., Giedd, J. N., Jacobsen, L. K., Hamburger, S. D., Krain, A. L., Rapoport, J. L., & Castellanos, F. X. (1998). Cerebellum in attention-deficit hyperactivity disorder: A morphometric MRI study. *Neurology, 50*, 1087–1093.

Burd, L., Kauffman, D. W., & Kerbeshian, J. (1992). Tourette syndrome and learning disabilities. *Journal of Learning Disabilities, 25*, 598–604.

Crowe, F. W., Schull, W. J., & Neel. J. V. (1956). *A clinical, pathological, and genetic study of multiple neurofibromatosis*. Springfield, IL: Charles C Thomas.

Cutting, L. E., Cooper, K. L., Koth, C. W., Mostofsky, S. H., Kates, W. R., Denckla, M. B., & Kaufmann, W. E. (in press). Megalencephaly in NF1: Predominantly white matter contribution and mitigation by ADHD. *Neurology*.

Cutting, L. E., Huang, G., Zeger, S., Koth, C. W., & Denckla, M. B. (2002). Specific cognitive functions remain "spared" and "impaired" over time in children with neurofibromatosis type–1: Growth curve analyses of neuropsychological profiles. *Journal of the International Neuropsychological Society, 8*, 838–846.

Cutting, L. E., Koth, C. W., Burnette, C. P., Abrams, M. T., Kaufmann, W. E., & Denckla, M. B. (2000). The relationship of cognitive functioning, whole brain volumes, and T–2 weighted hyperintensities in neurofibromatosis type 1. *Journal of Child Neurology, 15*, 157–160.

Cutting, L. E., Koth, C. W., & Denckla, M. B. (2000). How children with neurofibromatosis type 1 differ from "typical" learning disabled clinic attenders: Nonverbal learning disabilities revisited. *Developmental Neuropsychology, 17*, 29–47.

Cutting, L. E., Koth, C. W., Mahone, E. M., & Denckla, M. B. (in press). Evidence for Unexpected Weaknesses in Learning in Children with attention deficit hyperactivity disorder without reading disabilities. *Journal of Learning Disabilities*.

Davis, C. J., Knopik, V. S., Olson, R. K., Wadsworth, S. J., & DeFries, J. C. (2001). Genetic and environmental influences on rapid naming and reading ability: A twin study. *Annals of Dyslexia, 51*, 231–247.

DeFries, J. C., & Alarcón, M. (1996). Genetics of specific reading disability. *Mental Retardation and Developmental Disabilities Research Reviews, 2*, 39–47.

DeFries, J. C., Filipek, P. A., Fulker, D. W., Olson, R. K., Pennington, B. F., Smith, S. D., & Wise, B. W. (1997). Colorado Learning Disabilities Research Center. *Learning Disabilities: A Multidisciplinary Journal, 8*, 7–19.

Denckla, M. B., Hofman, K., Mazzocco, M. M., Melham, E., Reiss, A. L., Bryan, R. N., Harris, E. L., Lee, J., Cox, C. S., & Schuerholz, L. J. (1996). Relationship between T2-weighted hyperintensities (UBOs) and lower IQs in children with neurofibromatosis–1. *American Journal of Medical Genetics, 67,* 98–102.

Denckla, M. B., & Rudel, R. G. (1976). Rapid Automatized Naming Test (R. A. N.): Dyslexia differentiated from other learning disabilities. *Neuropsychologia, 14,* 471–479.

Denckla M. B., & Rudel R. G. (1978). Anomalies of motor development in hyperactive boys without learning disabilities. *Annals of Neurology, 3,* 231–233.

Dilts, C. V., Carey, J. C., Kircher, J. C., Hoffman, R. O., Creel, D., Ward, K., Clark, E., & Leonard, C. O. (1996). Children and adolescents with neurofibromatosis 1: A behavioral phenotype. *Developmental and Behavioral Pediatrics, 17,* 229–239.

DiMario, F. J., Jr., & Ramsby, G. (1998). Magnetic resonance imaging lesion analysis in neurofibromatosis type 1. *Archives of Neurology, 55,* 500–505.

DiPaolo, D. P., Zimmerman, R. A., Rorke, L. B., Zackai, E. H., Bilaniuk, L. T., & Yachnis, T. A. (1995). Neurofibromatosis type 1: Pathologic substrate of high-signal intensity foci in the brain. *Radiology, 195,* 721–724.

Eliason, M. J. (1986). Neurofibromatosis: Implications for learning and behavior. *Journal of Developmental Pediatrics, 7,* 175–179.

Fredericksen, K. A., Cutting, L. E., Kates, W. R., Mostofsky, S. H., Singer, H. S., Cooper, K. L., Lanham, D. C., Denckla, M. B., & Kaufmann, W. E. (2002). Disproportionate increases of white matter in right frontal lobe in Tourette syndrome. *Neurology, 58,* 85–89.

Friedman, J. M. (1999). Epidemiology of neurofibromatosis type 1. *American Journal of Medical Genetics, 89,* 1–6.

Geary, D. C. (1990). A componential analysis of an early learning deficit in mathematics. *Journal of Experimental Child Psychology, 49,* 363–383.

Geary, D. C. (1992). Counting knowledge and skill in cognitive addition: A comparison of normal and mathematically disabled children. *Journal of Experimental Child Psychology, 54,* 372–391.

Geary, D. C. (1993). Mathematical disabilities: Cognitive, neuropsychological, and genetic components. *Psychological Bulletin, 114,* 345–362.

Golden, G. S. (1984). Gilles de la Tourette's syndrome following methylphenidate administration. *Developmental Medicine and Child Neurology, 16,* 76–78.

Goldgar, D. E., Green, P., Parry, D. M., & Mulvhill, J. J. (1989). Multipoint linkage analysis in neurofibromatosis type 1: An international collaboration. *American Journal of Human Genetics, 44,* 6–12.

Gutman, D. H., & Collins, F. S. (1993). Neurofibromatosis type 1: Beyond positional cloning. *Archives of Neurology, 50,* 1185–1193.

Harris, E. L., Schuerholz, L. J., Singer, H. S., Reader, M. J., Brown, J. E., Cox, C., Mohr, J., Chase, G. A., & Denckla, M. B. (1995). Executive function in children with Tourette syndrome and/or attention deficit hyperactivity disorder. *Journal of*

the *International Neuropsychological Society, 1,* 511–516.

Hofman, K. J., Harris, E. L., Bryan, N., & Denckla, M. B. (1994). Neurofibromatosis type 1: The cognitive phenotype. *Journal of Pediatrics, 124,* S1–S8.

Hooper, S. R., Swartz, C. W., Wakely, M. B., de Kruif, R. E. L., & Montgomery, J. W. (2002). Executive functions in elementary school children with and without problems in written expression. *Journal of Learning Disabilities, 35,* 57–68.

Itoh, T., Magnaldi, S., White, R. M., Denckla, M. B., Hofman, K. J., & Naidu, S., & Bryan, R. (1994). Neurofibromatosis type 1: The evolution of deep gray and white matter MRI abnormalities. *American Journal of Neurology, 15,* 1–7.

Koth, C. W., Cutting, L. E., & Denckla, M. B. (2000). The association of neurofibromatosis type 1 and attention deficit hyperactivity disorder. *Child Neuropsychology, 6,* 185–194.

Kraut, M. A., Gerring, J. P., Cooper, K. L., Thompson, R. E., Denckla, M. B., & Kaufmann, W. E. (2002). *Longitudinal evolution of T2-weighted hyperintensities in children with neurofibromatosis Type 1.* Manuscript submitted for publication.

Leckman, J. F., & Cohen, D. J. (1999). Evolving models of pathogenesis. In J. F. Leckman & D. J. Cohen (Eds.), *Tourette's syndrome: Tics, obsessions, compulsions* (pp. 155–176). New York: Wiley.

Leckman, J. F., King, R. A., & Cohen, D. J. (1999). Tic and tic disorders. In J. F. Leckman & D. J. Cohen (Eds.), *Tourette's syndrome: Tics, obsessions, compulsions* (pp. 23–42). New York: Wiley.

Lyon, G. R. (1995). Toward a definition of dyslexia. *Annals of Dyslexia, 45,* 3–27.

Mackintosh, N. J. (1998). *IQ and human intelligence.* Oxford: Oxford University Press.

Mahone, E. M., Cirino, P. T., Cutting, L. E., Cerrone, P. M., Hagelthorn, K. M., Hiemenz, J. R., Singer, H. S., & Denckla. M. B. (in press). Validity of the Behavior Rating Inventory of Executive Function in children with ADHD and/or Tourette Syndrome. *Archives of Clinical Neuropsychology*

Mahone, E. M., Koth, C. W., Cutting, L. E., Singer, H. S., & Denckla, M. B. (2001). Executive function in fluency and recall measures among children with Tourette syndrome or ADHD. *Journal of the International Neuropsychological Society, 7,* 102–111.

Mazzocco, M. M. M. (2001). Math learning disability and math ld subtypes: Evidence from studies of Turner syndrome, fragile x syndrome, and neurofibromatosis type 1. *Journal of Learning Disabilities, 34,* 520–533.

Mazzocco, M. M. M., Turner, J. E., Denckla, M. B., Hofman, K. J., Scanlon, D. C., & Vellutino, F. R. (1995). Language and reading deficits associated with NF1: evidence for not-so-nonverbal learning disability. *Developmental Neuroscience, 11,* 503–522.

Moore, B. D., Slopis, J. M., Jackson, E. F., De Winter, A. E., & Leeds, N. E. (2000). Brain volume in children with neurofibromatosis type 1: Relation to neuropsychological status. *Neurology, 54,* 914–920.

Moore, B. D., Slopis, J. M., Schomer, D., Jackson, E. F., & Levy, B. M. (1996). Neuropsychological significance of areas of high signal intensity on brain MRIs of children with neurofibromatosis. *Neurology, 46,* 1660–1668.

Mostofsky, S. H., Cooper, K. L., Kates, W. R., Denckla, M. B., & Kaufmann, W. E. (in press). Smaller prefrontal and premotor volumes in boys with attention deficit/hyperactivity disorder. *Biological Psychiatry, 52,* 785–794.

Mostofsky, S. H., Lasker, A. G., Singer, H. S., Denckla, M. B., & Zee, D. S. (2001). Oculomotor abnormalities in boys with Tourette syndrome with and without ADHD. *Journal of the American Academy of Child and Adolescent Psychiatry, 40,* 1464–1472.

Mostofsky, S. H., Reiss, A. L., Lockhart, P., & Denckla, M. B. (1998). Evaluation of cerebellar size in attention deficit hyperactivity disorder. *Journal of Child Neurology, 13,* 434–439.

North, K. N., Joy, P., Yuille, D., Cocks, N., Mobbs, E., Hutchins, P., McHugh, K., & de Silva, M. (1994). Specific learning disability in children with neurofibromatosis type 1: Significance of MRI abnormalities. *Neurology, 44,* 878–883.

North, K. N., Riccardi, V., Samango-Sprouse, C., Ferner, R., Moore B., Legius E., Ratner, N., & Denckla, M. B. (1997). Cognitive function and academic performance in neurofibromatosis 1: consensus statement from the NF1 cognitive disorders task force. *Neurology, 48,* 1121–1127.

Ozonoff, S. (1999). Cognitive impairment in neurofibromatosis type 1. *American Journal of Medical Genetics, 89,* 45–52.

Reader, M. J., Harris, E. L., Schuerholz, L. J., & Denckla, M. B. (1994). Attention deficit hyperactivity disorder and executive dysfunction. *Developmental Neuropsychology, 10,* 493–512.

Riccardi, V. M. (1981). Von Recklinghausen neurofibromatosis. *New England Journal of Medicine, 305,* 1617–1627.

Said, S. M., Yeh, T. L., Greenwood, R. S., Whitt, J. K., Tupler, L. A., & Krishman, K. R. (1996). MRI morphometric analysis and neuropsychological function in patients with neurofibromatosis. *Neuroreport, 7,* 1941–1944.

Schuerholz, L. J., Baumgardner, T. L., Singer, H. S., Reiss, A. L., & Denckla, M. B. (1996). Neuropsychological status of children with Tourette's syndrome with and without attention deficit hyperactivity disorder. *Neurology, 46,* 958–965.

Schuerholz, L. J., Cutting, L. E., Mazzocco, M. M.,

Singer, H. S., & Denckla, M. B. (1997). Neuromotor functioning in children with Tourette syndrome with and without attention deficit hyperactivity disorder. *Neurology, 12,* 438–442.

Shaywitz, S. E., & Shaywitz, B. A. (1999). Dyslexia: From epidemiology to neurobiology. In D. D. Duane (Ed.), *Reading and attention disorders: Neurobiological correlates* (pp. 113–128). Timonium, MD: York Press.

Shue, K. L., & Douglas, V. I. (1992). Attention deficit hyperactivity disorder and the frontal lobe syndrome. *Brain and Cognition, 20,* 104–124.

Singer, H. S., Reiss, A. L., Brown, J. E., Aylward, E. H., Shih, B., Chee, E., Harris, E. L., Reader, M. J., Chase, G. A., & Bryan, R. N. (1993). Volumetric MRI changes in basal ganglia of children with Tourette's syndrome. *Neurology, 43,* 950–956.

Singer, H. S., Schuerholz, L. J., & Denckla, M. B. (1995). Learning difficulties in children with Tourette's syndrome. *Journal of Child Neurology, 10,* S58–S61.

Smith, S. D, Kelley, P. M., Askew, J. W., Hoover, D. M., Deffenbacher, K. E., Gayan, J., Brower, A. M., & Olson, R. K. (2001). Reading disability and chromosome 6p21. 3: Evolution of MOG as a candidate gene. *Journal of Learning Disabilities, 34,* 512–519.

Steen, R. G., Taylor, J. S., Langston, J. W., Glass, J. O., Brewer, V. R., Reddick, W. E., Mages, R., & Pivnick, E. K. (2001). Prospective evaluation of the brain in asymptomatic children with neurofibromatosis type 1: Relationship of macrocephaly to T1 relaxation changes and structural brain abnormalities. *American Journal of Neuroradiology, 22,* 810–817.

Stine, S. B., & Adams, W. V. (1989). Learning problems in neurofibromatosis patients. *Clinical Orthopaedics and Related Research, 245,* 43–48.

Stumpf, D. A., Alksne, J. F., & Annegers, J. F. (1988). Neurofibromatosis. *Archives of Neurology, 45,* 575–578.

Wang, P. Y., Kaufmann, W. E., Koth, C. W., Denckla, M. B., & Barker, P. B. (2000). Thalamic involvement in neurofibromatosis type 1: Evaluation with proton MR spectroscopic imaging. *Annals of Neurology, 47,* 477–487.

Weschler, D. (1974). *Weschler Intelligence Scale for Children—Revised.* New York: Psychological Corporation.

Wolf, M., & Bowers, P. G. (1999). The double-deficit hypothesis for the developmental dyslexias. *Journal of Educational Psychology, 91,* 415–438.

9

RAN's Contribution to
Understanding Reading Disabilities

Patricia Greig Bowers
Galit Ishaik

Much research evidence has accumulated demonstrating that phonological processing, especially sensitivity to the individual phonemes in oral language, plays an important role in learning to read not only English but other languages as well. A major issue for the field investigating cognitive bases for reading disabilities is that of the sufficiency of this factor in explaining reading difficulties. Are other cognitive differences (e.g., working memory and naming speed) which characterize reading disabled versus normally achieving readers just correlates of the phonological problems or consequences of poor reading? Or, are they somewhat independent correlates or causes of reading difficulties? This chapter addresses one variable for which this question has been debated, the rapid naming of highly familiar visual symbols. Is slow naming a marker for underlying problems associated with reading acquisition not explained by phonological difficulties (Bowers & Wolf, 1993; Wolf & Bowers, 1999)? Or, is slow naming speed a type of phonological problem partially distinct from phoneme awareness but still tapping a similar underlying deficit (e.g., Wagner, Torgesen, & Rashotte, 1994)? Although the debate about the nature of the deficit un-

derlying slow naming has not been resolved, the results of the many studies in this area have enriched our knowledge about reading acquisition and reading fluency. The perspective taken in this chapter is that slow naming speed marks a second core deficit associated with reading disabilities whose effects are reflected in a particular profile of reading skills.

The possibility that naming simple visual stimuli and reading tap similar processes was first suggested by Geschwind (1965a, 1965b). However, Denckla (1972) and Denckla and Rudel (1974, 1976) provided evidence that it was the speed rather than the accuracy of naming such stimuli (letters, digits, color patches, and pictures of simple objects) that was related to reading skill. They reported that naming speed for stimulus arrays (five highly familiar items repeated 10 times in semirandom order) distinguished children with reading disabilities from children with other learning disabilities as well as from normally achieving children. They called the test they devised Rapid Automatized Naming (RAN). (Figure 9.1 displays the RAN Digits format.) Number and letter arrays are usually the more sensitive discriminators of reading

2	6	4	9	7	2	6	4	7	9
9	7	2	6	4	7	2	9	4	6
7	4	6	2	9	4	6	2	9	7
4	6	2	7	9	2	4	9	7	6
6	2	7	9	4	7	6	2	4	9

FIGURE 9.1. RAN Digits. Adapted from Denckla and Rudel (1974).

skill (e.g., Wolf, Bally, & Morris, 1986), but in samples containing young children or severely dyslexic participants, time to name color and object arrays also distinguish groups well (e.g., Meyer, Wood, Hart, & Felton, 1998).

The RAN format has been adopted by many researchers. However, other formats have also been used. For example, as early as 1974, Spring and Capps reported that the speed of naming 50 single digits on one line was associated with reading disability. Recently, a rapid naming test with a slightly different format has been included in the Comprehensive Test of Phonological Processing (Wagner, Torgesen, & Rashotte, 1999), with published normative information. Denckla and Wolf (in press) are publishing RAN stimuli closer to the original set and format with normative data. The terms "RAN," "rapid naming," and "naming speed" are often used interchangeably to indicate serial list measures, with performance reported either by the time to name whole lists or by items per second, a metric with better psychometric properties. Wolf (1986) has developed a "Rapid Alternating Stimuli" (RAS) serial list, which alternates numbers and letters or numbers, letters, and colors. RAS discriminates dyslexics from controls well but is not further reviewed here.

During the 1980s, Blachman (1984), Mann (1984), Wolf (1982), Bowers, Steffy, and Swanson (1986), and Wagner and Torgesen (1987) independently pursued the role naming speed played in the emerging picture of the correlates and precursors of reading disability or dyslexia. Research in the 1990s investigated a variety of topics, such as rapid naming's relationships to various reading subskills and its degree of independence from other cognitive processes related to dyslexia. Other questions addressed were whether speed of processing deficits were limited to the language domain and whether the relationship between naming speed and reading was found in languages other than English. Naming speed's role in predicting response to remediation attempts and the type of remediation particularly relevant to children with naming-speed deficits have been investigated more recently. A theoretical basis for the empirical relationships between naming speed and reading has been much more difficult to establish, but some progress along these lines is described later in the chapter.

Our lab's contribution to this literature has been to help establish the parameters of the RAN–reading relationship and to explore theoretical issues concerning its basis. Our empirical work has been conducted using children in grades 2 through 5 in normal, publicly funded classrooms in several small cities in Ontario. Sampling strategies have varied. Some studies report results from the whole range of abilities found in such classrooms, whereas other studies screen subjects from those classrooms to fit subtypes based on rapid naming and phonemic awareness (PA) measures. PA is typically assessed by a phoneme deletion measure, the Auditory Analysis Test (Rosner & Simon, 1971). Another strategy is selecting children considered reading disabled, chronological age controls, and sometimes reading age controls. Children are called reading disabled or poor readers if they score at or below the 25th percentile on standardized tests of word recognition. Because speed of naming simple items increases with age for all children, with gains diminishing by grade 5 for normal readers (Flowers, Meyer, Lovato, Felton, & Wood, 2001), we have preferred to study children in a small age range to minimize the impact of age-related variance. In our samples, the reliability of rapid naming tests is impressive: test–retest reliabilities are above .90 and stability over 1- and 2-year periods above .85. Our work over the years reflects the three broad themes outlined below, which are then reviewed in greater depth.

Our initial focus was to investigate the independence of rapid naming's contribution to reading from that of phonological awareness, memory span, and verbal ability. The early work revealed that controlling for memory span or verbal ability in samples from either clinic (Bowers, Steffy, & Tate, 1988) or classroom (e.g., Bowers & Swanson, 1991) did not appreciably affect the moderately strong relationships found between rapid naming and reading. Determining the extent of the independent versus overlapping contributions of phoneme awareness and naming speed to a variety of different skills in reading was a much more complex task.

A second focus of research involved a fruitful and continuing collaboration with Maryanne Wolf of Tufts University. During a sabbatical at Tufts in 1990–1991, Bowers and Wolf joined forces to try to understand the implications of work on rapid naming done in our respective labs (and those of others) for theories of dyslexia, especially delayed growth of orthographic skill. While our initial conceptualization was published in Bowers and Wolf (1993), the University of Waterloo lab has continued to explore the association between orthographic processing and rapid naming (e.g., Bowers, Golden, Kennedy, & Young, 1994; Bowers, Sunseth, & Golden, 1999). In addition, both Wolf and Bowers have pursued the implications of the separable contributions to reading of phonological awareness and naming speed by positing subtypes of readers with no, only one, or "double" deficits in the two cognitive skills. Wolf has explored effects of interventions for severely dyslexic children, typically those with double deficits. She and her colleagues (Wolf, Miller, & Donnelly, 2000) developed a remediation program, "Retrieval, Automaticity, Vocabulary Elaboration, Orthography (RAVE-O)," as a supplement to phonological training; it targets remediation of the fluency and orthographic skill deficits associated with slow RAN.

A third focus of our work has been to understand the "why" of the association between rapid naming and reading (e.g., Bowers, 2001; Bowers & Wolf, 1993; Wolf & Bowers, 1999). Specifically, what types of processes relevant to reading are being tapped by this simple test? We explored this issue in the early years by comparing different formats for rapid naming and later by devising measures to test theoretical links between RAN and specific aspects of reading skill.

Focus 1: Independent Contributions of RAN to Reading

Should rapid naming be considered one of several phonological skills as suggested by Wagner and colleagues (1994)? Or, are the phonological aspects of rapid naming only part of its complex nature, with individual differences in the ability to rapidly integrate several processes the more distinctive attribute of the test (Wolf, 1991; Wolf, Bowers, & Biddle, 2000)? Many studies have used factor-analytic techniques to determine the factor structure of various reading-related tasks (e.g, DeJong & van der Leij, 1999, in Dutch; Wagner et al., 1994, in English-speaking samples; Wagner & Torgesen, 1987). Measures of these variables form three factors reflecting phonemic awareness, phonological memory, and RAN, with the first two factors being more strongly correlated with each other than with rapid naming. Recent work in our lab (Ishaik, Bowers, & Steffy, 2001) suggests that measures of verbal working memory (involving both storage and manipulation of verbal material) overlap considerably with phoneme deletion and sound categorization, common measures of phoneme awareness, but are distinct from rapid naming when predicting reading accuracy.

An early concern in our lab was whether phonemic awareness and rapid naming were related to different types of reading skill. Average and poor readers were selected in grade 2 and followed until grade 4, providing evidence about the concurrent and predictive relationships between these variables and a variety of reading skills (Bowers, 1995; Bowers & Swanson, 1991). Controlling for oral vocabulary skill, both phonemic awareness and rapid naming typically contributed shared and unique variance to word recognition, with phonemic awareness playing a larger role. Rapid naming's unique contribution to nonword decoding was small relative to the strong contribution of phonemic awareness. However, RAN's strong, unique contribution to the latency of correct identification of regular and exception words, whether of high or moderate frequency, as well as to reading comprehension, contrasted with the insignificant unique contribution of phonemic awareness to these measures. Naming speed's contribution to reading comprehension was fully explained through its association with latency of word recognition. Levy (2001) reviewed work highlighting the central importance of word recognition speed to reading fluency and comprehension and confirmed the special relationship of RAN to such speed.

The pattern of differential relationships of phonemic awareness and naming speed to types of reading skill found in the early study in our lab has been replicated in several other studies (e.g., Carver, 1997; Cornwall, 1992; Manis, Doi, & Bhadha, 2000; Manis, Seidenberg, & Doi, 1999; Torgesen, Wagner, Rashotte, Burgess, & Hecht, 1997). Table 9.1 (excerpted from Manis et al., 2000) highlights this finding. It is based on 85 children tested at the end of grade 2 who were representative of the full range of reading abilities in classrooms of two public elementary schools. Only children with limited English were excluded from the study. For the Commonality Analyses presented here, Wechsler Intelligence Scale for Children—III (WISC-III; Wechsler, 1991) Vocabulary was entered at Step 1 to control for general verbal ability. Then a measure of RAN and of phoneme awareness was entered at Steps 2 or 3 to provide estimates of the common and unique variance contributed to various reading measures. Both RAN Digits and Letters were administered and PA was measured by both Sound Deletion and Sound Blending. In general, stronger relations were evident for RAN Letters and for Sound Deletion, and these are presented here. However, the pattern was similar for both measures of each construct. That the pattern of relationship strength differs for PA and RAN is evident from Table 9.1. Other researchers do not always find such strong relationships (e.g., Torgesen et al., 1997), but the patterns are replicated. Reflecting a profile opposite to that of phonemic awareness, RAN is more related to recognition of exception words and to knowledge of orthographic patterns than to phonological decoding.

Levy (2001) underlines an important distinction between factors associated with learning to read unfamiliar words and factors associated with speeding the processing of print by automatizing access to representations of words already somewhat familiar to the child. RAN is related to both factors but perhaps in different ways. To study each of these factors, different designs are required. Study of automatizing access to print, as indexed by text reading speed, presupposes a high level of reading accuracy. If text is too difficult, poor readers' decoding deficits will affect speed and obscure the view of other factors also affecting fluency. Therefore, careful choice of text is imperative to a study of determinants of fluent reading (Young & Bowers, 1995). Noting the strong relationship between rapid naming and latency of correct word recognition, researchers in our lab and others have looked at predictors of reading fluency before and after practice with text. The children in the longitudinal study reported earlier (i.e., Bowers & Swanson, 1991) took part each year in a study of repeated reading of text chosen to be at a level of difficulty appropriate to each child's reading skill (Bowers, 1993). Not surprisingly, their text

TABLE 9.1. Hierarchical Regression Analyses Predicting Reading Subskills: Unique and Common Variance for RAN-Letters (RAN) and Sound Deletion (PA)

Variable	Word Identification	Nonwords	Word Attack	Comprehension	Orthographic Choice	Letter String Choice	Exception Words
Vocabulary	13.6***	8.1**	5.7*	23.4***	1.6	0.5	11.8**
Common RAN–PA	16.8	12.9	12.4	9.7	10.9	9.5	16.0
RAN unique	17.1***	7.1**	5.5**	9.3***	12.8***	11.0**	21.7***
PA unique	13.9***	18.7***	27.7***	12.3***	7.6**	4.2*	9.6***

Note. From Manis, Doi, and Bhadha (2000, Table 3, p. 329) Copyright 2000 by Pro-Ed, Inc. Adapted with permission.
*$p < .05$; **$p < .01$; ***$p < .001$.

reading speed on the first reading of the text was associated with their digit naming speed. However, the fluency of those children with better naming speed increased more after repeated reading of text than did the fluency of slower naming children, even after controlling for initial fluency. A subsequent study of practice with words and nonwords reported in Bowers and Kennedy (1993) and a study of text reading by Young (1997) with grade 5 children with reading disabilities produced a similar pattern of results. That is, rapid naming was associated not only with initial fluency but also with gains in fluency after practice, suggesting greater automatizing skill of those with faster naming speed. Not all studies have confirmed the details of these results. For example, Levy, Abello, and Lysynchuk (1997) found word and text practice as successful in increasing word recognition speed for slow RAN poor readers as it was for faster RAN poor readers.

Although the connection between reading speed and RAN is especially strong, word recognition accuracy is also associated with RAN, as evident in Table 9.1. Measured in kindergarten or grade 1, RAN predicts reading accuracy in grades 1 to 3 (Wagner et al., 1997; Wolf et al., 1986) and even in grade 5 (Kirby, Parrila, & Pfeiffer, 2001). Differences in naming speed between children with reading disabilities and normally achieving children are found at many ages (e.g., Lovett, 1987). Even adult dyslexics continue to be characterized by slow naming speed (e.g., Felton, Naylor, & Wood, 1990). Success in learning to read English as a second language is predicted by phonological awareness and naming speed (Geva, Yaghoub-Zadeh, & Schuster, 2000), just as is learning to read English when it is one's native language.

Variability on RAN within poor reader groups is associated with reading performance as well. McBride-Chang and Manis (1996) found that both rapid naming and phonemic awareness contributed independently to variability in reading accuracy within a poor reader group, but variance in oral vocabulary did not. On the other hand, within an average-and-above reader group, rapid naming contributed no independent variance to reading, but both phonemic awareness and oral vocabulary did. Similar-

ly, Meyer and colleagues (1998) report that variance in rapid naming in grade 3 poor readers was related predictively to grade 8 reading skill, whereas in grade 3 average readers, it was unrelated to grade 8 skill. Davis, Knopik, Olson, Wadsworth, and De-Fries (2001) found that the correlation between RAN and reading in a group of twins, at least one of whom had a reading disability ("low range group"), was higher than in the group of control twins, neither of whom had a reading disability ("normal range group"). Not all studies have found stronger correlations between RAN and reading in samples composed of just poor readers (e.g., Torgesen et al., 1997). Nevertheless, an implication of findings may be that RAN contributes variance to reading accuracy measures in the lower ranges of skill, while only its relationship to reading fluency may persist at higher levels.

RAN deficits are heritable to some extent (e.g., Compton, Davis, DeFries, Gayan, & Olson, 2001; Davis et al., 2001). Compton and colleagues (2001) report separable heritabilities for phonemic awareness and rapid naming in their sample of monozygotic and dizygotic twins. Furthermore, "subjects with deficits in alphanumeric RAN skill tend to have deficits in word reading skills that are influenced, in part, by a common set of genes" (Compton et al., 2001, p. 285). Grigorenko and colleagues (2001) have suggested locations on chromosome 1 and 6 for reading impairments associated with rapid naming, a linkage especially strong for those with deficits in both rapid naming and phonemic awareness.

Research investigating the role of RAN in reading achievement in languages other than English has been especially informative. Compared to its role in English-speaking samples, RAN plays a relatively larger role in prediction of reading in languages such as German (Wimmer, 1993) and Dutch (Van den Bos, 1998). In those languages, phonological demands are more easily met than in English due to the higher regularity of symbol/sound correspondence. Accuracy of word recognition of German-speaking dyslexics is quite high by grade 2 (as is phonemic awareness). Nevertheless, slow reading and poor spelling are persistent bottlenecks to performance (Wimmer, Mayringer, & Landerl, 2000) and, consistent with English-language research, are associated with slow RAN. As well, Chinese dyslexics are characterized by RAN deficits even more strongly than by phonological awareness deficits (Ho, 2001), presumably because Chinese orthography does not require as much reliance on the phoneme level of analysis of words as does English. Phonological memory (i.e., immediate repetition of digits and of syllables presented auditorially) discriminated Chinese dyslexics from both chronological-age and reading-age controls, and rapid naming, whether on continuous lists or discrete item presentations, discriminated Chinese dyslexics from age controls (Ho & Lai, 2000).

The degree to which RAN deficits are specific to reading difficulties as distinct from other learning and attention problems has been another area of concern. Denckla and Rudel (1976) reported such specificity in comparison to other learning disorders. More recently, researchers have distinguished samples of children diagnosed as attention-deficit/hyperactivity disorder (ADHD) with and without reading disability (RD) and those with RD alone or no diagnosis; they found that RAN was associated with RD, not ADHD (Felton, Wood, Brown, & Campbell, 1987; Nigg, Hinshaw, Carte, & Treuting, 1998). Several researchers have reported an interesting distinction between the more automatized RAN digits and letters and the less automatized RAN colors and objects. It appears ADHD and control children do not differ on RAN Digits or Letters but do differ on RAN objects or colors (Carte, Nigg, & Hinshaw, 1996; Semrud-Clikeman, Guy, & Griffin, 2000; Tannock, Martinussen, & Frijters, 2000). The specificity of the relationship between naming speed for the more automatized symbols and reading disabilities compared to the more general relationship of naming speed for stimuli requiring more controlled processing is a fascinating pattern worthy of further study. Although the literature is sparse, RAN deficits may be associated with arithmetic computation difficulties as well as reading disabilities (Hecht, Torgesen, Wagner, & Rashotte, 2001), perhaps associated with the commonly found covariance between disabilities in math and reading. Greater research focus on math disability is needed

before conclusions can be drawn with confidence.

In summary, slow naming speed forms a factor separate from factors for phonemic awareness or working memory. It is highly related to fluent reading and has a profile of relationships to measures of reading subskill accuracy different from that of phonemic awareness. For example, unlike phoneme deletion, RAN is related more strongly to orthographic skill than to phonemic decoding. RAN is more highly related to reading in samples of readers of low skill, such as beginning readers or children with RD than in higher-skilled samples. RAN deficits are heritable somewhat separately from phonemic awareness deficits. RAN's role in reading proficiency varies according to the characteristics of the orthography of the language. For example, in languages in which decoding is "easy" due to the high regularity of symbol–sound correspondence, RAN plays a larger role in distinguishing dyslexics from normally achieving readers than it does in English. RAN alphanumeric deficits do not characterize ADHD children without a reading disorder but may be associated with arithmetic computation difficulties.

Focus 2: The Double-Deficit Hypothesis

The fact of independent contributions to reading skill by phonemic awareness and rapid naming, and the differential profile of contributions to reading subskills, led to the hypothesis that children with deficits in both skills would be the poorest readers (Bowers & Wolf, 1993; Wolf & Bowers, 1999). This pattern of data was demonstrated by reanalysis of several data sets in the Wolf and the Bowers labs, as well as labs of Manis and of Lovett (Lovett, Steinbach, & Frijters, 2000; Manis et al., 2000; Wolf, Bowers, & Biddle, 2000). In several types of samples, it was possible to select children without deficits in either skill, with only a deficit in one but not the other skill, and those with double deficits. The no-deficit and double-deficit groups were the best and worst readers across many measures, with single-deficit children having variable profiles, sometimes similar to each other on reading tasks and sometimes different.

Many studies have adopted a subtyping strategy but have varied the selection criteria when studying children with these deficit patterns. Work in our lab has typically screened full class samples to select children with strengths and/or weaknesses in RAN and phoneme deletion skill (Baker, 2002; Bowers et al., 1999; Sunseth & Bowers, 2002), a strategy also used by Manis and colleagues (2000). Reading scores are free to vary with such a strategy. Other studies have first selected poor readers (e.g., Lovett et al., 2001; Meyer et al., 1998; Morris et al., 1998) and then defined subgroups by RAN and PA scores among other variables. In another variation, children who are poor readers (e.g., Levy, Bourassa, & Horn, 1999) have been subdivided into those with relatively slow or fast RAN. The children in both groups have poor phonological skills, and therefore represent a single-phonological-deficit group and a double-deficit group.

Varied selection methods have led to somewhat varied details of the findings. Results from sampling full classrooms are discussed first. Subtypes based on RAN and PA screening of children from full grade 3 classes (Bowers et al., 1999; Sunseth & Bowers, 2002), have found single-naming-speed-deficit children (above 50th percentile for their grade in phonemic awareness and below 30th percentile in rapid naming) scoring in the average range on word identification tasks but being slow readers on easy text and poor spellers. They had especially poor performance on a spelling recognition test in which the correct spelling of a word needed to be chosen from several foils. Single-phonological-deficit children (above the 50th percentile in rapid naming and below the 30th percentile on phonemic awareness) were low average in word recognition but read the easy text reasonably quickly; they had similarly poor spelling skill. Both groups scored below the level of no-deficit children on all spelling tasks.

TABLE 9.2. Performance of Subtypes of Grade 3 Children

Measures	Double asset ($n = 17$)	Phonological deficit ($n = 17$)	Naming speed deficit ($n = 18$)	Double deficit ($n = 16$)
Defining variables				
AAT	23.2 (3.2)[a]	11.4 (2.4)[b]	22.4(2.6)[a]	11.3 (2.7)[b]
RAN:D items/sec	2.1 (.3)[a]	2.1 (.2)[a]	1.5 (.1)[b]	1.4 (.2)[b]
Reading Accuracy Standard Scores (*WJ-R tests*; Woodcock & Johnson, 1989)				
Word Identification	116.9 (16.0)[a]	92.2 (9.1)[bc]	100.3 (16.3)[c]	83.8 (6.9)[b]
Word Attack	120.1 (22.2)[a]	88.4 (7.8)[b]	100.2 (11.9)[c]	82.3 (6.5)[b]
Reading speed and accuracy on GORT III "easy" passage (Wiederholt & Bryant, 1992)				
Seconds	15.3 (4.6)[a]	21.3 (4.8)[b]	31.5 (13.8)[c]	37.1 (11.1)[c]
Errors	0.1 (.3)[a]	.4 (.8)[ab]	1.3 (2.7)[ab]	2.1 (1.8)[b]
Spelling Standard Scores				
Dictation (Test of Written Spelling III; Larsen & Hammill, 1994)				
Predictable words	103.5 (10.5)[a]	89.4 (10.2)[b]	91.7 (6.0)[b]	84.9 (6.6)[b]
Unpredictable	97.5 (14.5)[a]	88.2 (9.0)[b]	88.2 (10.7)[b]	80.9 (6.8)[b]
Recognition (Peabody Individual Achievement Test—Revised; Markwardt Jr., 1989)	96.5 (13.7)[a]	85.8 (7.0)[b]	81.4 (8.5)[bc]	78.9 (5.5)[c]

Note. Values sharing superscripts do not differ from each other. Data from Sunseth & Bowers (2002).

However, whether they differed significantly from double-deficit children was less predictable. Table 9.2 highlights some of the results reported by Sunseth and Bowers (2002).

Sunseth and Bowers (2002) found that the single-deficit groups did not differ in the percent of children categorized as poor readers, despite the better word identification scores of single-naming-speed-deficit children on average. (Note however the large standard deviation on Word Identification of these children.) Approximately 30% of either single-deficit group could be considered poor readers using the 25th percentile cutoff definition on a Word Identification test, while over 90% of double-deficit (DD) children were so categorized. Similarly, Bowers and Newby-Clark (2002) report single-deficit groups having 20% poor readers and a DD group with 81% poor readers.

Subtyping full class samples based on kindergarten phonological processing and RAN scores has revealed later reading achievement differences between groups. Kirby and colleagues (2001) found that the grade 5 reading achievement of the DD group lagged behind the no-deficit group by almost 2 years. Interestingly, they also found that unlike the subtyping based on grade 3 scores, the single-RAN-deficit group scored almost as poorly as did the DD group, while the single-PA-deficit group fared much better. That many kindergarten children's PA deficits can be remedied by phonics training, with rapid naming deficits being less affected by interventions, may account for the difference between results of Kirby and colleagues and Sunseth and Bowers.

Another method for categorizing subtypes relevant to the DD hypothesis selects poor readers first and then categorizes them. Most children in such samples (in English-speaking countries) do have a phonological deficit, but there is more variability in rapid naming. Morris and colleagues (1998) found that a subtype defined by cluster analysis that had both PA and RAN deficits was one of the most severely impaired reader groups. Using a simpler strategy, Levy and colleagues (1999) and Levy (2001) divided grade 2 poor readers into groups above and below the median of a poor reader sample on RAN. Called fast

and slow RAN poor readers, their comparably low scores on PA tasks suggest they are equally well described as single phonological deficit (PD) and DD children, respectively. Groups differed initially on relative reading skill, with the slow RAN children worse readers than the faster RAN children. Also in the Levy laboratory, samples of grade 2 poor readers selected by Conrad (2002) found that the slow and fast poor reader groups had similarly poor word identification and phonemic awareness scores. However, the slow RAN group had poorer scores on a careful revision for this age group of the Olson, Kliegl, Davidson, and Foltz (1985) Orthographic Choice test. Choice of the correct spelling of a word from its homophone foil (e.g., truk vs. truck) on this task requires word-specific orthographic knowledge, with decoding skill unhelpful.

Differential response of the deficit groups to instruction has also been studied. Levy and colleagues (1999) investigated effects of training slow and fast RAN (i.e., DD and PD) poor readers. Twenty sessions of word practice were given, varying the unit in the word made salient to participants. That is, words were segmented in both visual and aural presentations based on phonemes or onset/rime, or were presented as whole words. For example, in the onset/rime condition, "band" would be pronounced in a segmented fashion by the examiner as b/and as well as shown visually, with "b" colored differently from "and." Controlling for their initially less skilled reading, DD children made less progress over time than did the children with faster RAN under all conditions of training. Although segmented practice was associated with better progress for all readers, it made a greater difference for the slow RAN (i.e., DD) poor readers, for whom whole word practice was particularly disadvantageous. Levy (2001) pursued this issue by providing whole word practice to comparable DD children in which the phonological information was always at the unsegmented whole word level, but the visual information either did or did not make the rime unit salient. Under whole word conditions in which the rime unit was emphasized visually by training the words in blocks with the same rime, rather than in randomly mixed order, the DD children learned about as well as DD children had in the previous study with words segmented both aurally and visually. These children seem to need extra orthographic support to notice the visual similarities between words.

Lovett and colleagues (2000) reported that in a sample of severely dyslexic children, both single- and double-deficit children made sizable gains after instruction. However, the DD children did not transfer their knowledge to uninstructed words as well as did single-deficit children. Although they used multiple regression procedures rather than a subtyping strategy, Torgesen and colleagues (1999) also found effects of slow RAN on later reading. In their sample of kindergarten children with weak letter naming accuracy and phonemic awareness skill, slower RAN was associated with less response to remediation over a 2½-year period.

In summary, a subtyping scheme based on relative strengths and weaknesses in phonemic awareness and rapid naming has proved robust and useful in distinguishing characteristics of reading in children in full class samples and in samples of children with RD. Children with double deficits typically read more poorly than did children in the other subgroups. Furthermore, within poor reader groups, children with double deficits respond less well to remediation efforts than children with single phonological deficits, even after controlling for any initial differences in reading skill.

Focus 3: Why is Rapid Naming Related to Reading?: Theoretical Explorations

Bowers and Wolf (1993) and Bowers and colleagues (1994) were impressed by evidence for RAN–orthographic skill relationships. Orthographic skill (knowledge and use of the specific letter patterns found in words) is known to be associated with phonological skill and print exposure (Cunningham & Stanovich, 1990). However, RAN contributes additional variance to orthographic skill (e.g., Bowers et al., 1999; Conrad, 2002; Manis & Freedman, 2001; Manis et al., 2000; Sunseth & Bowers, 2002). Bowers and Wolf hypothesized that the rapid naming deficit was associated with reading skill through the processes underlying rapid naming affecting a child's ability

to form orthographic codes for commonly seen letter strings. Many theories of skilled reading posit interacting phonological and orthographic "routes" to word recognition. Perhaps a neat correspondence could be found between a child having double deficits and impairment in both orthographic and phonological routes. Demonstrating clearly such a correspondence has proved difficult.

Several strategies have been employed in an attempt to unravel the mystery of RAN–reading relationships. These include varying the format of the test to explore effects on reading and devising tests tapping hypothesized mediating links between RAN and reading. Although no definitive solution has been found, researchers in our lab and in many others have learned much about the parameters an eventual explanation will need to accommodate.

Initially, Lynn Swanson asked whether the format of the rapid naming test (discrete item vs. serial list) mattered to the association with reading (Bowers, 1995; Bowers & Swanson, 1991; Swanson, 1989). If only the serial list format is predictive of reading, the more limited identification and name retrieval required by report of a single isolated number or letter may not be focal to the relationship. Instead, other processes involved in managing a list of items, including attentional ones, may be more important. Bowers and Swanson (1991) reported that grade 2 average and poor readers differed on both discrete trial naming latencies and serial list items per second. This conclusion was confirmed in the grade 4 data of these children (Bowers, 1995) and replicated recently in Chinese children (Ho & Lai, 2000). Bowers (1995) reported that the two methods of measuring rapid naming correlated highly. However, the serial list had the stronger relation with reading skill, and the contribution to reading of discrete trial latencies was entirely accounted for by the serial list measure. Something "extra" was contributed by the need to name one item and then name the next on the list in quick succession. However, results suggested that preprocessing of the next item on the list did not account for this "extra" variance. Following Swanson (1989), children were presented with a computer task in which five numbers (or letters) were displayed, with an arrow pointing to the one item they were to name, always the item in the second position. Conditions varied the relevance of the items to the right. In the relevant condition block of trials, the item to the immediate right of the target would be the next target to be named; in the irrelevant condition block, it would not be. If faster serial list performance reflected some preprocessing of the items to the right of the target, differences between these conditions, especially for faster RAN children, would be expected. Instead, no differences were found. In summary, although serial list presentation is not necessary to naming speed's association with reading skill, it does provide additional reading-related variance. However, the extra ingredient may not be the preprocessing of subsequent items on the list.

There have been other attempts to understand processes associated with RAN by analyzing serial list performance. Obregon and Wolf (1995) analyzed the responses of children as they named items on the RAN, timing various aspects of the response. Slow and fast RAN children differed only in the length of their pauses between naming items, not in the articulation time for items or in time managing the start of a new row of items. Similarly, Neuhaus, Foorman, Francis, and Carlson (2001) reported that in first- and second-grade students, RAN pause durations for numbers, letters, and objects were differentially related to reading, while articulation duration was rarely related to reading. The RAN letters pause time was the most robust predictor of several reading measures and predicted reading even after controlling for pause time for objects.

Scarborough and Domgaard (1998) tested several hypotheses about the source of the variance in RAN related to reading by devising many different serial list tasks, systematically altering just one variable (e.g., the number of different items in a list). Interestingly, most alterations did not affect the RAN–reading relationship. The one condition crucial to the task was actually naming letters rather than giving a yes/no decision about whether the symbol (printed in different fonts) had a particular name. The decision task reduces the demand to locate a new name because one name is always kept in mind as decisions are made.

This result highlights the crucial role in the RAN–reading relationship played by differential access time to symbol names, consistent with the previously reported correlation with reading of pause duration on serial lists, and latency of response on discrete trials.

How general are the processes that underlie RAN performances? The answer to this question is unclear. Carver (1997) and Kail, Hall, and Caskey (1999) argue that the association reflects general cognitive processing speed. Kail and colleagues found that rapid naming was uniquely predicted by general speed of processing measures (i.e., Visual Matching and Cross-Out tasks from the Woodcock–Johnson Tests of Cognitive Ability). Controlling for age, RAN and print exposure contributed unique variance to reading recognition, but processing speed no longer did. They interpret this pattern of findings to mean that RAN's relationship to reading overlapped with the slightly smaller variance contributed to reading by more general processing speed. They argue that "naming and reading are linked because skilled performance in both naming and reading depends, in part, on the rapid execution of the underlying processes" (p. 312). In a sample of normally achieving children in grades 1 to 3, Cutting and Denckla (2001) report that scores on these same processing speed measures are indirectly related to reading, through variance shared not only with RAN but also with phonemic awareness, memory span, and orthographic knowledge. In our lab, Baker (2002) found that grade 2 DD readers differed from other subgroups on Cross Out and Number Comparison processing speed tasks similar to those used by Kail and colleagues.

This "domain general" view of processing speed's association with reading is contrasted with the "domain specific" view espoused by Wimmer and Mayringer (2001), who used a different set of visual processing tasks. They found that latency of response for visual discrimination tasks not involving familiar letters or numbers did not distinguish German children with rate or accuracy and rate reading problems from normal reading controls, despite RAN deficits discriminating both groups quite well. Conflicting results provide no basis presently for strong conclusions about whether RAN represents domain general versus domain-specific processing speed associated with reading.

A large literature about perceptual processing speed of dyslexics does not focus on RAN performance but seems relevant to constructs that may be tapped by RAN. Farmer and Klein (1995) and Wolf, Bowers, and Biddle (2000) review evidence concerning visual and auditory reaction time and other basic perceptual process findings associated with dyslexia. Their reviews suggest that differences between dyslexics and controls appear when stimuli are presented at faster speeds and in series. Breznitz (2001) has provided evidence that dyslexic children and adults have slower event-related potentials (ERP) to visual and auditory stimuli. Her hypothesis that it is the greater asynchrony of the responses that undermines the amalgamation of phonological and orthographic knowledge for dyslexics will be discussed more fully later. Keen and Lovegrove (2000) report that dyslexics have a "sluggish" visual processing system. Fawcett and Nicolson (2001) have reviewed their findings suggesting that dyslexics show poorer automatization of many skills, both linguistic and nonlinguistic. Nicolson and Fawcett (2001) provide a framework in which cerebellar problems underlie both articulatory and automatizing deficits relevant to literacy. Stein (2001) also cites dyslexia-related difficulties in cerebellar functioning that can be indexed by motion detection tests.

Bowers and Wolf's (1993) argument for a special relationship between orthographic skill and RAN was not centered on how general processing speed factors might be reflected in RAN but, rather, on how factors associated with slow RAN would affect reading acquisition. Thus this position is unaffected by the outcome of the domain-general/domain-specific debate. Our hypothesis asserted that processes reflected in RAN underlie letter recognition speed in text. If letter identification proceeds too slowly, letter representations in words would not be activated in sufficiently close temporal proximity to induce sensitivity to commonly occurring orthographic patterns. In essence, Bowers and colleagues (1994) predicted that the variance in RAN associated with reading would be mediated through resulting variability in orthographic sensitivity. Cutting and Denckla (2001) provide some support for this position, as the shared variance of processing speed and RAN was related to orthographic skill in their normally achieving young reader sample. However, unlike our hypothesis, RAN was also directly related to reading apart from the shared variance with processing speed and orthographic skill.

Manis and colleagues (1999) have suggested a different basis for the RAN–orthographic skill correlation, arguing that both RAN and orthographic skill reflect the ability to learn arbitrary associations. Still others consider it more likely that rapid naming and orthographic skill are separate deficits (e.g., Badian, 1997; Berninger, Abbott, Billingsley, & Nagy, 2001). Further empirical work exploring these theoretical issues has led to a revision of the original hypothesis which places less stress on the mediating role of orthographic skill while continuing to highlight the impact of letter string processing deficits (Bowers, 2001).

To explore the hypothesized link between letter string processing efficiency, reading skill, and RAN, Bowers (1996) devised the Quick Spell Test (QST). It had three subtests, four letter simple words (e.g., went), pseudowords (e.g., meft), and all-consonant illegal nonwords (e.g., dlhw) which were presented to each child in mixed order on a computer screen for 250 ms, with the child's task simply to name the letters seen. There were 10 letter strings in each subtest and number of strings correctly reported was scored. Bowers and colleagues (1999) found that naming speed was a strong correlate of QST performance in grade 2 and grade 3 children. Although the association of RAN with accuracy of processing briefly presented letter strings was confirmed, the pattern of results did not clearly implicate orthographic skill as the route through which RAN was associated with reading. When comparing single- and double-deficit children on these subtests, the most consistent discriminator of groups was the illegal nonwords. The double-deficit children were particularly poor at reporting letters in these strings; single-deficit children were intermediate in their performance and no-deficit children were reasonably accurate. All groups exhibited a "word superiority effect" such that the performance was best for words, next for pseudowords, and worse for nonwords. If the original hypothesis was correct, RAN deficit and DD children would have smaller effects of orthographic structure than other children.

The data reported in Table 9.3 are from a subsequent study of grade 3 children (Sunseth & Bowers, 2002). (Some data from this study were reported in Table 9.2.) As indicated earlier, children were divided into groups based on their strengths and weaknesses in phonemic awareness and naming speed, with strengths defined as above the 50th percentile and weaknesses as below the 30th percentile. Again, QST nonword letter strings discriminated double-deficit from single-deficit children. Although all deficit groups performed more poorly than the double-asset group on strings with greater orthographic structure, they did not differ significantly from one another on these strings. In that study, Sunseth and Bowers also administered an embedded word test devised by Hultquist (1997) as a measure of orthographic skill. The same double-deficit children showed more errors detecting words embedded in strings of consonant letters (e.g., pjgirlwjwz) than single-deficit children, even when controlling for their poorer performance reading similar isolated words (e.g., rock). Thus DD children were more affected by the surrounding consonant strings.

Rueffer (2000) revised the QST by adding a list of nonwords with high bigram frequency to assess just how sensitive children were to the presence of orthographic patterns even in illegal all-consonant strings.

Both good and poor grade 4 readers made more correct identifications of letters in letter strings with high bigram frequency (e.g., blbs) compared to the original low bigram frequency letter strings (e.g., dlhw). In this sample, only the original nonword strings significantly differentiated good and poor readers, with differences between groups narrowed by the sensitivity to common patterns even in nonwords.

Summarizing the results of several studies using the QST, Bowers (2001) reported that poor reader and double-deficit groups differed most from other groups on the letter strings with the least orthographic structure, and each group's accuracy benefited similarly from each additional increase in orthographic structure. Van der leij and Van Daal (1999) present further evidence that dyslexics are particularly slow at processing nonwords with low frequency clusters and benefit from presentation of nonwords with higher frequency clusters. Much earlier, Horn and Manis (1985) showed that dyslexics used orthographic structure in visual search and lexical decision tasks as well as did normally reading controls. These results were in the context of dyslexics' lesser overall accuracy in visual search and slower latency in lexical decision tasks.

This pattern of data suggested a more complex route for RAN effects than proposed by the original hypothesis. Bowers (2001) interpreted the findings to mean that naming speed may affect sight word skill mainly through its association with a baseline for speed of visual letter string identification, upon which orthographic knowledge adds perceptual facilitation effects. In

TABLE 9.3. Performance on QST and Embedded Words by Subtypes of Grade 2 Children

	Double asset	Phonological deficit	Naming speed deficit	Double deficit
Quick Spell Test: Number correct/10				
Word	9.7 (.8)[a]	8.1 (1.8)[b]	7.3 (1.1)[b]	6.4 (2.1)[b]
Pseudoword	9.2 (1.0)[a]	6.2 (1.6)[b]	5.8 (1.3)[b]	4.7 (2.2)[b]
Nonword	8.8 (1.5)[a]	4.8 (1.7)[b]	4.7 (1.2)[b]	2.9 (1.4)[c]
Hultquist Embedded Word Test: % correct				
Embedded	95.3 (5.1)[a]	69.8 (13.1)[b]	78.5 (14.9)[b]	56.7 (13.1)[c]
Nonembedded	99.0 (2.3)[a]	84.6 (11.3)[b]	89.2 (13.1)[ab]	75.3 (14.3)[b]

Note. Values sharing superscripts do not differ from each other. Data from Sunseth & Bowers (2002).

our studies, this baseline is independently affected by PA as well as naming speed. (One might suppose that the memory component of PA might be associated with this baseline because the strings are not pronounceable.) Orthographic knowledge once attained helps speed the perceptual processes involved in letter recognition in strings with high orthographic structure, but baseline effects persist. Acquiring orthographic knowledge may be impeded by the slow baseline but also by other factors. Certainly orthographic skill requires much practice with common sublexical patterns, especially for double-deficit poor readers. Levy (2001) showed how special efforts to make sublexical patterns visually salient improved the word recognition of even these poor readers.

The focus on RAN effects on baseline letter string recognition with additive effects of orthographic knowledge coming from several sources may be more consistent with studies suggesting three deficits: phonological awareness, naming speed, and orthographic awareness (e.g., Badian, 1997). But it is also unsurprising that naming speed is particularly associated with "sight" word (orthographic) codes, as individual differences in processing strings of unrelated letters forms the baseline on which orthographic knowledge speeds recognition of real words.

Recent work by Conrad (2002) is consistent with this newer interpretation. She did find that double-deficit poor readers (compared to those poor readers with faster RAN performance, i.e., single-phonological-deficit poor readers) had significantly poorer performance on several tests of orthographic accuracy, replicating the RAN–orthographic skill association. However, her studies also suggest the separate effects of RAN and orthographic skill on reading. Using a probe task at letter, letter cluster, and word levels, she concluded that the DD children "have difficulty processing individual letters in a string, whether or not the string is orthographically regular." Yet she also replicated our finding that even DD children make use of orthographic structure to aid word processing. Most intriguing is the finding that the letter processing deficit of DD children occurs not only at relatively brief presentation rates (one second for the

letter string followed by a probe) but also at longer ones, up to 2½ seconds. The baseline difficulties in processing are not overcome by just more time to inspect targets.

We may need to interpret our findings about RAN-related difficulties in processing strings of letters with low or high orthographic structure within a broader framework of processing speed effects on the amalgamation of phonological and orthographic codes. Breznitz (2001) focuses attention on the degree of asynchrony in time between the auditory (phonological) and visual (orthographic) processing of print. She has found that normally reading children and adults have a natural asynchrony based on the different speed of visual and auditory information processing, as indexed by ERP responses to appropriate stimuli. However, the "gap" is not particularly large, and presumably within a space of time that can be resolved, such that connections between the two systems can be forged. However, dyslexics have ERP latencies (both P200 and P300) that are longer to both auditory and visual stimuli, especially the auditory ones. This finding can be interpreted to mean that dyslexics take longer to perceive/classify and integrate into working memory various types of simple stimuli, even nonlinguistic material. The most sensitive association between reading skill and speed of processing indices for children was between reading and a "gap" score devised by subtracting the visual from the auditory ERP latencies for graphemes and phonemes. Her data suggest that the link in time between the visual and verbal systems rather than the processing time for one of them is central. Retrieving verbal labels must be integrated with visual pattern recognition. Is it a sluggish visual system or an inefficient verbal system that acts as bottleneck to the integration? Or is the verbal–visual connection system itself not performing at an optimal rate? The efficiency of the integration of two systems remains the core of what is being measured. Work not only by Breznitz but also by Wimmer and Mayringer (2001), Berninger and colleagues (2001), and Levy (2001) emphasizes the importance of bringing these processes into synchrony, and the penalties incurred when slow processing of one or more elements impedes their integration. To rapidly name items on a RAN task requires the visual identification and phonological naming systems to be suitably synchronized.

This perspective might resonate with the second hypothesis described by Wolf and Bowers (1999), which emphasizes the different processing stages in word recognition in which speed requirements are crucial. Visual naming speed as indexed by RAN can be considered to reflect the rapid integration of lexical access and retrieval processes with lower-level visual, auditory, and motoric (articulatory) processes.

> We believe that this unique combination of (a) actual subprocesses used in reading and (b) similar efficiency or processing speed requirements needed in subprocess integration has made naming speed tasks one of the two best predictors of reading achievement (along with phonemic awareness tasks) across all languages studied to date. At the same time, the multicomponential nature of naming speed suggests that naming speed deficits could result from multiple, underlying sources. (Wolf & Bowers, 1999, p. 430)

Berninger and Abbott (1994) also emphasize the multiple connections between aspects of visible language needed for accurate and fluent reading. Berninger and colleagues (2001) suggest that "the time score for RAN reflects both the efficiency (speed) and automaticity (direct access) of integrating the orthographic and phonological layers . . ." (p. 402). Moreover, they agree that different individuals may be slow on RAN for different reasons.

In summary, the effort to understand the basis for the RAN–reading relationship has led to a rather complex set of findings. Our current interpretation of those findings suggest that RAN may reflect the relative ease of amalgamation of visual–orthographic and name retrieval processes. The degree to which asynchrony of the two processes impedes their amalgamation is reflected in both RAN and reading. The search for clues in the format of the RAN for the nature of the association has highlighted the pause times between naming items as the aspect of the serial list related to reading. That latency to name an isolated symbol is also associated with reading suggests that greater access time to the symbol's name is reflected in the pauses. Attempts to understand the as-sociation of RAN with orthographic skill has led to the hypothesis that RAN reflects a baseline speed of identifying letter strings on which orthographic knowledge builds perceptual facilitation effects. Thus, we hypothesize that RAN reflects the efficient *integration* of verbal and visual information at a fairly basic level, which in turn may be related to the degree of asynchrony of processing speed for visual and auditory information.

An Alternative View

The hypothesis just described is consistent with much data but still awaits confirmation. An alternative view about slow RAN and related deficits in reading is that they reflect underspecified or immature phonological representations whose effects are seen in slow naming and poor verbal short-term memory, as well as the more obvious deficit in PA (Pennington, Cardoso-Martins, Green, & Lefly, 2001). In this view, speed of processing does not play a direct role in reading skill but, rather, is another way in which poor phonological processing is revealed. Perhaps this interpretation coincides with that of Wagner and colleagues (1994), who describe rapid naming as one of the phonological processing abilities. "Time will tell" which view is more accurate.

Implications for Remediation

Because even children with RAN deficits can speed perceptual processes relevant to reading using their knowledge of orthographic constraints, a focus on ways to boost that knowledge may be key to remediation efforts. Although the baseline for perceptual identification of letter strings may change only through maturational processes, compensation for deficits in these lower-level processes is possible through the effects of print exposure and decoding skill on orthographic knowledge. Practice with commonly occurring letter patterns may indeed need to be extraordinarily intense to overcome baseline differences associated with RAN. The RAVE-O (Wolf, Miller, & Donnelly, 2000) program of remediation focuses on increasing the fluency of the several (orthographic, phonological, and semantic) components of reading skill and may provide this training. By directly teaching orthographic patterns and gradually building up the speed of access to them through practice with timed games, RAVE-O (in conjunction with systematic phonics) has boosted the reading performance of severely dyslexic children (Lovett, 2001). Levy (2001) has shown that double-deficit children need extra support to learn sublexical orthographic patterns. Once having learned those patterns, they benefit from the increased processing efficiency derived from orthographic knowledge.

Interventions targeted to the particular deficit profile of dyslexic children are recommended, with remediation focused on fluency and/or accuracy of decoding as needed. No one method is apt to address the difficulties of the variety of children with RD in our schools. Careful integration of remediation efforts, informed by the idea that dyslexics, especially those with double deficits in PA and RAN, require much greater support to develop and use orthographic knowledge, may lead to more successful remediation programs.

References

Badian, N. (1997). Dyslexia and the double-deficit hypothesis. *Annals of Dyslexia, 47,* 69–87.

Baker, K. (2002). *Visual processes and the double-deficit hypothesis for reading disabilities.* Unpublished doctoral dissertation, University of Waterloo, Waterloo, Ontario, Canada.

Berninger, V., & Abbott, R. (1994). Multiple orthographic and phonological codes in literacy acquisition: An evolving research program. In V. Berninger (Ed.), *The varieties of orthographic knowledge I: theoretical and developmental issues* (pp. 277–317). Dordrecht, The Netherlands: Kluwer Academic.

Berninger, V., Abbott, R. D., Billingsley, F., & Nagy, W. (2001). Processes underlying timing and fluency: Efficiency, automaticity, coordination and morphological awareness. In M. Wolf (Ed.), *Dyslexia, fluency and the brain* (pp 383–414). Timonium, MD: York Press.

Blachman, B. A. (1984). Relationship of rapid naming ability and language analysis skills to kindergarten and first-grade reading achievement. *Journal of Educational Psychology, 76,* 610–622.

Bowers, P. (1993). Text reading and rereading: Predictors of fluency beyond word recognition. *Journal of Reading Behavior, 25,* 133–153.

Bowers, P. G. (1995). Tracing symbol naming speed's unique contributions to reading disabilities over time. *Reading and Writing: An Interdisciplinary Journal, 7,* 189–216.

Bowers, P. (1996, April). *The effects of single and double deficits in phonemic awareness and naming speed on new tests of orthographic knowledge.* Paper presented at the annual meeting of the Society for the Scientific Study of Reading, New York.

Bowers, P. G. (2001). Exploration of the basis for rapid naming's relationship to reading. In M. Wolf (Ed.), *Dyslexia, fluency and the brain* (pp. 41–63). Timonium, MD: York Press.

Bowers, P. G., Golden, J. O., Kennedy, A., & Young, A. (1994). Limits upon orthographic knowledge due to processes indexed by naming speed. In V. W. Berninger (Ed.), *The varieties of orthographic knowledge: Theoretical and developmental issues* (pp. 173–218). Dordrecht, The Netherlands: Kluwer Academic.

Bowers, P. G., & Kennedy, A. (1993). Effects of naming speed differences on fluency of reading after practice. *Annals of the New York Academy of Sciences, 682,* 318–320.

Bowers, P. G., & Newby-Clark, E. (2002). The role of naming speed within a model of reading acquisition. *Reading and Writing: An International Journal, 15,* 109–126.

Bowers, P., Steffy, R., & Swanson, L. (1986). Naming speed, memory and visual processing in reading disability. *Canadian Journal of Behavioral Science, 18,* 209–223.

Bowers, P. G., Steffy, R., & Tate, E. (1988). Comparison of the effects of IQ control methods on memory and naming speed predictors of reading disability. *Reading Research Quarterly, 23,* 304–319.

Bowers, P.G., Sunseth, K., & Golden, J. (1999). The route between rapid naming and reading progress. *Scientific Studies of Reading, 3,* 31–53.

Bowers, P. G., & Swanson, L. B. (1991). Naming speed deficits in reading disability: Multiple measures of a singular process. *Journal of Experimental Child Psychology, 51,* 195–219.

Bowers, P. G., & Wolf, M. (1993). Theoretical links between naming speed, precise timing mechanisms and orthographic skill in dyslexia. *Reading and Writing: An Interdisciplinary Journal, 5,* 69–85.

Breznitz, Z. (2001). The determinants of reading fluency: A comparison of dyslexic and average readers. In M.Wolf (Ed.), *Time, fluency and developmental dyslexia* (pp. 245–276). Timonium, MD: York Press.

Carte, E. T., Nigg, J. T., & Hinshaw, S. P. (1996). Neuropsychological functioning, motor speed, and language processing in boys with and without ADHD. *Journal of Abnormal Child Psychology, 24,* 481–498.

Carver, R. P. (1997). Reading for one second, one minute, or one year from the perspective of reading theory. *Scientific Studies of Reading, 1,* 3–43.

Compton, D. L., Davis, C. J., DeFries, J. C., Gayan,

J., & Olson, R. K. (2001). Genetic and environmental influences on reading and RAN: An overview of results from the Colorado Twin Study. In M. Wolf (Ed.), *Time, fluency and developmental dyslexia* (pp. 277–303). Timonium, MD: York Press.

Conrad, N. J. (2002). *Letter processing in children with naming speed deficits*. Unpublished doctoral dissertation, McMaster University, Hamilton, Ontario, Canada.

Cornwall, A. (1992). The relationship of phonological awareness, rapid naming, and verbal memory to severe reading and spelling disability. *Journal of Learning Disabilities, 25*, 532–538.

Cunningham, A. E., & Stanovich, K. E. (1990). Assessing print exposure and orthographic processing skill in children: A quick measure of reading experience. *Journal of Educational Psychology, 82*, 733–740.

Cutting, L. E., & Denckla, M. B. (2001). The relationship of rapid serial naming and word reading in normally developing readers: An exploratory model. *Reading and Writing: An Interdisciplinary Journal, 14*, 673–705.

Davis, C. J., Knopik, V. S., Olson, R. K., Wadsworth, S. J., & DeFries, J. C. (2001). Genetic and environmental influences on rapid naming and reading ability: A twin study. *Annals of Dyslexia, 51*, 231–248.

DeJong, P. F., & Van der Leij, A. (1999). Specific contributions of phonological abilities to early reading acquisition: Results from a Dutch latent variable longitudinal study. *Journal of Educational Psychology, 91*, 450–476.

Denckla, M. B. (1972). Color-naming defects in dyslexic boys. *Cortex, 8*, 164–176.

Denckla, M. B., & Rudel, R. G. (1974). Rapid "automatized" naming of pictured objects, colors, letters and numbers by normal children. *Cortex, 10*, 186–202.

Denckla, M. B., & Rudel, R. G. (1976). Rapid automatized naming (RAN): Dyslexia differentiated from other learning disabilities. *Neuropsychologia, 14*, 471–479.

Denckla, M. B., & Wolf, M. (in press). *Rapid automatic naming (RAN) and Rapid alternating stimuli naming (RAS)*. Austin, TX: Pro-Ed.

Farmer, M. E., & Klein, R. M. (1995). The evidence for a temporal processing deficit linked to dyslexia: A review. *Psychonomic Society, 2*, 460–493.

Fawcett, A. J., & Nicolson, R. I. (2001). Speed and temporal processing in dyslexia. In M. Wolf (Ed.), *Time, fluency and developmental dyslexia* (pp. 23–40). Timonium, MD: York Press.

Felton, R. H., Naylor, C. E., & Wood, F. B. (1990). Neuropsychological profile of adult dyslexics. *Brain and Language, 39*, 485–497.

Felton, R. H., Wood, F. B., Brown, I. S., & Campbell, S. K. (1987). Separate verbal memory and naming deficits in attention deficit disorder. *Journal of Learning Disabilities, 22*, 3–13.

Flowers, L., Meyer, M., Lovato, J., Felton, R., & Wood, F. (2001). Does third grade discrepancy status predict the course of reading development? *Annals of Dyslexia, 51*, 49–71.

Geschwind, N. (1965a). Disconnection syndrome in animals and man (Part I). *Brain, 88*, 237–294.

Geschwind, N. (1965b). Disconnection syndrome in animals and man (Part II). *Brain, 88*, 585–644.

Geva, E., Vaghoub-Zadeh, Z., & Schuster, B. (2000). Understanding individual differences in word recognition skills of ESL children. *Annals of Dyslexia, 50*, 123–154.

Grigorenko, E. L., Wood, F. B., Meyer, M. S., Pauls, J. E. D., Hart, L. A., & Pauls, D. L. (2001). Linkage studies suggest a possible locus for developmental dyslexia on chromosome 1p. *American Journal of Medical Genetics (Neuropsychiatric Genetics), 105*, 120–129.

Hecht, S. A., Torgesen, J. K., Wagner, R. K., & Rashotte, C. A. (2001). The relations between phonological processing abilities and emerging individual differences in mathematical computation skills: A longitudinal study from second to fifth grades. *Journal of Experimental Child Psychology, 79*, 192–227.

Ho, C. S-H. (2001, June). *The cognitive profile and multiple-deficit hypothesis in Chinese developmental dyslexia*. Paper presented to annual meetings of the Society for the Scientific Study of Reading, Boulder, CO.

Ho, C. S-H., & Lai, D. N.-C. (2000). Naming speed deficits and phonological memory deficits in Chinese developmental dyslexia. *Learning and Individual Differences, 11*, 173–186.

Horn, C. C., & Manis, F. R. (1985). Normal and disabled readers' use of orthographic structure in processing print. *Journal of Reading Behavior, 17*, 143–161.

Hultquist, A. M. (1997). Orthographic processing abilities of adolescents with dyslexia. *Annals of Dyslexia, 47*, 89–109.

Ishaik, G., Bowers, P., & Steffy, R. (2001, June). *Phonological awareness tasks dissected*. Poster presented at the annual meeting of the Society for the Scientific Study of Reading, Boulder, CO.

Kail, R., Hall, L. K., & Caskey, B. J. (1999). Processing speed, exposure to print, and naming speed. *Applied Psycholinguistics, 20*, 303–314.

Keen, A. G., & Lovegrove, W. J. (2000). Transient deficit hypothesis and dyslexia: examination of whole-parts relationship, retinal sensitivity, and spatial and temporal frequencies. *Vision Research, 40*, 705–715.

Kirby, J. R., Parrila, R. K., & Pfeiffer, S. L. (2001, June). *Naming speed and phonological awareness as predictors of reading development*. Paper presented at the annual meeting of the Society for the Scientific Study of Reading, Boulder, CO.

Larsen, S. C., & Hammill, D. D. (1994). *Test of Written Spelling: Third edition*. Austin, TX: Pro-Ed.

Levy, B. A. (2001). Moving the bottom: Improving reading fluency. In M. Wolf (Ed.), *Time, fluency and developmental dyslexia* (357–379). Timonium, MD: York Press.

Levy, B. A., Abello, B., & Lysynchuk, L. (1997). Beginning word recognition: Benefits of training by segmentation and whole word methods. *Scientific Studies of Reading, 3,* 129–157.

Levy, B. A., Bourassa, D. C., & Horn, C. (1999). Fast and slow namers: Benefits of segmentation and whole word training. *Journal of Experimental Child Psychology, 73,* 115–138.

Lovett, M. W. (1987). A developmental approach to reading disability: Accuracy and rate criteria in the subtyping of dyslexic children. *Brain and Language, 22,* 67–91.

Lovett, M. (2001, November). *Reading disabilities can be remediated: Lessons from research at the Hospital for Sick Children.* Workshop presentation at the Research Into Practice Conference of the Learning Disabilities Association of Ontario, Toronto, Canada.

Lovett, M. W., Steinbach, K. A., & Frijters, J. C. (2000). Remediatiing the core deficits of developmental reading disability: A double-deficit perspective. *Journal of Learning Disabilities, 33,* 334–358.

Manis, F. R., Doi, L. M., & Bhadha (2000). Naming speed, phonological awareness and orthographic knowledge in second graders. *Journal of Learning Disabilities, 33,* 325–333.

Manis, F. R., & Freedman, L. (2001). The relationship of naming speed to multiple reading measures in disabled and normal readers. In M. Wolf (Ed.), *Dyslexia, fluency and the brain* (pp. 65–92). Timonium, MD: York Press.

Manis, F. R., Seidenberg, M. S., & Doi, L. M. (1999). See Dick RAN: Rapid naming and the longitudinal prediction of reading subskills in first and second graders. *Scientific Studies of Reading, 3*(2), 129–157.

Mann, V. (1984). Review: Reading skill and language skill. *Developmental Review, 4,* 1–15.

Markwardt Jr., F. C. (1989). *The Peabody Individual Achievement Test—Revised (PIAT-R).* Circle Pines, MN: American Guidance Service.

McBride-Chang, C., & Manis, F. R. (1996). Structural invariance in the associations of naming speed, phonological awareness, and verbal reasoning in good and poor readers: A test of the double deficit hypothesis. *Reading and Writing: An Interdisciplinary Journal, 8,* 323–339.

Meyer, M. S., Wood, F. B., Hart, L. A., & Felton, R. H. (1998). The selective predictive values in rapid automatized naming within poor readers. *Journal of Learning Disabilities, 31,* 106–117.

Morris, R., Stuebing, K., Fletcher, J., Shaywitz, S., Lyon, R., Shankweiler, D., Kata, L., Francis, D., & Shaywitz, B. (1998). Subtypes of reading disability: A phonological core. *Journal of Educational Psychology, 90,* 1–27.

Neuhaus, G., Foorman, B. R., Francis, D. J., & Carlson, C. D. (2001). Measures of information processing in Rapid Automatized Naming (RAN) and their relation to reading. *Journal of Experimental Child Psychology, 78,* 359–373.

Nicolson, R. I. & Fawcett, A. (2001). Dyslexia, learning and the cerebellum. In M. Wolf (Ed.), *Dyslexia, fluency and the brain* (pp.159–188). Timonium, MD: York Press.

Nigg, J. T., Hinshaw, S. P., Carte, E. T., & Treuting, J. J. (1998). *Journal of Abnormal Psychology, 107,* 468–480.

Obregon, M., & Wolf, M. (1995, April). *A fine-grained analysis of serial naming duration patterns in developmental dyslexia.* Poster presented at the annual meeting of the Society for Research in Child Development, Indianapolis, IN.

Olson, R. K., Kliegl, R., Davidson, B. J., & Foltz, G. (1985). Individual and developmental differences in reading disability. In G. E. MacKinnon & T. G. Waller (Eds.), *Reading research: Advances in theory and practice* (Vol. 4, pp. 1–64). Orlando, FL: Academic Press.

Pennington, B. F., Cardoso-Martins, C., Green, P. A., & Lefly, D. L. (2001). Comparing the phonological and double deficit hypotheses for developmental dyslexia. *Reading and Writing: An Interdisciplinary Journal, 14,* 707–755.

Rosner, J., & Simon, D. P. (1971). The Auditory Analysis Test: An initial report. *Journal of Learning Disabilities, 4*(7), 384–392.

Rueffer, K. A. (2000). *An examination of the factors underlying the development of skilled reading.* Unpublished master's thesis, University of Waterloo, Waterloo, Ontario, Canada.

Scarborough, H. S., & Domgaard, R. M. (1998, April). *An exploration of the relationship between reading and rapid serial naming.* Paper presented at the annual meeting of the Society for the Scientific Study of Reading, San Diego, CA.

Semrud-Clikeman, M., Guy, K., & Griffin, J. D. (2000). Rapid naming deficits in children and adolescents with reading disabilities and attention deficit hyperactivity disorder. *Brain and Language, 74,* 70–83.

Spring, C., & Capps, C. (1974). Encoding speed, rehearsal, and probed recall of dyslexic boys. *Journal of Educational Psychology, 66,* 780–786.

Stein, J. (2001). The neurobiology of reading difficulties. In M. Wolf (Ed.), *Dyslexia, fluency and the brain* (pp. 3 –22).Timonium, MD: York Press,

Sunseth, K., & Bowers, P. G. (2002). Rapid naming and phonemic awareness: Contributions to reading, spelling, and orthographic knowledge. *Scientific Studies of Reading, 6,* 401–429.

Swanson, L. B. (1989). *Analyzing naming speed-reading relationships in children.* Unpublished doctoral dissertation, University of Waterloo.

Tannock, R., Martinussen, R., & Frijters, J. (2000). Naming speed performance and stimulant effects indicate effortful, semantic processing deficits in attention-deficit/hyperactivity disorder. *Journal of Abnormal Child Psychology, 28,* 237–252.

Torgesen, J. K., Wagner, R. K., Rashotte, C. A., Burgess, S., & Hecht, S. (1997). Contributions of phonological awareness and rapid automatic naming ability to the growth of word-reading skills in second to fifth-grade children. *Scientific Studies of Reading, 1*(2), 161–185.

Torgesen, J. K., Wagner, R. K., Rashotte, C. A., Rose, E., Lindamood, P., Conway, T., & Garvan,

C. (1999). Preventing reading failure in young children with phonological processing disabilities: Group and individual responses to instruction. *Journal of Educational Psychology, 91,* 579–593.

Van den Bos, K. P. (1998). IQ, phonological awareness, and continuous naming speed related to Dutch children's poor decoding performance on two word identification tests. *Dyslexia, 4,* 73–89.

Van der Leij, A., & Van Daal, V. H. P. (1999). Automatization aspects of dyslexia: speed limitations in word identification, sensitivity to increasing task demands, and orthographic compensation. *Journal of Learning Disabilities, 32,* 417–428.

Wagner, R. K., & Torgesen, J. K. (1987). The nature of phonological processing and its causal role in the acquisition of reading skills. *Psychological Bulletin, 101,* 192–212.

Wagner, R. K., Torgesen, J. K., & Rashotte, C. A. (1994). Development of reading-related phonological processing abilities: New evidence of bidirectional causality from a latent variable longitudinal study. *Developmental Psychology, 30,* 73–87.

Wagner, R. K., Torgesen, J. K., & Rashotte, C. A. (1999). *Comprehensive Test of Phonological Processing.* Austin, TX: Pro-Ed.

Wagner, R. K., Torgesen, J. K., Rashotte, C. A., Hecht, S. A., Barker, T. A., Burgess, S. R., Donahue, J., & Garon, T. (1997). Changing causal relations between phonological processing abilities and word-level reading as children develop from beginning to fluent readers: A five-year longitudinal study. *Developmental Psychology, 33,* 468–479.

Wechsler, D. (1991). *Wechsler Intelligence Scale for Children—Third edition.* San Antonio, TX: The Psychological Corporation.

Wiederholt, J. L., & Bryant, B. R. (1992). *Gray Oral Reading Tests, third edition.* Austin, TX: Pro-Ed.

Wimmer, H. (1993). Characteristics of developmental dyslexia in a regular writing system. *Applied Psycholinguistics, 14,* 1–34.

Wimmer, H., & Mayringer, H. (2001). Is the reading–rate problem of German dyslexic children caused by slow visual processes? In M. Wolf (Ed.), *Dyslexia, fluency and the brain* (pp. 93–102). Timonium, MD: York Press.

Wimmer, H., Mayringer, H., & Landerl, K. (2000). The double-deficit hypothesis and difficulties in learning to read a regular orthography. *Journal of Educational Psychology, 92,* 668–680.

Wolf , M. (1982). The word-retrieval process and reading in children and aphasics. In K. Nelson (Ed.), *Children's language* (pp. 437–493). Hillsdale, NJ: Erlbaum.

Wolf, M. (1986). Rapid alternating stimulus (RAS) naming: A longitudinal study in average and impaired readers. *Brain and Language, 27,* 360–379.

Wolf, M. (1991). Naming speed and reading: The contribution of the cognitive neurosciences. *Reading Research Quarterly, 26,* 123–141.

Wolf, M., Bally, H., & Morris, R. (1986). Automaticity, retrieval processes, and reading: A longitudinal study in average and impaired readers. *Child Development, 57,* 988–1000.

Wolf, M., & Bowers, P. G. (1999). The double-deficit hypothesis for the developmental dyslexias. *Journal of Educational Psychology, 91,* 415–438.

Wolf, M., Bowers, P. G., & Biddle, K. (2000). Naming-speed processes, timing, and reading. A conceptual review. *Journal of Learning Disabilities, 33,* 387–407.

Wolf, M., Miller, L., & Donnelly, K. (2000). Retrieval, Automaticity, Vocabulary Elaboration, Orthography (RAVE-O): A comprehensive, fluency-based reading intervention program. *Journal of Learning Disabilities, 33,* 375–386.

Woodcock, R. W., & Johnson, M. B. (1989). *Woodcock–Johnson Psycho-Educational Battery—Revised.* Allen, TX: DLM Teaching Resources.

Young, A. (1997, March). *Relationship of phonological analysis and naming speed to training effects among dyslexic readers.* Paper presented at the annual meeting of the Society for the Scientific Study of Reading, Chicago.

Young, A., & Bowers, P. G. (1995). Individual difference and text difficulty determinants of reading fluency and expressiveness. *Journal of Experimental Child Psychology, 60,* 428–454.

10

Basic Cognitive Processes
and Reading Disabilities

Linda S. Siegel

This chapter reviews the literature on the normal course of the development of reading and also examines what happens when reading skills fail to develop adequately in children with reading disabilities.

The chapter discusses the development of reading by analyzing it in terms of a theoretical approach that is focused on the basic cognitive processes. First, however, it considers some important conceptual and methodological issues in this field.

Controversies and Methodological Issues

A great deal of inconsistency and controversy exist in the research on reading and reading disabilities. Therefore, any discussion of reading and reading disabilities must start with a clarification of some basic definitional issues and assumptions. The confusion in the field results from lack of clear, theoretically motivated, and consistent operational definitions of two major constructs, reading and reading disability. Although the question of what reading means may sound trivial, hundreds of tests are called reading tests, and reading is defined in a different way in each one and hence each yields a different

measure. This inconsistency constitutes a fundamental problem with the definition of this critical variable. The lack of integration in this field is a result of the lack of clarity in regard to the basic operational definitions. Siegel and Heaven (1986) reviewed these definitional issues, but one of the most significant issues is the difference between reading comprehension and word recognition. Tests of reading comprehension typically involve the reading of text and multiple-choice questions about the text; tests of word reading involve the reading of single words. Reading comprehension tests are timed; word reading tests are not. Although reading comprehension may appear to be the fundamental aspect of reading and is clearly the ultimate goal of reading, the measurement of reading comprehension is a methodologically complex issue full of pitfalls. The issues in the measurement of reading comprehension were examined in detail by Siegel and Heaven, Siegel and Ryan (1989b), and Tal and Siegel (1996); but the fundamental problem is that measures of reading comprehension are confounded by a number of other processes, such as background knowledge, vocabulary, and reading speed, and available tests of reading comprehension usually involve not making an inference from the text material but merely finding a verbatim answer in the text. In contrast, tests of word recognition measure more basic processes and responses are not confounded with differences in reading speed, background knowledge, and test-taking strategies. In addition, the use of reading comprehension scores as the independent variable or the basis of the definition of reading disability can yield different results from the use of word recognition scores (e.g., Siegel & Ryan, 1989a, 1989b; Stanovich, Nathan, & Zolman, 1988).

Also, from a theoretical perspective, word recognition is fundamental to comprehension (e.g., Gough & Tunmer, 1986; Stanovich, 1982a, 1982b). The ability to read isolated words is highly correlated with text comprehension (e.g., Shankweiler & Liberman, 1972). The problems of the beginning reader or the disabled reader are clearly at the level of the word. Problems at the word level interfere with the reading of connected text (Shankweiler & Liberman, 1972). Because word decoding is critical to comprehension and is the basic process in reading, the discussion in this chapter concentrates on the development of word recognition.

Definitional Issues: A Digression

Continuum versus Dichotomy

Another critical issue involves what constitutes the appropriate definition of a reading disability. Throughout this chapter, I use the term "reading disability" instead of "dyslexia." The terms "reading disability" and "dyslexia" are actually synonymous, but certain considerations have led to the widespread avoidance of the term "dyslexia" in many parts of the world, particularly by, although not limited to, the educational community. I do not understand why the term "dyslexia" is often viewed as if it were a four-letter word not to be uttered in polite company. However, I will speculate briefly. Dyslexia is often taken to imply an illness, such as measles, when, in fact, in the words of Ellis (1985), it is more similar to a problem such as obesity. As Ellis has written, "For people of any given age and height

there will be an uninterrupted continuum from painfully thin to inordinately fat. It is entirely arbitrary where we draw the line between 'normal' and 'obese,' but that does not prevent obesity being a real and worrying condition, nor does it prevent research into the causes and cures of obesity being both valuable and necessary" (p. 172). Ellis also wrote, "Therefore, to ask how prevalent dyslexia is in the general population will be as meaningful, and as meaningless, as asking how prevalent obesity is. The answer will depend entirely upon where the line is drawn" (p. 172). No virus, or specific brain lesion, or biochemical disturbance, has been shown to be the cause of dyslexia, so it is not an illness in the traditional medical sense. Because a reading disability is an educational problem and not a medical one, and because it cannot be treated by any of the traditional medical means, professionals are often reluctant to use the term "dyslexia." However, it is a real condition that deserves study and treatment.

Reading problems are best conceptualized as a continuum with varying degrees of severity. Clearly, a problem at any level deserves attention and treatment, but the dividing line between a reading problem and no problem is arbitrary. Fear and disdain of the term "dyslexia" is common in North America but seems less common in other parts of the world. I can offer no empirical evidence to support these speculations, but I suspect that the sociopolitical context has influenced the terminology. The egalitarian philosophy and the cultural ethos of North America may lead to the perception that a label, such as dyslexia, applied to a child may reduce access to educational opportunities. Therefore, for these considerations, and for those who find the term "dyslexia" offensive, I generally use the term "reading disability," although, as far as I am concerned, their meaning is identical.

Subtypes

One of the issues that has been raised in the study of reading disability is whether or not individuals with reading disabilities can be separated into subtypes. However, no reliable evidence supports the concept of subtypes and no clear subtypes have been delineated (see Siegel & Heaven, 1986; Siegel,

Levey, & Ferris, 1985; Siegel & Metsala, 1992, for a review of studies and methodological issues). On the contrary, children with a reading disability show a remarkable homogeneity in the profiles of their cognitive abilities (e.g., Siegel & Ryan, 1989b), and, when heterogeneity is found, it seems to result from the particular definition used in the study.

Evidence indicates that the definition of reading disability used in a study can influence the conclusions made about the heterogeneity of the population. For example, Siegel and Ryan (1989b) have shown that if reading disability is defined as a deficit in word reading skills, all the children with reading problems have deficits in phonological processing, working memory and short-term memory, and syntactic awareness. The pattern is similar if a deficit in pseudo-word reading skills is used as the basis for defining reading disability. However, if reading disability is defined on the basis of a deficit in reading comprehension, the group that emerges is heterogeneous and does not show deficits in phonological processing and syntactic skills but does show deficits in working memory and short-term memory. Thus, if and when subtypes appear within the population with reading disabilities, they may be artifacts of the definition used.

IQ and Reading

When issues related to reading disabilities are examined, the question is always raised as to the role of IQ and whether any differences in cognitive processes between individuals with reading disabilities and normal readers are merely a result of differences in IQ. However, no reliable evidence indicates that IQ level plays a causative role in the development of reading skills. On the contrary, evidence from a number of sources indicates that reading is not strongly related to intelligence as measured by IQ tests. Children with reading disability at all IQ levels show equal difficulty with phonological processing tasks such as pseudo-word reading, recognizing the visual form of a pseudo-word, and pseudo-word spelling (Siegel, 1988). Therefore, the presence of a reading disability, not a particular IQ, determines the pattern of cognitive strengths and weaknesses in regard to language, memory, and phonological skills.

Often, the individual with reading disabilities is defined as a person whose reading score is significantly lower than would be predicted from his or her IQ. (Individuals who fit this definition have traditionally been labeled "dyslexic.") If an individual has a lower reading score but it is *not* significantly lower than would be predicted by his or her IQ, the individual is not defined as dyslexic. This definition is referred to as the discrepancy definition. However, a number of investigators have provided evidence that a discrepancy between IQ and reading is not necessary for an individual to have reading disabilities. For example, I have compared (Siegel, 1992) dyslexics, defined as children whose reading scores were low (standard scores < 90) and significantly (1 standard deviation) below their IQ scores, and poor readers, whose reading scores were low (standard scores < 90) but not below the level predicted from their IQ. These two groups did not differ on any reading, spelling, or phonological processing tasks and on most language and memory tasks, in spite of the fact that the mean IQ score of the dyslexics was 25 points higher than that of the poor readers. Both these groups had scores on the reading, spelling, phonological processing, language, and memory tasks that were significantly below normal readers. The critical variable was the presence or absence of a reading disability.

Indeed, if the relative contributions of IQ and pseudo-word reading are compared, IQ contributes little independent variance beyond that contributed by pseudo-word reading to the prediction of word reading and reading comprehension scores (Siegel, 1993). Most of the variance is contributed by phonological processing as measured by pseudo-word reading. In summary, intelligence as measured by IQ scores seems irrelevant to the definition and analysis of reading disability.

Definitions

Throughout this chapter children who have low scores on reading tests are called poor readers, whether or not their reading scores are significantly lower than shat would be predicted by their IQ scores. Typically, a reading score at or below the 20th or 25th percentile is used. Good or average readers are defined as having scores on reading tests at or above the 30th, 35th or 40th percentile (depending on the study). For the aforementioned reasons, word reading tests, as opposed to reading comprehension tasks, yield the clearest definition of normal and atypical reading. Comparisons between disabled and normal readers are typically based on chronological age, and most of the studies reviewed in this chapter use chronological age to make these comparisons. However, another type of design is possible. This design involves what is called a reading-level match.

An alternative to studying both the development of reading skills and the differences and similarities between disabled and normal readers is to match disabled and normal readers on reading age, also called reading level (e.g., Backman, Mamen, & Ferguson, 1984). This type of design is used in an attempt to identify differences between reading disabled and normal readers that are merely consequences of differential experience with print. The theory underlying this type of comparison is that children who are poor readers probably read less and therefore do not have the same exposure to print. If so, a chronological age match confounds differences that reflect experience with print and differences that reflect factors that cause reading disability.

Basic Cognitive Processes in Reading

Theoretical Approach

I have postulated five processes that are possibly significant in the development of reading skills in the English language (Siegel, 1993). The processes involve phonology, syntax, working memory, semantics, and orthography. This chapter reviews the role of all these processes in the development of reading skills. Unfortunately, most of the information that is available about the development of reading is based on studies conducted with English, a language that has the highest degree of irregularity of the correspondence between letters, more properly graphemes, and phonemes, the sounds represented by letters and letter combinations. Some studies have addressed the prevalence of reading problems in other

languages, specifically, Stevenson, Stigler, Lucker, Hsu, and Kitamura (1982) for Chinese and Japanese and Lindgren, De Renzi, and Richman (1985) for Italian. However, in both of these studies, deficit in reading comprehension was used as the measure of a reading problem, and as discussed previously, this definition does not address the cognitive deficits that underlie severe reading problems, specifically phonological processing.

Liberman, Liberman, Mattingly, and Shankweiler (1980) outlined the complexities of studying the relationship between the acquisition of reading skills and different orthographies:

> Orthographies vary considerably in the demands they make on the beginning reader. This variation has two essentially independent aspects: first, the depth of the orthography, its relative remoteness from the phonetic representation; and second, the particular linguistic unit—morpheme, syllable, or phoneme—that is overtly represented. A deep orthography, like that of English, demands greater phonological development on the reader's part than a shallow orthography, like that of Vietnamese. Logographies (such as the Chinese writing system), syllabifies (such as old Persian cuneiform), and alphabetic systems (such as English) demand successively increasing degrees of linguistic awareness. (p. 146)

Clearly, the consideration of other languages is important and I include evidence from other languages when it is available, though such evidence is meager.

Phonological processing involves a variety of skills, but in the context of the development of reading skills, the most significant is the association of sounds with letters (i.e., the understanding of grapheme–phoneme conversion rules and the exceptions to these rules). This skill is the basis of decoding print, and although other routes can be used to obtain meaning from print, the phonological route is clearly an important one and critical in the early development of reading skills (e.g., Jorm, 1979; Stanovich, 1988a, 1988b).

Syntactic awareness, also called grammatical sensitivity, refers to the ability to understand the syntax of the language. This ability appears to be critical for fluent and efficient reading of text, and it requires making predictions about the words that come next in the sequence. Syntactic factors may influence the difficulty of reading single words, such as function words, prepositions, and auxiliary verbs, which are difficult to integrate in a semantic network. Ehri and Wilce (1980) have shown that beginning readers acquire information about the syntactic properties of function words when they have been trained to read these words in the context of a sentence. Therefore, the ability to process syntax may be an important aspect of word learning.

Working memory refers to the retention of information in short-term storage while processing incoming information and retrieving information from long-term storage. Working memory is relevant to reading because the reader must decode and/or recognize words while remembering what has been read and retrieving information such as grapheme–phoneme conversion rules. Working memory may also be critical to the reading of individual words, particularly in the beginning of the acquisition of word reading skills because the grapheme–phoneme conversion rules for each segment of the word must be held in memory while the remaining segments of the word are processed. Longer words, in terms of the number of syllables, place increasing demands on working memory. In addition, the complexity of a particular rule will influence the difficulty of word recognition because the number of possible alternative grapheme–phoneme pronunciations may have an influence on ease or difficulty of reading a particular word. Given more alternative pronunciations, reading will be slower and less accurate until the individual items are mastered. More rules might be searched and applied to the word being read. For example, "c" and "g" have multiple pronunciations at the beginning of English words, and, therefore, words or pseudo-words starting with these letters may be more difficult than words or pseudo-words beginning with other letters, especially for beginning readers.

Semantic processing refers to the understanding of meaning. Theoretically, word meanings are coded in semantic networks and are retrieved through these networks. In the context of reading, semantic processing is relevant to the retrieval of words. For example, the ease of retrieving the meaning of a word may depend, at least partially, on

the connections that it has with other words in a semantic network.

Orthographic processing refers to the understanding of the writing conventions of the language in question and knowledge of the correct and incorrect spellings of words. All alphabetic systems include legal and illegal and more and less probable sequences of letters, and a fluent reader uses knowledge of these sequences to some extent. Positional constraints and probabilities that letters will occur in certain positions are additional aspects of orthographic knowledge used by the skilled reader.

The following sections provide details of the growth of these skills in children who are normal readers and also in children with reading disabilities.

Phonological Processing

Current theories of the development of reading skills in English stress that phonological processing is the most significant underlying cognitive process. Stanovich (1988a, 1988b) outlined arguments for this position. Phonological processing involves a variety of functions, but in the context of the development of reading skills, the most significant is the association of sounds with letters or combinations of letters. This function is referred to as the understanding of grapheme–phoneme conversion rules, and because of the irregular nature of the correspondences in English, learning these rules is a complex process. The child who is learning to read must map oral language onto written language by decomposing the word into phonemes and associating each letter (or combination of letters) with these phonemes.

DUAL-ROUTE THEORIES

The development of phonological processing and the development of reading can be understood in the context of "dual-route" theories of reading. These theories have a variety of manifestations, but their basic premise is that two possible routes are involved in gaining access to the meaning of print (e.g., Coltheart, 1978; Forster & Chambers, 1973; Meyer, Schvanevelt, & Ruddy, 1974). One of these routes involves direct lexical access—that is, visually reading a word without any intermediate phonological processing. The orthographic configuration of a word is directly mapped onto an internal visual store in lexical memory. The other route, the phonological route, involves the use of grapheme–phoneme conversion rules to gain lexical access to a print stimulus. Grapheme–phoneme conversion rules are used to translate a graphemic code into a phonemic one. This route is referred to as nonlexical because the application of the rules does not rely on word-specific pronunciations. Instead, grapheme–phoneme conversion rules are presumed to be stored explicitly and used to determine a word's pronunciation. According to this model, pseudo-words can be read only by means of a nonlexical route, as, by definition, a pseudo-word cannot have a lexical representation.

Dual-route theories have been challenged. For example, the reading of nonwords is influenced by their similarity to real words, and regular words that have irregular orthographic neighbors are read more slowly than regular consistent ones, indicating reciprocal influences of these two routes. If pseudo-words were read only by grapheme–phoneme conversion rules, then the reading of pseudo-words should not be influenced by their similarity to real words, and regular words should not be influenced by the characteristics of their orthographic neighbors. Furthermore, multiple-level models (e.g., Brown, 1987) and connectionist models (e.g., Seidenberg & McClelland, 1989) that have been proposed involve a variety of postulated units and processes but not two distinct routes. (For an extended discussion of these issues, see Besner, Twilley, McCann, & Seergobin, 1990; Glushko, 1979; Humphreys & Evett, 1985; Metsala & Siegel, 1992). However, in spite of a certain ambiguity about the validity of dual-route theories, conceptualizations of reading in terms of dual-route theory represent one way of examining the development of reading skills and the performance of children with a reading disability. I will discuss tasks used to measure both these kinds of processing, the direct lexical access and the use of grapheme–phoneme conversion rules and the performance of reading disabled and normal readers on these types of tasks.

MEASUREMENT OF PHONOLOGICAL PROCESSING SKILLS

The task of the beginning reader is to extract these grapheme–phoneme conversion rules. The alternative is simply to memorize each word as a visual configuration and to associate a meaning with it. This kind of learning may occur, but it is inefficient and makes tremendous demands on visual memory. In English, no one-to-one correspondence exists between a letter (or letters) and a sound. The same letter represents different sounds and the same sound may be represented by different letters.

In an alphabetic language such as English, the best measure of phonological processing skills is the reading of pseudo-words, that is, pronounceable combinations of letters that can be read by the application of grapheme–phoneme conversion rules, but that are, of course, not real words in English. Examples include pseudo-words, such as "shum," "laip," and "cigbet." Pseudo-words can be read by anyone who is familiar with the grapheme–phoneme conversion rules of English even though they are not real words and have not been encountered in print or in spoken language before.

The development of the ability to read pseudo-words has been studied extensively (e.g., Calfee, Lindamood, & Lindamood, 1973; Hogaboam & Perfetti, 1978; Siegel & Ryan, 1988; Venezky & Johnson, 1973). Ample evidence indicates that children with dyslexia have a great deal of difficulty reading pseudo-words. Studies such as those of Bruck (1988), Ehri and Wilce (1983), Snowling (1980), Siegel and Ryan (1988), and Waters, Bruck, and Seidenberg (1985) have shown that disabled readers have more difficulty reading pseudo-words than do normal readers matched on either chronological age or reading level. For example, Siegel and Ryan studied the development of the ability to read pseudo-words in normal and disabled readers ages 7 to 14 years old. By the age of 9, the normal readers were quite proficient and performed at almost a perfect level for even the most difficult pseudo-words, with, in some cases, as many as three syllables. Similarly, Backman, Bruck, Hebert, and Seidenberg (1984) showed that 10-year-olds perform as well as adults on tasks involving the reading of pseudo-words. However, Siegel and Ryan found that the performance of the children with reading disabilities was quite different. These children appear to acquire these reading skills late in development and even children with reading disabilities at the age of 14 were performing no better than normal readers at the age of 7.

To control, at least partially, for experience with print, Siegel and Ryan (1988) used a comparison of disabled and normal readers matched on reading grade level. Even when the disabled readers and the normal readers were matched on reading level (hence the disabled readers were considerably older than the normal readers), the performance of those with reading disabilities on a task involving the reading of pseudo-words was significantly poorer than that of the normal readers.

Thus, difficulties with phonological processing seem to be the fundamental problem of children with reading disability, and this problem continues to adulthood. Many adults with a reading disability become reasonably fluent readers but still have difficulty reading pseudo-words or read them slowly (e.g., Barwick & Siegel, 1996; Bruck, 1990; Shafrir & Siegel, 1994).

For children learning to read English, the learning of grapheme–phoneme conversion rules is a result of systematic instruction, and the extraction of the rules is a result of repeated encounters with print. No evidence is available as to how much of the development of decoding skills is a result of specific instruction in the grapheme–phoneme conversion rules and how much is a result of experience with print. In any case, the understanding of the grapheme–phoneme conversion rules develops rapidly in the first years of experience with print under normal conditions.

DEVELOPMENTAL STAGES OF
PHONOLOGICAL PROCESSING

No conclusive evidence exists as to the process by which these skills develop. Before the child learns to apply phonological skills to print, the child must develop phonological awareness skills. Phoneme awareness refers to the ability to segment spoken vowels into component parts called phonemes. This ability develops reciprocally with learning to

read and write (Vandervelden & Siegel, 1995). Several general accounts of the process by which the child learns to read have been proposed. Ehri and Wilce (1983) postulated three phases in this process. In phase 1, unfamiliar words become familiar and the child pays attention to the component letters of a word. In phase 2, words come to be recognized as wholes with deliberate processing of grapheme–phoneme correspondences, and the meanings of words are accessed automatically. In phase 3, the speed of processing increases significantly. However, less skilled readers do not show this automaticity or the growth of speed in identifying words and nonwords.

Harris and Coltheart (1986) proposed four phases in learning to read. Initially, children learn to read a small set of words through the direct access or visual route; that is, they recognize words without sounding them out. Then children learn a small set of words on which they have been instructed. Then, around 5 or 6 years of age children rely on partial cues and relate printed words to items stored in memory. Phonological recoding occurs at the next stage and grapheme–phoneme conversion rules are used extensively. But grapheme–phoneme conversion rules are inadequate for many languages in which the correspondence between letters and phonemes is not perfect; hence, an orthographic stage, with no phonological recoding of words, is the final stage.

Gough and Juel (1991) also proposed a series of stages by which the child learns to read. In the first stages, the child learns to pair sounds with a printed word in an associative process. According to Gough and Juel, the child selects one cue from the printed word and the response is associated with that one cue. To illustrate this process, Gough reported an unpublished study in which children 4–5 years old were asked to learn four words on cards. One of the cards had a thumbprint in the lower left corner. The children learned the word on the card with the thumbprint much faster than those on the other three but often could not identify the word unless the thumbprint was on the card, and would, in the presence of the thumbprint, incorrectly label a word with the word that had been on the card with the thumbprint. Thus, the children appeared to be learning the word–sound association based on the overall visual stimulus without attention to individual letters. That is, they were learning a sound–picture association and incorrectly using part of the visual stimulus, in this case an irrelevant element. In terms of the dual-route theory, these children were apparently using the direct access or visual route but doing so inefficiently.

Gough (in Gough & Juel, 1991) provided an additional demonstration of this use of partial cues. He taught children 4–5 years old to read four words and then determined whether they could recognize a word when half of it was hidden. Some of the children could recognize the word if the first part was hidden ("du" in duck) but not if the second part was hidden, and some could recognize the word when the second part was hidden but not the first. They appeared to be using only partial visual cues.

According to Gough and Juel (1991), in the next stage the child must map spoken language onto printed words using a process called cryptanalysis, that is, learning the correspondences of sounds and letters (the orthographic cipher). Gough and Juel distinguished between this cipher and what is called phonics. They characterized the rules of English phonics as explicit and the cipher as a larger set of regularities that may be learned as rules or that may be represented by analogies. They asserted that the use of phonics rules is a slow and laborious process of associating each sound with a letter, holding the sound in memory, and blending all the individual sounds to make a word.

Gough and Juel (1991) noted that the test of mastering the cipher is the reading of pseudo-words. They obtained a correlation of .55 between the reading of real words and pseudo-words. Siegel and Ryan (1988) obtained a correlation of .86 for English and, for Portuguese, Da Fontoura and Siegel (1995) obtained a correlation of .63. Children who are "using the cipher," in their terminology, will make more reading errors that are nonwords than children who are not using it; that is, the child not using it will be more likely to guess another word. A number of studies have shown that children who cannot read well make just these sorts of errors (e.g., Johnston, 1982; Siegel, 1985;

Sprenger-Charolles, 1991). These studies are discussed in detail later in this chapter. In contrast, the child using the cipher will make errors indicating a misapplication of rules.

ACQUISITION OF GRAPHEME–PHONEME CONVERSION RULES

Although we have evidence about the inadequate phonological skills of children with reading disabilities, little is known about the precise manner in which the complex grapheme–phoneme conversion rules of the English language are acquired. The studies reported previously have involved global measures of pseudo-word reading. This type of measure is an important first step, but in order to understand the process of reading, a more detailed analysis is needed. Venezky and Johnson (1973) said, "A single 'word attack' score has little diagnostic value, especially for those children who fall in the middle ranges between mastery and complete failure" (pp. 109–110). The ascertainment of the order and nature of the acquisition of these rules is an important step in the understanding and treatment of reading skills. A number of investigators have begun to work on the problem of specifying the order of acquisition of these grapheme–phoneme conversion rules with the expectation that the rules are acquired in a relatively fixed and predictable order in a manner similar to the way syntactic structures develop in oral language (e.g., Guthrie & Seifert, 1983; Siegel & Faux, 1989; Snowling, 1980). To study these issues, we showed disabled and normal readers words and pseudo-words that involved a variety of grapheme–phoneme conversion rules, such as consonant blends, r-influenced vowels, and inconsistent vowels (Siegel & Faux, 1989). We found that complexity, as measured by the number of syllables in a pseudo-word, was a significant determinant of the difficulty of reading the pseudo-word. Pseudo-words with two or more syllables were quite difficult for older disabled readers (11–13 years) even though normal readers had become quite proficient by the age of 9 to 10. Even simple vowels and consonant blends were not mastered by the oldest children with reading disabilities in the study (ages 11–14) when they were required to read pseudo-words such as "mog," "lun," and "spad," although most of the 7-

and 8-year-old normal readers had no difficulty with these features in words or pseudo-words.

In most cases, even when the disabled readers appeared to demonstrate mastery of grapheme–phoneme conversion rules when they read a word, they were unable to read a pseudo-word with the same rule. The reading disabled experienced unusual difficulty when reading pseudo-words. Even when they could read words with particular grapheme–phoneme correspondences in consonant-vowel/consonant words, such as "ran," "wet," and "sit," they could not read pseudo-words such as "han," "fet," and "rit," and although they could read words involving consonant blends, such as "hunt," "spot," and "help," they could not read pseudo-words of a similar structure, such as "lunt," "grot," and "melp."

This superiority of words over pseudo-words suggests that the children with reading disabilities were using some sort of direct lexical access which, of course, they could use when they read words but which was not possible in the reading of pseudo-words. This direct lexical access probably involves processing each word as a picture (visual representation) rather than a series of letters with sounds. This visual representation is retrieved from long-term memory.

One relatively simple rule of English, with few exceptions, is that a final e in a one-syllable word makes the vowel long. This rule was not mastered by the oldest children with reading disabilities in this study. That is, the older disabled readers could correctly read the words that reflected the rule (e.g., "like," "cute," and "nose") but not the comparable pseudo-words (e.g., "rike," "fute," and "mose"). This difficulty is quite surprising because this rule is repeatedly stressed in reading instruction and is normally mastered early in the development of reading skills. In many instances, the scores of the children with reading disabilities were significantly lower than those of normal readers who were matched on reading grade level. For example, the disabled readers had significantly lower scores than did the normal readers of the same reading age on the following tasks: reading one-syllable pseudo-words at grade-level 3; two-syllable pseudo-words at grade-level 4–5; multisyllable pseudo-words at grade-level 6; and

pseudo-words with consonant blends at grade levels 2, 3, and 6. In some cases, the reading disabled and normal readers did not differ; however, these cases often resulted from floor or ceiling effects.

English orthography is characterized by unpredictable correspondences between graphemes and phonemes. That is, when reading a given grapheme, one often cannot predict its pronunciation. Some words are regular (e.g., "paid," "gave," and "heat") and can be read using the rules of pronunciation of their component graphemes. Other words are irregular or exceptions, and they violate grapheme–phoneme conversion rules and have no rhymes with similar spelling patterns (e.g., "said," "have," and "great"). Words in another category also have irregular grapheme–phoneme correspondences but also have unusual spellings that do not occur in many other words, such as "aisle," "ache," and "tongue." Waters, Seidenberg, and Bruck (1984) found that younger normal and poor readers were sensitive to the effects of irregular spelling and irregular grapheme–phoneme correspondence and took longer to read words with these characteristics. The children also showed the effects of frequency, in that the regular exception differences were greater with low-frequency words, such as "pint" and "wool." Because children with reading disabilities have poor phonological skills, they are more likely to rely on context when reading (e.g., Bruck, 1988).

Other studies have shown that poor readers have difficulty with exception words (Manis & Morrison, 1985; Seidenberg, Bruck, Fornarolo, & Backman, 1985). However, still others have not revealed any difference between regular and irregular words for disabled readers (Frith & Snowling, 1983; Seymour & Porpodos, 1980; Siegel & Ryan, 1988). If regular words with regular pronunciations are not read more easily than irregular words, grapheme–phoneme conversion rules are apparently not being used. In addition, disabled readers are much less likely than normal readers to regularize the vowels in irregular words (Seidenberg et al., 1985).

One set of hypotheses that has been advanced is that the development of reading skills is accompanied by increasing reliance on the visual/orthographic route. At the early stages of acquisition, readers rely heavily on phonological information, but good readers learn to recognize high-frequency words automatically. Words are largely recognized by direct access through the visual route. Doctor and Coltheart (1980) found that good readers relied more on phonological mediation when judging the meaningfulness of sentences. They used four types of meaningless: sentences that sounded correct, but in print had an incorrect real word (e.g., "I have know time"); meaningless sentences with a pseudo-word ("I have bloo time"); meaningless sentences containing real words ("I have blue time"); meaningful sentences with a pseudohomophone (e.g., "I have noe time"). The children were required to read these sentences and were asked whether the sentences made sense. Sentences that sounded correct when phonologically recoded (e.g., "I have know time" and "I have noe time") produced more incorrect responses than did sentences that were meaningless when phonologically recoded (e.g., "I have blue time" and "I have bloo time"). However, the difference decreased with age, and the investigators concluded that young readers rely on phonological encoding and older readers rely on visual encoding through the direct route.

Backman and colleagues (1984) found that beginning readers appear to be using the visual route for high-frequency words but they are also learning more about grapheme–phoneme conversion rules. Young readers and poor readers had difficulty reading homographic patterns, that is orthographic patterns with multiple pronunciations such as "ose" in "hose," "lose," and "dose." Backman and colleagues showed good and poor readers regular words (e.g., "hope"), exception words ("said"), regular inconsistent words, that is, words with regular pronunciations but with irregular orthographically similar neighbors (e.g., "paid" and "said"), ambiguous words (e.g., "clown" because "own" can be pronounced as in "down" or "blown"), and pseudo-words constructed to test these orthographic features. Young normal readers read the regular words that were of high frequency quite well but made more errors on exception, regular inconsistent, and ambiguous words. Older good readers performed at a level comparable to high school comparison subjects.

Although most errors on the exception words involved regularizations (e.g. "come" pronounced as "coam") rather than errors that were not ("come" pronounced as "came"), younger children made fewer regularizations than did older children and high school students. However, fewer errors involved giving regular inconsistent words an irregular pronunciation (e.g., "bone" read as "bun" like "done"). Poor readers were not as skilled at using grapheme–phoneme conversion rules and had more difficulty with orthographic patterns that had multiple pronunciations. Poor readers also had more difficulty than normal readers with the exception, inconsistent, and ambiguous words and tended to make fewer regularization errors. Poor readers also had more difficulty with pseudo-words. Under normal circumstances, as children get older they become more skilled at reading the irregular and unpredictable aspects of English orthography. Poor readers, however, continue to have difficulty with the orthographic features that are not predictable but do well with high-frequency regular words. This pattern of findings is consistent with the findings by Doctor and Coltheart (1980) about a shift from phonological recoding to direct visual access.

Seidenberg and colleagues (1985) also found that poor and disabled readers took longer and were less accurate in reading words with homographic patterns (e.g., "one," as in "done" and "gone") than normal readers. Exception words were the hardest for good readers, but they read regular inconsistent, ambiguous, and regular words equally well. This pattern suggests that they were significantly influenced by grapheme–phoneme conversion rules because exception words, by definition, violate these rules and these words were the most difficult to read. Poor and disabled readers made more errors on exception, regular inconsistent, and ambiguous than on regular words. Manis and colleagues (1987) found that children with reading disabilities had more difficulty than normal readers in a task that required learning to associate symbols with words or symbols with other symbols, particularly when the rule was inconsistent. This type of rule learning is analogous to the grapheme–phoneme conversion rules of English. However, the disabled and normal readers did not differ in learning the association when no rule was applicable. Therefore, children with reading disabilities do not appear to have a deficit in visual memory that does not involve linguistic stimuli.

Relatively few detailed studies of the acquisition of specific grapheme–phoneme conversion rules have been conducted. Venezky and Johnson (1973) studied the acquisition of reading the letter "c," pronounced as "k" or "s," and the letter "a," pronounced short (ae) or long (e) using pseudo-words such as "cipe," "acim," and "bice." They found that for normal readers, the rules for the long and short "a" appeared early in reading acquisition, but the rule for the "c" pronounced as "s" appeared much later. The initial "c" as "s" was learned more slowly than the pronunciation of "c" in the medial position. Venezky and Johnson speculated that the child may not be exposed to as many words with "ce," "ci," and "cy" and the teaching may not emphasize the multiple pronunciations of "c." Although Venezky and Johnson did not specifically test poor readers, they noted that the scores on their reading task were correlated with reading comprehension scores.

VOWELS

English vowels tend to have more complex and irregular pronunciations than English consonants. The grapheme–phoneme correspondences of English vowels are unpredictable. At this time, the understanding of the relationship between the nature of English vowel orthography and the development of reading skills and problems cannot be determined because, as Shankweiler and Liberman (1972) have noted:

> This generalization applies to English. We do not know how widely it may apply to other languages. We would greatly welcome the appearance of cross–language studies of reading acquisition, which could be of much value in clarifying the relations between reading and linguistic structure. That differences among languages in orthography are related to the incidence of reading failure is often taken for granted, but we are aware of no data that directly bear on this question. (p. 310)

More vowel spellings correspond to a particular vowel phoneme than consonant spellings to a particular consonantal phoneme. Consequently, misreadings of vowels occur more frequently than misreadings of consonants (Fowler, Shankweiler, & Liberman, 1979; Weber, 1970). Unlike consonants, which are more likely to be misread in the final than initial position, the position of a vowel has no effect on the probability that it will be misread. Unlike consonant errors, vowel errors are unrelated to their target sound, that is, they are random in regard to phonetic features. According to Fowler, Liberman, and Shankweiler (1977), vowels are less clearly defined and are more subject to individual and dialect variation. Vowels are the foundation of the syllable and code the prosodic features, and consonants carry the information.

English vowels have the property that their pronunciation can change depending on the context. An example is the rule that an "e" at the end of a word usually makes the vowel long. The reading of vowels is "context free" if this rule is ignored and the vowel is pronounced with the short vowel sound (e.g., "cape" read as "cap"), and the reading is *context dependent* if the rule is followed (Fowler et al., 1979). Fowler and colleagues (1979) administered pseudo-words to young normal readers and found that most of the responses to vowels were not random but were either context dependent or context free, that is, the children were using the possible sounds for that vowel. Context-dependent responses increased with increasing age, indicating an awareness of the context in which the possible spellings of phonemes occur. Even the youngest readers, who had received only 1 year of reading instruction, could apply their knowledge of orthographic regularities to pseudo-words.

As noted earlier, disabled readers are less likely to regularize the vowels in irregular words. Bryson and Werker (1989) administered a pseudo-word reading task to disabled readers to determine whether they would be more likely to read vowels as context dependent. As normal readers gained reading skills, they made more context-dependent responses. Some of the children with reading disabilities (those with significantly higher performance than verbal IQ scores) made more context-free responses than age- and reading-level matched controls. Some of the children with reading disabilities did not make context-free errors. However, it should be noted that these children were defined on the basis of below-grade-level scores on a reading comprehension and/or text reading test. As noted earlier, children with low scores on these types of reading tests may *not* have poor word recognition or decoding skills; therefore, these children may not have been reading disabled in the sense used in this chapter.

Bryson and Werker (1989) noted that poor readers and younger normal readers, when attempting to read double vowels, either sounded out the first letter and ignored the second or sounded out each individual letter. Often, the poor readers sounded out the final silent "e," therefore adding a phoneme. They appeared to be reading letter by letter.

Seidenberg and colleagues (1985) found that both poor readers and clinically diagnosed, probably dyslexic readers made more vowel than consonant errors. Most of these errors involved the incorrect lengthening or shortening of the vowel. The more severely disabled readers produced errors that involved substitution of a totally different vowel (e.g., "lake" for "like"); poor readers produced mispronunciations of the target vowel on the exception words; good readers tended to regularize them ("come" pronounced to rhyme with "home"). The reading disabled and poor readers were less likely to make these kinds of errors. Poor and disabled readers were less likely to regularize a pseudo-word that could be pronounced like a regular or an exception word (e.g., "naid" that could be pronounced to rhyme with "said" or "paid"). Using pseudo-words, Smiley, Pasquale, and Chandler (1976) also found that poor readers made more errors on vowels, especially long vowels, than did good readers. Shankweiler and Liberman (1972) conducted detailed analyses of the errors that were actually made in misreading vowels. Vowels that have many orthographic representations—such as /u/, which is represented by *u, o, oo, ou, oe, ew,* and *ie*—were the most difficult to read.

Guthrie and Seifert (1977) found that long vowel sounds were learned later than short vowel sounds. What they called special rule word production, with such vowel sounds as in "food," "join," and "bulk," were learned even later. Typically, the poor readers' mastery of these complex rules was slower and less adequate than that of the good readers.'

The increased likelihood of vowel errors does not appear to be a result of inadequate perception of sounds or difficulties with speaking. When children were asked to repeat the words that they had been asked to read, Shankweiler and Liberman (1972) found that fewer errors occurred on vowels than consonants and that the errors were evenly distributed between the initial and final positions.

In languages other than English, vowels have more regular patterns with fewer representations of each vowel sound. One such language is Hebrew, in which the orthography is transparent, that is, the grapheme–phoneme conversion rules are predictable. Children learning to read both English and Hebrew can be tested to compare these two very different orthographies. In a comparison of English-speaking children learning to read Hebrew as a second language, we (Geva & Siegel, 2000) found that the incidence of errors in reading vowels was significantly higher in English than in Hebrew. Other children who had reading disabilities (in both languages) made many vowel errors in English but few in Hebrew. Younger children with reading disabilities made vowel errors in both languages. However, other types of errors were more common in Hebrew. Hebrew has many visually similar letters and more errors were made involving visually confusable letters in Hebrew than in English. In addition, because Hebrew has a transparent orthography, one can decode it syllable by syllable and pronounce it properly and read the word without the proper stress. Failure to read the word with the stress on the correct syllable was more common in Hebrew than in English. In English, a syllable-by-syllable decoding would usually result in vowel errors (e.g., pronouncing the vowel as a short vowel when the word ends in "e" and perhaps even pronouncing the final silent "e"). Order errors, in which a consonant was omitted or the order of the consonants was confused, were more common in English than Hebrew, possibly because Hebrew words can be decoded in a linear manner from right to left and the linear strategy does not always work successfully in English.

CONSONANTS

Consonants in English are more regular than vowels in that particular consonantal phonemes are represented in fewer ways. Consequently, consonants are less likely to be misread. Shankweiler and Liberman (1972) and Fowler and colleagues (1977) found that consonants in the initial position were more likely to be read correctly than consonants in the final position. (In the Shankweiler and Liberman study, the positions of the vowels and the particular consonants used were not counterbalanced; but this methodological problem was corrected in the Fowler and colleagues study.) The reason for this positional effect is not clear. It could result from guessing a word on the basis of the initial letter rather than trying to apply grapheme–phoneme conversion rules to the word because of poor reading ability and underdeveloped phonological skills. Fowler and colleagues noted that the initial segment is easiest to isolate and unlike the final one does not require analysis of the syllable. Therefore, children with inadequate phonological skills might be expected to be able to process the first consonant but not the later ones.

Consonant errors were closely related to their target sound but vowel errors were not. For example, "b" and "p" were more likely to be substituted for each other than "b" and "s." Consonants with more complex orthographies (i.e., the ones that can be represented by more than one letter), were more difficult, but this effect cannot explain the initial–final consonant difference.

The error patterns were not the same for vowels and consonants (vowel errors were independent of position, consonant errors were not; vowel errors were not closely related to the target, consonant errors were). The errors evidently do not reflect visual difficulties because visual difficulties should not work differently with vowels and consonants. In addition, visual difficulties do not appear to be characteristic of beginning readers. Word and letter reversals accounted

for only a small portion of the errors made in reading words in the Shankweiler and Liberman (1972) study, even though they used lists designed to elicit these errors. Furthermore, sequence reversals such as "saw" read as "was" were uncorrelated with letter reversals such as "b" read as "d." However, consonant errors were more common than vowel errors.

Werker, Bryson, and Wassenberg (1989) examined the reading of consonants and found that both disabled and normal readers made more phonetic feature substitution errors than orientation reversal substitutions. Also, children with a reading disability made more consonant addition errors. Most errors were not reversal errors. Although some reversals are found in young children regardless of reading ability (Taylor, Satz, & Friel, 1979; Vellutino, Steger, & Kandel, 1972), these reversal errors may be linguistic rather than perceptual because reversals of orientation ("b" read as "d") are not correlated with reversal of sequencing ("was"–"saw"). Reversals occur with words but not with single letters presented tachistoscopically, and consonants are confused when they differ by a single phonetic feature regardless of visual similarity. Seidenberg and colleagues (1985) found that disabled readers make more substitution errors ("belt" for "best") and insertion errors ("grave" for "gave") than slow readers, who make more errors than normal readers.

Werker and colleagues (1989) noted that Seidenberg and colleagues (1985) confounded phonetic feature and orientation reversal substitutions by calling them both reversals ("deed" for "beed") and inversions ("deed" for "deep"). Werker and colleagues studied orientation reversal errors in which one letter was read as another differing in left/right or up/down orientation, such as "b" for "d," and phonetic feature errors in which one letter was misread as another differing in a single phonetic feature such as voicing "b" versus "p" and place of articulation ("b" and "d" are both voiced but "b" is bilabial and "d" is alveolor). They found that normal and disabled readers were equally likely to make orientation reversal errors. All groups made more phonetic feature than orientation reversal errors. Therefore, errors were the result of phonetic and not visual similarities. The order of types of errors was as follows: phonetic > addition > omission > sequencing. The children with reading disabilities made more errors than normal readers that involved adding a consonant. The normal readers made more phonetic feature substitutions than any other type of error. Disabled readers seemed to be reading letter by letter. The most common type of addition errors involved homorganic errors, that is, closing a syllable with the consonant sound already existing (e.g., "ap" to "pap"). Reading disabled, not normal readers, made these errors. Intrasyllable additions, reading "ope" as "olpe," were less common but did occur especially among the disabled readers and typically involved the addition of the liquids, "r" and "l." Werker and colleagues speculated that errors result from knowledge of individual letters but that the disabled readers have trouble knowing and retrieving the rules when they must combine letters. In addition, they may rely on articulatory information when sounding out words so that they retrieve the pronunciation of letters that are close in place of articulation to the target letter.

Smiley and colleagues (1976) found that disabled readers made more errors on the variable consonants (e.g., "c" and "g"). The reading disabled group had particular difficulty with the "s" pronunciation of "c," the "j" pronunciation of "g," the initial "ch" sound, and two-syllable words ending in "y." The good readers made more plausible (similar to the correct answer) errors than did poor readers.

ANALOGY VERSUS RULES

Other kinds of tasks have been used to measure the development of the understanding of grapheme–phoneme conversion rules. The reading of pseudo-words that can be read by analogy or by grapheme–phoneme rules, such as "puscle," "fody," and "risten," has been studied (Manis, Szeszulski, Howell, & Horn, 1986). For example, "puscle" can be pronounced as if it rhymed with "muscle" or with the "cl" pronounced, and "fody" can be pronounced like "body" or with a long "o." Children with a reading disability had a great deal of difficulty with these pseudowords. The children with reading disabilities were significantly less able than normal readers of the same chronological age to read

these words correctly. Even when matched with normal readers of the same reading level, the disabled readers made significantly more errors than did the normal readers. Compared to the normal readers, the younger children with a reading disability were significantly less likely to use a rule-based strategy and more likely to use an analogy strategy. This pattern suggests a greater reliance on the visual route.

OTHER PHONOLOGICAL SKILLS

Pseudo-word reading is not the only task that distinguishes poor from normal readers. Another task is the spelling of pseudo-words. Obviously, pseudo-words can be spelled only by using phoneme–grapheme conversion strategies as no lexical entry exists. Disabled readers had significantly lower scores on a task that involved the spelling of pseudo-words, even when the disabled readers were at the same reading level as younger normal readers (Siegel & Ryan, 1988).

One type of evidence of phonological processing skills is the use of phonological recoding in short-term memory such that rhyming (confusable) stimuli are more difficult to remember than nonrhyming stimuli. A number of studies have shown that younger poor readers are less disrupted by rhyming stimuli (e.g., Byrne & Shea, 1979; Mann, Liberman, & Shankweiler, 1980; Shankweiler, Liberman, Mark, Fowler, & Fischer, 1979; Siegel & Linder, 1983). However, Johnston (1982) and Siegel and Linder (1983) found that older dyslexic children do show phonetic confusability, although their short-term memory for letters was significantly poorer than that of age-matched controls. This latter finding is not surprising as phonological recoding skills are likely to be involved in any verbal memory task and the dyslexics' poor verbal memory may be a function of inadequate phonological abilities.

Performance on a variety of phonological tasks distinguishes disabled from normal readers. Children with reading disabilities were slower than normal readers in deciding whether two aurally presented words rhymed, presumably because of inadequate use of phonological recoding in memory (Rack, 1985). Phonemic awareness, the ability to recognize the basic phonemic segments of the language, is obviously an important component of phonological processing. Difficulties with phonemic awareness predict subsequent reading problems (e.g., Bradley & Bryant, 1983; Mann, 1984; Wallach & Wallach, 1976). Poor readers also have deficits in phonological production tasks, for example, naming objects represented by multisyllable words and repeating multisyllabic words and difficult phrases with alliteration. Pratt and Brady (1988) found differences between good and poor readers on the ability to segment words into phonemes and delete sounds from words. Good readers were more accurate in judging the length of a word or pseudo-word. Good readers were more disrupted than poor readers by misspellings in text that were phonologically inappropriate ("robln" for "robin"), indicating that the good readers were using phonological cues (Snowling & Frith, 1981).

Children with a reading disability also have difficulty recognizing the visual code of sounds (Siegel & Ryan, 1988). In the Gates McKillop test, children hear pseudo-words such as "wiskate" and are asked to select the correct version of the word from among four printed choices: "iskate," "wiskay," "wiskate," and "whestit." Poor readers had significantly lower scores than normal readers on this task. Although this task involves skills that are relevant to spelling, aspects of it are relevant to phonological processing, including the segmentation involved in analyzing the pseudo-word and in decoding the alternatives.

THE DEVELOPMENT OF PHONOLOGICAL SKILLS
IN OTHER LANGUAGES

We have been discussing only English up to this point. Children who have difficulty learning to read Portuguese have difficulty reading pseudo-words (Da Fontoura & Siegel, 1995) and children learning Hebrew as a second language also have difficulty with pseudo-words (Geva & Siegel, 2000). English is an alphabetic language with a significant amount of irregularity; Chinese is a morphemic orthography in which the characters have meaning and in which phonological information about pronunciation is sometimes coded in a character but is not

essential. Even in Chinese (Cantonese), children with reading problems have difficulty with tone and rhyme discrimination and have significantly lower scores than do normal readers on tasks measuring these phonological skills (So & Siegel, 1997).

SYNTACTIC AWARENESS

Syntactic awareness is the ability to understand the basic grammatical structure of the language in question. Siegel and Ryan (1988) have investigated the development of these skills in disabled and normal readers using an Oral Cloze task, a Sentence Correction task, and the Grammatical Closure subtest of the Illinois Test of Psycholinguistic Abilities. In the Oral Cloze task, a sentence is read aloud to the child and the child is required to fill in the missing word. Examples include the following: "Jane _____ her sister ran up the hill"; "Betty _____ a hole with her shovel"; "The girl_____ is tall plays basketball." In the sentence correction task, a sentence that is syntactically incorrect is read aloud to the child, who is then required to correct the sentence. Examples include the following: "Animal are kept in zoos"; "Can you read them book?"; and "It was very cold outside tomorrow." In the Illinois Test of Psycholinguistic Abilities Grammatic Closure subtest, the child is required to supply the missing word in a sentence that is read aloud while the examiner points to pictures illustrating the sentence. For example, "Here the thief is stealing the jewels. Here the jewels have been _____." In this example, the child must understand the irregular past tense of the verb "to steal" in order to supply the correct word. When the disabled and the normal readers were compared on these three tasks, the children with a reading disability performed at a level that was significantly lower than the normal readers. More difficult tasks might have yielded differences between the older dyslexics and the normal readers but the differences were certainly significant in the elementary school years. Brittain (1970) found that performance on a test of the production of morphology (similar to the ITPA Grammatic Closure) was related to reading ability in grade 1 and 2 children.

Other evidence suggests that children with reading problems have difficulty with syntactic awareness. Guthrie (1973) found that disabled readers performed at a lower level than both chronological-age- and reading-level-matched normal readers on a reading cloze task that measured syntax comprehension, even though the disabled readers had an adequate sight reading vocabulary to perform this task. Although reading disabled children were not studied, Goldman (1976) found that the understanding of complex syntax (e.g., sentences such as "John tells Bill to bake the cake" and "John promises Bill to bake the cake") was related to performance on a reading comprehension test. Cromer and Wiener (1966) found that poor readers made more errors than normal readers that indicated a lack of awareness of syntax on text reading tasks. Glass and Perna (1986) found that performance on an oral-language sentence comprehension test was poorer for children with a reading disability than for normal readers. Willows and Ryan (1981) found that less skilled readers were not as accurate as normal readers at substituting a missing word in a reading cloze procedure. Although difficulties in the processing of syntax may be an artifact of working-memory problems, this possibility is relatively unlikely as we have found that children with reading disabilities, except at the ages of 7 to 8, are as likely to show correct verbatim recall of sentences of varying length and grammatical complexity (Siegel & Ryan, 1988). Byrne (1981) has also shown that poor readers had more difficulty than good readers only with certain types of syntactic structures; the complexity of sentence structure, not the length of the sentence, was a determinant of performance.

Some evidence from other languages indicates that children with reading difficulties experience syntactic difficulties. Children with reading problems in Chinese (Cantonese) demonstrated poorer performance in an oral cloze test involving syntactic awareness of Chinese (So & Siegel, 1997). Similar results were found for Canadian children who spoke Portuguese as a first language, received instruction in reading in English, and attended a Portuguese Heritage Language Program in Portuguese (Da Fontoura & Siegel, 1995). The children who had low scores on Portuguese word and pseudo-word reading tests had significantly lower scores on Portuguese oral cloze than did children who were good readers of Portuguese. Testing native speakers of Hebrew, Bentin, Deutsch, and Liberman (1990) found that disabled readers in Hebrew were less accurate at judging whether the syntax of a sentence was correct and correcting a sentence with incorrect syntax. In addition, good readers were more influenced by context in identifying unclear words and made more errors than disabled readers that involved substituting a syntactically correct word but one that was not the word they had heard.

Working Memory

Working memory is the ability to retain information in short-term memory while processing incoming information. In reading, working memory means the decoding or recognizing of words or phrases while remembering what has been read. Siegel and Ryan (1989a) studied working memory in normal and disabled readers and dyslexics, using a task based on one developed by Daneman and Carpenter (1980). In the modified version of this task, the child is read aloud two, three, four, or five sentences and is asked to fill in a missing word at the end of each sentence. The child is then required to remember the missing words. Examples include the following: "In the summer it is very _____. People go to see monkeys in a _____. With dinner we sometimes eat bread and _____." The child was then required to repeat the three words that he or she selected in the order of presentation of the sentences. The disabled readers performed significantly more poorly than did the normal readers on this task, indicating significant difficulties with working memory in the disabled readers. Similar difficulties with working memory have been noted in Chinese (So & Siegel, 1997), Hebrew (Geva & Siegel, 2000), and Portuguese (Da Fontoura & Siegel, 1995).

Semantic Processing

The three basic cognitive processes described previously are important for the development of reading skill and are significantly disrupted in disabled readers. Two other processes, semantic and orthographic, are also involved in reading, but children with reading disabilities do not seem to experience the same degree of difficulties with these processes as with the preceding three.

READING ERRORS

Two types of analyses indicate that the semantic processing skills of poor readers are relatively intact. One type is analysis of errors made in word-reading tasks and the other is analysis of sentence processing. The analysis of errors made in reading single words can reveal important information about the reading process. A number of studies indicate that some children with severe reading problems make semantic errors in the reading of single words. An important point is that these errors are made in reading single words with *no context cues*. Johnston (1982) reported the case of an 18-year-old girl who made semantic errors such as "down" read as "up," "chair" read as "table," and "office" read as "occupation," and who could not read any pseudo-words. I have shown that a small group of children with reading disabilities make semantic substitutions while reading single isolated words (Siegel, 1985). All these children had very poor, or nonexistent, phonological processing skills and were unable to read a single pseudo-word. These types of semantic errors indicate that phonological processing is not used at all because none of the sounds implicit in the stimulus word is produced in the response. In addition, the printed equivalent of the response is not visually similar to the target word. However, this type of error indicates that some semantic processing is occurring and that although the word is not being read correctly, some semantic information is being processed. This type of error is made only in the early stages of reading acquisition. Normal readers do not appear to make this type of error. The types of errors that normal readers typically make involve the substitution of a visually and/or phonologically similar word (e.g., "look" as "book," "chicken" as "children," and "away" as "way").

Temple (1988) reported the case of a 9-year-old poor reader who could not read pseudo-words and who made some semantic substitutions when reading single words, such as "eye" read as "blue" and "mother"

read as "mommy." Temple, among others, argued that these errors may have been due to chance. This explanation seems unlikely for several reasons. Normal readers do not make these errors. The substitutions all make sense in terms of having similar meaning and no pairings are random. Given the total speaking vocabulary of 10,000–20,000 words of children this age, these particular errors seem unlikely to occur by chance.

In the one report of semantic errors in single-word reading among French-speaking children, Sprenger-Charolles (1991) administered a task in which children were required to read words or pseudo-words that were attached to pictures. Some pictures were correctly named; others were given a name related to the correct name but not synonymous (e.g., "limace," slug, was written under a picture of a snail); and others were given pseudo-word names that differed in a single letter from the real name (e.g., "falise" instead of "valise" or "pantalin" instead of "pantalon"). The children were required to say whether or not the correct name was attached to the picture. Semantic errors (e.g., "locobotive" read as "train," "binyclette," a nonword similar to the real word "bicyclette," read as "velo" [bike]) were quite common for a group of poor readers, average age 10, but virtually never occurred in the group of good readers.

Normal readers at the earliest stages of reading may sometimes appear to make these semantic errors. Seymour and Elder (1986) studied 4½–5½-year-old children who had received reading instruction that emphasized a sight vocabulary and that did not involve systematic instruction in grapheme–phoneme conversion rules. When reading single words, these children made semantic errors such as "boat" read as "yacht," "milk" read as "tea," "little" read as "wee." Thus, semantic coding of words appears to be the first aspect of words to be acquired, and semantic coding will be used if the child lacks an understanding of spelling–sound correspondences either because these correspondences have not been taught or because they have not been acquired because of cognitive factors, as in reading disability. These types of errors indicate that grapheme–phoneme conversion rules are not being used at all and that the phonological processing is virtually nonexistent.

Other evidence exists of the accuracy of semantic processing in disabled readers. Frost (1998) found that dyslexics could respond as quickly and as accurately as normal readers when required to make decisions about whether two words belonged to the same semantic category but were significantly slower on a phonological task that involved making a decision about whether two orthographically dissimilar words rhymed.

SENTENCE PROCESSING

Skills involved in processing the semantic aspects of sentences appear to be adequate in children with a reading disability. In the sentence correction task described earlier, some of the sentences were syntactically correct but meaningless. Examples include the following: "There are flowers flying in the garden"; "In the summer, it snows"; and "The moon is very big and bright in the morning." The reading disabled did not have any difficulty correcting these sentences and performed at a level similar to that of the normal readers. This finding contrasts with their performance on sentences where the correction of syntax was required. Therefore, the children with reading disabilities have a deficit in the processing of syntactic information, but this deficit does not extend to processing of semantic information. Lovett (1979) found that reading competence in young readers was not related to the ability to remember the semantic aspects of what had been read. Lovett required children to read short passages and then to recognize whether a sentence had been in the passage when the sentence was identical or differed slightly in semantic, syntactic, or lexical context. The children at all reading levels were easily able to recognize changes in the semantic content, were less able to recognize syntactic changes, and had much more difficulty in recognizing lexical changes (e.g., "picked up" changed to "lifted up"). Even when the children were required to read material between reading the sentence and remembering it, semantic information remained available, but syntactical and lexical information

were less so. These data indicate that semantic processing is primary for reading and at the earliest stages, or with disabled readers, semantic processing is operating even when other processes are much less efficient.

Waller (1976) studied good and poor readers and found that poor readers were as likely as good readers to remember many of the semantic aspects of what they had read but were less likely to remember whether a lexical item was singular or plural and whether a past or present tense was used. This pattern of errors indicates relatively intact semantic processing but difficulties with the syntactic processing.

Some evidence indicates that children with reading disabilities may even be superior to normal readers in their use of semantic context. Frith and Snowling (1983) administered a task in which reading disabled and normal readers, matched on reading level, were required to read sentences with homographs (with the correct pronunciation) such as "He had a pink bow" and "He made a deep bow." The performance of the children with reading disabilities was *superior* to that of the normal readers, indicating that the disabled readers were better able to make use of semantic/syntactic cues.

Orthographic Processing

Orthographic processing involves the awareness of the structure of the words in a language. For example, in English one does not find "v" at the end of a word or any words that start with "dl" or have "zxg" in them. Olson, Kliegl, Davidson, and Foltz (1985) have developed two tasks that provide a direct contrast of the visual (orthographic) and phonological processing routes. In the Visual task, the child is shown a real word and a pseudo-word (e.g., "rain"–"rane," and "boal"–"bowl") and has to select the correct spelling. In the Phonological task, the child has to specify which of two pseudo-words, presented visually, sounds like a real word (e.g., "kake"–"dake" and "joap"–"joak"). Each of these tasks is designed so that only one process can operate. That is, in the Visual task both choices sound exactly the same, so that visual memory for the orthography of a word must be used; phonological processes are not helpful in this case because sounding out the words would produce the identical response to each word. For the Phonological task, recall of the visual pattern would not be useful because neither alternative is a correct orthographic pattern in the English language. However, one of the alternatives, when sounded out, does produce an English word, although it is obviously not the correct orthographic form.

These tasks were administered to disabled and normal readers, ages 7 to 16 years. Not surprisingly, the disabled readers performed more poorly on the Phonological task than age-matched and reading-level-matched normal readers and did not catch up to the normal readers until the age of 13. They also performed more poorly on the Visual task than age-matched normal readers until age 13. However, the disabled readers performed at a significantly higher level on the Visual task than did the reading-level-matched normal readers at reading level 2. This finding indicates good visual memory skills in the disabled readers relative to their level of word reading. It indicates that the reading disabled were paying attention to the visual aspects of a word rather than the phonological aspects.

Another aspect of the awareness of orthographic structures is the ability to recognize legal and illegal orthographic combinations of English letters. Siegel, Share, and Geva (1995) developed a task to assess this ability. Children were shown 17 pairs of pronounceable pseudo-words, one containing a bigram that never occurs in an English word in a particular position and the other containing a bigram that occurs in English. Examples are "filv"–"filk," "moke"–"moje," "vism"–"visn," and "powl"–"lowp." This task was administered to disabled and normal readers, ages 7 to 16 years.

The performance of the poor and normal readers did not differ except at the youngest ages. At 7–8, the children with reading disabilities made significantly more errors than normal readers of the same chronological age, but an important point is that the children with reading disabilities did not perform more poorly than the age-matched normal readers at ages 9 to 16. However, when matched on reading level, the disabled readers performed at a significantly *higher*

level than the normal readers. Therefore, in comparison to the data on phonological processing, the orthographic processing of the reading disabled is quite good. These data indicate that orthographic processing is not as impaired in dyslexics as is phonological processing. These data indicate that semantic and orthographic processing occur in reading but that the use of these processes can disrupt normal reading and cause errors.

The preceding discussion has been based on what might be called orthographic awareness skills. Some evidence suggests that disabled readers are more sensitive to the visual aspects of printed stimuli than better readers. For example, Steinhauser and Guthrie (1974) found that poor readers were *faster* than good readers of the same reading level on a task that involved circling individual letters in a text. However, poor readers were worse than good readers when required to circle phonemes. A visual matching procedure can be used to circle individual letters, but phonemes probably require some phonological coding. These data suggest that individuals with reading disabilities are paying attention to the visual aspects of printed stimuli, but because of differences in phonological skills, they have more difficulty with these aspects of print. Snowling (1980) also found that children with a reading disability were *more accurate* than normal readers of the same reading level on a task involving selecting the visual form of an aurally presented pseudo-word. This superiority of the group with reading disabilities occurred only at the lowest reading level studied (age 7). However, the children with reading disabilities performed significantly more poorly than reading-level-matched normal readers on a task involving recognition of the auditory form of a visually presented pseudo-word. Clearly, this latter task involves phonological processing skills and the Auditory to Visual task relies on visual skills that are operating normally, or perhaps in a superior manner. The children with reading disabilities did not differ from normal readers in the Auditory–Auditory task in which they had to judge whether two aurally presented pseudo-words were the same or different, so the difficulties of poor readers were not due to problems in auditory discrimination.

The reading disabled did not show an improvement with age on the Visual–Visual task, but the normal readers did, suggesting that the disabled readers did not use a phonemic code in the visual matching task and that the normal readers were probably converting the visual stimuli to a phonemic code. The normal readers performed at the same level on the Visual–Visual, Auditory–Visual, and Visual–Auditory tasks. However, the children with reading disabilities performed significantly better on the Visual–Visual task than on the two crossed-modality tasks, suggesting again that the visual stimuli (pseudo-words) were not phonologically recoded. All the studies imply that the direct or visual access route is relatively intact in the reading disabled, but that the phonological route is impaired.

Evidence from adults with reading disability indicates that phonemic coding does not occur, at least not to the same extent as in normal readers. We (Shafrir & Siegel, 1991) found that adults with reading disabilities reported using a visual scanning strategy, rather than phonological recoding, in reading tasks that involved matching words and pseudo-words. The adults with reading disabilities who did use a phonological recoding strategy in the word task showed significantly *longer latencies* than those who used a phonological recoding strategy, suggesting that the visual strategy may be more efficient for disabled readers.

Evidence from spelling tasks indicates that adults with reading disabilities have an adequate knowledge of English orthography and, in some cases, a greater degree of knowledge than do normal readers. Pennington and colleagues (1986) scored the spelling errors of adults with reading disabilities and normal reading adults according to a simple system in which any orthographically illegal sequence occurred (e.g., "ngz" in "angziaty" for "anxiety") and a complex system in which errors indicating a lack of knowledge of more subtle aspects of orthography were scored, for example, knowing that vowel clusters can be represented by one vowel ("iou" in "precious" is the sound of /u/) or knowing that "phys" occurs in many words (e.g., "physics" and "physician") and represents the same sound in all of them. The reading disabled and normal readers did not differ in the preservation of simple orthographic features.

However, the reading disabled were significantly *more* accurate in the complex aspects of English orthography than normal readers of the same spelling level.

We (Lennox & Siegel, 1993) found that the spelling errors of children who were poor spellers were *more* similar visual matches to the correct word than were those of good spellers of the same spelling age. However, the misspellings of poor spellers were less phonologically accurate than those of good spellers of the same spelling age. These findings indicate that the poor spellers were more likely to use visual memory than phonological strategies in spelling.

These results suggest that individuals with a reading disability may be able to compensate for their difficulties in phonological processing. Rack (1985) found that children with reading disabilities make use of an orthographic code in memory. Reading disabled and normal readers, ages 8 to 14, were presented four lists of words to learn. The words in a list were orthographically similar and rhyming (e.g., "farm"–"harm"), orthographically similar and not rhyming (e.g., "farm"–"calm"), orthographically dissimilar and rhyming (e.g., "farm"–"warm"), and orthographically dissimilar and not rhyming (e.g., "farm"–"pond"). Whether the presentation was visual or auditory, orthographic similarity improved the performance of reading disabled more than normal readers, indicating that the disabled readers were more sensitive to orthographic effects. Phonetic similarity did not predict recall for the disabled readers but it did for the normal readers. Children with reading disabilities remembered *more* orthographically similar targets than did the normal readers and *fewer* rhyming targets, indicating that they were making more use of an orthographic rather than a phonetic code. Normal readers of the same reading age did not show this effect. Children with reading disabilities took longer to say yes for rhyming pairs that were orthographically dissimilar ("farm"–"calm") than for those that were orthographically similar ("head"–"lead"). Reading-level-matched normal readers did not show this effect.

However, Katz (1977) found that poor readers were not as accurate as good readers in recognizing which serial position an individual letter occurred in most frequently. In this study, good and poor readers were shown two pseudo-words, one containing a letter in its most frequent serial position and the other containing the letter in its least frequent serial position. Poor readers made more errors than good readers. Thus, poor readers had less orthographic knowledge about *single* letters, in contrast to groups of letters, than did good readers

Conclusions

The period of rapid acquisition of reading skills, three processes—phonological, syntactic, and working memory—show significant increases in development. These processes are significantly disrupted in children who are reading disabled, but semantic and orthographic processes are not disrupted to the same extent. However, the underutilization of phonological processing and the reliance almost entirely on semantics and orthographic or visual processes disrupts reading. A deficit in three fundamental cognitive processes—phonological processing, syntactic awareness, and working memory—constitutes the basic characteristics of reading disability. It is important that assessment for learning disabilities reflect an understanding of these processes and systematically measure them.

Acknowledgments

The preparation of this chapter was partially supported by a grant from the Natural Sciences and Engineering Research Council of Canada and was written while I was a Scholar in Residence at The Peter Wall Institute for Advanced Studies. I wish to thank Sarah Kontopoulos and Stephanie Vyas for their secretarial assistance.

References

Backman, J., Bruck, M., Hebert, M., & Seidenberg, M. (1984). Acquisition and use of spelling–sound correspondences in reading. *Journal of Experimental Child Psychology, 38,* 114–133.

Backman, J. E., Mamen, M., & Ferguson, H. B. (1984). Reading level design: Conceptual and methodological issues in reading research. *Psychological Bulletin, 96,* 560–568.

Barwick, M. A., & Siegel, L. S. (1996). Learning difficulties in adolescent clients of ashelter for runaway and homeless street youths. *Journal of Research on Adolescence, 6,* 649–670.

Bentin, S., Deutsch, A., & Liberman, I. Y. (1990). Syntactic competence and reading ability in children. *Journal of Experimental Psychology, 49*(1), 147–172.

Besner, D., Twilley, L., McCann, R., & Seergobin, K. (1990). On the association between connectionism and data: Are a few words necessary? *Psychological Review, 97,* 1–15.

Bradley, L., & Bryant, P. E. (1983). Categorizing sounds and learning to read: A causal connection. *Nature, 301,* 419–421.

Brittain, M. M. (1970). Inflectional performance and early reading achievement. *Reading Research Quarterly, 1,* 34–48.

Brown, A. D. (1987). Resolving inconsistency: A computational model of word naming. *Journal of Memory and Language, 26,* 1–23.

Bruck, M. (1988). The word recognition and spelling of dyslexia children. *Reading Research Quarterly, 23,* 51–68.

Bruck, M. (1990). Word-recognition skills of adults with childhood diagnosis of dyslexia. *Developmental Psychology, 26,* 439–454.

Bryson, S. E., & Werker, J. F. (1989). Toward understanding the problem in severely disabled readers: I. Vowel errors. *Applied Psycholinguistics, 10,* 1–12.

Byrne, B. (1981). Deficient syntactic control in poor readers: Is a weak phonetic memory code responsible? *Applied Psycholinguistics, 2,* 201–212.

Byrne, B., & Shea, P. (1979). Semantic and phonemic memory in beginning readers. *Memory and Cognition, 7,* 333–341.

Calfee, R. C., Lindamood, P., & Lindamood, C. (1973). Acoustic–phonetic skills and reading: Kindergarten through twelfth grade. *Journal of Educational Psychology, 64,* 293–298.

Coltheart, M. (1978). Lexical access in simple reading tasks. In G. Underwood (Ed.), *Strategies of information processing* (pp. 151–216). London: Academic Press.

Cromer, W., & Wiener, M. (1966). Idiosyncratic response patterns among good and poor readers. *Journal of Consulting Psychology, 30,* 1–10.

Da Fontoura, H. A., & Siegel, L. S. (1995). Reading, syntactic, and working memory skills of bilingual Portuguese–English Canadian children. *Reading and Writing: An Interdisciplinary Journal, 7,* 139–153.

Doctor, E. A., & Coltheart, M. (1980). Children's use phonological encoding when reading for meaning . *Memory and Cognitive, 8,* 195–209.

Ehri, L. C., & Wilce, L. S. (1980). The influence of orthography on readers' conceptualization of the phonemic of words. *Applied Psycholinguistics, 1,* 371–385.

Ehri, L. C., & Wilce, L. S. (1983). Development of word identification speed in skilled and less-skilled beginning readers. *Journal of Educational Psychology, 75,* 3–18.

Ellis, A. W. (1985). The cognitive neuropsychology of developmental (and acquired) dyslexia: A critical survey. *Cognitive Neuropsychology, 2,* 169–205.

Forster, K. I., & Chambers, S. (1973). Lexical access and naming time. *Journal of Verbal Learning and Verbal Behavior, 12,* 627–635.

Fowler, C., Liberman, I., & Shankweiler, D. (1977). On interpreting the error pattern in beginning reading. *Language and Speech, 20,* 162–173.

Fowler, C., Shankweiler, D., & Liberman, I. (1979). Apprehending spelling patterns for vowels: A developmental study. *Language and Speech, 22,* 243–251.

Frith, U., & Snowling, M. (1983). Reading for meaning and reading for sound in autistic and dyslexic children. *British Journal of Developmental Psychology, 1,* 329–342.

Frost, R. (1998). Toward a strong phonological theory of virtual word recognition: True issues and false trails. *Psychological Bulletin, 123*(1), 71–99.

Geva, E., & Siegel, L. S. (2000). Orthographic and cognitive factors in the concurrent development of basic reading skill in two languages. *Reading and Writing: An Interdisciplinary Journal, 12,* 1–30.

Glass, A. L., & Perna, J. (1986). The role of syntax in reading disability. *Journal of Learning Disabilities, 19,* 354–359.

Glushko, R. J. (1979). The organization and activation of orthographic knowledge in reading aloud. *Journal of Experimental Psychology: Human Perception and Performance, 5,* 674–691.

Goldman, S. R. (1976). Reading skills and the minimum distance principle: A comparison of listening and reading comprehension. *Journal of Experimental Child Psychology, 22,* 123–142.

Gough, P. B., & Juel, C. (1991). The first stages of word recognition. In L. Rieben & C. A. Perfetti (Eds.), *Learning to read: Basic research and its implications* (pp. 47–56). Hillsdale, NJ: Erlbaum.

Gough, P. B., & Tunmer, W. E. (1986). Decoding, reading, and reading disability. *Remedial and Special Education, 7,* 6–10.

Guthrie, J. T., & Seifert, M. (1977). Letter–sound complexity in learning to identify words. *Journal of Educational Psychology, 69*(6), 686–696.

Guthrie, J. T., & Seifert, M. (1983). Profiles of reading activity in a community. *Journal of Reading, 26,* 498–508.

Harris, M., & Coltheart, M. (1986). *Language processing in children and adults: An introduction.* London: Routledge & Kegan Paul.

Hogaboam, T. W., & Perfetti, C. A. (1978). Reading skill and their role of verbal experience in decoding. *Journal of Educational Psychology, 5,* 717–729.

Humphreys, G. W., & Evett, L. J. (1985). Are there independent lexical and nonlexical routes in the word processing? An evaluation of the dual-route theory of reading. *Behavioral and Brain Sciences, 8,* 689–740.

Johnston, R. (1982). Phonological coding in dyslexic readers. *British Journal of Psychology, 73,* 455–460.

Jorm, A. F. (1979). The nature of reading deficit in developmental dyslexia: A reply to Ellis. *Cognition, 1,* 421–433.

Katz, L. (1977). Reading ability and single-letter orthographic redundancy. *Journal of Educational Psychology, 69,* 653–659.

Lennox, C., & Siegel, L. S. (1993). Visual and phonological spelling errors in subtypes of children with learning disabilities. *Applied Psycholinguistics, 14,* 473–488.

Liberman, I. Y., Liberman, A. M., Mattingly, I., & Shankweiler, D. (1980). *Orthography and the beginning reader.* Unpublished manuscript.

Lindgren, S. D., De Renzi, E., & Richman, L. C. (1985). Cross–national comparisons of developmental dyslexia in Italy and the United States. *Child Development, 56,* 1404–1417.

Lovett, M. W. (1979). The selective encoding of sequential information in normal reading development. *Child Development, 50,* 897–900.

Manis, F. R., & Morrison, F. J. (1985). Reading disability: A deficit in rule learning? In L. S. Siegel & F. J. Morrison (Eds.), *Cognitive development in atypical children: Progress in cognitive development research* (pp. 1–26). New York: Springer–Verlag.

Manis, F. R., Savage, P. L., Morrison, F. J., Horn, C. C., Howell, M. J., Szesulski, P. A., & Holt, L. K. (1987). Paired associate learning in reading-disabled children: Evidence for a rule-learning deficiency. *Journal of Experimental Child Psychology, 43,* 25–43.

Manis, F. R., Szeszulski, P. A., Howell, M. J., & Horn, C. C. (1986). A comparison of analogy- and rule-based decoding strategies in normal and dyslexic children. *Journal of Reading Behavior, 18,* 203–213.

Mann, V. A. (1984). Longitudinal prediction and prevention of early reading difficulty. *Annals of Dyslexia, 34,* 117–136.

Mann, V. A., Liberman, I. Y., & Shankweiler, D. (1980). Children's memory for sentences and word strings in relation to reading ability. *Memory and Cognition, 8,* 329–335.

Metsala, J., & Siegel, L. S. (1992). Patterns of atypical reading development: Attributes and underlying reading processes. In S. Segalowitz & I. Rapin (Eds.), *Handbook of neuropsychology* (Vol. 7, pp. 187–210). New York: Elsevier.

Meyer, D. E., Schvanevelt, R. W., & Ruddy, M. G. (1974). Functions of graphemic and phonemic codes in visual word-recognition. *Memory and Cognition, 2,* 309–321.

Olson, R. K., Kliegl, R., Davidson, B. J., & Foltz, G. (1985). Individual and developmental differences in reading disability. In G. E. MacKinnon & T. G. Waller (Eds.), *Reading research: Advances in theory and practice* (Vol. 4, pp. 1–64). New York: Academic Press.

Pennington, B. F., McCabe, L. L., Smith, S. D., Lefly, D. L., Bookman, M. O., Kimberling, W. J., & Lubs, H. A. (1986). Spelling errors in adults with a form of familial dyslexia. *Child Development, 57*, 1001–1013.

Pratt, A. C., & Brady, S. (1988). Relations of phonological awareness to reading disability in children and adults. *Journal of Educational Psychology, 80*, 319–323.

Rack, J. P. (1985). Orthographic and phonetic coding in developmental dyslexia. *British Journal of Psychology, 76*, 325–340.

Seidenberg, M. S., Bruck, M., Fornarolo, G., & Backman, J. (1985). Word recognition processes of poor and disabled readers: Do they necessarily differ? *Applied Psycholinguistics, 6*, 161–180.

Seidenberg, M. S., & McClelland, J. L. (1989). Visual word recognition and pronunciation: A computational model of acquisition, skilled performance, and dyslexia. In A. M. Galaburda (Ed.), *From reading to neurons. Issues in the biology of language and cognition* (pp. 255–303). Cambridge, MA: MIT Press.

Seymour, P. H. K., & Elder, L. (1986). Beginning reading without phonology. *Cognitive Neuropsychology, 3*, 1–36.

Seymour, P. H. K., & Porpodos, C. D. (1980). Lexical and nonlexical processing of spelling in dyslexia. In U. Frith (Ed.), *Cognitive processes in spelling* (pp. 443–473). New York: Academic Press.

Shafrir, U., & Siegel, L. S. (1991). Preference for visual scanning strategies versus phonological rehearsal in university students with reading disabilities. *Journal of Learning Disabilities, 27*, 583–588.

Shafrir, U., & Siegel, L. S. (1994). Subtypes of learning disabilities in adolescents and adults. *Journal of Learning Disabilities, 27*, 123–134.

Shankweiler, D., & Liberman, I. (1972). Misreading: A search for causes. In J. Kavanaugh & I. Mattingly (Eds.), *Language by ear and by eye: The relationship between speech and reading* (pp. 293–317). Cambridge, MA: MIT Press.

Shankweiler, D., Liberman, I. Y., Mark, L. S., Fowler, C. A., & Fischer, F. W. (1979). The speech code and learning to read. *Journal of Experimental Psychology: Human Learning and Memory, 5*, 531–545.

Siegel, L. S. (1985). Psycholinguistic aspects of reading disabilities. In L. S. Siegel & F. J. Morrison (Eds.), *Cognitive development in atypical children* (pp. 45–65). New York: Springer-Verlag.

Siegel, L. S. (1988). Evidence that IQ scores are irrelevant to the definition and analysis of reading disability. *Canadian Journal of Psychology, 42*, 201–215.

Siegel, L. S. (1992). An evaluation of the discrepancy definition of dyslexia. *Journal of Learning Disabilities, 25*, 618–629.

Siegel, L. S. (1993). Phonological processing deficits as the basis of a reading disability. *Developmental Review, 13*, 246–257.

Siegel, L. S., & Faux, D. (1989). Acquisition of certain grapheme–phoneme correspondences in normally achieving and disabled readers. *Reading*

and Writing: An Interdisciplinary Journal, 1, 37–52.

Siegel, L. S., & Heaven, R. K. (1986). Categorization of learning disabilities. In S. J. Ceci (Ed.), *Handbook of cognitive, social and neuropsychological aspects of learning disabilities* (Vol. 1, pp. 95–121). Hillsdale, NJ: Erlbaum.

Siegel, L. S., Levey, P., & Ferris, H. (1985). Subtypes of developmental dyslexia: Do they exist? In F. J. Morrison, C. Lord, & D. P. Keating (Eds.), *Applied developmental psychology* (Vol. 2, pp. 169–190). New York: Academic Press.

Siegel, L. S., & Linder, B. A. (1983). Short-term memory processes in children with reading and arithmetic learning disabilities. *Developmental Psychology, 20*, 200–207.

Siegel, L. S., & Metsala, J. (1992). An alternative to the food processor approach to subtypes of learning disabilities. In N. N. Singh & I. Beale (Eds.), *Current perspectives in learning disabilities: Nature, theory, and treatment* (pp. 44–60). New York: Springer-Verlag.

Siegel, L. S., & Ryan, E. B. (1988). Development of grammatical sensitivity, phonological, and short-term memory in normally achieving and learning disabled children. *Developmental Psychology, 24*, 28–37.

Siegel, L. S., & Ryan, E. B. (1989a). The development of working memory in normally achieving and subtypes of learning disabled children. *Child Development, 60*, 973–980.

Siegel, L. S., & Ryan, E. B. (1989b). Subtypes of developmental dyslexia: The influence of definitional variables. *Reading and Writing: An Interdisciplinary Journal, 2*, 257–287.

Siegel, L. S., Share, D., & Geva, E. (1995). Evidence for superior orthographic skills in dyslexics. *Psychological Science, 6*(4), 250–254.

Smiley, S. S., Pasquale, F . L., Chandler, C. L. (1976). The pronunciation of familiar, unfamiliar and synthetic words by good and poor adolescent readers. *Journal of Reading Behavior, 8*(3), 289–297.

Snowling, M. J. (1980). The development of grapheme–phoneme correspondence in normal and dyslexic readers. *Journal of Experimental Child Psychology, 29*, 294–305.

Snowling, M., & Frith, U. (1981). The role of sound, shape, and orthographic cues in early reading. *British Journal of Psychology, 72*, 83–87.

So, D., & Siegel, L. S. (1997). Learning to read Chinese: Semantic, syntactic, phonological and working memory skills in normally achieving and poor Chinese readers. *Reading and Writing: An Interdisciplinary Journal, 9*, 1–21.

Sprenger-Charolles, L. (1991). Word–identification strategies in a picture context: Comparisons between "good" and "poor" readers. In L. Rieben & C. A. Perfetti (Eds.), *Learning to read: Basic research and its implications* (pp. 175–188). Hillsdale, NJ: Erlbaum.

Stanovich, K. E. (1988a). Explaining the differences between the dyslexic and garden variety poor reader. The phonological–core variance–difference model. *Journal of Learning Disabilities, 21,* 590–604, 612.

Stanovich, K. E. (1988b). The right and wrong places to look for the cognitive locus of reading disability. *Annals of Dyslexia, 38,* 154–177.

Stanovich, K. E., Nathan, R. G., & Zolman, J. E. (1988). The developmental lag hypothesis in reading: Longitudinal and matched reading–level comparisons. *Child Development, 59,* 71–86.

Steinhauser, R., & Guthrie, J. T. (1974). Scanning times through prose and word strings for various targets by normal and disabled readers. *Perceptual and Motor Skills, 39,* 931–938.

Stevenson, H. W., Stigler, J. W., Lucker, G. W., Hsu, C. C., & Kitamura, S. (1982). Reading disabilities: The case of Chinese, Japanese, and English. *Child Development, 53,* 1164–1181.

Tal, N. F., & Siegel, L. S. (1996). Pseudoword reading errors of poor , dyslexic and normally achieving readers on multisyllable pseudo-words. *Applied Psycholinguistics, 17,* 215–232.

Taylor, H. G., Satz, P., & Friel, J. (1979). Developmental dyslexia in relation to other childhood reading disorders: Significance and clinical utility. *Reading Research Quarterly, 15,* 84–101.

Temple, C. M. (1988). Red is read but eye is blue: A case study of developmental dyslexia and follow-up report. *Brain and Language, 34,* 13037.

Vandervelden, M. C., & Siegel, L. S. (1995). Phonological recoding and phonemic awareness in early literacy: A developmental approach. *Reading Research Quarterly, 30,* 854–875.

Vellutino, F. R., Steger, J. A., & Kandel, G. (1972). Reading disability: An investigation of the perceptual deficit hypotheses. *Cortex, 8,* 106–118.

Venezky, R. L., & Johnson, D. (1973). Development of two letter–sound patterns in grades one through three. *Journal of Educational Psychology, 64,* 109–115.

Wallach, M., & Wallach, L. (1976). *Helping disadvantaged children learn to read by teaching them phoneme identification skills.* Paper presented at the Learning Research and Development Center, Pittsburgh University, Pittsburgh.

Waller, G. (1976). Children's recognition memory for written sentences: A comparison of good and poor readers. *Child Development, 47,* 90–95.

Waters, G. S., Bruck, M., & Seidenberg, M. (1985). Do children use similar processes to read and spell words? *Journal of Experimental Child Psychology, 39,* 511–530.

Waters, G. S., Seidenberg, M. S., & Bruck, M. (1984). Children's and adults' use of spelling–sound information in three reading tasks. *Memory and Cognition, 12,* 293–305.

Weber, R. (1970). A linguistic analysis of first-grade reading errors. *Reading Research Quarterly, 5,* 427–451.

Werker, J. F., Bryson, S. E., & Wassenberg, K. (1989). Toward understanding the problem in severely disabled readers. Part II: Consonant errors. *Applied Psycholinguistics, 10,* 13–30.

Willows, D. M., & Ryan, E. B. (1981). Differential utilization of syntactic and semantic information by skilled and less skilled readers in the intermediate grades. *Journal of Educational Psychology, 73,* 607–615.

11

Memory Difficulties in Children and Adults with Learning Disabilities

H. Lee Swanson
Leilani Sáez

Memory reflects the ability to encode, process, and retrieve information to which one has been exposed. As a skill, it is inseparable from intellectual functioning and learning. Individuals deficient in memory skills, such as children and adults with learning disabilities (LD), would be expected to have difficulty on a variety of academic and cognitive tasks. Memory is linked to performance in several academic (e.g., reading) and cognitive areas (e.g., problem solving), and therefore, it is a critical area of focus in the field of LD for three reasons.

1. It reflects *applied* cognition; that is, memory functioning reflects all aspects of learning.
2. Several studies suggest that the memory skills used by students with LD do not appear to exhaust, or even tap, their abilities; therefore, we need to discover instructional procedures that can capitalize on this underdeveloped potential.
3. Several cognitive intervention programs that attempt to enhance the overall cognition of persons with learning disabilities rely on principles derived from memory research (see Swanson, Cooney, & O'Shaughnessy, 1998, for a review).

This chapter selectively reviews previous and current working memory (WM) research conducted by the first author (H. L. S.). The reader is also referred to Swanson (1989, 1991) for a comprehensive review of short-term memory (STM) serial recall and neuropsychological studies spanning 10 years of research. In addition, a comprehensive review of memory research as applied to LD has been provided elsewhere (e.g., Cooney & Swanson, 1987; Swanson et al., 1998). Before reviewing some of these studies, we provide the theoretical framework and definitional criteria used for participant selection in most of the investigations.

Theoretical Framework

The research reported within this chapter draws heavily on the tripartite view of WM put forth by Baddeley (e.g., Baddeley, 1986, 1996; Baddeley & Logie, 1999). This view characterizes WM as comprising a central executive controlling system that interacts with a set of two subsidiary storage systems: the speech-based phonological loop and the visual–spatial sketch pad. The phonological loop is responsible for the temporary storage of verbal information; items are held within a phonological store of limited duration, maintained through the process of subvocal articulation. The visual–spatial sketch pad is responsible for the storage of visual–spatial information over brief periods and plays a key role in the generation and manipulation of mental images. The central executive is involved in the control and regulation of the WM system. According to Baddeley and Logie (1999), it coordinates the two subordinate systems, focusing and switching attention, in addition to activating representations within long-term memory (LTM). Correlates in the neuropsychological literature complement the tripartite structure, showing functional independence among the three systems (e.g., Smith & Jonides, 1999).

Although assumptions we make about the WM model are consonant with Baddeley's tripartite structure, we also incorporate the notion that the central executive system includes a mental workspace, distinct from the two subordinate systems, with limited resources. This assumption is also consistent with Daneman and Carpenter's model (1980), which views WM as reflecting a combination of processing and storage components.

Within the aforementioned theoretical context, Swanson and Siegel (2001a) delineated a causal model of LD drawing from Swanson's studies on WM, as well as those of others (e.g., Bull, Johnston, & Roy, 1999; Chiappe, Hasher, & Siegel, 2000; De Beni, Palladino, Pazzaglia, & Cornoldi, 1998; de Jong, 1998; Passolunghi, Cornoldi, & De Liberto, 1999; Siegel & Ryan, 1989). The model states:

> Limitations in WM capacity have a neurological/biological base. These limitations are multifaceted as to the psychological operations they influence. Limitations in WM capacity cause LD. However, these limitations disrupt only certain cognitive operations (a cognitive operation involves manipulating, representing, storing, and/or allocating of attentional resources) when high demands are placed on processing. When performance demands on various tasks directly tax the WM capacity of individuals with LD, deficiencies related to the accessing of speech-based information and/or the monitoring of attentional processes emerge. These two areas of deficiencies are re-

lated to components of WM referred to in Baddeley's model (Baddeley & Logie, 1999) as the phonological loop and the executive system. Individuals with LD do *not* suffer all aspects of the phonological loop (e.g., they have relatively normal abilities in producing spontaneous speech and have few difficulties in oral language comprehension) or the executive system (e.g., they have normal abilities in planning and sustaining attention across time). Those aspects of the phonological system that appear particularly faulty for individuals with LD relates to accurate and speedy access of speech codes and those aspects of the executive system that appear faulty are related to the concurrent monitoring of processing and storage demands and the suppression of conflicting (e.g., irrelevant) information. Deficiencies in these operations influence performances in academic domains (reading comprehension, mathematics) that draw heavily upon those operations. Deficiencies in these operations are not due to academic achievement or psychometric IQ because problems in WM capacity remain when achievement and IQ are partialed out or controlled in a statistical analysis. In addition, our results show that these limitations in WM are *independent* of limitations in phonological processing. Children with LD do well in some academic domains because (a) those domains do not place heavy demands on WM operations, and/or (b) they compensate for WM limitations by increasing domain specific knowledge and/or their reliance on environmental support. (pp. 107–108)

Definition of LD

In our studies we define LD samples by their primary academic difficulties in reading and mathematics and then attempt to isolate problems in psychological processes. Participants with LD are operationally defined as those children and adults who have general IQ scores on standardized tests above 85 and who have scores below the 25th percentile on a standardized reading and/or mathematics achievement measure. In some studies, the criterion we have used for defining low achievement is much lower than a cutoff score below the 25th percentile (i.e., < 8th percentile). In general, the majority of the studies we cite involve LD samples with primarily reading deficits, particularly word recognition accuracy and reading comprehension. However, we recognize that reading problems are strongly correlated with other problems, such as mathematics. Thus, LD samples with reading problems may suffer problems in other academic domains that share a common resource (e.g., language).

Executive System

This section reviews studies that have implicated deficits in executive processing for children with LD. There are a number of cognitive activities assigned to the central executive, including subsidiary memory systems coordination, control of encoding and retrieval strategies, attention switching during manipulation of material held in the verbal and visual–spatial systems, and LTM knowledge retrieval (e.g., Baddeley, 1996). We hypothesize that the crucial component of the central executive as it applies to LD is controlled attention. Controlled attention is defined as the capacity to maintain and hold relevant information in "the face of interference or distraction" (Engle, Kane, & Tuholski, 1999, p. 104). Executive processing constraints for participants with LD is inferred from three outcomes: (1) poor performance on complex divided attention tasks, (2) weak monitoring ability, as exhibited in the failure to suppress (inhibit) irrelevant information, and (3) depressed performance across verbal and visual–spatial tasks that require concurrent storage and processing.

Complex Divided Attention

An early study by Swanson (1984) showed that the mental allocation of attentional resources of students with LD was more limited than that of their nonlearning disabled (NLD) counterparts. Elementary-age students were given anagram problems to solve (the primary task). Upon the determination of an answer, LD and NLD participants were asked to recall words related to their anagram solution (the secondary task). A significant group × cognitive effort interaction emerged in the results. That is, no matter what the organizational characteristics of words (i.e., semantic, nonsemantic, or phonetic) were, words were better recalled by skilled than by readers with LD under high-effort conditions. However, recall of

readers with LD was at a statistically comparable level to that of skilled readers in low-effort conditions. Furthermore, in the lower-effort condition, a trend, in which readers with LD recalled *more* words than did skilled readers. The results suggest that after a difficult primary task, secondary task performance is easier for skilled readers than it is for LD readers.

Two additional experiments (Swanson, 1984) replicated these findings. However, the experiments primarily required the processing of words. Thus, three additional experiments were designed to reflect attentional demands on both the verbal and visual–spatial system. In Experiment 1 (Swanson, 1993a), a concurrent memory task, adapted from Baddeley, Lewis, Eldridge, and Thomas (1984) was administered to LD and skilled readers. The task required subjects to remember digit strings (e.g., 9, 4, 1, 7, 5, and 2) while they concurrently sorted blank cards, cards with pictures of nonverbal shapes, and cards with pictures of items that fit into semantic categories (e.g., vehicles—car, bus, truck; clothing—dress, socks, belt). Demands on the central executive capacity system were manipulated through the level of difficulty (three- vs. six-digit strings) and type of sorting required (e.g., nonverbal shapes, semantic categories, and blank cards). The results showed that LD readers could perform comparably to chronological age (CA)–matched peers on verbal and visual–spatial sorting conditions that involved low demands (i.e., three-digit strings), and that only when the coordination of tasks became more difficult (e.g., six-digit strings) did ability group differences emerge. More important, the results for the high-memory load condition indicated less recall for LD readers than CA-matched (and achievement-matched) peers during both verbal and nonverbal sorting. Because recall performance was not restricted to a particular storage system (i.e., verbal storage), one can infer that processes other than a language-specific system accounted for the results.

Monitoring Activities

Our earlier work also investigated how capacity limits in the allocation of attention resources were strategically handled. We investigated whether children with LD had greater trade-offs and weaker inhibition strategies than average achievers on divided attention tasks. Swanson (1989a) compared the performance of slow learners, children with LD, average achievers, and intellectually gifted children on a primary and secondary recall task. Children were asked to select one of two nouns (e.g., foot or dress) presented in the context of two different types of sentences, "base" sentences (e.g., The woman wore a pretty _____) and "elaborative" sentences (e.g., The woman wore a pretty _____ at the dance). The missing word varied as a function of the mental effort needed to ascertain a correct response. For example, consider the base sentence "The _____ went to school." The response set included either an easy- or low-effort choice (e.g., children vs. house) or a hard- or high-effort choice (e.g., friends vs. children). Thus, children were provided with two words from which to choose the best word for sentence completion (the primary task). Recall for chosen words, nonselected words, and targeted adjectives was measured (the secondary task). The results produced three noteworthy findings. To simplify the reporting of the results, only findings related to LD and average achievers will be highlighted.

First, as found in the previous studies (Swanson, 1984), no differences occurred between ability groups in secondary recall for the low-effort condition. However, high-effort conditions favored the recall of secondary words by average-achieving children when compared to children with LD.

Second, recall insertions (the proportion of nontargeted words incorrectly recalled between the secondary and the central task) were significantly higher in children with LD than in average achievers. Thus, children with LD had greater difficulty inhibiting nontargeted words than did average achievers.

Finally, clear differences emerged between ability groups in the prioritization of resources (i.e., in the direction of the correlations between the primary and secondary tasks). Trade-offs, in the form of low positive or negative correlations, emerged for students with LD between the primary and secondary task, whereas there was a sharing of resources (i.e., positive correlations) for average children.

In our laboratory we have also explored selective attention to word features within and across the cerebral hemispheres for children with LD. An abundance of experimental evidence points to an association between left and right cerebral hemispheres and variations in capacity demands. For example, the targeting of information in one ear is assumed to consume resources that would normally be used in processing information in the competing ear (e.g., see Friedman & Polson, 1981). Given this assumption, Swanson and Cochran (1991) compared 10-year-old average-achieving children and same-age peers with LD on a dichotic listening task.

Participants were asked to recall words organized by semantic (e.g., red, black, green, and orange), phonological (e.g., sit, pit, and hit), and orthographic (e.g., sun, same, seal, and soft) features presented to either the left or right ear. The study included two experiments. Experiment 1 compared free recall with different orienting instructions to word lists. For example, in the orienting condition, children were told about the organizational structure of the words to be presented, such as to remember all of the words heard, "but to specifically remember words that go with _____" (e.g., colors–semantic feature orientation), or "words that rhyme with _____" (e.g., it–phonological feature orientation), or "words that start with the letter _____" (e.g., s–orthographic feature orientation). For the nonorienting condition, children were told to remember all words, but no mention was made of the distinctive organizational features of the words. Experiment 2 extended Experiment 1 by implementing a cued-recall condition. In both experiments, children were told they would hear someone talking through a set of earphones but that they should only pay attention to what was said in one of the ears (i.e., the targeted ear). The children were told that when they stopped hearing the information in both ears, they were to tell the experimenter all the words they could remember.

In both experiments, NLD children had higher levels of targeted and nontargeted recall compared to children with LD. More important, ability group differences emerged in how specific word features were selectively attended to. The selective attention index focused on the targeted words in comparison to the background words (targeted word recall minus background word recall from other lists *within* the targeted ear), as well as background items in the contralateral ear. Regardless of word features, whether competing word features were presented (within-ear or across-ear conditions), or whether retrieval conditions were cued or noncued, selective attention scores of readers with LD were smaller (the difference score between targeted items and nontargeted items was closer to zero) than that of NLD readers. Thus, when compared with children with LD, NLD children were more likely to ignore irrelevant information in the competing conditions. Taken together, the results of this study, as well as those of three earlier dichotic listening studies (Swanson, 1986; Swanson & Mullen, 1983) suggest that children with disabilities suffer processing deficits related to resource monitoring, regardless of the type of word features, retrieval conditions, or ear presentation.

Combined Processing and Storage Demands

Recent studies (e.g., Swanson, 1994; Swanson & Ashbaker, 2000; Swanson, Ashbaker, & Lee, 1996; Swanson & Sachse-Lee, 2001b) on executive processing have included tasks that follow the format of Daneman and Carpenter's Sentence Span measure, a task strongly related to student achievement (see Daneman & Merikle, 1996, for a review). These studies have consistently found readers with LD to be more deficient than skilled readers in WM performance using this task format, which presumably taps central executive processes related to "updating" (Miyake, Friedman, Emerson, Witzki, & Howerter, 2000). Updating requires monitoring and coding of information for relevance to the task at hand and then appropriately revising items held in WM. A cross-sectional study (Swanson & Sachse-Lee, 2001a) compared skilled readers and readers with LD across a broad age span. The study compared six age groups (7, 10, 13, 20, 35, 55) on phonological, semantic, and visual–spatial WM measures administered under conditions referred to in Swanson and colleagues (1996): initial (no probes or cues), gain (cues that bring performance to an asymptotic level), and maintenance conditions (asymptotic conditions

without cues). The study also explored whether ability groups vary in their WM spans as a function of the type of WM task across age.

This study included two verbal WM measures that required the processing of acoustically familiar rhyming words (phonological task, e.g., car, star, bar, and far) or the processing of semantically related words (semantic task, e.g., pear, apple, prune; car, bus, and truck), and a visual–spatial WM measure (visual-matrix task) that required the sequencing of dots on a matrix. The general findings of the Swanson and Sachse-Lee (2001a) study were that (1) young adults (i.e., 20 and 35 years old) performed better than did children and older adults (i.e., 55-year-olds), (2) skilled readers performed better than readers with LD in all processing conditions, and (3) the gain condition improved span performance from initial conditions, but performance declined when maintenance conditions were administered. However, these findings were qualified by age × ability group interactions related to memory conditions (initial, gain, maintenance) and type of WM task (verbal vs. visual–spatial). Both skilled readers and those with LD showed continuous growth in verbal and visual–spatial WM that peaked at approximately 20 and 35 years of age. The results clearly showed that the readers with LD had less WM recall than did skilled readers across a range of age groups on tasks that involved the processing of phonological, visual–spatial, and semantic information. Although WM performance levels of skilled readers and those with LD were comparable at some adult ages on the phonological and visual–spatial WM measures, comparable performance levels were not sustained across all adult age groups. Thus, the study provided little evidence that WM skills of readers with LD "catch up" with skilled readers as they age, suggesting that a deficit model rather than a developmental lag model best captures such readers' age-related performance.

From the foregoing findings, as well as others (Swanson, 1992, 1993d; Swanson et al., 1996), we have found evidence of domain-general processing deficits in children and adults with LD, suggestive of executive system involvement. Because of the potential for misinterpretations related to these findings (e.g., the paradox between domain-specific deficits commonly attributed to LD with the finding that they have domain general processing deficits), we will clarify our interpretation of the results (also see Swanson & Siegel, 2001a, p. 111, for discussion). The perplexity in adequately linking a domain-general processing deficit to LD is related to the confusion in the literature as to what such a system entails. Cognitive operations independent of, or not directly moderated by, verbal or visual–spatial skills have been referred to as domain-general processes or the central executive system. This system reflects a diversity of activities (12 are listed in Swanson & Siegel, 2001b, such as planning, allocating attention, accessing information from LTM, etc.). These processes draw from several regions of the brain but are associated primarily with the prefrontal cortex (e.g., Smith & Jonides, 1999). Thus, domain-general processing is perhaps a *misnomer* because operations that cut across verbal and visual spatial skills are multifaceted.

We have addressed some of the alternative explanations to our findings on executive processing—for example, deficits are due to attention-deficit/hyperactivity disorder (ADHD), low intelligence, domain-specific knowledge, low-order processes (such as phonological coding), and so on (see Swanson & Siegel, 2001a, for a review of studies). We find (as do independent laboratories) that (1) children with normal IQ can have executive processing deficits, (2) some readers with LD suffer executive processing deficits that do not overlap with the deficits attributed to children with ADHD (e.g., WM deficits emerge in readers with LD but not in children with ADHD of normal intelligence), (3) significant differences in WM remain between LD and NLD participants when achievement, domain-specific knowledge, and psychometric intelligence are partialed from the analysis, and (4) the causal basis of attention between children with LD and ADHD (as well as manifestations) differs.

Of course, the foregoing comments raise the issue of whether deficits in a domain-general system can operate independently of deficits in a specific system, such as the phonological loop (to be discussed later). When we have partitioned variance related to a general system from that related to a specific WM system we have found results, which substantiate the notion of between-systems independence (Swanson & Alexander, 1997; Wilson & Swanson, 2001). For example, Wilson and Swanson (2001) statistically controlled the domain-specific variance from verbal and visual–spatial WM performance of participants with math disabilities and participants without math disabilities across a broad age span. We partitioned the variance in WM performance, via structural equation modeling, by creating two first-order factors (the verbal WM tasks reflected factor 1 and the visual–spatial WM tasks reflected factor 2) to capture unique variance, and a single second higher-order factor that reflected shared variance or domain-general performance among all the tasks. When the ability groups were compared on these factor scores, groups without math disabilities were superior to those with math disabilities on factor scores that included variance partitioned into domain-general WM, verbal WM, and visual–spatial WM. Thus, it appears, at least in the area of mathematics, that ability group differences emerge in domain-specific systems *and* in a general executive system of WM.

In terms of interdependence among domain-general and isolated processes, Swanson and Alexander (1997) examined the interrelationship among cognitive processes in predicting word recognition and reading comprehension performance of readers with LD. The correlation among phonological, orthographic, semantic, metacognitive, verbal/visual–spatial WM measures, and reading performance were examined in readers with LD and skilled readers, ages 7 to 12. The study yielded the following important results: (1) readers with LD were deficient in all cognitive processes when compared to skilled readers, but these differences were not a reflection of IQ scores; (2) readers with LD were deficient compared to skilled readers in a general factor primarily composed of verbal and visual–spatial WM measures and unique components, suggesting that reading ability group differences emerge in *both* general and specific (modular) processing; (3) the general WM factor best predicted reading comprehension for both skilled and LD readers' groups; and (4) phonological awareness best predicted skilled readers' pseudo-word reading, whereas the general WM factor best predicted pseudo-word performance of readers with LD. Overall, Swanson and Alexander's study showed that verbal and visual–spatial WM tasks share variance with a common system but also have some unique variance related to a specific system. Furthermore, both the general system and specific phonological system predicted reading.

Summary

We have selectively reviewed studies suggesting that WM deficits of children with LD may, depending on the task and materials, reflect problems in the executive system. These problems appear to be related to attention allocation, and the shifting and updating of information in WM. These problems are not isolated to the verbal domain.

It is important to note that students with LD are not deficient on all executive processing activities. For example, although planning (such as mapping out a sequence of moves) is considered a component of the executive system (however, see, e.g., Miyake et al., 2000, p. 90), we have not found ability group differences between LD and NLD students on such tasks (see Swanson, 1988, 1993c, for studies that examine performance on other executive processing tasks, such as the Tower of Hanoi, Combinatorial, Picture Arrangement or Pendulum tasks).

The Phonological System

In Baddeley's model (1986), the articulatory or phonological loop is specialized for the retention of verbal information over short periods. It is composed of both a phonological store, which holds information in phonological form, and a rehearsal process, which maintains representations in the phonological store (see Baddeley, Gathercole, & Papagano, 1998, for an extensive review). A substantial number of studies support the notion that children with LD experience memory deficits in processes related to the phonological loop (e.g., see Siegel, 1993, for a review of studies showing deficits in readers with LD related to phonological representations). That is, diffi-

culty in forming and accessing phonological representations impairs the ability to retrieve verbal information. Interestingly, this phonological impairment does not appear to have broad effects on general ability apart from the developmental consequences on language-related functions (Hohen & Stevenson, 1999). One language function alluded to in the literature is verbal memory. Before reviewing the evidence on verbal memory, the overlap and distinctions between verbal STM and verbal WM must be addressed. Most studies that compare the performance of skilled readers and those with LD assume that verbal STM measures capture a subset of WM performance (i.e., the use and/or operation of the phonological loop). Some authors have even suggested that the phonological loop may be referred to as verbal STM (e.g., Dempster, 1985) because it involves two major components discussed in the STM literature: a speech-based phonological input store and a rehearsal process (see Baddeley, 1986, for review). Our research has addressed some of this confusion. We briefly review our research here, which suggests that some distinction between the two concepts is necessary.

STM-A Review

A 1998 meta-analysis was conducted to quantitatively summarize the experimental literature (O'Shaughnessy & Swanson, 1998) for studies within the last 30 years that met the following criteria: (1) directly compared readers with LD with average readers, as identified on a standardized reading measure and at least one STM measure; (2) reported standardized reading scores, which indicated that students with LD were at least 1 year below grade level; and (3) reported intelligence scores for students with LD that were in the average range (i.e., 85–115). Although the search resulted in approximately 155 articles on immediate memory and learning disabilities, only 38 studies (24.5%) met the criteria for inclusion. For comparisons in this synthesis, an effect size (ES) magnitude of −0.20, was considered small, −0.50 was moderate, and −0.90 was considered a large ES difference in favor of NLD when compared to LD participants. A summary of the results follows:

1. The group with LD performed poorly on STM tasks requiring memorization of verbal information compared to the NLD group (ES = –0.68). STM tasks that employed stimuli that could not easily be named, such as abstract shapes, did not produce large differences between NLD and LD readers (ES = –0.15).

2. STM tasks requiring readers with LD to recall exact sequences of verbal stimuli, such as words or digits, immediately after a series presentation yielded a much greater overall mean ES (ES = –0.80) than nonverbal serial recall tasks (ES = –0.17). Thus, serial recall performance with verbal material of students with LD was over three-quarters of a standard deviation below that of average readers. However, when memory performance with nonverbal stimuli was compared, the difference equaled less than one-quarter of a standard deviation in favor of the average readers.

3. The overall mean ES for studies that provided instructions in mnemonic strategies (e.g., rehearsal and sorting items into groups) prior to recall and used verbal stimuli was –0.54; the overall mean ES for studies using verbal stimuli without mnemonic strategy instruction was –0.71. These results indicate a lingering difference in memory performance between LD and NLD students in spite of mnemonic training. That is, although the memory performance of students with reading disabilities improved with training in mnemonic strategies, 70.5% of average readers still scored above the mean of the group with LD.

4. STM tasks that involved auditory presentation of verbal stimuli resulted in an overall mean ES of –0.70, whereas those that involved visual presentation of verbal stimuli resulted in an overall mean ES of –0.66. Thus, the inferior verbal STM performance of readers with LD appears to be unrelated to the modality in which a stimulus is received.

5. STM tasks that involved the visual presentation of nonverbal stimuli, such as abstract shapes, resulted in an overall mean ES of –0.15.

The largest overall ES was exhibited in studies that used both word recognition and reading comprehension as a means of distinguishing between subjects with LD (ES =

–0.68). That is, studies that used either word recognition alone or reading comprehension alone resulted in similar effect sizes of ES = –0.59 and ES = –0.56, respectively. Thus, studies that used *both* word recognition and reading comprehension as the criteria for assessing reading skills resulted in a sample of subjects with LD who demonstrated more severe immediate memory problems.

In summary, this quantitative analysis of the literature clearly showed that children and adults with LD are inferior to their counterparts on measures of STM in which familiar items such as letters, words, and numbers, and unfamiliar items such as abstract shapes were recalled.

Verbal STM versus Verbal WM

Are verbal STM deficits synonymous with deficits in verbal WM? Results from our lab have suggested that the tasks differ in subtle ways. Simply stated, some children with LD perform poorly on tasks that require accurate and/or speedy recognition/recall of letter and number strings or real words and pseudo-words. Tasks, such as these, which have a "read in and read out" quality to them (i.e., place few demands on LTM to infer or transform the information) reflect STM. One common link among these tasks is the ability to store and/or access the sound structure of language (phonological processing). However, some children with LD also do poorly on tasks that place demands on attentional capacity. Everyday examples of verbal WM processing include holding a person's address in mind while listening to directions regarding location, listening to a sequence of events in a story while trying to understand what the story means, and locating a sequence of landmarks on a map while determining the correct route.

We tested whether the operations related to STM and WM operated independently of one another. A study by Swanson and Ashbaker (2000) compared readers with LD and skilled readers and younger achievement-matched children on a battery of WM and STM tests to assess executive and phonological processing. Measures of the executive system were modeled after Daneman and Carpenter's (1980) WM tasks (i.e., tasks demanding the coordination of both processing and storage), whereas measures of the phonological system included those that related to articulation speed, digit span, and word span. The Swanson and Ashbaker study yielded two important results. First, although the reading group with LD was inferior to skilled readers in WM, verbal STM, and articulation speed, the differences in verbal STM and WM revealed little relation with articulation speed. That is, reading-related differences on WM and STM measures remained when articulation speed was partialed from the analysis. These reading-group differences were pervasive across verbal and visual–spatial WM tasks, even when the influence of verbal STM was removed, suggesting that reading-group differences are domain general. Second, WM tasks and verbal STM tasks contributed unique, or independent, variance to word recognition and reading comprehension beyond articulation speed. These results are consistent with those of Daneman and Carpenter (1980) and others (e.g., Engle, Tuholski, Laughlin, & Conway, 1999), who have argued that verbal STM tasks and WM tasks are inherently different, and although phonological coding might be important to recall in STM, it may not be a critical factor in WM tasks.

The foregoing findings from Swanson and Ashbaker's study are consistent with early work on samples with LD (Swanson, 1994; Swanson & Berninger, 1995). In a 1994 study, Swanson tested whether STM and WM contributed unique variance to academic achievement in children and adults with learning disabilities. Swanson found that STM and WM tasks loaded on different factors. Further, both of these factors contributed unique variance to reading and mathematics performance. A study by Swanson and Berninger also examined potential differences between STM and WM by testing whether STM and WM accounted for different cognitive profiles in readers with LD. Swanson and Berninger used a double-dissociation design to compare children deficient in reading comprehension (based on scores from the Passage Comprehension subtest of the Woodcock Reading Mastery Test) and/or word recognition (based on scores from the Word Identification subtest of the Woodcock Reading Mastery Test) on WM and phonological STM

measures. Participants were divided into four ability groups: High Comprehension/High Word Recognition, Low Comprehension/High Word Recognition, High Comprehension/Low Word Recognition, and Low Comprehension/Low Word Recognition. The results were straightforward: WM measures were related primarily to reading comprehension, whereas phonological STM measures were related primarily to reading recognition. Most critically, because no significant interaction emerged, the results further indicated that the comorbid group (i.e., children low in both comprehension and word recognition) had combined memory deficits. That is, WM deficits were reflective of the poor comprehension–only group and STM deficits were reflective of the poor recognition–only group.

Why the distinction between STM and WM? We argue that WM tasks require the active monitoring of events. Monitoring of events within memory is distinguishable from simple attention to stimuli held in STM. There are many mnemonic situations in which a stimulus in memory is attended to and the other stimuli exist as a background—that is, they are not the center of current awareness. These situations, in our opinion, do not challenge monitoring. Monitoring within WM implies attention to the stimulus that is currently under consideration together with active consideration (i.e., attention) of several other stimuli whose current status is essential for the decision to be made.

Summary

There is evidence that participants with LD suffer deficits in the phonological system. A substrate of this system may contribute to problems in verbal WM that are independent of problems in verbal STM. In addition, these problems in verbal WM are not removed by partialing out the influence of verbal articulation speed, reading comprehension, or IQ scores.

Visual–Spatial Processing

In Baddeley's (1986) model, the visual–spatial sketch pad is specialized for the processing and storage of visual material, spatial material, or both, and for linguistic information that can be recoded into imaginal forms. The literature linking LD to visual–spatial memory deficits is mixed. For example, several studies in the STM literature suggest that visual STM of children with LD is intact (see Swanson et al., 1998, for a comprehensive review). Some studies have found that visual–spatial WM in students with LD is intact when compared with their same-age counterparts (e.g., Swanson et al., 1996, Experiment 1), whereas others suggest problems in various visual–spatial tasks (Swanson et al., 1996, Experiment 2). Most studies indicate, however, that greater problems in performance are more likely to occur on verbal than visual–spatial WM tasks. For example, Swanson, Mink, and Bocian (1999) found by partialing out the influence of verbal IQ via regression analysis, that students with reading disabilities were inferior in performance to slow learners (i.e., garden-variety poor readers) on visual–spatial and verbal WM measures. That is, although children with a specific reading disability demonstrated a greater deficit on the verbal WM task than the visual–spatial WM task, performance on both types of tasks was inferior to other poor learning groups when verbal IQ was statistically controlled.

It may *not* be the case, however that differentiation occurs between reading and math subgroups when visual–spatial WM measures are used (Swanson, 1993b, 1993d). For example, Swanson (1993d) found that 10-year-old children with LD who suffered either math problems or reading problems could not be clearly differentiated by performance for verbal or visual–spatial WM measures. This study included six tasks that assessed verbal WM (Rhyming, Story Retelling, Auditory Digit Sequence, Phrase Sequencing, Semantic Association, Semantic Categorization) and five tasks that assessed visual–spatial WM (Visual Matrix, Picture Sequence, Mapping & Directions, Spatial Organization, Nonverbal Sequencing). In general, Swanson found that children with arithmetic disabilities performed as low as children with reading disabilities across verbal and visual–spatial WM tasks.

In a later study, Swanson and colleagues (1996) tested whether there might be potential performance advantages for readers with LD on visual–spatial WM tasks relative to verbal WM tasks. The Swanson and colleagues results showed demonstrations of deficiency in both verbal and visual–spatial WM performance for readers with LD for gain and maintenance conditions (i.e., after receiving cues to aid recall) that were not evident for initial condition performance (i.e., without cue assistance). Furthermore, these performance differences held up when verbal STM scores (see Experiment 2) were partialed from the analysis, providing additional support for a general system involvement that cuts across both verbal and visual–spatial WM tasks, which influences the performance of readers with LD when processing demands are high.

Summary

The evidence for whether children with LD have any particular advantage on visual–spatial WM tasks, when compared to their normal-achieving counterparts, appears to fluctuate with processing demands. Swanson (2000) proposed a model that may account for these mixed findings.

WM and Achievement

The importance of the executive and phonological system in predicting reading performance is related to age. As children age, the executive system may play a more primary role in separating good and poor readers than at the younger ages. Furthermore, difficulties in the executive system may develop independent of the specific difficulties in reading of readers with LD. That is, based on the foregoing observations, we speculate that as children age, skilled readers have relatively higher WM capacity than do readers with LD, and therefore will have more available resources related to the executive system with which to perform tasks, regardless of the nature of the task. We hold that people are poor readers because they have a small WM capacity, and this capacity is *not* entirely specific to reading. That is, poor readers have more limited WM than skilled readers, not as a consequence of poor reading skills but because they have less WM capacity available for performing reading and nonreading tasks. Of course, individuals will vary in the efficiency (e.g., speed of activation) of their mental operations on some specific tasks, but other things being equal, it is our belief that high-WM-capacity individuals still have more attentional resources available to them than do low-WM-capacity individuals.

Our research shows that WM plays an important role in predicting academic performance. In general, we find that both the executive system and the phonological loop predict performance for complex domains (e.g., reading comprehension) and low-order domains (e.g., calculation). We briefly review studies here that support these conclusions in the areas of reading comprehension, problem solving, writing, and computation.

Complex Cognition

READING COMPREHENSION

Several of our studies have shown that WM accounts for significant variance in comprehension performance of readers with LD (e.g., Swanson, 1999a; Swanson & Alexander, 1997; Swanson & Sachse-Lee, 2001b). One study (Swanson, 1999a) in particular identifies those components of WM that are most important to reading comprehension. In this study, Swanson (1999a) found significant differences between students with LD and peers matched for age and nonverbal IQ on measures of phonological processing accuracy (i.e., phonemic deletion, digit recall, phonological choice, and pseudo-word repetition), phonological processing speed (i.e., timed responses from phonemic deletion, digit recall, phonological choice, and pseudo-word repetition task), LTM accuracy (i.e., orthographic choice, semantic choice, and vocabulary), LTM time (i.e., timed response from orthographic choice, semantic choice, and vocabulary), and executive processing (i.e., Sentence Span, Counting Span, and Visual-matrix tasks). The results showed that the CA-matched group outperformed the reading group with LD, whereas the readers with LD were comparable to reading level–matched children. The important findings, however, were that the significant relationship between executive processing and reading comprehension was maintained when LTM and phonological processing composite scores were partialed

from the analysis. Furthermore, the attenuating effect of executive processing on reading comprehension did not appear to be due to phonological processing speed or LTM.

Swanson was also interested in determining whether there were some fundamental processing differences between readers with LD and skilled readers that superseded their problems in reading comprehension. He analyzed the processing variables as a function of reading conditions by reframing the comparison groups in terms of the regression-based design outlined by Stanovich and Siegel (1994). When reading comprehension was statistically controlled, the results indicated significant differences in WM and processing speed for phonological information between LD and skilled readers, independent of their reading comprehension levels.

WRITING

Unfortunately, only one of our studies focuses specifically on the relationship between WM and writing in samples with LD. In this study (Swanson & Berninger, 1996), children from a university clinic were administered a standardized WM battery (Swanson Cognitive Performance Test [S-CPT]; Swanson, 1995), Test of Written Language, Wide Range Achievement Test, and Peabody Achievement Test. The correlation analysis yielded three important outcomes. First, visual–spatial and verbal WM were significantly correlated with writing, reading recognition, and reading comprehension (r ranged from .39 to .79 across measures). Second, the influence of both visual–spatial and verbal WM was pervasive across all writing tasks. These relationships remained even when the influence of vocabulary was removed from the analysis. Finally, the contribution of WM tasks to writing was not a function of reading ability. That is, the correlations between WM and writing were maintained when reading was entered first into a regression equation.

WORD PROBLEM SOLVING

There is limited information on the contribution of WM to the problem-solving accuracy for students with LD. In one of the few studies conducted (Swanson & Sachse-Lee, 2001b), children with LD, approximately

12 years of age, were compared with CA-matched and younger achievement-matched (matched for reading comprehension and math computation skill) children on measures of verbal and visual–spatial WM, phonological processing, components of problem solving, and word problem-solving accuracy. In this study, children were presented arithmetic word problems orally and asked a series of questions about the various processes they would use to solve the task. They also solved problems that required them to apply algorithms related to subtraction, addition, and multiplication. The study produced a number of important findings. First, phonological processing, verbal WM, and visual WM each contributed unique variance to solution accuracy. More important, both verbal and visual–spatial WM performance predicted solution accuracy when phonological processing was controlled by entering it first in the regression model. Furthermore, the results showed that performance on phonological, verbal WM, and visual–spatial WM measures were statistically comparable in their contribution to ability group differences in solution accuracy.

Low-Order Tasks: Arithmetic Computation

Wilson and Swanson (2001) examined the relationship between verbal and visual–spatial WM and mathematical computation skill in children and adults. Participants, skilled and disabled in mathematics, ranged in age from 11 to 52 years. Our major finding was that groups without math disabilities were superior to those with math disabilities on factor scores that included variance partitioned into domain-general and domain-specific verbal and visual–spatial WM. These results were the same when both the linear and quadratic components of age were partialed from the analysis. The results also showed that both the verbal and visual–spatial WM composite scores predicted mathematics performance. Furthermore, these results held when reading ability was partialed from the analysis.

Lifespan WM Development and Achievement

The interrelationship between phonological and executive processes, as well as related

processes (i.e., semantic and orthographic), may be qualitatively different in predicting academic performance of participants with LD in some age groups (Swanson & Alexander, 1997). We summarize our observations across various age ranges as follows:

For skilled readers and those with LD, ages 6 to 75: (1) both domain-general WM and domain-specific WM are related to word recognition (Swanson, 1996; Swanson & Sachse, 2001a, 2001b); (2) age-related changes in WM in skilled readers are best explained by a capacity rather than a processing-efficiency model (Swanson, 1999b); (3) readers with LD, defined by word-recognition deficits, experience WM deficits into adulthood (Swanson & Sachse-Lee, 2001a); and (4) WM performance of readers with LD is changeable via probing or cued procedures; however, significant differences remain between reading groups because of greater domain-general capacity limitations in readers with LD (Swanson et al., 1996; Swanson & Sachse-Lee, 2001b).

For children ages 9 to 15, we find that (1) domain-general WM differences between skilled readers and those with LD are not eliminated when reading comprehension is partialed from the analysis (Swanson, 1999a); (2) phonological and executive processes are equally important in predicting reading comprehension, as well as problem solving (Swanson, 1999a; Swanson & Alexander, 1997; Swanson & Sachse-Lee, 2001b); (3) deficits in executive processing and reading comprehension are only partially mediated by the phonological system or LTM (Swanson, 1999a); (4) domain-specific deficits emerge on verbal WM tasks on initial (noncued) conditions, but deficits in both verbal and visual–spatial WM emerge as processing demands increase under gain (cued) and maintenance (high demand) conditions (Swanson et al., 1996); and (5) WM deficits related to poor readers are best attributed to a capacity, not processing-efficiency, model (Swanson, 1994; Swanson & Sachse-Lee, 2001a).

Based on these observations, it appears to us that the phonological system may play its primary role in predicting reading recognition and comprehension (accuracy and fluency) for early elementary school learning. Between the ages of 9 and 16, the executive system and the phonological system play equal, as well as independent, roles in predicting word reading and reading comprehension accuracy and fluency (Swanson, 1999a; Swanson & Alexander, 1997). We also suggest that for adult poor readers (drawing on our pilot work, and Engle, Cantor, & Carullo, 1992), executive processes play a more important role in predicting reading, especially reading comprehension, than does the phonological system. That is, we find with older participants (junior high through adult ages) that a general WM system, not specific to reading, separates skilled readers and those with LD (Swanson, 1999a; Swanson et al., 1999). Our previous research with older samples shows that skilled readers have relatively higher WM capacity than do readers with LD, even when reading comprehension (Swanson, 1999a), word recognition (Swanson et al., 1999), word recognition and IQ (Ransby & Swanson, 2001; Swanson & Sachse-Lee, 2001b), and articulation speed (Swanson & Ashbaker, 2000) are removed from analysis. Depending on age and reading fluency, we assume that although the executive system plays a role relaying the results of lower-level phonological analyses upward through the language system, it also serves as a monitoring system independent of those skills (e.g., Baddeley, 1986).

Summary

We have selectively reviewed studies related to various components of WM. There is evidence in the literature indicating both the phonological loop and the executive system as sources of deficit for participants with LD. Either one or both of these components play a significant role in predicting complex cognitive activities such as reading comprehension, arithmetic problem solving, and writing, as well as some basic skills (e.g., arithmetic computation).

Independent Researchers

There is empirical support, independent from our lab, that an LD may reflect a fundamental deficit in WM for both children and adults (e.g., Bull et al., 1999; Chiappe et al., 2000; De Beni et al., 1998; de Jong, 1998; Passolunghi et al., 1999; Siegel & Ryan, 1989). For example, Stanovich and Siegel (1994) showed that readers with LD (as well as poor readers) suffer deficits in both verbal WM and verbal STM, even after reading ability was controlled. In their study, Stanovich and Siegel amalgamated a sample that consisted of more than 1,500 children from 7 to 16 years of age. Children were classified into poor readers who also had low IQs (< 86), poor readers who had average IQs (> 90), and those children who had average scores in IQ and reading. They compared these groups on various processing measures when reading scores were entered first into a regression model. The processing variables of interest were performance on STM rhyming and nonrhyming tasks and WM tasks that included words or numbers. The STM tasks included letter strings that rhymed (e.g., B, C, D, G, P, T, and V) and those that did not rhyme (e.g., H, K, L, Q, R, S, and W). The verbal WM task (WM sentences) included an oral presentation of sentences, which increased in set size. Children were asked to supply missing words (e.g., People go see monkeys in a _____) and later recall those words supplied. The number WM task required children to count yellow dots from a series of blue and yellow dots arranged in irregular patterns. The patterns were on cards, and the number of cards within each set increased in number. For each set, the child was to recall the count of yellow dots for each card after all cards had been presented. When readers with LD (those children with a discrepancy between IQ and reading) and poor readers (those children whose IQ matched their low reading level) were compared to skilled readers, a significant advantage was found in favor of skilled readers' recall on the verbal WM and STM tasks. No differences in recall were found between the two poor reading groups.

Further support that readers with LD suffer problems in both verbal STM and verbal WM is found in a life-span study of Siegel (1994). Her study included some 1,200 individuals, ages 6 to 49. These individuals were presented tasks related to word recognition, pseudo-word decoding, reading comprehension, and WM, as well as a STM task requiring the recall of rhyming and nonrhyming letters. The results indicated gradual growth in WM skills from ages 6 to 19, with a gradual decline after adolescence. On the memory tasks, across most age levels, individuals with reading disabilities performed at a significantly lower level than individuals with normal reading skills. Thus, readers with LD experienced deficits on WM and verbal STM tasks across childhood, adolescence, and adulthood.

Practical Applications

Prior to 1989, memory research in LD was strongly influenced by the hypothesis that variations in memory performance are rooted in the children's acquisition of mnemonic strategies (Cooney & Swanson, 1987; Swanson et al., 1998). Strategies are deliberate, consciously applied procedures that aid in the storage and subsequent retrieval of information. Research in the last 10 years has moved in a different direction, toward an analysis of nonstrategic processes that are not necessarily consciously applied. The major motivation behind this movement has been that important aspects of memory performance are often disassociated with changes in mnemonic strategies. The most striking evidence has come from strategy-oriented research, which shows that differences between children with and without learning disabilities remain after the use of an optimal strategy (i.e., a strategy shown to be advantageous in the majority of studies).

It is clear from our synthesis of the literature (Swanson et al., 1998), however, that children with LD can benefit from mnemonic instruction when training is sufficiently rigorous. However, strategy training does not eliminate ability group differences between students with LD and their peers with disabilities in a multitude of situations. Some of the causes of strategy ineffectiveness or utilization deficiencies may be related to individual differences in information processing capacity (i.e., children without LD benefit more from the strategy than do children with LD) and/or a particular level of strategy effectiveness may have different causes in different children. A child with LD, for example, may be unable to benefit from a strategy because of his or her limited capacity, whereas another child may be constrained by his or her lack of knowledge relevant to the task. Thus, different children may follow different developmental routes to overcome their utilization deficiencies.

Some practical concepts and principles from memory research can serve as guidelines for the instruction of students with learning disabilities (see Swanson et al., 1998, for a review of eight instructional principles). Three major principles are particularly germane to our discussion.

Strategy Instruction Must Operate on the Law of Parsimony

Because of capacity demands, particular attention must be paid to developing strategies that are parsimonious and not placing excessive demands on children's attentional resources. A number of multiple-component packages of strategy instruction have been suggested to improve functioning of children with LD. These components have usually encompassed some of the following: skimming, imagining, drawing, elaborating, paraphrasing, using mnemonics, accessing prior knowledge, reviewing, orienting to critical features, and so on. No doubt, there are some positive aspects to these strategy packages in that:

1. These programs are an advance over some of the studies that are seen in the LD literature as rather simple or "quick-fix" strategies (e.g., rehearsal or categorization to improve performances).
2. These programs promote a domain skill and have a certain metacognitive embellishment about them.
3. The best of these programs involved (a) teaching a few strategies well rather than superficially, (b) teaching students to monitor their performance, (c) teaching students when and where to use the strategy to enhance generalization, (d) teaching strategies as an integrated part of an existing curriculum, and (e) teaching that included a great deal of supervised student practice and feedback.

The difficulty of such packages, however, at least in terms of theory, is that little is known about which components best predict student performance, nor do they readily permit one to determine why the strategy worked. The multiple-component approaches that are typically found in a number of strategy intervention studies on LD must be carefully contrasted with a component-analysis approach that involves the systematic combination of instructional components known to have an additive effect on performance.

Memory Strategies in Relation to a Student's Knowledge Base and Capacity

Memory capacity seems to increase with development; a number of factors have the potential to contribute to this overall effect. With development, the number of component processes increase in speed, with faster processes generally consuming less effort than slower processes, thereby increasing capacity (i.e., there is a functional gain in capacity with increasing efficiency of processing). Older children are likely to have more and better organized prior knowledge, which can reduce the total number of information chunks to be processed and decrease the amount of effort to retrieve information from LTM. Because of these developmental relationships, as well as the constraints that underlie development, this could play a role in strategy effectiveness.

Comparable Memory Strategy May Not Eliminate Performance Differences

Several studies have indicated that residual differences remain between ability groups even when groups are instructed and/or prevented from strategy use (Swanson et al., 1998, for a review). For example, Swanson (1983) found that the recall of a group with LD did not improve from baseline level when trained with rehearsal strategies. They recalled less than normally-achieving peers, although the groups were comparable in the various types of strategies used. The results support the notion that groups of children with different learning histories may continue to learn differently, even when the groups are equated in terms of strategy use.

Conclusions

Our conclusions from approximately two decades of research are that WM deficits are fundamental problems of children and adults with LD. Further, these WM problems are related to difficulties in reading, mathematics, and perhaps writing. Students with LD in reading and/or math demonstrate WM deficits related to the phonological loop, a component of WM that specializes in the retention of speech-based information. This system is of service in complex cognition, such as reading comprehension, problem solving, and writing. Research over the last decade also finds that children and adults with LD are clearly disadvantaged in situations that place high demands on a limited-capacity system. These constraints on the limited capacity of children and adults with LD mainifest themselves as deficits in controlled attentional processing (e.g., monitoring limited resources, suppressing conflicting information, and updating information). Further, these deficits are sustained when articulation speed, phonological processing, and verbal STM are removed from analyses.

Acknowledgments

This chapter draws primarily from Swanson (1991, 1992), Swanson and Siegel (2001a, 2001b), Swanson, Cooney, and O'Shaughnessy (1998), and Swanson and Sachse-Lee (2001b), and the reader is referred to those sources for more complete information. Appreciation is given to Joel Levin for his critique of this earlier work.

References

Baddeley, A. D. (1986). *Working memory*. London: Oxford University Press.

Baddeley, A. D. (1996). Exploring the central executive. *Quarterly Journal of Experimental Psychology: Human Experimental Psychology, 49*(1), 5–28.

Baddeley, A. D., Gathercole, S. E., & Papagano, C. (1998). The phonological loop as a language learning device. *Psychological Review, 105*(1), 158–173.

Baddeley, A. D., & Logie, R. H. (1999). Working memory: The multiple component model. In A. Miyake & P. Shah (Eds.), *Models of working memory: Mechanisms of active maintenance and executive control* (pp. 28–61). New York: Cambridge University Press.

Baddeley, A. D., Lewis, V., Eldridge, M., & Thomson, N. (1984). Attention and retrieval from long-term memory. *Journal of Experimental Psychology: General, 113*(4), 518–540.

Bull, R., Johnston, R. S., & Roy, J. A. (1999). Exploring the roles of the visual–spatial sketch pad and central executive in children's arithmetical skills: Views from cognition and developmental neuropsychology. *Developmental Neuropsychology, 15*(3), 421–442.

Chiappe, P., Hasher, L., & Siegel, L. S. (2000). Working memory, inhibitory control, and reading disability. *Memory and Cognition, 28*(1), 8–17.

Cooney, J. B., & Swanson, H. L. (1987). Memory and learning disabilities: An overview. In H. L. Swanson (Ed.), *Advances in learning and behavioral disabilities: Memory and learning disabilities* (Suppl. 2, pp. 1–40). Greenwich, CT: JAI Press.

Daneman, M., & Carpenter, P. A. (1980). Individual differences in working memory and reading. *Journal of Verbal Learning and Verbal Behavior, 19*(4), 450–466.

Daneman, M., & Merikle, P. M. (1996). Working memory and language comprehension: A meta-analysis. *Psychonomic Bulletin and Review, 3*(4), 442–433.

De Beni, R., Palladino, P., Pazzaglia, F., & Cornoldi, C. (1998). Increases in intrusion errors and working memory deficit of poor comprehenders. *Quarterly Journal of Experimental Psychology: Human Experimental Psychology, 51*(2), 305–320.

de Jong, P. (1998). Working memory deficits of reading disabled children. *Journal of Experimental Child Psychology, 70*(2), 75–95.

Dempster, F. (1985). Short-term memory development in childhood and adolescence. In C. Brainerd & M. Presseley (Eds.), *Basic processes in memory* (pp. 209–248). New York: Springer-Verlag.

Engle, R. W., Cantor, J., & Carullo, J. J. (1992). Individual differences in working memory and comprehension: A test of four hypotheses. *Journal of Experimental Psychology: Learning, Memory and Cognition, 18*(5), 972–992.

Engle, R. W., Kane, M. J., & Tuholski, S. (1999). Individual differences in working memory capacity and what they tell us about controlled attention, general fluid intelligence, and functions of the prefrontal cortex. In A. Miyake & P. Shah (Eds.), *Models of working memory: Mechanisms of active maintenance and executive control* (pp. 102–134). Cambridge, UK: Cambridge University Press.

Engle, R. W., Tuholski, S. W., Laughlin, J. E., & Conway, A. R. (1999). Working memory, short-term memory, and general fluid intelligence: A latent-variable approach. *Journal of Experimental Psychology: General, 128*(3), 309–331.

Friedman, A., & Polson, M. V. (1981). Hemispheres as independent resource systems: Limited-capacity processing and cerebral specialization. *Journal of Experimental Psychology: Human Perception and Performance, 7*(5), 1031–1058.

Miyake, A., Friedman, N. P., Emerson, M. J., Witzki, A. H., & Howerter, A. (2000). The unity and diversity of executive functions and their contributions to complex "frontal lobe" tasks: A latent variable analysis. *Cognitive Psychology, 41*(1), 49–100.

O'Shaughnessy, T., & Swanson, H. L. (1998). Do immediate memory deficits in students with learning disabilities in reading reflect a developmental lag or deficit? A selective meta-analysis of the literature. *Learning Disability Quarterly, 21*(2), 123–148.

Passolunghi, M. C., Cornoldi, C., & De Liberto, S. (1999). Working memory and intrusions of irrelevant information in a group of specific poor problem solvers. *Memory and Cognition, 27*(5), 779–790.

Ransby, M., & Swanson, H. L. (2001). *Reading comprehension skills of young adults with childhood diagnosis of dyslexia.* Unpublished manuscript, University of California, Riverside.

Siegel, L. S. (1993). Phonological processing deficits as a basis for reading disabilities. *Developmental Review, 13*(3), 246–257.

Siegel, L. S. (1994). Working memory and reading: A life-span perspective. *International Journal of Behavioral Development, 17*(1), 109–124.

Siegel, L. S., & Ryan, E. B. (1989). The development of working memory in normally achieving and subtypes of learning disabled children. *Child Development, 60*(4), 973–980.

Smith, E. E., & Jonides, J. (1999). Storage and executive processes in the frontal lobes. *Science, 283*(5408), 1657–1661.

Stanovich, K. E., & Siegel, L. (1994). Phenotypic performances profile of children with reading disabilities: A regression-based test of the phonological-core variable-difference model. *Journal of Education Psychology, 86*(1), 24–53.

Swanson, H. L. (1984). Effects of cognitive effort and word distinctiveness on learning disabled readers' recall. *Journal of Educational Psychology, 76*(5), 894–908.

Swanson, H. L. (1986). Do semantic memory deficiencies underlie disabled readers encoding processes? *Journal of Experimental Child Psychology, 41*(3), 461–488.

Swanson, H. L. (1989). Verbal coding deficits in learning disabled readers: A multiple stage model. *Educational Psychology Review, 1*(3), 235–277.

Swanson, H. L. (1991). Learning disabilities, distinctive encoding and hemispheric resources: An information processing perspective. In J. E. Obrzut & G. W. Hynd (Eds.), *Neurological foundations of learning disabilities: A handbook of issues, methods, and practice* (pp. 241–280). San Diego, CA: Academic Press.

Swanson, H. L. (1992). Generality and modification of working memory among skilled and less skilled readers. *Journal of Educational Psychology, 84*(4), 473–488.

Swanson, H. L. (1993a). Executive processing in learning disabled readers. *Intelligence, 17*(2), 117–149.

Swanson, H. L. (1993b). Individual differences in working memory: A model testing and subgroup analysis of learning-disabled and skilled readers. *Intelligence, 17*(3), 285–332.

Swanson, H. L. (1993c). Working memory in learning disability subgroups. *Journal of Experimental Child Psychology, 56*(1), 87–114.

Swanson, H. L. (1994). Short-term memory and working memory: Do both contribute to our understanding of academic achievement in children and adults with learning disabilities? *Journal of Learning Disabilities, 27*(1), 34–50.

Swanson, H. L. (1995). *Swanson Cognitive Processing Test (S-CPT): A dynamic assessment measure* (p. 122). Austin, TX: Pro-Ed.

Swanson, H. L. (1996). Individual and age-related differences in children's working memory. *Memory and Cognition, 24*(1), 70–82.

Swanson, H. L. (1999a). Reading comprehension and working memory in skilled readers: Is the phonological loop more important than the executive system? *Journal of Experimental Child Psychology, 72*(1), 1–31.

Swanson, H. L. (1999b). What develops in working memory? A life span perspective. *Developmental Psychology, 35*(4), 986–1000.

Swanson, H. L. (2000). Are working memory deficits in readers with learning disabilities hard to change? *Journal of Learning Disabilities, 33*(6), 551–566.

Swanson, H. L., & Alexander, J. (1997). Cognitive processes as predictors of word recognition and reading comprehension in learning disabled and skilled readers: Revisiting the specificity hypothesis. *Journal of Educational Psychology, 89*(1), 128–158.

Swanson, H. L., & Ashbaker, M. (2000). Working memory, Short-term memory, articulation speed, word recognition, and reading comprehension in learning disabled readers: Executive and/or articulatory system? *Intelligence, 28*(1), 1–30.

Swanson, H. L., Ashbaker, M., & Lee, C. (1996). Working-memory in learning disabled readers as a function of processing demands. *Journal of Child Experimental Psychology, 61*(3), 242–275.

Swanson, H. L., & Berninger, V. W. (1995). The role of working memory in skilled and less skilled readers' word comprehension. *Intelligence, 21,* 83–108.

Swanson, H. L., & Berninger, V. W. (1996). Individual differences in children writing: A function of working memory or reading or both processes? *Reading and Writing: An Interdisciplinary Journal, 8*(4), 357–383.

Swanson, H. L., & Cochran, K. (1991). Learning disabilities, distinctive encoding, and hemispheric resources. *Brain and Language, 40*(2), 202–230.

Swanson, H. L., Cooney, J. B., & O'Shaughnessy, T. (1998). Memory and learning disabilities. In B. Y. Wong (Ed.), *Understanding learning disabilities* (2nd ed.) San Diego, CA: Academic Press.

Swanson, H. L., Mink, J., & Bocian, K. M. (1999). Cognitive processing deficits in poor readers with symptoms of reading disabilities and ADHD: More alike than different? *Journal of Educational Psychology, 91*(2), 321–333.

Swanson, H. L., & Mullen, R. (1983). Hemisphere specialization in learning disabled readers' recall as a function of age and level of processing. *Journal of Experimental Child Psychology, 35*(3), 457–477.

Swanson, H. L., & Sachse-Lee, C. (2001a). *Learning disabled readers' working memory: What does or does not develop?* Unpublished manuscript, University of California, Riverside.

Swanson, H. L., & Sachse-Lee, C. (2001b). Mathematical problem solving and working memory in children with learning disabilities: Both executive and phonological processes are important. *Journal of Experimental Child Psychology,79*(3), 294–321.

Swanson, H. L., & Siegel, L. (2001a). Elaborating on working memory and learning disabilities: A reply to commentators. *Issues in Education: Contributions from Educational Psychology, 7*(1), 107–129.

Swanson, H. L., & Siegel, L. (2001b). Learning disabilities as a working memory deficit . *Issues in Education: Contributions from Educational Psychology, 7*(1), 1–48.

Wilson, K., & Swanson, H. L. (2001). Are mathematics disabilities due to a domain-general or domain-specific working memory deficit? *Journal of Learning Disabilities, 34*(3), 237–248.

12

Learning Disabilities in Arithmetic: Problem-Solving Differences and Cognitive Deficits

David C. Geary

The complexity of the field of mathematics makes the study of any associated learning disability daunting. In theory, a mathematical learning disability can result from deficits in the ability to represent or process information used in one or all of the many areas of mathematics (e.g., arithmetic and geometry), or in one or a set of individual domains (e.g., theorems vs. graphing) within each of these areas (Russell & Ginsburg, 1984). One approach that can be used to focus the search for any such learning disability (LD) is to apply the models and methods used to study mathematical development in academically normal children to the study of children with poor achievement in mathematics (e.g., Geary & Brown, 1991). Unfortunately, for most mathematical domains, such as geometry and algebra, not enough is known about the normal development of the associated competencies to provide a systematic framework for the study of LD. Theoretical models and experimental methods are, however, sufficiently well developed in the areas of number, counting, and simple arithmetic to provide such a framework (Briars & Siegler, 1984; Geary, 1994; Gelman & Meck, 1983; Siegler, 1996; Siegler & Shrager, 1984).

The use of these models and methods to guide the study of children with LD has revealed a consistent pattern of cognitive strengths and weaknesses. These studies suggest that most children with LD are normal (i.e., performance is similar to academically normal peers) or only slightly delayed in the development of number concepts (Geary, Hamson, & Hoard, 2000; Gross-Tsur, Manor, & Shalev, 1996). At the same time, several studies have shown that many children with LD do not understand certain counting concepts (Geary, Bow-Thomas, & Yao, 1992; Geary, Hoard, & Hamson, 1999), and many studies have revealed that these children have a variety of deficits in simple arithmetic (Ackerman & Dykman, 1995; Barrouillet, Fayol, & Lathuli(re, 1997; Bull & Johnston, 1997; Garnett, & Fleischner, 1983; Geary, Brown, & Samaranayake, 1991; Geary, Widaman, Little, & Cormier, 1987; Jordan & Hanich, 2000; Jordan, Levine, & Huttenlocher, 1995; Jordan & Montani, 1997; Ostad, 1997, 1998a; Räsänen & Ahonen, 1995; Rourke, 1993; Svenson & Broquist, 1975). The deficits in the basic arithmetical competencies of children with LD (hereafter, arithmetical disability, or AD) have been found in studies conducted in the United States (e.g., Garnett & Fleischner, 1983), Israel (Shalev, Manor, & Gross-Tsur, 1993), and several European nations (Ostad, 2000; Svenson & Broquist, 1975). The difficulties children with AD have solving simple arithmetic problems are the focus of the next section. The second section provides an overview of research on the cognitive and potential neural mechanisms contributing to these deficits.

Arithmetical Learning Disability

The first part presents background information on the diagnosis, prevalence, and etiology of AD; the second provides an overview of our research program in AD.

Background

DIAGNOSIS

Unfortunately, measures that are specifically designed to diagnose AD are not available. As a result, most researchers rely on standardized achievement tests, often in combination with measures of intelligence (IQ). A score lower than the 20th or 25th percentile on a mathematics achievement test combined with a low-average or higher IQ score are typical criteria for diagnosing AD (e.g., Geary, Hamson, & Hoard, 2000; Gross-Tsur et al., 1996). There are, however, two difficulties with these criteria.

First, if applied in only a single academic year, the criteria often lead to a number of false positives, that is identifying children as AD who in fact have no cognitive deficits and typically show improved achievement scores in later grades (Geary, 1990; Geary et al., 1991): We have found that most children who meet these criteria across two successive grades do appear to have some form of cognitive deficit and AD. Second, the cutoff of the 25th percentile on a mathematics achievement test does not fit with the estimation, described below, that between 5 and 8% of children have some form of AD. The discrepancy results from the nature of standardized achievement tests and the often rather specific deficits of children with AD. By design, standardized achievement tests sample a broad range of arithmetical and mathematical topics, whereas children with AD often have severe deficits in some of these areas and average or better competencies in others. The result of averaging across these topics is a level of performance (e.g., at the 20th percentile) that overestimates competencies in some areas and underestimates them in others.

PREVALENCE AND ETIOLOGY

Large-scale epidemiological studies of the prevalence of AD have not been conducted, although several smaller-scale studies that included more than 300 children from a well-defined population have (e.g., all fourth-graders in an urban school district). Measures, designed from neuropsychological studies of number and arithmetic deficits following brain injury, are more sensitive to AD than are standard achievement tests have been used in these studies. They have been conducted in the United States (Badian, 1983), Europe (Kosc, 1974), and Israel (Gross-Tsur et al., 1996; Shalev et al., 2001). The findings across studies suggest that 5 to 7% of school-age children exhibit some form of AD. Ostad (1998a) described several related studies of elementary-school children conducted in Norway during the 1950s. These studies revealed that 8% of the children likely had some form of AD. Thus, the best estimate, at this time, is that between 5 and 8% of children have some form of AD.

Some children with AD exhibit comorbid attention-deficit/hyperactivity disorder (ADHD) or reading disability (RD). The most comprehensive of these studies indicated that 26% of the children with AD had symptoms of ADHD, and 17% had RD (Gross-Tsur et al., 1996). Badian (1983), in contrast, found that nearly half of the children with AD also showed comorbid reading difficulties, and Ostad (1998a) found that just over half of the children with AD had a comorbid spelling disability (SD). At this time, it appears that children with AD constitute at least two different subgroups, those with only difficulties in arithmetic and those with comorbid learning disabilities in other areas. The latter most typically involve language-related deficits, that is RD and (or) SD (for related discussion, see Geary, 1993; Geary & Hoard, 2001).

As with other forms of LD, twin and familial studies suggest both genetic and environmental contributions to both forms of AD. In a twin study, Light and DeFries (1995) provided evidence that the same genes may contribute to AD and RD and thus their comorbidity in many children. Shalev and her colleagues (2001) studied familial patterns of AD, excluding children with comorbid ADHD or RD. The results showed that family members (e.g., parents and siblings) of children with AD are 10 times more likely to be diagnosed with AD than are members of the general population.

Research Program

As noted, performance on standardized achievement tests does not provide information on the strengths and weaknesses of individual children within the broad domain of mathematics, only relative performance averaged across all the assessed mathematical subareas. The only means to better understand learning in mathematics, as well as learning disabilities, is to focus research efforts on circumscribed mathematical domains and to use methods that enable a fine-grained assessment of performance in each domain. To this end, our initial efforts were focused on simple addition and were guided by Ashcraft's (e.g., Ashcraft & Battaglia, 1978) information-processing studies of cognitive arithmetic and later by Siegler's (1996; Siegler & Shrager, 1984) strategy choice model of cognitive development.

INFORMATION PROCESSING

Beginning with Svenson and Broquist's (1975) study more than 25 years ago and continuing today, the information-processing approach has guided much of the cognitive research on children with AD. In our first study of children with AD (Geary et al., 1987), we employed the reaction time (RT) techniques developed by Groen and Parkman (1972) and later elaborated by Ashcraft and his colleagues (for a review, see Ashcraft, 1995). Here, simple arithmetic problems, such as $3 + 2 = 4$ or $9 + 5 = 14$, are presented on a computer monitor. The child indicates by button push whether the presented answer is correct. The resulting RTs are then analyzed by means of regression equations. Here, statistical models representing the approaches potentially used while problem solving, such as counting or memory retrieval, are fit to RT patterns. As an example, if children counted both addends in the problem, starting from one, then RTs should increase linearly with the sum of the problem, and the value of the raw regression slope should be consistent with estimates of the speed with which children count implicitly (for general discussion, see Geary, Widaman, & Little, 1986; Widaman, Geary, Cormier, & Little, 1989).

In the first study in which we used these techniques, second-, fourth-, and sixth-grade children with AD were compared to their academically normal peers (Geary et al., 1987). The RT patterns suggested that children with AD differed from other children in terms of the form and frequency of counting strategies used to solve simple addition problems. For a problem such as $9 + 5$, academically normal second-grade children typically stated "nine" and then counted, "ten, eleven, twelve, thirteen, fourteen" (termed the counting-on procedure; Fuson, 1982). Children with AD tended to count, starting from one (the counting-all procedure). Cross-sectional comparisons suggested that most academically normal children gradually switched from counting to direct retrieval of the answer, whereas most children with AD did not make this transition (Geary et al., 1987). Rather, they still counted to solve addition problems, although many of these children appeared to use the more efficient counting-on procedure in later grades. The same pattern has recently been reported in a study that contrasted the subtraction competencies of children with AD with those of other children (Ostad, 2000).

STRATEGY CHOICE

Soon after beginning data collection for this first study (i.e., Geary et al., 1987), I read Siegler and Shrager's (1984) strategy-choice model of arithmetical and later more general cognitive development (Siegler, 1996). The approach was based on a combination of the RT methods used by cognitive psychologists, such as Ashcraft (1995), and direct observation of problem solving used by educational researchers, such as Carpenter and Moser (1984). The goal was not only to describe the types of strategies children used to solve simple arithmetic problems but also to determine the mechanisms that governed whether a child would use one strategy (e.g., counting) or another (e.g., retrieval) to solve each particular problem. A related goal was (and still is) to understand developmental change in the mechanisms governing strategy choices. Although the model has been elaborated over the years, the basic mechanisms are the same (Siegler, 1996).

In all domains that have been studied, including arithmetic, children use a mix of strategies during problem solving. In solving arithmetic problems, children will sometimes retrieve the answer to solve one problem and count to solve the next problem. Memory retrieval is assumed to be based on an associative relationship between the presented problem and all potential answers to the problem. These associations appear to develop as children use other types of strategies during problem solving. Counting on to solving 5 + 3, for instance, appears to result in the formation of a long-term memory association between this problem and the answer generated by the count. Each time the problem is solved through counting, the strength of the association between 5 + 3 and the generated answer (typically 8) increases. Eventually children automatically retrieve 8, or whatever answer has been most frequently generated, when presented with 5 + 3. So, if an answer is not readily retrieved, due to a low associative strength between the problem and potential answers, children resort to some form of backup strategy to complete problem solving; Table 12.1 provides a description of retrieval and the primary backup strategies used to solve simple addition problems (Geary, 1994).

Our first study that followed Siegler and Shrager's (1984) method replicated and extended their basic findings (e.g., the relation between RTs and strategy choices) by demonstrating that individual differences in strategy choices were related to individual performance differences on standard arithmetical achievement and ability tests (Geary & Burlingham-Dubree, 1989). Strong performance on the strategy-choice task (e.g., fast and accurate strategy execution) was predictive of above-average performance on the achievement and ability measures (see

TABLE 12.1. Strategies Used to Solve Simple Addition Problems

Strategy	Description	Example
Finger counting: Counting all	A number of fingers representing the augend and addend are lifted and then counted starting from 1.	To solve 2 + 3, two fingers are lifted on one hand and three on the other. All uplifted fingers are then counted.
Finger counting: Counting on	A number of fingers representing the augend and addend are lifted and then counted starting from the larger number.	To solve 2 + 3, two fingers are lifted on one hand and three on the other. The count starts with "three" and proceeds "four, five."
Verbal counting: Counting all	As above, but counting is done without the use of fingers.	To solve 2 + 3, the child counts (explicitly or implicitly), "one, two, three, four, five."
Verbal counting: Counting on	As above, but counting is done without the use of fingers.	To solve 2 + 3, the child states "three" and then counts "four, five."
Retrieval	Direct retrieval of a basic fact from long-term memory.	The child states an answer quickly and without signs of counting; typically stating "just knew it."
Decomposition	Retrieval of a partial sum and counting on.	To solve 2 + 3, the child first retrieves the answer to 2 + 2 and then counts up to "five"

Note. See Geary (1994) for further discussion and illustration.

also Siegler, 1988). The results also indicated that the methods and theoretical model proposed by Siegler and Shrager would likely provide an excellent framework for guiding the study of children with AD. The approach was followed in an initial study of first-grade children with AD (Geary, 1990), many of whom were reassessed in second grade (Geary et al., 1991), and another study of fourth-graders that included children with AD as well as gifted children (Geary & Brown, 1991).

All these studies involved the use of a variant of Siegler and Shrager's (1984) strategy assessment task for simple addition, which provides information on problem-solving strategies, accuracy of strategy use, and accompanying RTs. Here, simple addition problems, such as 5 + 6, are presented one at a time on a computer monitor. The child is instructed to solve the problem using whatever means is easiest for him or her. With the completion of problem solving, the child immediately speaks the answer into a voice-activated relay which triggers an internal timing device in the computer (for recording RTs). The child's problem solving, such as whether fingers are used, is monitored and recorded by the experimenter. The child is then asked to describe how he or she got the answer. High-levels of agreement between experimenter observation and child reports (typically > 90% of trials), along with a consistency between these reports and associated RTs patterns, attest to the utility of the method (e.g., Geary, 1990; Siegler, 1987).

In the first study based on this approach, first-grade children with AD were divided into two groups: improved and no change

(Geary, 1990). The children in the improved group had below-average mathematics achievement scores at the end of kindergarten but average or better scores at the end of first grade. Children in the no-change group had below-average scores at both assessments. There were no differences comparing children in the improved group to children in an academically normal control group in terms of strategy choices, error rates, or RTs. This pattern was subsequently replicated (Geary, Hamson, & Hoard, 2000), which bolstered the conclusion that the initial low mathematics achievement of children in the improved group was not likely to be due to any form of cognitive deficit or AD. Their initial poor performance may have been due to inattention during test taking or poor early math instruction. In any case, the improved group is not considered further.

An unexpected finding was that children with AD (i.e., the no-change group) did not differ from their academically normal peers in terms of the mix of strategies used to solve simple addition problems, as shown in Table 12.2. Differences were, however, found in percentage of retrieval and counting errors and in the use of the counting-on procedure, all favoring the academically normal group. Error and RT patterns for problems on which an answer was retrieved also differed comparing the academically normal and AD groups. For children with AD, the distribution of RTs was unusual. The pattern was not similar to that found in younger, academically normal children and seemed to reflect a highly variable speed of fact retrieval. The interpretation of this pat-

TABLE 12.2. Addition Strategy Characteristics Comparing Academically Normal Children and Children with AD

Strategy	Trials on which strategy used (%)		Errors (%)		Counting on (%)	
	Normal	AD	Normal	AD	Normal	AD
Counting fingers	5	6	21	50	100	69
Verbal counting	60	64	7	31	100	86
Retrieval	35	26	5	22	—	—

Note. Data based on Geary (1990).

tern was that it suggested "an anomalous long-term memory representation of addition facts" (Geary, 1990, p. 379). Further analyses revealed greater variability in the speed with which children with AD executed other numerical processes, such as number articulation, in comparison to their academically normal peers.

A year later, many of these children were reassessed on the strategy-choice task and were administered a numerical digit span task (Geary et al., 1991). In keeping with models of arithmetical development (Ashcraft, 1982), the academically normal children showed an across-grade shift from reliance on verbal counting (56% to 44% across years) to retrieval (39% to 51% across years). The academically normal children also showed faster retrieval times and fewer retrieval errors (6% to 2%), comparing grade 1 to grade 2 performance. As with the previously described cross-sectional study (Geary et al., 1987), the children with AD showed no developmental change in the mix of problem-solving strategies (e.g., 26% to 25% retrieval across years) or in retrieval accuracy (e.g., 18% to 16% retrieval errors).

The children with AD did, however, show improvement in how effectively they used counting to solve addition problems. In grade 2, they almost always used the counting-on procedure when using a counting strategy to problem solve and showed a marked reduction in the proportion of counting errors (e.g., from 49% to 10% for finger counting). Analyses of RTs indicated that the academically normal children showed faster counting comparing grade 2 to grade 1, but the children with AD showed no change in counting speed. Again, the distribution of retrieval RTs of children with AD differed from that of their academically normal peers. An important discovery was that the pattern of retrieval RTs of children with AD was similar to that found with children who had suffered from an early (before 8 years of age) lesion to the left hemisphere or subcortical regions (Ashcraft, Yamashita, & Aram, 1992).

This pattern of developmental change suggested that the children with AD were developmentally delayed in terms of their ability to use counting to solve arithmetic problems and were fundamentally different from normal children in the mechanisms

supporting fact retrieval (see also Garnett & Fleischner, 1983). Subsequent studies using the same model and methods have been conducted in the United States by Jordan and her colleagues (Jordan & Hanich, 2000; Jordan et al., 1995; Jordan & Montani, 1997) and by Ostad and others in Europe (e.g., Barrouillet et al., 1997; Ostad, 1997, 1998b, 2000). These studies have confirmed the differences in counting-strategy use and retrieval deficit and extended the domain of study to subtraction, multiplication, and word problems, among others (e.g., Hanich, Jordan, Kaplan, & Dick, 2001; Ostad, 1998b). Subsequent research has also led to the discovery of at least two different forms of AD (Jordan & Montani, 1997)—that is, AD with no comorbid forms of LD and AD with comorbid RD or other forms of language-related disorder (e.g., SD). Subsequent research has further demonstrated that the differences comparing children with AD to other children cannot be attributed to differences in IQ (Geary et al., 1999; Geary, Hamson, & Hoard, 2000; McLean & Hitch, 1999).

Cognitive Mechanisms and Deficits

The aforementioned studies led to attempts to discern the nature of the cognitive deficits underlying some children's developmental delay in the use of counting procedures and their difficulties in representing and/or retrieving basic facts from long-term memory. Cognitive studies combined with research on arithmetical difficulties associated with brain injury (i.e., dyscalculia) and with behavioral genetic studies of individual differences in mathematical abilities provided clues as to possible sources of the problem-solving characteristics of children with AD. The integration of these literatures resulted in a taxonomy of three general subtypes of mathematical disability (MD), procedural, semantic memory, and visuospatial (Geary, 1993). Table 12.3 shows the defining characteristics of these subtypes.

The development delay in the use of counting procedures while solving arithmetic problems is subsumed under the more general procedural subtype of MD. Deficits in the retrieval of basic arithmetic facts is the defining feature of the semantic memory

TABLE 12.3. Subtypes of Learning Disabilities in Mathematics

Procedural subtype

Cognitive and performance features
  A. Relatively frequent use of developmentally immature procedures (i.e., the use of procedures that are more commonly used by younger, academically normal children)
  B. Frequent errors in the execution of procedures
  C. Poor understanding of the concepts underlying procedural use
  D. Difficulties sequencing the multiple steps in complex procedures

Neuropsychological features
  Unclear, although some data suggest an association with left-hemispheric dysfunction and in some cases (especially for feature D above) a prefrontal dysfunction

Genetic features
  Unclear

Developmental features
  Appears, in many cases, to represent a developmental delay (i.e., performance is similar to that of younger, academically normal children, and often improves across age and grade)

Relation to RD
  Unclear

Semantic memory subtype

Cognitive and performance features
  A. Difficulties retrieving mathematical facts, such as answers to simple arithmetic problems
  B. What facts are retrieved, there is a high error rate
  C. For arithmetic, retrieval errors are often associates of numbers in the problem (e.g., retrieving 4 to 2 + 3 = ?; 4 is the counting-string associate that follows 2, 3)
  D. RTs for correct retrieval are unsystematic

Neuropsychological features
  A. Appears to be associated with left-hemispheric dysfunction, possibly the posterior regions for one form of retrieval deficit and the prefrontal regions for another
  B. Possible subcortical involvement, such as the basal ganglia

Genetic features
  Appears to be a heritable deficit

Developmental features
  Appears to represent a developmental difference (i.e., cognitive and performance features differ from that of younger, academically normal children, and do not change substantively across age or grade)

Relation to RD
  Appears to occur with phonetic forms of RD

Visuospatial subtype

Cognitive and performance features
  A. Difficulties in spatially representing numerical and other forms of mathematical information and relationships
  B. Frequent misinterpretation or misunderstanding of spatially represented information

Neuropsychological features
  Appears to be associated with right-hemispheric dysfunction, in particular, posterior regions of the right hemisphere, although the parietal cortex of the left hemisphere may be implicated as well

Genetic features
  Unclear, although the cognitive and performance features are common with certain genetic disorders (e.g., Turner's syndrome)

Developmental features
  Unclear

Relation to RD
  Does not appear to be related

Note. Adapted from Geary (1993, 2000).

subtype. Still, semantic memory deficits should affect other mathematical competencies that are based on the retrieval of facts, such as recalling prime numbers. In any case, the respective sections that follow describe research on the arithmetical problem solving of children with AD in terms of the three forms of MD subtype, and as related to the cognitive and neural systems that may underlie their problem-solving characteristics (e.g., the retrieval deficit).

Procedural Deficits

Much of the research on children with AD has focused on their use of counting procedures to solve simple arithmetic problems. As described, when they solve such problems, children with AD often commit more errors than do their academically normal peers, and they often use problem-solving procedures, such as counting all, that are more commonly used by younger children (Geary, 1990; Jordan et al., 1995; Jordan & Montani, 1997). The errors result when these children miscount, typically undercounting or overcounting by 1 (Geary, 1990). As a group, children with AD also rely on finger counting, as contrasted with verbal counting, more frequently and use this strategy for more years than do academically normal children. A few studies have assessed the procedural competencies of children with AD during the solving of multistep arithmetic problems, such as 45 × 12 or 126 + 537. Russell and Ginsburg (1984) found that fourth-grade children with AD committed more errors than did their IQ-matched academically normal peers when solving such problems. These errors involved (1) the misalignment of numbers while writing down partial answers or (2) errors while carrying or borrowing from one column to the next. The following sections discuss these procedural characteristics of children with AD in terms of working memory, conceptual knowledge, and neural correlates.

WORKING MEMORY

Although the relationship between working memory and difficulties in executing arithmetical procedures is not yet fully understood, it is clear that children with AD have some form of working-memory deficit

(Hitch & McAuley, 1991; McLean & Hitch, 1999; Siegel & Ryan, 1989: Swanson, 1993). There are several ways in which a working-memory deficit could affect the procedural competencies of children with AD.

As an example, children with AD (and younger, academically normal children) appear to use finger counting as a working-memory aid, in that fingers appear to help these children to keep track of the counting process (Geary, 1990). In particular, representing the problem addends on fingers and then using fingers to note the counting sequence should greatly reduce the working-memory demands of the counting process. Working memory may also contribute to the tendency of children with AD to undercount or overcount during the problem-solving process. Such miscounting can occur if the child loses track of where he or she is in the counting process, that is, how many fingers he or she has counted and how many remain to be counted. Working memory is also implicated in the difficulties that children with AD have during the solving of more complex arithmetic problems. The procedural errors for the children with AD assessed by Russell and Ginsburg (1984) appeared to result from difficulties monitoring and coordinating the sequence of problem-solving steps, which, in turn, suggest compromised executive functions.

At a more basic level, a working-memory deficit could result from difficulties with representing information in the basic phonetic/articulatory or visuospatial working memory systems, or from a deficit in accompanying executive processes, such as attentional or inhibitory control (see McLean & Hitch, 1999). In theory, difficulties with representing and manipulating information in the phonetic buffer could disrupt the representation of number words and their articulation during the counting process. Attentional and other executive difficulties could result in problems keeping track of the counting process and sequencing the multiple steps involved in executing complex procedures (Geary, 1993).

CONCEPTUAL KNOWLEDGE

In addition to working memory, a poor understanding of the concepts underlying a procedure can also contribute to a developmental delay in the adoption of more sophisticated procedures and reduce the ability to detect procedural errors.

For instance, delayed use of the counting-on procedure and frequent counting errors of children with AD appear to be related, in part, to immature counting knowledge. In our first study in the area of counting, we found that first-grade children with AD and RD understood most of the essential features of counting, such as cardinality—that is, that the last stated number word represents the total number of items in the counted set (Geary et al., 1992; for discussion of counting, see Briars & Siegler, 1984; Gelman & Gallistel, 1978). However, these children consistently made errors on tasks that assessed other features of counting, in particular order irrelevance. Many of the children with AD believed that a correct but nonsequential counting of items (e.g., skipping items and then coming back to count them) resulted in an incorrect count. The pattern suggests that although most children with AD know the standard counting sequence and understand some counting concepts, they nonetheless appear to view counting as a rote, mechanical activity.

Children, including many children with AD, who do not understand the order-irrelevance concept use the counting-on procedure during problem solving much less frequently than do other children (Geary et al., 1992; Geary, Hamson, & Hoard, 2000). It is possible that the switch from use of the counting-all procedure to the counting-on procedure requires an understanding that counting does not have to start from one and proceed in the standard sequential order. The immature counting knowledge of children with AD may also contribute to their frequent counting errors, in particular a failure to detect and thus self-correct these errors. In other words, conceptual knowledge not only guides procedural use, it may also provide a frame for evaluating the accuracy with which procedures are executed.

NEURAL CORRELATES

Given the similarity between the deficits associated with AD and those associated with acquired dyscalculia, neuropsychological studies of dyscalculia provide insights as to the potential neural systems contributing to the procedural deficits of children with AD (Geary, 1993; Geary & Hoard, 2001). As is found with children with AD, individuals with acquired or developmental dyscalculia are generally able to count arrays of objects, recite the correct sequence of number words during the act of counting (e.g., counting from 1 to 20), and understand many basic counting concepts (e.g., cardinality; Hittmair-Delazer, Sailer, & Benke, 1995; Seron et al., 1991; Temple, 1989). Individuals with dyscalculia caused by damage to the right hemisphere sometimes show difficulties with the procedural component of counting, specifically, difficulties with systematically pointing to successive objects as they are enumerated (Seron et al., 1991). However, the relation between this feature of dyscalculia and the procedural deficits of children with AD is not clear.

Difficulties solving complex arithmetic problems are also common with acquired and developmental dyscalculia (Semenza, Miceli, & Girelli, 1997; Temple, 1991). As an example, in an extensive assessment of the counting, number, and arithmetic competencies of a 17-year-old—M.M.—with severe congenital damage to the right frontal and parietal cortices, Semenza and his colleagues reported deficits similar to those reported by Russell and Ginsburg (1984) for children with AD. Basic number and counting skills were intact, as was the ability to retrieve basic facts (such as 8 for 5 + 3) from memory. However, M.M. had difficulty solving complex division and multiplication problems, such as 32 × 67. Of particular difficulty was tracking the sequence of partial products. Once the first step was completed (2 × 7), difficulties placing the partial product (4) in the correct position and carrying to the next column were evident. Thus, the primary deficit of M.M. appeared to involve difficulties sequencing the order of operations and monitoring the problem-solving process, as is often found with damage to the frontal cortex (Luria, 1980); Temple (1991) reported a similar pattern of procedural difficulties for an individual with neurodevelopmental abnormalities in the right frontal cortex. It remains to be seen if a compromised right frontal cortex contributes to aspects of the procedural deficits of children with AD.

Semantic Memory Deficits

As described earlier, many children with AD do not show the shift from procedural-based problem solving to memory-based problem solving that is commonly found in academically normal children (Geary et al., 1987; Ostad, 1997). The pattern suggests that children with AD have difficulties storing or accessing arithmetic facts in or from long-term memory. Indeed, disrupted memory-based processes are consistently found with comparisons of children with AD and other children (Barrouillet et al., 1997; Bull & Johnston, 1997; Garnett & Fleischner, 1983; Geary, 1993; Geary & Brown, 1991; Geary et al., 1987; Jordan & Montani, 1997; Ostad, 1997). Disruptions in the ability to retrieve basic facts from long-term memory might, in fact, be considered a defining feature of AD (Geary, 1993). Most of these individuals can, however, retrieve some facts, and disruptions in the ability to retrieve facts associated with one operation (e.g., multiplication) are sometimes found with intact retrieval of facts associated with another operation (e.g., subtraction), at least when retrieval deficits are associated with overt brain injury (Pesenti, Seron, & Van Der Linden, 1994).

As described in Table 12.3, when they retrieve arithmetic facts from long-term memory, children with AD commit many more errors than do their academically normal peers and show error and RT patterns that often differ from the patterns found with younger, academically normal children (Geary, 1993; Geary, Hamson, & Hoard, 2000). The RT patterns are similar to the patterns found with children who have suffered from an early (before age 8 years) lesion to the left hemisphere or associated subcortical regions (Ashcraft et al., 1992), as noted earlier. Although this pattern does not indicate that children with AD have suffered from some form of overt brain injury, it does suggest that the memory-based deficits of many of these children may reflect the same mechanisms underlying the retrieval deficits associated with dyscalculia (Geary, 1993; Rourke, 1993).

However, the cognitive and neural mechanisms underlying these deficits are not completely understood. On the basis of Siegler's strategy-choice model, solving arithmetic problems by means of counting should eventually result in associations forming between problems and generated answers (Siegler, 1996; Siegler & Shrager, 1984). Because counting typically engages the phonetic and semantic (e.g., understanding the quantity associated with number words) memory systems, any disruption in the ability to represent or retrieve information from these systems should, in theory, result in difficulties in forming problem/answer associations during counting (Geary, 1993; Geary, Bow-Thomas, Fan, & Siegler, 1993). Although not definitive with respect to this hypothesis, the work of Dehaene and his colleagues suggests that the retrieval of arithmetic facts is indeed supported by a system of neural structures that appear to support phonetic and semantic representations and are engaged during incrementing processes, such as counting. These areas include the left basal ganglia and the left parieto–occipito–temporal areas (Dehaene & Cohen, 1995, 1997). Damage to either the subcortical or cortical structures in this network is associated with difficulties accessing previously known arithmetic facts (Dehaene & Cohen, 1991, 1997). However, it is not currently known if the retrieval deficits of children with AD are the result of damage to or neurodevelopmental abnormalities in the regions identified by Dehaene and Cohen (1995, 1997).

More recent studies of children with AD suggest a second form of retrieval deficit, specifically, disruptions in the retrieval process due to difficulties in inhibiting the retrieval of irrelevant associations. This form of retrieval deficit was first discovered by Barrouillet and colleagues (1997), based on the memory model of Conway and Engle (1994), and was recently confirmed in our laboratory (Geary, Hamson, & Hoard, 2000; see also Koontz & Berch, 1996). In the Geary and colleagues (2000) study, one of the arithmetic tasks required children to use only retrieval—the children were instructed not to use counting strategies—to solve simple addition problems (see also Jordan & Montani, 1997). Children with AD, as well as children with RD, committed more retrieval errors than did their academically normal peers, even after controlling for IQ. The most common of these errors was a counting-string associate of one of the addends. For instance, common retrieval errors for the problem 6 + 2 were 7 and 3, the numbers following 6 and 2, respectively, in the counting sequence. Hanich and colleagues (2001) found a similar pattern, although the proportion of retrieval errors that were counting-string associates was lower than that found by Geary and colleagues.

The pattern in these more recent studies (e.g., Geary, Hamson, & Hoard, 2000) and that of Barrouillet and colleagues (1997) is in keeping with Conway and Engle's (1994) position that individual differences in working memory and retrieval efficiency are related, in part, to the ability to inhibit irrelevant associations. In this model, the presentation of a to-be-solved problem results in the activation of relevant information in working memory, including problem features—such as the addends in a simple addition problem—and information associated with these features. Problem solving is efficient when irrelevant associations are inhibited and prevented from entering working memory. Inefficient inhibition results in activation of irrelevant information, which functionally lowers working-memory capacity. In this view, children with AD make retrieval errors, in part because they cannot inhibit irrelevant associations from entering working memory. Once in working memory, these associations either suppress or compete with the correct association for expression. Whatever the cognitive mechanism, these results suggest that the retrieval deficits of some children with AD may spring from either delayed development of those areas of the prefrontal cortex that support inhibitory mechanisms, or neurodevelopmental abnormalities in these regions (Bull, Johnston, & Roy, 1999; Welsh & Pennington, 1988). The results also suggest that inhibitory mechanisms should be considered potential contributors to the comorbidity of AD and ADHD in some children.

Visuospatial Deficits

The relation between visuospatial competencies and AD has not been fully explored. In theory, visuospatial deficits should affect performance in some mathematical domains, such as certain areas of geometry and the solving of complex word problems, but not other domains, such as fact retrieval

or knowledge of geometric theorems (e.g., Dehaene, Spelke, Pinel, Stanescu, & Tsivkin, 1999; Geary, 1993, 1996). Many children with the procedural and/or semantic memory forms of AD, at least as related to simple arithmetic, do not appear to differ from other children in basic visuospatial competencies (Geary, Hamson, & Hoard, 2000; Morris et al., 1998). There is, however, evidence that some children with AD who show broader performance deficits in mathematics may have a deficit in visuospatial competencies.

McLean and Hitch (1999) found that children with AD showed a performance deficit on a spatial working-memory task, although it is not clear if the difference resulted from an actual spatial deficit or from a deficit in executive functions (e.g., the ability to maintain attention on the spatial task). In any case, Hanich and her colleagues (2001) found that children with AD differed from their peers on an estimation task and in the ability to solve complex word problems. Although performance on both of these tasks is supported by spatial abilities (Dehaene et al., 1999; Geary, 1996; Geary, Saults, Liu, & Hoard, 2000), it is not clear whether the results of Hanich and colleagues were due to a spatial deficit in children with AD.

Conclusion

The theoretical models and experimental methods used to study the development of number, counting, and arithmetical competencies in academically normal children have provided a much needed framework for guiding the study of children with AD. We now understand the problem-solving functions and deficits of children with AD, at least as related to the solving of simple arithmetic problems (e.g., 4 + 7) and simple word problems (Geary, Hamson, & Hoard, 2000; Hanich et al., 2001; Ostad, 2000). Most of these children use problem-solving procedures that are more commonly used by younger, academically normal children, and tend to commit more procedural errors. Over the course of the elementary-school years, the procedural competencies of many children with AD tend to improve, and thus their early deficits seem to represent a developmental delay and not a fundamental cognitive deficit. At the same time, many children with AD have difficulties retrieving basic arithmetic facts from long-term memory, a deficit that often does not improve and thus may represent a developmental difference. Some insights have also been gained regarding the cognitive and neural mechanisms contributing to the procedural and retrieval characteristics of children with AD, including compromised working memory and executive functions.

Much remains to be accomplished, however. In comparison to simple arithmetic, relatively little research has been conducted on the ability of children with AD to solve more complex arithmetic problems (but see Russell & Ginsburg, 1984), and even less has been conducted in other mathematical domains. Even in the area of simple arithmetic, the cognitive and neural mechanisms that contribute to the problem-solving characteristics of children with AD are not fully understood and are thus in need of further study. Other areas that are in need of attention include the development of diagnostic instruments for AD; cognitive and behavioral genetic research on the comorbidity of AD and other forms of LD and ADHD; and, of course, the development of remedial techniques. If progress over the past 10 years is any indication, we should see significant advances in many of these areas over the next 10 years.

Acknowledgments

I thank Cathy DeSoto and Mary Hoard for comments on an earlier draft. Preparation of the chapter was supported by grant R01 HD38283 from the National Institute of Child Health and Human Development.

References

Ackerman, P. T., & Dykman, R. A. (1995). Reading-disabled students with and without comorbid arithmetic disability. *Developmental Neuropsychology, 11,* 351–371.

Ashcraft, M. H. (1982). The development of mental arithmetic: A chronometric approach. *Developmental Review, 2,* 213–236.

Ashcraft, M. H. (1995). Cognitive psychology and simple arithmetic: A review and summary of new directions. *Mathematical Cognition, 1,* 3–34.

Ashcraft, M. H., & Battaglia, J. (1978). Cognitive arithmetic: Evidence for retrieval and decision processes in mental addition. *Journal of Experimental Psychology: Human Learning and Memory, 4,* 527–538.

Ashcraft, M. H., Yamashita, T. S., & Aram, D. M. (1992). Mathematics performance in left and right brain-lesioned children. *Brain and Cognition, 19,* 208–252.

Badian, N. A. (1983). Dyscalculia and nonverbal disorders of learning. In H. R. Myklebust (Ed.), *Progress in learning disabilities* (Vol. 5, pp. 235–264). New York: Stratton.

Barrouillet, P., Fayol, M., & Lathulière, E. (1997). Selecting between competitors in multiplication tasks: An explanation of the errors produced by adolescents with learning disabilities. *International Journal of Behavioral Development, 21,* 253–275.

Briars, D., & Siegler, R. S. (1984). A featural analysis of preschoolers' counting knowledge. *Developmental Psychology, 20,* 607–618.

Bull, R., & Johnston, R. S. (1997). Children's arithmetical difficulties: Contributions from processing speed, item identification, and short-term memory. *Journal of Experimental Child Psychology, 65,* 1–24.

Bull, R., Johnston, R. S., & Roy, J. A. (1999). Exploring the roles of the visual–spatial sketch pad and central executive in children's arithmetical skills: Views from cognition and developmental neuropsychology. *Developmental Neuropsychology 15,* 421–442.

Carpenter, T. P., & Moser, J. M. (1984). The acquisition of addition and subtraction concepts in grades one through three. *Journal for Research in Mathematics Education, 15,* 179–202.

Conway, A. R. A., & Engle, R. W. (1994). Working memory and retrieval: A resource-dependent inhibition model. *Journal of Experimental Psychology: General, 123,* 354–373.

Dehaene, S., & Cohen, L. (1991). Two mental calculation systems: A case study of severe acalculia with preserved approximation. *Neuropsychologia, 29,* 1045–1074.

Dehaene, S., & Cohen, L. (1995). Towards an anatomical and functional model of number processing. *Mathematical Cognition, 1,* 83–120.

Dehaene, S., & Cohen, L. (1997). Cerebral pathways for calculation: Double dissociation between rote verbal and quantitative knowledge of arithmetic. *Cortex, 33,* 219–250.

Dehaene, S., Spelke, E., Pinel, P., Stanescu, R., & Tsivkin, S. (1999). Sources of mathematical thinking: Behavioral and brain-imaging evidence. *Science, 284,* 970–974.

Fuson, K. C. (1982). An analysis of the counting-on solution procedure in addition. In T. P. Carpenter, J. M. Moser, & T. A. Romberg (Eds.), *Addition and subtraction: A cognitive perspective* (pp. 67–81). Hillsdale, NJ: Erlbaum.

Garnett, K., & Fleischner, J. E. (1983). Automatization and basic fact performance of normal and learning disabled children. *Learning Disabilities Quarterly, 6,* 223–230.

Geary, D. C. (1990). A componential analysis of an early learning deficit in mathematics. *Journal of Experimental Child Psychology, 49,* 363–383.

Geary, D. C. (1993). Mathematical disabilities: Cognitive, neuropsychological, and genetic components. *Psychological Bulletin, 114,* 345–362.

Geary, D. C. (1994). *Children's mathematical development: Research and practical applications.* Washington, DC: American Psychological Association.

Geary, D. C. (1996). Sexual selection and sex differences in mathematical abilities. *Behavioral and Brain Sciences, 19,* 229–284.

Geary, D. C. (2000). Mathematical disorders: An overview for educators. *Perspectives, 26,* 6–9.

Geary, D. C., Bow-Thomas, C. C., Fan, L., & Siegler, R. S. (1993). Even before formal instruction, Chinese children outperform American children in mental addition. *Cognitive Development, 8,* 517–529.

Geary, D. C., Bow-Thomas, C. C., & Yao, Y. (1992). Counting knowledge and skill in cognitive addition: A comparison of normal and mathematically disabled children. *Journal of Experimental Child Psychology, 54,* 372–391.

Geary, D. C., & Brown, S. C (1991). Cognitive addition: Strategy choice and speed-of-processing differences in gifted, normal, and mathematically disabled children. *Developmental Psychology, 27,* 398–406.

Geary, D. C., Brown, S. C., & Samaranayake, V. A. (1991). Cognitive addition: A short longitudinal study of strategy choice and speed-of-processing differences in normal and mathematically disabled children. *Developmental Psychology, 27,* 787–797.

Geary, D. C., & Burlingham-Dubree, M. (1989). External validation of the strategy choice model for addition. *Journal of Experimental Child Psychology, 47,* 175–192.

Geary, D. C., Hamson, C. O., & Hoard, M. K. (2000). Numerical and arithmetical cognition: A longitudinal study of process and concept deficits in children with learning disability. *Journal of Experimental Child Psychology, 77,* 236–263.

Geary, D. C., & Hoard, M. K. (2001). Numerical and arithmetical deficits in learning-disabled children: Relation to dyscalculia and dyslexia. *Aphasiology, 15,* 635–647.

Geary, D. C., Hoard, M. K., & Hamson, C. O. (1999). Numerical and arithmetical cognition: Patterns of functions and deficits in children at risk for a mathematical disability. *Journal of Experimental Child Psychology, 74,* 213–239.

Geary, D. C., Saults, S. J., Liu, F., & Hoard, M. K. (2000). Sex differences in spatial cognition, computational fluency, and arithmetical reasoning. *Journal of Experimental Child Psychology, 77,* 337–353.

Geary, D. C., Widaman, K. F., & Little, T. D. (1986). Cognitive addition and multiplication: Evidence for a single memory network. *Memory and Cognition, 14,* 478–487.

Geary, D. C., Widaman, K. F., Little, T. D., & Cormier, P. (1987). Cognitive addition: Comparison of learning disabled and academically normal elementary school children. *Cognitive Development, 2,* 249–269.

Gelman, R., & Gallistel, C. R. (1978). *The child's understanding of number.* Cambridge, MA: Harvard University Press.

Gelman, R., & Meck, E. (1983). Preschooler's counting: Principles before skill. *Cognition, 13,* 343–359.

Groen, G. J., & Parkman, J. M. (1972). A chronometric analysis of simple addition. *Psychological Review, 79,* 329–343.

Gross-Tsur, V., Manor, O., & Shalev, R. S. (1996). Developmental dyscalculia: Prevalence and demographic features. *Developmental Medicine and Child Neurology, 38,* 25–33.

Hanich, L. B., Jordan, N. C., Kaplan, D., & Dick, J. (2001). Performance across different areas of mathematical cognition in children with learning difficulties. *Journal of Educational Psychology, 93,* 615–626.

Hitch, G. J., & McAuley, E. (1991). Working memory in children with specific arithmetical learning disabilities. *British Journal of Psychology, 82,* 375–386.

Hittmair-Delazer, M., Sailer, U., & Benke, T. (1995). Impaired arithmetic facts but intact conceptual knowledge—A single-case study of dyscalculia. *Cortex, 31,* 139–147.

Jordan, N. C., & Hanich, L. B. (2000). Mathematical thinking in second-grade children with different forms of LD. *Journal of Learning Disabilities, 33,* 567–578.

Jordan, N. C., Levine, S. C., & Huttenlocher, J. (1995). Calculation abilities in young children with different patterns of cognitive functioning. *Journal of Learning Disabilities, 28,* 53–64.

Jordan, N. C., & Montani, T. O. (1997). Cognitive arithmetic and problem solving: A comparison of children with specific and general mathematics difficulties. *Journal of Learning Disabilities, 30,* 624–634.

Koontz, K. L., & Berch, D. B. (1996). Identifying simple numerical stimuli: Processing inefficiencies exhibited by arithmetic learning disabled children. *Mathematical Cognition, 2,* 1–23.

Kosc, L. (1974). Developmental dyscalculia. *Journal of Learning Disabilities, 7,* 164–177.

Light, J. G., & DeFries, J. C. (1995). Comorbidity of reading and mathematics disabilities: Genetic and environmental etiologies. *Journal of Learning Disabilities, 28,* 96–106.

Luria, A. R. (1980). *Higher cortical functions in man* (2nd ed.). New York: Basic Books.

McLean, J. F., & Hitch, G. J. (1999). Working memory impairments in children with specific arithmetic learning difficulties. *Journal of Experimental Child Psychology, 74,* 240–260.

Morris, R. D., Stuebing, K. K., Fletcher, J. M.,

Shaywitz, S. E., Lyon, G. R., Shankweiler, D. P., Katz, L., Francis, D. J., & Shaywitz, B. A. (1998). Subtypes of reading disability: Variability around a phonological core. *Journal of Educational Psychology, 90*, 347–373.

Ostad, S. A. (1997). Developmental differences in addition strategies: A comparison of mathematically disabled and mathematically normal children. *British Journal of Educational Psychology, 67*, 345–357.

Ostad, S. A. (1998a). Comorbidity between mathematics and spelling difficulties. *Log Phon Vovol, 23*, 145–154.

Ostad, S. A. (1998b). Developmental differences in solving simple arithmetic word problems and simple number-fact problems: A comparison of mathematically normal and mathematically disabled children. *Mathematical Cognition, 4*, 1–19.

Ostad, S. A. (2000). Cognitive subtraction in a developmental perspective: Accuracy, speed-of-processing and strategy-use differences in normal and mathematically disabled children. *Focus on Learning Problems in Mathematics, 22*, 18–31.

Pesenti, M., Seron, X., & Van Der Linden, M. (1994). Selective impairment as evidence for mental organisation of arithmetical facts: BB, a case of preserved subtraction? *Cortex, 30*, 661–671.

Räsänen, P., & Ahonen, T. (1995). Arithmetic disabilities with and without reading difficulties: A comparison of arithmetic errors. *Developmental Neuropsychology, 11*, 275–295.

Rourke, B. P. (1993). Arithmetic disabilities, specific and otherwise: A neuropsychological perspective. *Journal of Learning Disabilities, 26*, 214–226.

Russell, R. L., & Ginsburg, H. P. (1984). Cognitive analysis of children's mathematical difficulties. *Cognition and Instruction, 1*, 217–244.

Semenza, C., Miceli, L., & Girelli, L. (1997). A deficit for arithmetical procedures: Lack of knowledge or lack of monitoring? *Cortex, 33*, 483–498.

Seron, X., Deloche, G., Ferrand, I., Cornet, J.-A., Frederix, M., & Hirsbrunner, T. (1991). Dot counting by brain damaged subjects. *Brain and Cognition, 17*, 116–137.

Shalev, R. S., Manor, O., & Gross-Tsur, V. (1993). The acquisition of arithmetic in normal children: Assessment by a cognitive model of dyscalculia. *Developmental Medicine and Child Neurology, 35*, 593–601.

Shalev, R. S., Manor, O., Kerem, B., Ayali, M., Badichi, N., Friedlander, Y., & Gross-Tsur, V. (2001). Developmental dyscalculia is a familial learning disability. *Journal of Learning Disabilities, 34*, 59–65.

Siegel, L. S., & Ryan, E. B. (1989). The development of working memory in normally achieving and subtypes of learning disabled children. *Child Development, 60*, 973–980.

Siegler, R. S. (1987). The perils of averaging data over strategies: An example from children's addition. *Journal of Experimental Psychology: General, 116*, 250–264.

Siegler, R. S. (1988). Individual differences in strategy choices: Good students, not-so-good students, and perfectionists. *Child Development, 59*, 833–851.

Siegler, R. S. (1996). *Emerging minds: The process of change in children's thinking.* New York: Oxford University Press.

Siegler, R. S., & Shrager, J. (1984). Strategy choice in addition and subtraction: How do children know what to do? In C. Sophian (Ed.), *Origins of cognitive skills* (pp. 229–293). Hillsdale, NJ: Erlbaum.

Svenson, O., & Broquist, S. (1975). Strategies for solving simple addition problems: A comparison of normal and subnormal children. *Scandinavian Journal of Psychology, 16*, 143–151.

Swanson, H. L. (1993). Working memory in learning disability subgroups. *Journal of Experimental Child Psychology, 56*, 87–114.

Temple, C. M. (1989). Digit dyslexia: A category-specific disorder in developmental dyscalculia. *Cognitive Neuropsychology, 6*, 93–116.

Temple, C. M. (1991). Procedural dyscalculia and number fact dyscalculia: Double dissociation in developmental dyscalculia. *Cognitive Neuropsychology, 8*, 155–176.

Welsh, M. C., & Pennington, B. F. (1988). Assessing frontal lobe functioning in children: Views from developmental psychology. *Developmental Neuropsychology, 4*, 199–230.

Widaman, K. F., Geary, D. C., Cormier, P., & Little, T. D. (1989). A componential model for mental addition. *Journal of Experimental Psychology: Learning, Memory, and Cognition, 15*, 898–919.

13

Language Processes: Keys to Reading Disability

Virginia A. Mann

Introduction and Statement of the Problem

What makes a poor reader a poor *reader*? Some 4 to 10% of children encounter severe difficulty in learning to read, and it is the objective of this chapter to review one of the most prevalent causes of their problems. Since the early 1970s, an ever-growing body of evidence has linked developmental reading problems to inadequacies in one or more areas of spoken language.

The focus of this review is reading difficulty as it is manifest in the elementary grades. It includes but is not limited to developmental dyslexia. Developmental dyslexia is a syndrome defined by discrepancy between a child's intelligence level and his or her level of reading ability. Individuals with dyslexia read significantly below the level that would be expected based on their IQ scores alone. Although learning to read is a complex learning task that correlates about 0.6 with IQ (Rutter, 1978), there nevertheless exist children who possess a seemingly adequate IQ (typically 90 or higher) but nonetheless encounter reading problems. Such children are said to have a specific reading difficulty, as their actual reading ability lags between 1

and 2 years behind that which is predicted on the basis of their age, IQ, and social standing.

Recent reviews have seriously discredited the use of a discrepancy between IQ and reading ability as a definitive characteristic that sets children with dyslexia apart from other "garden-variety" poor readers (see Fletcher, Francis, Rourke, Shaywitz, & Shaywitz, 1992; Francis et al., 1996; Shankweiler et al., 1995). Rather than forming into two separate groups, dyslexic and garden-variety poor readers seem to form a continuous distribution (see Stanovich, 1988). Both types of readers with disabilities have problems with the language skills that are of primary interest in this chapter. Most of the differences between the groups seem to involve "real-world knowledge" and "strategic abilities": The children with dyslexia possess superior skills in these "nonlinguistic" areas; hence the discrepancy between their IQ and their reading ability, whereas the garden-variety poor readers may show inadequacies in these skills as well as in their language skills (see Stanovich, 1988, for a discussion).

Over the course of this chapter, my intent is to introduce and justify a language-based approach to reading disability. This approach owes largely to the work of I. Y. Liberman and her husband and colleague, Alvin Liberman. Their synergistic insights and their erudition with respect to education, psychology, linguistics, and the speech sciences were a necessary catalyst to the realization that many instances of reading problems are rooted in spoken language.

A Theoretical Perspective: English Transcribes Phonemes and Morphemes

Two insights underscore the role of language problems in poor reading. One is theoretical and historical; the other is research driven. The theoretical and historical insight concerns the relation between the units of written languages and spoken language, how the one is designed to map onto the other. The research-based insight concerns the active role of language skills in skilled reading. We often think of reading as a "visual" skill, yet visual perception is only the tip of the reading iceberg. For readers to successfully decode the words and uncover the sentences and paragraphs on the page, seeing is not enough. Readers must successfully map the units of their written language onto the units of their spoken language. Spoken language comes first in both the history of the individual and the history of our species; it is both universal and natural. Writing and reading are parasitic upon speaking and listening and operate by virtue of some of the very same skills that allow us to be speakers and hearers of our language.

How Writing Systems Represent Spoken Language

A writing system, or "orthography," writes language by representing certain units of a spoken language. All writing systems represent units of a spoken language, but there are differences that turn on the type of linguistic units that are being represented. For example, ideographies such as American Indian petroglyphs or the universal set of road signs that a driver encounters in a daily commute represent language at the level of "ideas." Logographies such as the Chinese

writing system and Japanese Kanji represent language in terms of units of smaller units of meaning called morphemes. Syllabaries such as Hebrew and Japanese Kana represent language at the syllables. Alphabets such as Spanish, German, French, Italian, and English represent units that are called phonemes (e.g., consonants and vowels).

Each type of writing system places certain demands on a reader (for discussion, see Hung & Tzeng, 1981; Watt, 1989). As first noted by the Libermans and their colleagues (see, e.g., Liberman, Liberman, Mattingly, & Shankweiler, 1980; Mattingly, 1972) one of the most important demands involves language awareness. A reader of a writing system needs to be aware of the unit the writing system is representing. Otherwise it will be difficult to understand how written words relate to the spoken language.

Alphabets are a case in point. Because alphabets represent phonemes, someone wishing to learn to read an alphabet needs to be sensitive to the fact that spoken language can be broken down into phonemes. In contrast, a reader of a syllabary need only be aware of syllables. This sensitivity to the phonemes within words is referred to as phoneme awareness and is an important trait of successful beginning readers and a definitive problem for many young children and poor readers, in particular, as we shall see in the section "Reading Problems, Phoneme Awareness, and Morpheme Awareness."

The English Writing System

The English alphabet represents a special case because it is not a pure alphabet as much as an alphabet with logographic overtones. It does not provide the consistent one-to-one mapping of letter to phonemes that one finds in Spanish or German, for example. Rather, it provides a "deeper," more abstract level of representation that goes beyond phonemes and sounds to the morphemes and meanings of words. As such it has been, referred to as a morphophonological transcription because it combines the transcription of morphemes and phonemes As noted by Chomsky (1964), English alphabetic transcription corresponds not so much to the consonants and vowels that speakers and hearers think they pronounce and perceive as much as it to the way theoretical linguistics assumes that words are abstractly represented in the ideal speaker/hearer's mental dictionary, or "lexicon." Words in the mental lexicon are represented in terms of morphemes (e.g., root words, prefixes, and suffixes) as well as in terms of phonemes. When speakers of English produce or perceive language, they convert the morphophonological representations of the words in their lexicon to less abstract, "phonetic" representations by using an ordered series of phonological rules that alter, insert, or delete phonemes. These same rules can help them to pronounce words spelled according to their morphophonological representations.

If a writing system correctly represents words in a deep manner it will sometimes fail to represent the more superficial phonetic representations with which we are most familiar. Witness, for example, the spellings of words in pairs such as "atom" versus "atomic," "heal" versus "health," and "relate" versus "relation." In each of these word pairs, the similar spelling of the base and derived form captures the relatedness of their meanings. But the similar spelling comes at the cost of having a letter or letter sequence represent different phonemes in different words (e.g., the two pronunciations of "o," "ea," and "t"). Preservation of common roots and common word ancestries is one of the reasons the English vowel system is so complicated and one of the reasons English uses nearly 120 spelling patterns for 40 phonemes. It is also the source of homophones such as *to-two-too* and *their-there-they're*. The different spellings of these homonyms reflects their different meanings (e.g., morphology); the common pronunciation is what makes their usage so hard. The important point to be remembered is that the English alphabet represents phonemes and morphemes and there is a certain trade-off between then two types of representation.

Why have a writing system that transcribes both phonemes and morphemes? Each unit has certain advantages. Economy of characters is a clear benefit of transcribing phonemes. By transcribing phonemes, the alphabet can get away with 26 letters and 120 spelling patterns where a logographic orthography requires 2,000 to 3,000 characters for a newspaper and over 10,000 for scholarly works. Phoneme transcription is also highly productive. By embodying a highly "rule-governed" relationship between written and spoken words, it allows the reader to read not only highly familiar words but also less familiar ones such as "skiff," and even nonsense words such as "ifts" or "polypluckable." A reader of a logography may have difficulty pronouncing an unfamiliar word even when he or she has memorized thousands of distinct characters.

The benefit that accrues from the transcription of morphemes involves clues to word meaning and function. By transcribing a "deep," relatively abstract level of phonological structure where units of meaning are represented, the English writing system helps convey cues to meaning as well as to sound. Recognizing "joy" in "enjoy," "heal" in "health," "atom" in "atomic," or "relate" in "relation" can facilitate the recovery of that word's meaning. Recognizing suffixes such as *–ly, -ing,* and *-ness* can provide cues to a word's function in a sentence. The transcription of morphemes can also offer a common denominator to people who speak with different accents. Rather than specifying each surface phoneme, it leaves it to the speaker to apply his or her accent to the morphophonological representation available on the page. A final advantage of morphophonological spelling is that it can disambiguate homonyms. Indeed, one of the most common justifications of the use of a logography in Chinese concerns the number of homophones in the Chinese language.

Ultimately, the utility of a given orthography rests on the nature of the spoken language it transcribes. A logography is appropriate for Chinese because it allows people to read the same text even though they cannot understand each other's speech. For Japanese, the Kana syllabaries are quite well suited to the 100 or so syllables in the Japanese language. English, however, has a less profound dialectical variation than Chinese, and the English language employs more than 1,000 syllables. Hence, an alphabet is appropriate, and historical change and language infusions have made that alphabet morphophonemic. It would be less efficient and even a disservice to present the English writing system otherwise.

A Research-Based Perspective: Language Processes Support Skilled Reading

We have reviewed the way in which the English alphabet transcribes spoken English language as a form of deductive evidence about the importance of spoken language skills to reading. Now let us turn to a complementary source of empirical evidence, namely, investigations of the process of skilled reading. Studies of adult readers show a clear involvement of certain spoken language processes in the skilled reading of words, sentences, and paragraphs. They confirm that reading is really quite "parasitic" upon spoken language processes.

Language Skills and Word Recognition

Whether words must be recoded into some type of "silent speech" has preoccupied psychological studies of skilled reading. It especially preoccupied studies of the "lexical access" processes that make it possible for us to decode and recognize the words of our vocabulary (for recent reviews of how readers gain lexical access, see Berent & Perfetti, 1995; Frost, 1998; van Orden, 1987). Under some circumstances, silent speech does not appear necessary for word recognition; some words may be directly perceived as visual units, instead of being decoded into a string of phonemes. But there is clear evidence implicating at least some "speech code" involvement in word perception, making many psychologists favor a "dual access" or "parallel race horse" model in which both phonetic and visual access occur in parallel. Others believe that a "speech code" or "phonetic" route may be most heavily used in the case of less frequent words and unfamiliar ones (Seidenberg, 1985), and still others regard the speech code as playing an early, dominant role in all lexical access (Frost, 1998; Rayner, Sereno, Lesch, & Pollatsek, 1995; van Orden, 1987).

As for the recognition of morphemic units within spoken words, various authors have investigated the role of morpheme-size units in fluent reading. Use of such methodologies as letter cancellation tasks (Drenowski & Healy, 1980) and lexical decision (Taft, 1984; Taft & Forster, 1975) has given some support to the view that stems and affixes are recognized as units within words and may play a part in the reading of English. However, it is not clear whether the recognition of morphemic units mediates word recognition for all words as opposed to morphologically complex ones.

Language Skills and the Reading of Sentences and Paragraphs

From the point of word perception onward, the involvement of speech processes in reading is quite clear. First, there is considerable evidence that temporary working or "short-term" memory for written material involves a speech code. This speech code is sometimes referred to as silent speech, or phonetic representation, and it is used whether the to-be-remembered material is spoken or written or whether it is isolated letters, printed nonsense syllables, or printed words. Both the nature of the errors that subjects make in recalling such material and the experimental manipulations that help or hurt their memory performance have shown us that a phonetic representation is being used. That is, subjects are temporarily remembering a sequence of written words in terms of the consonants and vowels within each word, rather than the visual shape of the letters, the shape of the words, and so on (cf., for example, Baddeley, 1978; Conrad, 1964, 1972; Levy, 1977). It is further the case that subjects appear to rely on phonetic representation when they are required to comprehend sentences written in either alphabetic (Kleiman, 1975; Levy, 1977; Slowiaczek & Clifton, 1980) or logographic orthographies (Tzeng, Hung, & Wang, 1977). Understanding a sentence often requires the reader to hold several words in memory until the structure of the sentence is apparent. This is one reason we may observe such significantly high correlations between reading and listening comprehension across a variety of languages and orthographies, including English (Daneman & Carpenter, 1980; Jackson & McClelland, 1979).

Thus, regardless of the way in which the reader recognizes each word on the page, the processes involved in reading sentences and paragraphs place certain obvious demands on temporary memory, and temporary memory for language appears to make use of phonetic representation in short-term memory. In the section "Reading Problems and Language Processing" we will see that problems with phonetic representation are often found among poor beginning readers, in the form of "short-term memory problems."

For morphemes as well as for speech coding, the study of sentences and paragraphs yield a clearer picture. For example, readers' eye movements tend to be guided by the morphemic structure of words within a text (Lima, 1987; Rayner & McConkie, 1976). It is also the case that whether or not words are automatically decomposed into their morphemic constituents prior to lexical access, their morphemic composition is essential to sentence comprehension. Adult skilled readers are able to use the morphemic structure of words to complete a sentence completion task, and they do so more extensively than do poor readers (Mahony, 1994; Tyler & Nagy, 1990), a finding elaborated on in the next section.

Reading Problems, Phoneme Awareness, and Morpheme Awareness

If reading is a language skill, why doesn't every speaker of English automatically becomes a successful beginning reader of English? The answer to this question is that "knowing" spoken English is a necessary but not a sufficient requirement for skilled reading. Would-be readers must go one step further than merely being a speaker/hearer of their language—they must be able to consciously analyze and manipulate the units that their writing system represents.

Phoneme Awareness

Phoneme awareness, as first discussed by Mattingly (1972), and later developed in several other places (A. M. Liberman, 1999; I. Y. Liberman, 1982; Liberman et al., 1980), is not something we use in the normal activities of speaking and hearing. We use it in certain "secondary language activities" such as appreciating verse (i.e., alliteration), making jokes (i.e., "Where do you leave your dog? In a barking lot . . ."), and talking in secret languages (i.e., Pig Latin). Such activities require that we consciously compare and manipulate the consonants and vowels that comprise spoken words. Taking the "t" off "cat," realizing that "clay" and "cream" start with the same sound, realizing that "shoe" and "toe" have the same number of sounds—are some other examples of activities that require phoneme awareness.

One slight problem with the term "phoneme awareness" is that it is often used interchangeably with several other terms: "phonemic awareness," "phonological awareness," "metalinguistic awareness" and "linguistic awareness," to name a few. By using the term "phoneme awareness" (or "phonemic awareness") we confine the issue to sensitivity about phonemes. "Phonological awareness" could also include sensitivity to rhyme, syllables, and morphemes and the phonological rules that operate on them; "linguistic awareness" and "metalinguistic" awareness would further include sensitivity to syntax (i.e., grammar), semantics (i.e., meaning), and their rules. To date, awareness of phonemes has been most often studied and deficient phoneme awareness is a major factor in reading disorders.

EVIDENCE FROM THE ANALYSIS OF
READING ERRORS

The errors a person makes can be informative about the difficulties that produce those errors, and oral reading errors can offer an important source of evidence about the cause of reading problems. A consideration of these errors has shown that a lack of phoneme awareness is responsible for making beginning reading difficult for all young children (Shankweiler & Liberman, 1972), including those with dyslexia (Fischer, Liberman, & Shankweiler, 1977). Such errors do not tend to involve visual confusions or letter or sequence reversals to any appreciable degree. What they instead reflect is a problem with integrating the phonological information that letter sequences convey. Hence, children often tend to be correct as to the pronunciation of the first letter in a word but to have more and more difficulty with subsequent letters, and a particular problem with vowels as opposed to consonants. For more detailed presentation of these findings and their implications, the reader is referred to work by

Shankweiler and Liberman (1972) and Fischer and colleagues (1977), and also Russell (1982), which suggests that deficient phoneme awareness may also account for the reading difficulties of adult dyslexics.

EVIDENCE FROM TASKS THAT MEASURE AWARENESS DIRECTLY

Most studies of phoneme awareness have concerned tasks that measure awareness directly. These tasks require children to play language "games" that manipulate the phonemes within a word in one way or another: counting them, deleting them, choosing words which contain the same phoneme, and so on. The use of these tasks has revealed that phoneme awareness develops later than phonetic perception and the use of phonetic representation, and it remains a chronic problem for those individuals who are poor readers.

The use of such tasks in the study of beginning readers began in the 1970s, when Liberman and her colleagues asked whether a sample of 4-, 5-, and 6-year-olds could learn to play syllable counting games and phoneme counting games. In each game the idea was to "tap" the number of syllables/phonemes in a spoken word and the child was given examples to illustrate the concept before being asked to play the game with a set of words (Liberman, Shankweiler, Fischer, & Carter, 1974). It was discovered that none of the nursery school children could tap the number of phonemes in a spoken word, although half of them managed to tap the number of syllables. Only 17% of the kindergarteners could tap phonemes, although, again, about half of them could tap syllables. At 6, 90% of the children could tap syllables, and 70% were able to tap phonemes. From such findings it is clear that the awareness of phonemes and syllables develops considerably between the ages of 4 and 6. It is also clear that awareness of phonemes is slower to develop than awareness of syllables. Finally, both types of awareness markedly improve at just the age when children are learning to read (Liberman et al., 1974).

Numerous experiments involving widely diverse subjects, school systems, and measurement devices have shown a strong positive correlation between a lack of awareness about phonemes and current problems in learning to read (to name but a few, see, e.g., Bradley & Bryant, 1985; Fox & Routh, 1976; Muter, Hulme, Snowling, & Taylor, 1997; Yopp, 1988; see also Adams, 1990; Brady & Shankweiler, 1991; Perfetti, 1985; Wagner & Torgesen, 1987, for reviews). Studies of kindergarten children provide evidence that problems with phoneme segmentation can presage and predict reading problems (see, e.g., Blachman, 1984; Mann, 1993; Wagner et al., 1997; see also Hulme & Joshi, 1998, for an expanded set of references). Two examples come to mind. Eighty-five percent of a population of kindergarten children who went on to become good readers in the first grade correctly counted the number of syllables in spoken words, whereas only 17% of the future poor readers could do so (Mann & Liberman, 1984). Sixty-six percent of first-grade variance in reading scores could be accounted for by a kindergarten battery of tests that assessed phoneme awareness (Stanovich, Cunningham, & Cramer, 1984).

FACTORS THAT UNDERLIE DEFICIENT PHONEME AWARENESS

Research is showing that the relation between phoneme awareness and reading is a complex two-way street. On the one hand, exposure to the alphabet and the alphabetic principle has a clear effect on the development of phoneme awareness. For example, illiterate adults are unable to manipulate the phonetic structure of spoken words (Morais, Cary, Alegria, & Bertelson, 1979; Read, Zhang, Nie, & Ding, 1986). It is also the case that the onset of phoneme awareness in the early grades follows exposure to alphabetic instruction: Children in Germany, who start to learn to read in first-grade, begin to develop phoneme awareness in the first grade where American children who begin learning to read in kindergarten show an earlier onset (Mann & Wimmer, 2002). It would seem that awareness of phonemes is enhanced by methods of reading instruction that direct the child's attention to the phonetic structure of words, and it may even depend on such instruction.

However, experience alone cannot be the

only factor behind some children's failure to achieve phoneme awareness, which is aptly shown by Bradley and Bryant's (1978) finding that among a group of 6-year-old skilled readers and 10-year-old readers with disabilities who were matched for reading ability, the readers with disabilities performed significantly worse on a phonological awareness task, even though they would be expected to have had more reading instruction than the younger children. Here it could be argued that some constitutional factor limited the ability of readers with disabilities to profit from instruction, and thus limited their attainment of phonological sophistication. Indeed, Pennington, Van Orden, Kirson, and Haith (1991) have offered some new and interesting evidence that deficient phoneme awareness is the primary trait of individuals who are "familial" dyslexics.

What might that constitutional factor be? Elbro (1996), Fowler (1991), and Walley (1993) have all in one way or another suggested that problems with phoneme awareness might reflect a deficiency in children's internal phonological representations. In Foy and Mann (2001), we recently attempted to investigate this possibility by examining putative measures of phonological strength (perception, production, naming) in relation to phonological awareness and reading development. The results did not validate strength of phonological representation as a unitary construct underlying phonological awareness. Instead they revealed a more selective pattern of associations between spoken-language tasks and rhyme and phoneme awareness as separable aspects of phonological awareness. Speech perception (to be discussed in the section "Reading Problems and Deficient Language Processing") was closely associated with the awareness of rhyme, even when age, vocabulary, and letter knowledge were controlled. Children with a less developed sense of rhyme also had a less mature pattern of articulation, independent of age, vocabulary, and letter knowledge. Phoneme awareness, per se, associated with phonological perception and production and children with low phoneme awareness skills showed a different pattern of speech perception and articulation errors than did children with strong abilities, but these differences appeared to be largely a function of age, letter knowledge, and especially vocabulary knowledge.

Morpheme Awareness

In word pairs such as *reduce-reduction, atom-atomic* and *personal-personality,* the presence of the derivational suffix (i.e. *-ion, -ic,* and *–ity*) changes the base or stem word's stress and pronunciation even though its spelling remains constant. Thus the simple one-to-one relationship between graphemes and phonemes is destroyed, and the solution is to take morpheme-size units into account. Some authors have noted that young readers must take advantage of morpheme-sized units if they are to succeed in the reading of multisyllabic words (Carlisle, 1995; Carlisle & Nomanbhoy, 1993; Fowler & Liberman, 1995). Only if they are aware of morpheme-size units may it becomes possible for them to realize that attaching certain suffixes to a word can alter the word's pronunciation in regular, predictable ways.

The literature to date does show some intriguing relationships between morpheme awareness and reading. Morphological word formation can be generalized into two types: inflectional and derivational, both of which are transcribed in the English orthography. Mastery of inflections (e.g., past tense and plural markers) is usually accomplished relatively early in life in a fixed manner and has been subtly linked to reading progress during the first and second grades (Carlisle, 1995; Carlisle & Nomanbhoy, 1993). Mastery of derivational morphology (e.g., suffixes that do not automatically apply to each member of a syntactic category) seems to involve a longer, more open-ended course (Tyler & Nagy, 1990) that coincides with the ages at which children are learning to become proficient readers. There are growing indications that the production of derived forms is related to the ability to read English in the first and second grades (Carlisle, 1995, 2000; Carlisle & Nomanbhoy, 1993) and middle elementary grades (Fowler & Liberman, 1995; Singson, Mahony, & Mann, 2000), as well as in the junior and high school years (Mahony, 1994)

One problem with the interpretation of studies that link morpheme awareness to reading is that many tests of morpheme awareness may presume phonological awareness. Performance on phoneme- and syllable-segmentation tasks is well documented to be related to reading ability, and there have been successful attempts to show that poor sensitivity to derivational morphology relates to reading simply because it also requires phonological awareness. Carlisle and Nomanbhoy (1993; see also Carlisle, 1995), for example, studied first-graders using separate measures of reading, phoneme awareness, and morpheme awareness. Their results indicated that the two skills were related to each other and to reading ability, but that once the contribution of phoneme awareness was considered, morpheme awareness made little additional contribution to the children's variance in reading ability. Using various phoneme and morpheme production tasks, Fowler and Liberman (1995) investigated the levels of phonological and morphological awareness in less-skilled readers ages 7½ to 9½ years to see whether a low level in each skill correlated with poor reading ability. Their conclusions pointed more to a phonologically based deficit in poor readers, rather than a morphological one. They reasoned that morphological production tasks often draw on a mixture of skills (ranging from orthographic knowledge to phonological sensitivity and receptive vocabulary) that are well documented to be underdeveloped in poor readers. In their view, the poor readers' low performance on morphological tasks is most likely a consequence of their deficiency in these other skills.

In yet another relevant study which administered separate phoneme- and morpheme-based tests to children with reading disabilities between 7½ and 9½ years of age, Shankweiler and colleagues (1995) conclude that phonological deficits and deficient production of morphologically related forms stem from a common weakness in the phonological components of language and not from separable problems with phonology and morphology. Taken together, these results suggest that any finding that morphological awareness is related to reading must be analyzed with the caveat that phonological awareness is an underlying factor.

We have made another approach to the question of morphological involvement by using a morphological measure that is exclusively focused on derivational morphology and by using recognition as opposed to production. We, too, have found that morpheme awareness significantly correlated with phoneme awareness. Our analysis further controlled for the effects of vocabulary knowledge whereas Shankweiler and colleagues (1995) studied controlled for age and IQ. Yet our results were similar. When we controlled for performance on the phonological awareness and vocabulary tasks, we found that morphological awareness accounted for 4% of decoding variance; Carlisle (1995) found 4%, and Shankweiler and colleagues found 5%. If what we had found was a mere statistical artifact, it would be hard to explain how at least three arrived at the same 4–5% contribution of morphological awareness to decoding ability. Rather, it would be more parsimonious to conclude that morphological awareness has a small but reliable contribution to decoding ability. When we extend our scope of study to children in the later elementary grades, we may find even higher, more reliable levels of contribution (see Carlisle, 2000; Singson et al., 2000) due to the fact that reading ability turns on the ability to decode and comprehend multisyllabic words.

Reading Problems and Deficient Language Processing

Without spoken English, there would be nothing for the English orthography to transcribe; the well-known difficulties of readers who are deaf attest to the importance of spoken language skills for successful reading. But children who are deaf are not the only ones for whom deficient language abilities are a cause of reading problems. As we shall see shortly, many of the children who hear and are poor readers also suffer from spoken language problems, and although their problems are considerably more subtle than those of children who are deaf, they are no less critical. The following paragraphs summarize various forms of evidence about the types of language processing skills that have been linked to reading disability. This evidence can be organized in terms of four levels of language processing: speech perception, vocabulary skills, linguistic short-term memory, and syntax and semantics.

Speech Perception

The possibility that some aspect of speech perception might be a special problem for poor readers is illustrated and supported by Brady, Shankweiler, and Mann (1983). In considering a group of beginning readers who did not differ from each other in age, IQ, or audiometry scores but strongly differed in reading ability, they asked the children to identify spoken words or environmental sounds under a normal listening condition and under a "noisy" condition. When the performances of the good and poor readers were compared, the good and poor readers were equally able to identify the environmental sounds, whatever the listening condition. They were also equivalent on the unmasked words. However, the poor readers made almost 33% more errors than did the good readers when they were asked to identify the spoken words in the "noisy" condition.

Other research has confirmed that children who are poor readers may have problems perceiving speech. They require a longer segment of a gated word to perceive it correctly (Metsala, 1997). At least some poor readers do not perceive synthetic speech as categorically as good readers do (Manis et al., 1997; Mody, Studdert-Kennedy, & Brady, 1997). Following Walley (1993), Metsala (1997) suggested that the perceptual problem associated with poor reading and the concomitant difficulty with phoneme awareness may have a common source. Both may follow from the fact that the mental representation of phonemes may gradually develop over childhood, as the growth of spoken vocabulary causes lexical representations to become more segmental. Similarly, Manis and his colleagues (1997) have proposed that if children cannot perceive clear distinctions between phonemes it will be hard for them to have representations that can be easily accessed. Problems with accessing phonological representations will in turn lead to difficulty segmenting and manipulating phonemes and in learning grapheme–phoneme relationships. Foy and Mann (2001) have confirmed a relationship between speech perception and early reading skill, but their data on preschool children reveal that speech perception is more closely tied to the awareness of rhyme than to the awareness of phonemes, per se (see section "Reading Problems, Phoneme Awareness, and Morpheme Awareness").

Vocabulary Skills

There are quite a few indications that reading ability is related to certain vocabulary skills, depending on how reading ability is measured and on what type of vocabulary skill is at issue. Reading ability can be measured in terms of the ability to read individual words (e.g., in terms of "decoding") or in terms of the ability to understand the meaning of sentences and paragraphs (e.g., in terms of "comprehension"). In the case of beginning readers, decoding and comprehension tests are correlated quite highly, implying that children who differ on one type of test will usually differ on the other as well. Still, there are cases in which the two types of tests identify different groups of good and poor readers that may lead researchers to different conclusions about the cause of poor reading (see Stanovich, 1988, for discussion). Vocabulary skills are a case in point; future research may uncover other cases as well.

Vocabulary skills can be tested with two basic types of test. "Recognition vocabulary" tests such as the Peabody Picture Vocabulary Test require the child to point to a picture that illustrates a word. Recognition vocabulary has sometimes been related to early reading ability (see Stanovich, Cunningham, & Feeman, 1984), although it is not always a significant predictor (see Mann, 1984; Wolf & Goodglass, 1986). The utility of this test may depend on how "reading ability" is measured, as the relationship seems stronger for tests of reading comprehension, such as the Reading Survey of the Metropolitan (see Stanovich, Nathan, & Zolman, 1988), than for tests of word recognition such as the Word Identification and Word Attack tests of the Woodcock (see Mann & Liberman, 1984).

"Naming" or "productive vocabulary" tests such as the Boston Naming Test require the child to produce the word that a picture illustrates. Productive vocabulary give clearer indications of a link between reading ability and vocabulary skill and there is evidence that this link exists whether reading skill is measured in terms of decoding or in terms of comprehension. Performance on the Boston Naming Test, for example, predicted both the word recognition and the reading comprehension ability of kindergarten children far more accurately than did performance on the Peabody Picture Vocabulary Test (Wolf & Goodglass, 1986). In one study of the naming speed among individuals with dyslexia, the performance of 17-year-olds was closest to that of 8-year-old normal children for colors, digits, letters, and pictures of common objects (Fawcett & Nicolson, 1994). Tests of continuous naming (sometimes called rapid automatized naming), which require children to name a series of repeating objects, letters, or colors, have also shown that children who are poor readers take longer to name the series than do good readers (see, e.g., Blachman, 1984; Denckla & Rudel, 1976; Wolf, 1984). Performance on these tests bears an interesting relationship to the success of certain remediation measures (Torgesen & Davis, 1996).

A causal link between naming problems and reading problems is indicated by the discovery that performance on naming tests can predict future reading ability (for a review, see Bowers & Wolf, 1993). Wolf (1984) has noted that whereas continuous naming tests using objects and colors are predictive of early problems with word recognition, problems with rapid letter recognition and retrieval can play a more prolonged role in the reading of severely impaired readers, compromising both decoding and reading comprehension. Using a test of letter-naming ability in our longitudinal studies of kindergarten children (e.g., Mann, 1984; Mann & Ditunno, 1990) my colleagues and I have consistently found that kindergarteners who take longer to name a randomized array of the capital letters are significantly more likely to perform poorly on word decoding tests and comprehension tests that are administered in first grade. It further seems that present letter naming predicts future reading ability more consistently than present reading ability predicts future letter naming ability (for relevant evidence, see Mann & Di-

tunno, 1990; see also Stanovich et al., 1988). Thus it is likely that something other than a lack of educational experience is preventing these children from naming the letter names as fast as other children can.

Should problems with letter naming to be viewed in the context of language and phonological representation, or do they owe to something outside the realm of language? One pertinent piece of evidence about the naming problems of poor readers comes from a study by Katz (1986), who found that children who perform poorly on a decoding test are particularly prone to difficulties in producing low frequency and polysyllabic names, and suggested that for such words, these children may possess less "phonologically complete" lexical representations than do good readers. On the basis of his research, he further suggests that because poor readers often have access to aspects of the correct phonological representation of a word, even though they are unable to produce that word correctly, their problem may be attributable to phonological deficiencies in the structure of the lexicon rather than to the process of lexical access per se. McBride-Chang (1996) similarly argues from her extensive studies of phonological skills among elementary-school-age children that naming speed owes its effect on reading to its relation with speech perception and phonological processing.

However, Wolf and her colleagues (Wolf & Bowers, 1999; Wolf, Bowers, & Biddle, 2000) have recently countered such proposals with a view that naming problems stem from a broader source than deficient phonological representation. In their view, naming speed deficiencies may reflect a more pervasive rate-of-processing problem that affects varied aspects of reading and other modalities as well. Their "double-deficit" account proposes that separate deficits can underlie problems in the phonological system and problems in rapid serial naming. It is the children who suffer from both deficits that become the poorest readers.

Phonetic Working Memory

One of the more fruitful lines of research in the field of reading disability stems from the observation that poor readers perform less well than do good readers on a variety of working memory or "short-term" memory tests. It has often been noted that poor readers tend to perform less well on the digit span test and are deficient in the ability to recall strings of letters, nonsense syllables, or words in order, whether the stimuli are presented by ear or by eye. Poor readers even fail to recall the words of spoken sentences as accurately as good readers do (for reviews, see Brady & Shankweiler, 1991; Jorm, 1979; Mann, Liberman, & Shankweiler, 1980; McBride-Chang, 1996; Shankweiler, Liberman, Mark, Fowler, & Fischer, 1979, for references to these effects). Evidence that these differences are not merely consequences of differences in reading ability has come from a longitudinal study which showed that problems with recalling a sequence of words can precede the attainment of reading ability and may actually serve to presage future reading problems (Mann & Liberman, 1984).

In searching for an explanation of this pattern of results, researchers were inspired by research indicating that linguistic materials such as letters, words, and so on, are held in short-term memory through use of phonetic representation. Liberman, Shankweiler, and their colleagues (Shankweiler et al., 1979) were the first to suggest that the linguistic short-term memory difficulties of poor readers might reflect a problem with using this type of representation. Several experiments have supported this hypothesis. These experiments show that when recalling letter strings (Shankweiler et al., 1979), word strings (Mann et al., 1980; Mann & Liberman, 1984), and sentences (Mann et al., 1980), poor readers are much less sensitive than good readers to a manipulation of the phonetic structure of the materials (i.e., the density of words that rhyme). Indeed, good readers can be made to appear as error-prone as poor readers when they are asked to recall a string of words in which all of the words rhyme (such as "bat, cat, rat, hat, mat"), whereas poor readers perform at the same level whether or not the words rhyme. This observation has led to the postulation that poor readers—and children who are likely to become poor readers—are for some reason less able to use phonetic structure as a means of holding material in short-term memory (Mann et al., 1980; Mann & Liberman, 1984; Shankweiler et al., 1979).

One might ask, at this point, whether poor readers are avoiding phonetic representation altogether or merely using it less well. We have obtained little evidence that poor readers employ a visual form of memory instead of a phonetic one (Mann, 1984). Evidence that poor readers are attempting to use phonetic representation has been found in the types of errors that they make as they attempt to recall or recognize spoken words in a short-term memory task (Brady et al., 1983; Brady, Mann, & Schmidt, 1987). These errors reveal that poor readers make use of many of the same features of phonetic structure as good readers do. They make the same sort of phonetically principled errors—they merely make more of them.

Syntax and Semantics

The observation that poor readers cannot repeat spoken sentences as accurately as good readers has led to some obvious questions about higher-level language skills and their involvement in reading problems. To date, quite a few studies have examined the syntactic abilities of poor readers. There is an accumulating body of evidence that poor readers do not comprehend sentences as well as good readers do (see Mann, Cowin, & Schoenheimer, 1989, for a review). It has been shown that good and poor readers differ in the ability to both repeat and comprehend spoken sentences that contain relative clauses such as "The dog jumped over the cat that chased the monkey" (Mann, Shankweiler, & Smith, 1986). They also perform less well on instructions from the Token Test, such as "Touch the small red square and the large blue triangle" (Smith, Mann, & Shankweiler, 1987). They also are less able to distinguish the meaning of spoken sentences such as "He showed her bird the seed" from "He showed her the birdseed," which use the stress pattern of the sentence (its "prosody") and the position of the article "the" to mark the boundary between the indirect object and the direct object.

In searching to explain these and other sentence comprehension problems that have been observed among the poor readers we have studied, my colleagues and I have been struck by the fact that a short-term memory problem could lead to problems with comprehending sentences whose processing somehow stresses short-term memory. When we examined the results of the aforementioned studies, we found little evidence that the poor readers were having trouble with the grammatical structures being used in the sentences that caused them problems. In fact, the structures were often ones which young children master within the first few years of life and ones which the poor readers could understand if the sentence was short enough (see Mann et al., 1989, for a discussion). Instead, we found much evidence that the comprehension problem was predominantly due to the phonetic working memory problem discussed in the previous section. It seems as if poor readers are just as sensitive to syntactic structure as good readers; they fail to understand sentences because they cannot hold an adequate representation of the sentence in short-term memory (see Gottardo, Stanovich, & Siegel, 1996; Mann et al., 1985, 1989; Smith, Macaruso, Shankweiler, & Crain, 1989).

Another task that at first glance seems to indicate a syntactic impairment on the part of poor readers is the sentence completion task used by Mahony (1994) and Singson and colleagues (2000). That task requires children to choose among derivational forms that complete a sentence, as in "He was blinded by the _____: bright, brighten, brightly, brightness." Poorer readers, both children and adults, perform less well on this test than do normal readers, whether they are reading the sentences or hearing them aloud, and whether the word that fills in the blank is a real word or an appropriately derived word such as "froodness." Here the poor readers' difficulty in distinguishing among nouns, verbs, and adjectives appears to be due to a problem with derivational morphology and not a problem with syntax.

At present, then, although it is clear that poor readers do have sentence comprehension problems, there is little reason to think that their difficulties reflect a problem with the syntax of language. Problems with working memory and problems with morphology seem a more likely source of the difficulty. But the issue of whether or not poor readers are deficient in syntactic skills is far from resolved and will have to await

further research. Such deficits as do exist are relatively subtle, with poor readers merely performing like somewhat younger children than do the good readers.

As for the question of semantic impairments among poor readers, here, there is no reason to presume that any real deviance exists. If anything, poor readers place greater reliance on semantic context and semantic representation than do good readers, perhaps in compensation for their other language difficulties (see Stanovitch, 1982, for a review; see also Simpson, Lorsbach, & Whitehouse, 1983).

Conclusion and Applications

The literature on the relation between language processing skills and reading problems indicates that poor readers—and children who are likely to become poor readers—tend to have problems with phoneme awareness, morpheme awareness, and three aspects of language processing skill: (1) speech perception under difficult listening conditions; (2) vocabulary, especially when measured in terms of naming ability; and (3) using phonetic representation in linguistic short-term memory. As Stanovich has noted, there is a logical interrelation between the behavioral difficulties of poor readers, for they all involve "phonological processes" that concern the sound pattern of language. Hence we may speculate that the cause of many instances of reading disability involves a certain dysfunction within the "phonological" system—a "phonological core deficit" (see Stanovich, 1988, and Stanovich & Beck, 2000, for further discussion).

The research surveyed by this chapter may be of helpful interest to those who are concerned with the remediation of reading problems. As we come closer and closer to identifying the linguistic problems associated with specific reading difficulty—and their causes—we should also come closer to being able to point the way toward more effective procedures for their remediation. As for remediation of deficient morpheme awareness and deficiencies in such processing skills as speech perception, naming, and phonetic representation, the jury is still out. It is certainly reasonable to think that explicit practice and training can benefit some, if not all, of these skills, but clearly more research is needed. In the meantime it would seem best to use clear enunciation, repetition, and drilling to compensate for the bottleneck created by spoken language problems.

Certainly the brightest prospects for remediation are offered by evidence that various types of training can facilitate phoneme awareness. The best favor we can do for all children is to promote their phoneme awareness so that we may let them in on the secrets of the alphabetic principle as early as possible. Some interesting and practical advice on how to facilitate phoneme awareness is currently available from the work of such researchers as Liberman, Blachman, Torgesen, and Bradley and their colleagues. A variety of word games, nursery rhymes, and other "prereading" activities exist that can help nurture a child's awareness of the way in which words break down into phonemes. Such activities will undoubtedly pave the way for "phonics"-oriented methods of instruction so obviously favored by current research and so obviously in keeping with this chapter's focus on the importance of phoneme awareness in early reading.

Cunningham's (1990) research on phoneme awareness training offers the caveat that we should pay attention not only to the activities that promote phoneme awareness but also to how we are integrating these into instruction. Children need to appreciate the value application and utility of phoneme awareness to reading, and activities that encourage phoneme awareness are the most beneficial when the children are shown how these activities are beneficial to reading. Other caveats come from Torgesen and Davis (1996), who have united screening and training to show how one predicts the success of the other. In their research, children who reveal a three-way deficiency in phoneme awareness, letter naming, and phonemic representation may require much longer, more explicit training than the typical 8–12-week course seen in the literature.

References

Adams, M. J. (1990). *Beginning to read: thinking and learning about print*. Cambridge, MA: MIT Press.

Baddeley, A. D. (1978). The trouble with Levels: A reexamination of Craik and Lockhardt's framework for memory research. *Psychological Review, 85*, 139–152.

Berent, I., & Perfetti, C. A. (1995). A rose is a REEZ: The two-cycles model of phonology assembly in reading English. *Psychological Review, 102*, 146–184.

Blachman, B. (1984). Relationship of rapid naming and language analysis skills to kindergarten and first-grade reading achievement. *Journal of Educational Psychology, 76*, 610–622.

Bowers, P. G., & Wolf, M. (1993). Theoretical links among naming, speed, precise timing mechanisms, and orthographic skills in dyslexia. *Reading and Writing, 5*, 69–85.

Bradley, L., & Bryant, P. E. (1978). Difficulties in auditory organization as a possible cause of reading backwards. *Nature, 271*, 746–747.

Bradley, L., & Bryant, P. (1985). *Rhyme and reason in reading and spelling*. Ann Arbor: University of Michigan Press.

Brady, S., Mann, V., & Schmidt, R. (1987). Errors in short-term memory for good and poor readers. *Memory and Cognition, 15*, 444–453.

Brady, S., & Shankweiler, D. (1991). *Phonological processes in literacy*. Hillsdale, NJ: Erlbaum.

Brady, S. Shankweiler, D., & Mann, V. (1983). Speech perception and memory coding in relation to reading ability. *Memory and Cognition, 35*, 345–367.

Carlisle, J. F. (1995). Morphological awareness and early reading achievement. In L. Feldman (Ed.), *Morphological aspects of language processing* (pp. 189–209). Hillsdale, NJ: Erlbaum.

Carlisle, J. F. (2000). Awareness of morphological structure and meaning: Impact on reading. *Reading and Writing, 12*, 169–190.

Carlisle, J. F., & Nomanbhoy, D. M. (1993). Phonological and morphological awareness in first graders. *Applied Psycholinguistics, 14*, 177–195.

Chomsky, N. (1964). Comments for project literacy meeting. In M. Lester (Ed.), *Reading in applied transformational grammar*. New York: Holt Rinehart & Winston.

Conrad, R. (1964). Acoustic confusions in immediate memory. *British Journal of Psychology, 55*, 75–84.

Conrad, R. (1972). Speech and reading. In J. F. Kavanaugh & I. G. Mattingly (Eds.), *Language by ear and by eye: The relationships between speech and reading* (pp. 205–240). Cambridge, MA: MIT Press.

Cunningham, A. E. (1990). Explicit versus implicit instruction in phoneme awareness. *Journal of Experimental Child Psychology, 50*, 429–444.

Daneman, M., & Carpenter, P. A. (1980). Individual differences in working memory and reading. *Journal of Verbal Learning and Verbal Behavior, 19*, 450–466.

Denckla, M. B., & Rudel, R. G. (1976). Naming of object drawings by dyslexic and other learning-disabled children. *Brain and Language, 3*, 1–15.

Drenowski, A., & Healy, A. F. (1980). Missing –ing in reading: Letter detection errors in word endings. *Journal of Verbal Learning and Verbal Behavior, 19,* 247–262.

Elbro, C. (1996). Early linguistic abilities and reading development: A review and a hypothesis. *Reading and Writing, 8,* 453–485.

Fawcett, A. J., & Nicolson, R. I. (1994). Naming speed in children with dyslexia. *Journal of Learning Disabilities, 27,* 641.646.

Fischer, F. W., Liberman, I. Y., & Shankweiler, D. (1977). Reading reversals and developmental dyslexia: A further study. *Cognition, 14,* 496–510.

Fletcher, J. M., Francis, D. J., Rourke, B. P., Shaywitz, S. E., & Shaywitz, B. A. (1992). The validity of discrepancy-based definitions of reading disabilities. *Journal of Learning Disabilities, 25,* 555–561.

Fowler, A. E. (1991). How early phonological development might set the stage for phoneme awareness. In S. Brady & D. Shankweiler (Eds.), *Phonological processes in literacy: A tribute to Isabelle Y. Liberman* (pp. 97–117). Hillsdale, NJ: Erlbaum.

Fowler, A., & Liberman, I. (1995). The role of phonology and orthography in morphological awareness. In L. Feldman (Ed.), *Morphological aspects of language processing* (pp. 157–188). Hillsdale, NJ: Erlbaum.

Fox, B., & Routh, D. K. (1976). Phonemic analysis and synthesis as word-attack skills. *Journal of Educational Psychology, 69,* 70–74.

Foy, J. G., & Mann, V. (2001). Does strength of phonological representations predict phonological awareness? *Applied Psycholinguistics, 22,* 301–325.

Francis, D. J., Shaywitz, S. E., Stuebing, K. K., Shaywitz, B. A., & Fletcher, J. M. (1996). Developmental lag versus deficit accounts of reading disability: A longitudinal, individual growth curves analysis. *Journal of Educational Psychology, 88,* 3–17.

Frost, R. (1998). Toward a strong phonological theory of visual word recognition: True issues and false trails. *Psychological Bulletin, 123,* 71–99.

Gottardo, A., Stanovich, K., & Siegel, L. (1996). The relationships between phonological sensitivity, syntactic processing, and verbal working memory in the reading performance of third-grade children. *Journal of Experimental Child Psychology, 63,* 563–582.

Hung, D. L., & Tzeng, O. J. L. (1981). Orthographic variations and visual information processing. *Psychological Bulletin, 90,* 377–414.

Hulme, C, & Joshi, R. M. (1998). *Reading and spelling: Development and disorders.* Mahwah, NJ: Erlbaum.

Jackson, M., & McClelland, J. L. (1979). Processing determinants of reading speed. *Journal of Experimental Psychology: General, 108,* 151–181.

Jorm, A. F. (1979). The cognitive and neurological basis of developmental dyslexia: A theoretical framework and review. *Cognition, 7,* 19–33.

Katz, R. B. (1986). Phonological deficiencies in children with reading disability: Evidence from an object naming task. *Cognition, 22,* 225–257.

Kleiman, G. (1975). Speech recoding in reading. *Journal of Verbal Learning and Verbal Behavior, 14,* 323–339.

Levy, B. A. (1977). Reading: Speech and meaning processes. *Journal of Verbal Learning and Verbal Behavior, 16,* 623–638.

Liberman, A. M. (1999). The reading researcher and the reading teacher need the right theory of speech. *Scientific Studies of Reading, 3,* 95–111.

Liberman, I. Y. (1982). A Language-oriented view of reading and its disabilities. In H. Mykelburst (Ed.), *Progress in learning disabilities* (Vol. 5, pp. 81–101). New York: Grune & Stratton.

Liberman, I. Y., Liberman, A. M., Mattingly, I. G., & Shankweiler, D. (1980). Orthography and the beginning reader. In J. Kavanaugh & R. Venezky (Eds.), *Orthography, reading and dyslexia* (pp. 137–154). Baltimore: University Park Press.

Liberman, I. Y., Shankweiler, D., Fischer, F. W., & Carter, B. (1974). Explicit syllable and phoneme segmentation in the young child. *Journal of Experimental Child Psychology, 18,* 201–212.

Lima, S. D. (1987). Morphological analysis in sentence reading. *Journal of Memory and Language, 26,* 84–99.

Mahony, D. L. (1994). Using sensitivity to word structure to explain variance in high school and college level reading ability. *Reading and Writing, 6,* 19–44.

Manis, F. R., McBride-Chang, C., Seidenberg, M. S., Keating, P., Doi, L. M., Munson, B., & Petersen, A. (1997). Are speech perception deficits associated with developmental dyslexia? *Journal of Experimental Child Psychology, 66,* 211–235.

Mann, V. A. (1984). Longitudinal prediction and prevention of early reading difficulty. *Annals of Dyslexia, 34,* 117–136.

Mann, V. A. (1993). Phoneme awareness and future reading ability. *Journal of Learning Disabilities, 26,* 259–269.

Mann, V. A., Cowin, E., & Schoenheimer, J. (1989). Phonological processing, language comprehension and reading ability. *Journal of Learning Disabilities, 22,* 76–89.

Mann, V. A., & Ditunno, P. (1990). Phonological deficiencies: effective predictors of future reading problems. In G. Pavlides (Ed.), *Dyslexia: Neuropsychological and learning perspectives* (pp. 105–131). New York: Wiley.

Mann, V. A., & Liberman, I. Y. (1984). Phonological awareness and verbal short-term memory: Can they presage early reading success? *Journal of Learning Disabilities, 17,* 592–598.

Mann, V. A., Liberman, I. Y., & Shankweiler, D. (1980). Children's memory for sentences and word strings in relation to reading ability. *Memory and Cognition, 8,* 329–335.

Mann, V. A., Shankweiler, D., & Smith, S. T. (1985). The association between comprehension of spoken sentences and early reading ability:

The role of phonetic representation. *Journal of Child Language, 11, 627–643.*

Mann, V. & Wimmer, H. (2002). Phoneme awareness and pathways to literacy: A comparison of German and American children. *Reading and Writing, 15, 653–682.*

Mattingly, I. G. (1972). Reading, the linguistic process, and linguistic awareness. In J. F. Kavanaugh & I. G. Mattingly (Eds.), *Language by ear and by eye: The relationship between speech and reading* (pp. 133–148). Cambridge, MA: MIT Press.

McBride-Chang, C. (1996). Models of speech perception and phonological processing in reading. *Child Development, 67, 1836–1856.*

Metsala, J. (1997). Spoken word recognition in reading disabled children. *Journal of Educational Psychology, 89*(1), 159–173.

Mody, M., Studdert-Kennedy, M., & Brady, S. (1997). speech perception deficits in poor readers: Auditory processing or phonological coding? *Journal of Experimental Child Psychology, 64, 199–231.*

Morais, J., Cary, L., Alegria, J., & Bertelson, P. (1979). Does awareness of speech as a sequence of phonemes arise spontaneously? *Cognition, 7, 323–331.*

Muter, V., Hulme, C., Snowling, M., & Taylor, S. (1997). Segmentation, not rhyming, predicts early progress in learning to read. *Journal of Experimental Child Psychology, 65, 370–396.*

Pennington, B. F., Van Orden, G., Kirson, D., & Haith, M. (1991). What is the causal relation between verbal STM problems and dyslexia? In S. A. Brady & D. P. Shankweiler (Eds.), *Phonological processing skills in literacy* (pp. 173–186). Hillsdale, NJ: Erlbaum.

Perfetti, C. A. (1985). *Reading skill.* Hillsdale, NJ: Erlbaum.

Rayner, K., & McConkie, G. W. (1976). What guides a readers' eye movements? *Vision Research, 16, 829–837.*

Rayner, K., Sereno, S. C., Lesch, M. F., & Pollatsek, A. (1995). Phonological codes are automatically activated during reading: Evidence from an eye movement priming paradigm. *Psychological Science, 6, 26–32.*

Read, C, Zhang, Y., Nie, H., & Ding, B. (1986). The ability to manipulate speech sounds depends on knowing alphabetic writing. *Cognition, 24, 31–44.*

Russell, G. (1982). Impairment of phonetic reading in dyslexia and its persistence beyond childhood—Research note. *Journal of Child Psychology and Child Psychiatry, 23, 459–475.*

Rutter, M. (1978). Prevalence and types of dyslexia. In A. L. Benton & D. Pearl (Eds.), *Dyslexia: An appraisal of current knowledge* (pp. 3–28) New York: Oxford University Press.

Shankweiler, D., & Liberman, I. Y. (1972). Misreading: A search for the causes. In J. F. Kavanaugh & I. G. Mattingly (Eds.), *Language by ear and by eye: The relationships between speech and reading* (pp. 293–318). Cambridge, MA: MIT Press.

Shankweiler, D., Liberman, I. Y., Mark, L. S., Fowler, C. A., & Fischer, F. W. (1979). The speech code and learning to read. *Journal of Experimental Psychology: Human Perception and Performance, 5, 531–545.*

Shankweiler, D., Crain, S., Katz, L., Fowler, A. E., Liberman, A. E., Brady, S. A., Thornton, R., Lundquist, E., Dreyer, L., Fletcher, J. M., Stuebing, K. K., Shaywitz, S. E., & Shaywitz, B. A. (1995). Cognitive profiles of reading-disabled children: Comparisons of language skills in phonology, morphology and syntax. *Psychological Science, 6, 149–156.*

Simpson, G. B., Lorsbach, T. C., & Whitehouse, D. (1983). Encoding and contextual components of word recognition in good and poor readers. *Journal of Experimental Child Psychology, 35, 161–171.*

Singson, M., Mahony, D., & Mann, V. (2000). The relation between reading ability and morphological skills: Evidence from derivational suffixes. *Reading and Writing, 12, 219–252.*

Slowiaczek, M. L., & Clifton, C. (1980). Subvocalization and reading for meaning. *Journal of Verbal Learning and Verbal Behavior, 19, 573–582.*

Smith, S. T., Macaruso, P., Shankweiler, D., & Crain, S. (1989). Syntactic comprehension in young poor readers. *Applied Psycholinguistics, 10, 429–454.*

Smith, S. T., Mann, V. A., & Shankweiler, D. (1986). Spoken sentence comprehension by good and poor readers: A study with the token test. *Cortex, 22, 627–632.*

Stanovich, K. (1982). Individual differences in the cognitive processes of reading: II. Text-level processes. *Journal of Learning Disabilities, 15, 549–554.*

Stanovich, K. (1988). Explaining the differences between the dyslexic and the garden-variety poor reader: The phonological-core variable difference model. *Journal of Learning Disabilities, 21, 590–604.*

Stanovich, K. E., & Beck, I. (2000). *Progress in understanding reading.* New York: Guilford Press.

Stanovich, K. E., Cunningham, A. E., & Cramer, B. B. (1984). Assessing phonological awareness in kindergarten children: Issues of task comparability. *Journal of Experimental Child Psychology, 38, 175–190.*

Stanovich, K. E., Cunningham, A. E., & Feeman, D. J. (1984). Intelligence, cognitive skills and early reading progress. *Reading Research Quarterly, 19, 278–303.*

Stanovich, K. E., Nathan, R. G., & Zolman, J. E. (1988). The developmental lag hypothesis in reading: Longitudinal and matched reading-level comparisons. *Child Development, 59, 71–86.*

Taft, M., & Forster, K. I. (1975). Lexical storage and retrieval of prefixed words. *Journal of Verbal Learning and Verbal Behavior, 14, 638–647.*

Taft, M. (1984). Evidence for an abstract lexical representation of word structure. *Memory and Cognition, 12, 264–269.*

Torgesen, J. K., & Davis, C. (1996). Individual difference variables that predict response to training in phonological awareness, *Journal of Experimental child Psychology, 63,* 1–21.

Tyler, A., & Nagy, W. (1990). Use of derivational morphology during reading. (1990). *Cognition, 36,* 17–34.

Tzeng, O. J. L., Hung, D. L., & Wang, W. (1977). Speech recoding in reading Chinese characters. *Journal of Experimental Psychology: Human Learning and Memory, 3,* 621–630.

van Orden, G. C. (1987). A rows is a rose: Spelling, sound, and reading. *Memory and Cognition, 15,* 181–198.

Walley, A. C. (1993). The role of vocabulary development in children's spoken word recognition and segmentation ability. *Developmental Review, 13,* 286–350.

Wagner, R. K., & Torgesen, J. K. (1987). The nature of phonological processing and its causal role in the acquisition of reading skills. *Psychological Bulletin, 101,* 192–212.

Wagner, R. K., Torgesen, J. K., Rashotte, C. A., Hecht, S. A., Barker, T. A., Burgess, S. R., Donahue, J., & Garon, T. (1997). Changing relations between phonological processing abilities and word-level reading as children develop from beginning to skilled readers: A 5-year longitudinal study. *Developmental Psychology, 33,* 468–479.

Watt, W. C. (1989). Getting writing right. *Semiotica, 75,* 279–315.

Wolf, M. (1984). Naming, reading and the dyslexias: A longitudinal overview. *Annals of Dyslexia, 34,* 87–115.

Wolf, M., & Bowers, P. G. (1999). The double-deficit hypothesis for the developmental dyslexia. *Journal of Educational Psychology, 91,* 415–438.

Wolf, M., Bowers, P. G., & Biddle, K. (2000). Naming-speed processes, timing, and reading: A conceptual review. *Journal of Learning Disabilities, 33,* 387–407.

Wolf, M., & Goodglass, H. (1986). Dyslexia, dysnomia and lexical retrieval: A longitudinal investigation. *Brain and Language, 28,* 159–168.

Yopp, H. K. (1988). The validity and reliability of phonemic awareness tests. *Reading Research Quarterly, 23,* 159–177.

14

Self-Concept and Students with Learning Disabilities

Batya Elbaum
Sharon Vaughn

A man cannot be comfortable without his own approval.
—Twain (1929, p. 17)

In the educational, psychological, and popular literature, self-concept has long been considered important both in and of itself and as a variable that mediates other significant outcomes, such as academic achievement (Carlock, 1999; Chapman, 1988; Cronin, 1994; Haager & Vaughn, 1997; Marsh & Yeung, 1997a; Purkey & Novak, 1996). Individuals who have a positive sense of self-worth tend to be happier than others (Swann, 1996) and to grapple more successfully with failure experiences and other adverse circumstances (Carlock, 1999). Once an individual develops negative self-perceptions, these perceptions can be extremely resistant to change (Swann, 1996), even when the individual achieves success (Achenbach & Zigler, 1963).

Self-concept has particular relevance to students with learning disabilities (LD). Learning disabilities have been consistently linked to poor self-concept (De Francesco & Taylor, 1985; Kloomok & Cosden, 1994; Vaughn & Elbaum, 1999). Children's experiences in school, particularly in the early grades, can have a powerful influence on their self-perceptions. Difficulties in reading, writing, and spelling make students with LD more vulnerable to failure experiences, which may lower self-esteem. These academic difficulties are often coupled with difficulties in the social domain. The effect of these academic and social challenges on the self-concept of students with LD can range in severity from minimal (or none) to quite pronounced. Clinical experience with students with LD indicates that "children with learning disorders appear to suffer psychologically more than their peers who do not have learning disorders. Their psychological suffering cannot be measured through manifest symptoms alone, as many do not display such symptoms" (Palombo, 2001, p. 3). Though few students with LD may require clinical treatment for problems relating to self-concept, many are affected to some degree by the negative perceptions they hold of themselves as readers, as students, or as members of their social group.

In this chapter, we first provide a brief overview of self-concept as it relates to students with LD. In doing so, we emphasize the dimensions of self-concept that are especially relevant to students with LD: academic self-concept, social self-concept, and global self-worth. We then describe the findings and implications of our own research in the area of self-concept. This research has focused on the impact of specific school factors—identification, educational placement, and school-based interventions—on the self-concept of students with LD.

Overview

Current conceptualizations of self-concept place it in the area of social cognition, which deals with the mental representations and processes that underlie self-awareness, perspective taking, and the understanding of social relations. Social cognition has been an area of serious psychological investigation since the 1960s (Lefrancois, 1990), though the importance of a positive evaluation of oneself has been noted by psychologists and philosophers for much longer than that (for a history of the study of self-concept, see Harter, 1996). Within the social cognitive perspective, self-concept was defined early as "the person known to himself, particularly the stable, important, and typical aspects of himself as he perceives them" (Gordon & Combs, 1958, p. 433).

Though the construction of self involves descriptive and narrative aspects (Palombo, 2001), it is usually the evaluative aspects that are at issue in considerations of psychological adjustment. The term "self-esteem" captures one's overall sense of self-worth; it is, in the words of Carlock (1999), "the way you feel about yourself" (p. 3). For the purpose of this discussion, we consider the term "self-concept" to be synonymous with "self-perception" and "self-esteem."

Self-concept is now established as a multidimensional construct, based on the evidence that individuals view themselves differently across different domains of functioning (Harter, 1985; Marsh, 1989; Shavelson, Hubner, & Stanton, 1976). That is, individuals may perceive that they are poor performers in some domains, are average in others, and excel in yet others. Harter (1985), for example, identified eight domains of self-perception: general cognitive competence, peer likeability, behavioral conduct, physical appearance, romantic appeal, close friendship, athletic competence, and job competence. Marsh (1988) further divided the general domain of academic competence into reading, mathematics, and general school competence.

The development of multidimensional models has enabled researchers investigating students with LD to ask important questions beyond whether students with LD have lower self-concept than do students without LD. These questions include the following: In which domains do students with LD have self-perceptions that differ from those of their peers without disabilities? How do self-perceptions in specific domains relate to perceptions of general self-worth? In the next sections, we briefly review what is known about academic, social, and global self-concept for students with and without LD.

Academic Self-Concept

A study by Caslyn and Kenny (1977) that included over 500 adolescents revealed that students' academic achievement was significantly associated with their self-concept. On the one hand, students with lower academic achievement subsequently exhibited lower self-concepts than did students with higher academic achievement, suggesting that low achievement may be one of the causes of low self-evaluations of competence. At the same time, low self-esteem itself may lead to lowered expectations for future success (Chapman & Boersma, 1979) and diminished motivation for academic tasks (McInerney, Roche, McInerney, & Marsh, 1997). For high school students, self-concept has also been demonstrated to be related to students' subsequent choices of coursework (Marsh & Yeung, 1997b) and their career interests (McInerney et al., 1997).

Because self-evaluations are based on comparisons we make between our own competencies and those of people around us, an individual's self-concept may also depend on the reference group used as a comparison group. (A complementary perspective is that individuals compare their own competencies across different domains [Marsh, 1990a].) For example, we perceive ourselves more favorably when we compare ourselves to others whose performance or physical features are less positive than ours. When students with LD compare themselves to other students with LD, their self-concept may be different than if they compare themselves to students without LD.

This point is supported by studies that reveal that students with LD demonstrated lower self-concepts when average- or high-achieving peers were used as reference groups but not when low-achieving peers were used as the reference group (Haager & Vaughn, 1995; Vaughn, Haager, Hogan, & Kouzekanani, 1992). Also, because students with LD often receive most of their education in the general education classroom, they are highly aware of how their academic performance compares with that of their classmates (e.g., Cooley & Ayers, 1988; Hiebert, Wong, & Hunter, 1982; Kistner, Haskett, White, & Robbins, 1987; Montgomery, 1994). When students consistently compare themselves to others unfavorably, their self-concept is negatively affected.

Renick and Harter (1989) found that perceptions of academic competence for students with LD who were placed in regular classrooms were more highly correlated with general self-worth than they were with perceptions of either social acceptance or athletic competence. According to Byrne (1996), these results suggest that for children with LD at least, perceptions of how well they perform academically may have an overriding effect on the extent to which they like themselves as persons in general.

In a meta-analysis of studies comparing the self-reports of children and adolescents with LD to those of their peers without LD (Prout, Marcal, & Marcal, 1992), the academic self-concept of students with LD was .71 of a standard deviation below that of their peers without disabilities. According to Hagborg (1996), 70% of students with LD demonstrated significantly lower academic self-concepts when compared with peers without LD. In a meta-analysis by Chapman (1988), the average difference between students with and without LD, with regard to academic self-concept, was .81 of a standard deviation, considered quite a large effect.

The lower self-concept of some students with LD in the academic area is of significant concern in that academic self-concept may mediate students' accomplishments related to important educational goals. Marsh and Yeung (1997b) reported that students with higher self-concepts in particular academic areas were more likely to pursue subsequent study in these areas. This finding suggests that having a strong academic self-concept may be related to the interest of students with LD in pursuing challenging coursework and participating more fully in the general education curriculum.

Social Self-Concept

One view of the origins and functioning of self-concept is based on the idea that human beings have a strong drive to maintain significant interpersonal relationships (Leary, 1999). According to this view, self-concept evolved as a mechanism that enables individuals to monitor the degree to which they are valued and accepted by others. Peer acceptance is an important index of social acceptance, and low perceived peer acceptance is often associated with low self-esteem. A positive social self-concept is associated with peer acceptance, self-confidence, effective coping, and psychosocial well-being (Bednar, Wells, & Peterson, 1989; Harter, 1993; Parker & Asher, 1987). Students with positive social self-concepts perceive that others like to be around them and want to have them as friends. In addition, they are able to make and maintain friendships without significant difficulties.

Students who lack a positive social self-concept are vulnerable to a host of emotional, social, and learning problems (Brendtro, Brokenleg, & Van Bockern, 1990), including long-term unhappiness (Bednar et al., 1989; Harter, 1993) and low peer acceptance (Li, 1985; Vaughn, McIntosh, & Spencer-Rowe, 1991). One consistent finding is the correlation between low self-concept or self-perception of acceptance and depression (Leahy, 1985; Wiest, Wong, & Kreil, 1998). Research conducted by Leahy (1985) suggests that students with low self-concept are more likely to experience depression.

As early as kindergarten, same-grade classmates perceive students later identified as having LD as low on social acceptance (Vaughn, Hogan, Kouzekanani, & Shapiro, 1990), and this low peer acceptance remains relatively stable over time (Vaughn & Haager, 1994). Heath and Wiener (1996) reported that students with LD who scored high on ratings of depression also rated themselves poorly on self-perceptions of social acceptance and that students with LD demonstrated higher levels of depression than did students without LD. The long-term impact of peer rejection (Alexander & Entwisle, 1988; Parker & Asher, 1987) and the contribution of peer rejection to depression (Heath & Wiener, 1996) may operate in part through links to poor social self-concept.

There is diverging evidence regarding the social self-concept of students with LD. Some studies have reported no difference in the social self-concept of students with and without LD (Berndt & Burgy, 1996; Clever, Bear, & Juvonen, 1992; Durrant, Cunningham, & Voelker, 1990; Hagborg, 1999), whereas others indicate that students with LD demonstrated lower social self-concept (Hosley, Hopper, & Gruber, 1998). A study of students with LD in the fourth and fifth grades indicated that participants demonstrated lower self-perceptions of social acceptance and global self-concept when compared to average-achieving students (La Greca & Stone, 1990). In contrast, second-, third-, and fourth-grade students with LD studied by Bursuck (1989) did not experience lowered self-concept. In a study of more than 100 students with LD, 70 students with behavior disorders (BD), and 200 average achievers in grades 9–12 (Harter, Whitesell, & Junkin, 1998), the students with LD and BD both differed from the average achievers with respect to their social self-perceptions, but only the students with BD had significantly lower self-perceptions of conduct. Both groups with disabilities exhibited lower scores on global self-worth than did average achievers without disabilities. In a study by Hagborg (1998), a smaller sample of high school students with LD did not differ from their peers without LD on this dimension.

The link between poor academic performance and low social self-concept is not clear. There is some evidence for a relation between students' achievement and their social status (Wentzel & Erdley, 1993). However, in the study by La Greca and Stone (1990), low-achieving students who were not identified as having LD perceived their social acceptance more positively than did students with LD. Thus, the low social acceptance and low social self-concept of some students with LD may be related to causes other than low academic achievement—for example, poor social skills or behavioral difficulties, which themselves may be a response to the learning disability (Palombo, 2001).

Global Self-Concept

Overall, students with LD display lower perceptions of self-worth than do average achieving students without disabilities (Vaughn & Elbaum, 1999). In a meta-analysis of studies comparing the self-reports of children and adolescents with LD to those of their peers without LD (Prout et al., 1992), students with LD demonstrated a general self-concept that was .43 of a standard deviation below that of their peers. However, this difference is unlikely to be due solely to the academic difficulties of students with LD. In fact, there is evidence that students' global self-worth is more influenced by nonacademic factors such as perceived physical appearance and social acceptance than it is by academic achievement (Cosden, Elliott, Noble, & Kelemen, 1999). Thus, whereas students with LD may be aware of their low academic performance (Grolnick & Ryan, 1990), a poor self-evaluation of academic performance may not by itself lead to a diminished sense of self-worth.

We now turn to a description of research that we have conducted, over the past decade, on self-concept and students with LD. The main goal of our research program has been to investigate the extent to which school factors, such as identification with a learning disability and educational placement, affect the self-concept of students with LD. Another important goal has been to investigate the extent to which school-based interventions can ameliorate the self-concept of students with LD.

Identification

Some researchers and advocates have argued that being identified as having a disability is itself detrimental to a student's self-concept (Brophy & Good, 1970; Good, 1982). Vaughn and colleagues (1992) followed students from kindergarten through fourth grade, assessing self-concept each year. Students identified as students with LD at the end of second grade did not differ from students not so identified with regard to self-concept. Other research that compared adults who had or had not received special education services found no difference in self-concept (Lewandowki & Arcangelo, 1994)

Whereas the popular perception is that being labeled as having a learning disability may lead to feelings of shame or humiliation, and hence to low self-concept, there is as yet no solid empirical evidence that identification with a learning disability results in a diminished sense of self-worth. Indeed, for some children, the knowledge that their reading or other academic difficulties are related to a disabling condition, and not to low intelligence or lack of effort, may help sustain positive perceptions of general intellectual competence and self-worth.

Placement

Over the past 25 years, there has been considerable debate surrounding the placement of students with LD in general education classrooms for most, or all, of their instruction. One of the arguments for general education placement for all of a student's instruction has been that students with LD placed in regular classrooms fare better, in terms of social acceptance, friendship relations, and self-concept, than students with LD educated in more segregated settings (Vaughn, Elbaum, & Boardman, 2001). Predictions based on social comparison theory would suggest that students with LD have higher self-concept in special education settings (resource rooms and self-contained classrooms), where all students experience similar academic challenges. However, empirical studies have shown mixed results.

To better understand the contrasting empirical findings, Elbaum (2002) conducted a meta-analysis of studies that compared the self-concept of groups of students with LD in more and less restrictive settings. A total of 38 studies published between 1975 and 1999 were located, yielding 65 placement comparisons. Each comparison was coded into one of five placement comparison categories. These categories, and the number of comparisons coded into each, were regular class versus resource room (16); regular class versus self-contained classroom (18); resource room versus self-contained classroom (26); self-contained classroom versus special school (3); and regular class versus special school (2).

The results of the meta-analysis indicated that there was no reliable association between self-concept and educational placement for any of the major comparison categories. The one exception, represented by three samples of students from a single study (Butler & Marinov-Glassman, 1994), was that students with LD who received instruction in self-contained classrooms in regular schools exhibited lower self-concept compared to students attending special schools. The findings of the meta-analysis suggest that educational placement is not the overriding determinant of self-concept students with LD. Rather, other factors operating within each context—for example, individual teachers' understanding and acceptance of students with disabilities—may have greater influence on the way students with LD feel about themselves in specific classroom settings. For example, Chapman (1988) reported a relation between children's academic self-concepts and teachers' feedback and level of academic achievement.

Social support also influences the social self-concept of students with LD. Marsh (1990b) notes that self-perceptions "are formed through experience with and interpretations of one's environment. They are especially influenced by evaluations by significant others, reinforcement, and attributions for one's own behavior" (p. 27). Forman (1988) reported that students with LD who had higher levels of perceived social support—particularly support from classmates—demonstrated higher self-concept regardless of school placement (resource room or self-contained special education setting).

School-Based Interventions

In light of the research indicating the many adverse concomitants and consequences of negative self-concept, considerable work has been focused on developing interventions to improve the self-concept of students with LD. Elbaum and Vaughn (2001) used meta-analysis to determine the overall effectiveness of interventions on the self-concept of students with LD. Sixty-four studies were located that met the following criteria: (1) the majority of the participants were students with LD, (2) a measure of self-concept was used as one of the outcome measures, (3) the intervention took place in a school setting, (4) the study included both a treatment and a comparison group, (5) the study was published or available between 1975 and 1997, and (6) sufficient data were provided to calculate an effect size.

Types of Interventions

Most, but not all, of the interventions included in the meta-analysis were designed for the primary purpose of enhancing the self-concept of students with LD. Others were designed primarily to accomplish another goal, such as improved academic skills or physical abilities; however, the researchers hypothesized that students participating in the intervention would also evidence higher self-concept than control students. Thus, the interventions ranged from what would be considered traditional counseling groups to cooperative learning curricula, fitness programs, and so on. For purposes of analysis, we classified the interventions into six general categories based on the focus of the intervention. The categories were counseling (33 studies), academic (18 studies), physical (5 studies), reinforcement (5 studies), sensory/perceptual (2 studies), and "other" (4 studies). The "other" category consisted of interventions using music, arts and crafts, education plans provided to the teacher, and a home-to-school facilitator.

Calculation of Effect Sizes

Effect sizes were calculated as the mean of the treatment group posttest score minus the mean of the comparison group posttest score divided by the pooled standard deviation. When means and standard deviations were not available, effect sizes were estimated from t, F, or p values. When statistical tests were reported as nonsignificant and no

other data were provided, we assumed an effect size of 0.

Findings

Aggregated across all categories of intervention, the mean intervention effect was quite modest, $d = 0.19$ (where d symbolizes the mean weighted effected size, interpreted in standard deviation units [Cooper, 1998]). When outcomes of interventions across all grade levels were aggregated, intervention type (e.g., counseling, academic, physical) was not reliably associated with intervention effect sizes. The mean weighted effect sizes for different categories of intervention ranged from $d = 0.12$ to $d = 0.31$.

However, differences in outcomes were found to be reliably associated with students' grade level. The mean weighted effect size for adolescents ($d = 0.42$) was significantly higher than that for elementary ($d = 0.12$) and high school students ($d = 0.17$). Within grade groupings, different types of interventions were found to be most effective. For elementary students, only academic interventions yielded effect sizes that were reliably different from 0 ($d = 0.17$); for middle and high school students, this was true only of counseling interventions ($d = 0.61$ and $d = 0.32$, respectively)

Based on the earlier review of the academic and social self-concept of students with LD, we were interested in the extent to which interventions had a differential impact on the academic and social domains of self-concept. Interventions had the greatest impact on academic self-concept ($d = 0.28$), followed by social self-concept ($d = 0.18$) and general self-concept ($d = 0.15$).

Analyses also revealed that effect sizes were not influenced by the self-concept measure used. The two most frequently used measures of self-concept, the Piers–Harris Children's Self-Concept Scale (PHC-SCS; Piers, 1984) and the Self-Esteem Inventory (SEI; Coopersmith, 1986) yielded almost identical effect sizes, $d = 0.21$ and $d = 0.22$, respectively.

In a subsequent study, Elbaum and Vaughn (in press) used a subset of the intervention studies from the previously described meta-analysis to investigate whether intervention effectiveness was associated with the level of self-concept that students demonstrated prior to intervention. The subset of studies consisted of those that used the PHCSCS and provided both pre- and postintervention scores for the intervention group. The 20 groups of students with LD for whom these data were available were divided into those whose self-concept scores, prior to intervention, were high (at or above the 75th percentile for this sample), low (at or below the 25th percentile), and midlevel (the middle 50%). Comparing the average scores for these groups to the mean normative score reported for the PHCSCS ($M = 51.84$; Piers, 1984), the high self-concept groups had an average score 0.45 standard deviations above the normative mean (57.74), the middle groups had an average score almost exactly identical to the normative mean (51.78), and the low groups had an average score approximately 1.3 standard deviations below the mean (34.36). When outcomes for these groups were compared meta-analytically, there was a statistically reliable association between self-concept level prior to intervention and intervention effect size. Groups of students with high self-concept prior to intervention gained an average of 14 points ($d = 1.22$); students with midlevel self-concept gained an average of 4 points ($d = 0.29$); and groups of students with low self-concept prior to intervention gained an average of 3 points ($d = 0.23$). An analysis of residualized gain scores suggested that the observed results could not be completely explained as an artifact of regression to the mean.

Taken together, the analyses of intervention outcomes suggest that students with LD who have truly low self-concept can benefit considerably from appropriate interventions. For these students, the most effective interventions, as delineated earlier, may differ according to students' age. The fact that the most effective interventions for younger students appear to be academic interventions suggests that improving these students' academic skills can have a collateral effect on their self-perceptions. Increased self-efficacy in the academic domain may confer a sense of empowerment that results in more positive self-evaluations.

For older students, the theory proposed by Leary (1999) may be especially relevant. In this view, the explanation for the beneficial effects of programs that enhance self-esteem is that these interventions "change people's perceptions of the degree to which they are socially valued individuals. Self-esteem programs always include features that would be expected to increase real or perceived social acceptance, for example, these programs include components aimed at enhancing social skills and interpersonal problem solving, improving physical appearance, and increasing self-control" (Leary, 1999, p. 35). This view accords with literature on the social functioning of students with LD which suggests that many students with LD demonstrate overall low social skills (e.g., Foss, 1991; Jarvis & Justin, 1992; Kavale & Forness, 1996; Merrell, 1991).

At the same time, the findings suggest that students with LD who have average-to-high levels of self-concept do not benefit from efforts to further enhance their self-esteem. Indeed, including such students in interventions that do not have an academic component, that focus exclusively on self-concept, and that use time during which students would otherwise be engaged in instructional activities, may actually be to their detriment in the long run.

Summary of Findings on the Self-Concept of Students with LD

Students with LD often demonstrate lower academic self-concept than do normally achieving students without disabilities, and sometimes demonstrate lower self-concepts in the social domain. In addition, students with LD may demonstrate low perceptions of general self-worth. We do not yet have a clear understanding of why some students with lower academic self-concept also have lower general self-perceptions, whereas others do not. It may be that a combination of low self-evaluations across multiple domains—academic, social, and physical, for example—is a better predictor of low self-worth than poor academic self-concept alone.

It is equally important to note that many students with LD have self-concept scores that are on par with those of students without disabilities (or, in some cases, even higher; cf. Bear & Minke, 1996; Clever et al., 1992; Kistner et al., 1987; Kistner & Osborne, 1987). Moreover, even when the self-concept scores of students with LD are below those of students without disabilities, they may still be within the normal range. Scores on measures of general self-worth which are substantially below those of typical students may indicate problems that require specialized attention. Students with LD who experience low perceptions of self-worth may or may not be those who are experiencing the greatest academic difficulties. Only by assessing students' self-perceptions in different domains is it possible to reach a more complete understanding of the source of overall low self-concept and to provide appropriate interventions.

Issues Related to the Measurement of Self-Concept

Research on the self-concept of students with LD, like other self-concept research conducted since the 1970s, has benefited from the availability of self-report questionnaires either designed from the outset (e.g., Bracken, 1992; Marsh, 1988, 1990b) or revised (e.g., Piers, 1984) to reflect evolving theory regarding the multidimensional nature of self-concept. However, as documented in considerable detail by Keith and Bracken (1996), many widely used instruments lack a compelling theoretical foundation and/or evidence of strong technical adequacy. For example, the PHCSCS, which was used more frequently than any other measurement instrument in the intervention studies we synthesized, was originally developed as a unidimensional measure of self-concept, albeit with content drawn from different domains. According to Keith and Bracken, the items were subsequently assigned to one or more cluster scales based on factor analysis; however, the cluster items are not mutually exclusive (i.e., some items loaded on two or more factors), hence the interpretation of subscales as representing discrete domains is somewhat hazardous. Moreover, whereas the internal consistency of the PHCSCS total scale is adequate (.88 to .93 for girls and boys in grades 6 and 10), the internal consistency of the subscales is much lower (.73–.81). This means that the subscales are much less reliable than the measure as a whole.

Hence, considerable caution must be used when comparing subscale scores of different groups of students, or when comparing the same students' scores on different subscales.

Another concern has to do with the accuracy of measuring change in self-concept over time. Again using the PHCSCS as an example, test–retest reliabilities for the total scale are in the .86–.96 range for intervals of 3–4 weeks, but in the .42–.51 range for intervals of 8–12 months; the median reported test–retest reliability is .725. For the studies we synthesized, the median duration of self-concept interventions was 10 weeks; test–retest reliability of the PHCSCS over this interval is likely to be considerably lower than the recommended level of .9. This is problematic from an analytic standpoint, in that the lower the reliability of the measurement instrument, the greater the amount of error, and, in pre–post designs, the greater the likelihood of artifacts due to regression to the mean (Campbell & Kenny, 1999). The problems illustrated here are not unique to the PHCSCS; similar concerns could be adduced with regard to many other commonly used self-concept instruments.

A third issue with regard to the measurement of self-concept in students with LD has to do with whether measures normed on samples of students without disabilities function similarly for students with LD. Only by comparing the performance of students with and without LD on the same instrument is it possible to verify whether students from these two populations respond similarly to item content and whether the subscales operate similarly for both populations. However, most instrument developers did not include students with LD in their original norming samples. The only currently available instrument that was specifically designed to assess both students with LD and students without disabilities is the Self-Perception Profile for Learning Disabled Students (SPPLD; Renick & Harter, 1988). According to Keith and Bracken (1996), the authors of the SPPLD developed its five academic subscales based on the finding that students with LD responded differentially to items that had all been part of a single academic subscale in an earlier instrument. That is, the newer instrument was developed based on the evidence suggesting that compared to students without LD, students with LD had more strongly differentiated perceptions of their competence in different academic domains. This fits with the typical profile of students with LD as students with severe deficits in reading (and sometimes also in mathematics) but not in other areas of the curriculum insofar as these are not reading dependent.

More recently developed measures of self-concept appear to address at least some of these concerns. For example, instruments developed by Marsh (1988, 1990b) and Bracken (1992) provide evidence of high reliability as well as construct and concurrent validity. Marsh's instruments may prove to be particularly useful in investigations involving students with LD in that they assess self-perceptions in three separate academic domains—Reading, Mathematics, and General School—and thus allow for a more nuanced understanding of students' academic self-concepts.

Implications for Future Research and Intervention

The first implication we draw for future research on the self-concept of students with LD is that researchers need to be extremely mindful of the issues discussed earlier surrounding the measurement of self-concept. In addition, given that self-concept is almost always assessed by means of written self-report instruments, consideration needs to be given to the reading level of the instrument and how it is administered. Reading the items aloud may be necessary to ensure adequate comprehension by all students.

Second, careful longitudinal studies are needed to investigate the extent to which students' self-concept may change in relation to their academic progress and to changes in their educational context (e.g., transitions between schools and changes in placement). In some developmental stages, particularly early adolescence, students' self-perceptions may range from high to low in the same day, depending on the valence of the day's everyday events—interactions with individual friends and family members,

grades received on school assignments, or being included or not included in the self-constituting clusters that characterize the social networks of students in schools (Vaughn et al., 2001).

Third, intervention researchers should gather and report much more comprehensive data on the students with LD who participate in intervention studies. In particular, it would be extremely useful to know students' individual placement histories and current level of academic performance (e.g., grade level in reading), as well as contextual factors such as the range of service delivery options used at the school(s). As well, where older children are concerned, it would be illuminating to obtain students' own perceptions of the usefulness of self-concept interventions in which they have participated.

Fourth, when selecting students with LD for an intervention aimed at improving their self-concept, it is essential to determine first whether they are likely to benefit from such intervention. Palombo (2001) cautions that with regard to problems of the self experienced by students with LD, there is no clear correlation between diagnosis and treatability. That is, there is more to the determination of likely benefit than the severity of the unease experienced by the child. In discussing the advisability of individual therapy for self-esteem problems, Palombo recommends consideration of the "psychological mindedness" of the child, that is, the ability of the child to think about his or her feelings and the relation between feelings, attitudes, and behaviors. This advice would appear to be equally relevant to school-based interventions based on group therapy models. Moreover, educators should realize that for some students, participating in a group that deals explicitly with painful personal issues may not be in the student's best interest. In addition, Baumeister, Smart, and Boden (1996) caution that when self-appraisals are overly (unrealistically) inflated, the result may be increased vulnerability to ego threats and increased evaluative dependency on others. Neither of these outcomes would be desirable for any students, especially students with persistent learning difficulties.

Finally, Ellis (1998) argues that an important means for contributing to the self-concepts of adolescents with LD is to provide them opportunities to control their destinies and positively influence others. He suggests that adolescents with LD require educational environments that challenge them and provide personally meaningful work. Furthermore, teachers can have a significant impact on students by providing positive feedback (Bear, Minke, Griffin, & Deemer, 1998). Appropriate, positive feedback is an easily administered intervention that classroom observations reveal is used infrequently by teachers (McIntosh, Vaughn, Schumm, Haager, & Lee, 1993).

Conclusion

According to Palombo (2001), improvements in the feelings students with LD have about themselves "occur when they can function adequately academically, have experienced real life successes, and have developed a good understanding of the reading disability. Children who reach this point can go on to be their own advocates as they progress within the educational system" (p. 134). Educators' main responsibility is to ensure that students with LD accomplish the first of these goals, that is, that they develop the ability to function adequately in school. The judicious use of adjunct services, including school-based interventions for some students, may further assist students with LD to develop and maintain the positive self-perceptions that enable them to be their own best advocates.

References

Achenbach, T., & Zigler, E. (1963). Social competence and self-image disparity in psychiatric and nonpsychiatric patients. *Journal of Abnormal and Social Psychology, 67,* 197–205.

Alexander, K. L., & Entwisle, D. R. (1988). Achievement in the first 2 years of school: Patterns and processes. *Monographs of the Society for the Research in Child Development, 53*(2), 157.

Baumeister, R. F., Smart, L., & Boden, J. M. (1996). Relation of threatened egotism to violence and aggression: The dark side of high self-esteem. *Psychological Review, 103*(1), 5–33.

Bear, G. G., & Minke, K. M. (1996). Positive bias in maintenance of self-worth among children with LD. *Learning Disability Quarterly, 19,* 23–32.

Bear, G. G., Minke, K. M., Griffin, S. M., & Deemer, S. A. (1998). Achievement-related perceptions of children with learning disabilities and normal achievement: Group and developmental differences. *Journal of Learning Disabilities, 31*(1), 91–104.

Bednar, R. L., Wells, M. G., & Peterson, S. R. (1989). *Self-esteem: Paradoxes and innovations in clinical theory and practice.* Washington, DC: American Psychological Association.

Berndt, T. J., & Burgy, L. (1996). Social self-concept. In B. A. Bracken (Ed.), *Handbook of self-concept* (pp. 171–209). New York: Wiley.

Bracken, B. A. (1992). *Multidimensional Self Concept Scale.* Austin, TX: Pro-Ed.

Brendtro, L. K., Brokenleg, M., & Van Bockern, S. (1990). *Reclaiming youth at risk: Our hope for the future.* Bloomington, IN: National Educational Service.

Brophy, J., & Good, T. L. (1970). Teachers' communication of differential expectations for children's classroom performance: Some behavioral data. *Journal of Educational Psychology, 20,* 941–952.

Bursuck, W. (1989). A comparison of students with learning disabilities to low achieving and high achieving students on three dimensions of social acceptance. *Journal of Learning Disabilities, 22*(3), 188–194.

Butler, R., & Marinov-Glassman, D. (1994). The effects of educational placement and grade level on the self-perceptions of low achievers and students with learning disabilities. *Journal of Learning Disabilities, 27,* 325–334.

Byrne, B. M. (1996). Academic self-concept: Its structure, measurement, and relation to academic achievement. In B. A. Bracken (Ed.), *Handbook of self-concept* (pp. 287–316). New York: Wiley.

Campbell, D. T., & Kenny, D. A. (1999). *A primer on regression artifacts.* New York: Guilford Press.

Carlock, C. J. (Ed.). (1999). *Enhancing self-esteem* (3rd ed.). Philadelphia: Taylor & Francis.

Caslyn, R. J., & Kenny, D. A. (1977). Self-concept of ability and perceived evaluation of others: Cause or effect of academic achievement. *Journal of Educational Psychology, 69*(2), 136–145.

Chapman, J. W. (1988). Learning disabled children's self-concepts. *Review of Educational Research, 58*(3), 347–371.

Chapman, J. W., & Boersma, F. J. (1979, April). *Self-perceptions of ability, expectations and locus of control in elementary learning disabled children.* Paper presented at the annual meeting of the American Educational Research Association. (ERIC Document Reproduction Service No. ED 169 738)

Clever, A., Bear, G. G., & Juvonen, J. (1992). Discrepancies between competence and importance in self-perceptions of children in integrated classrooms. *Journal of Special Education, 26,* 125–138.

Cooley, E. J., & Ayers, R. R. (1988). Self-concept

and success-failure attributions of nonhandicapped students and students with learning disabilities. *Journal of Learning Disabilities, 21*(3), 174–178.

Cooper, H. (1998). *Synthesizing research* (3rd ed.). Thousand Oaks, CA: Sage.

Coopersmith, S. A. (1986). *Self-esteem inventories.* Palo Alto, CA: Consulting Psychologists Press.

Cosden, M., Elliott, K., Noble, S., & Kelemen, E. (1999). Self-understanding and self-esteem in children with learning disabilities. *Learning Disability Quarterly, 22*(4), 279–290.

Cronin, E. M. (1994). *Helping your dyslexic child: A guide to improving your child's reading, writing, spelling, comprehension, and self-esteem.* Roseville, CA: Prima.

De Francesco, J. J., & Taylor, J. (1985). Dimensions of self-concept in primary and middle school learning disabled and nondisabled students. *Child Study Journal, 15,* 99–105.

Durant, J. E., Cunningham, C. E., & Voelker, S. (1990). Academic, social and general self-concepts of behavioral subgroups of learning disabled children. *Journal of Educational Psychology, 82,* 657–663.

Elbaum, B. (2002). The self-concept of students with learning disabilities: A meta-analysis of comparisons across different placements. *Learning Disabilities Research & Practice, 17*(4), 216–226.

Elbaum, B., & Vaughn, S. (2001). School-based interventions to enhance the self-concept of students with learning disabilities: A meta-analysis. *Elementary School Journal, 101*(3), 303–329.

Elbaum, B., & Vaughn, S. (in press). For which students with learning disabilities are self-concept interventions effective? *Journal of Learning Disabilities.*

Ellis, E. S. (1998). Watering up the curriculum for adolescents with learning disabilities—Part 2. *Remedial and Special Education, 19*(2), 91–105.

Forman, E. A. (1988). The effects of social support and school placement on the self-concept of LD students. *Learning Disability Quarterly, 11,* 115–124.

Foss, J. M. (1991). Nonverbal learning disabilities and remedial interventions. *Annals of Dyslexia, 41,* 128–140.

Good, T. L. (1982). How teachers' expectations affect results. *American Education, 18*(10), 25–32.

Gordon, I. J., & Combs, A. W. (1958). The learner: Self and perception. *Review of Educational Research, 28,* 433.

Grolnick, W. S., & Ryan, R. M. (1990). Self-perceptions, motivation, and adjustment in children with learning disabilities: A multiple group comparison. *Journal of Learning Disabilities, 23,* 177–184.

Haager, D., & Vaughn, S. (1995). Parent, teacher, peer and self-reports of the social competence of students with learning disabilities. *Journal of Learning Disabilities, 28*(4), 205–215.

Haager, D., & Vaughn, S. (1997). Assessment of social competence in students with learning disabil-

ities. In D. Chard, E. J. Kameenui, & J. W. Lloyd (Eds.), *Issues in educating students with learning disabilities* (pp. 129–152). Hillsdale, NJ: Erlbaum.

Hagborg, W. J. (1996). Self-concept and middle school students with learning disabilities: A comparison of scholastic competence subgroups. *Learning Disability Quarterly, 19,* 117–126.

Hagborg, W. J. (1998). School membership among students with learning disabilities and nondisabled students in a semirural high school. *Psychology in the Schools, 35*(2), 183–188.

Hagborg, W. J. (1999). Scholastic competence subgroups among high school students with learning disabilities. *Learning Disability Quarterly, 22*(1), 3–10.

Harter, S. (1985). *Manual for the Self-Perception Profile for Children.* Denver, CO: University of Denver.

Harter, S. (1993). Causes and consequences of low self-esteem in children and adolescents. In R. Baumeister (Ed.), *Self-esteem: The puzzle of low self-regard* (pp. 18–37). New York: Plenum Press.

Harter, S. (1996). Historical roots of contemporary issues involving self-concept. In B. A. Bracken (Ed.), *Handbook of self-concept* (pp. 1–37). New York: Wiley.

Harter, S., Whitesell, N. R., & Junkin, L. J. (1998). Similarities and differences in domain-specific and global self-evaluations of learning-disabled, behaviorally disordered, and normal achieving adolescents. *American Educational Research Journal, 35*(4), 653–680.

Heath, N. L., & Wiener, J. (1996). Depression and nonacademic self-perceptions in children with and without learning disabilities. *Learning Disability Quarterly, 19,* 34–44.

Hiebert, B., Wong, B., & Hunter, M. (1982). Affective influences on learning disabled adolescents. *Learning Disability Quarterly, 5,* 334–343.

Hosley, M., & Hopper, C., & Gruber, M. B. (1998). Self-concept and motor performance of children with learning disabilities. *Perceptual and Motor Skills, 87,* 859–862.

Jarvis, P. A., & Justin, E. M. (1992). Social sensitivity in adolescents and adults with learning disabilities. *Adolescence, 27*(108), 977–988.

Kavale, K., & Forness, S. R. (1996). Social skill deficits and learning disabilities: A meta-analysis. *Journal of Learning Disabilities, 29*(3), 226–237.

Keith, L. K., & Bracken, B. A. (1996). Self-concept instrumentation: A historical and evaluative review. In B. A. Bracken (Ed.), *Handbook of self-concept* (pp. 91–170). New York: Wiley.

Kistner, J. A., Haskett, M., White, K., & Robbins, R. (1987). Perceived competence and self-worth of LD and normally achieving students. *Learning Disability Quarterly, 10,* 37–44.

Kistner, J. A., & Osborne, M. (1987). A longitudinal study of learning disabled children's self-evaluations. *Learning Disability Quarterly, 12,* 133–140.

Kloomok, S., & Cosden, M. (1994). Self-concept in

children with learning disabilities: The relationship between global self-concept, academic "discounting," nonacademic self-concept, and perceived social support. *Learning Disability Quarterly, 17,* 140–153.

La Greca, A., & Stone, W. (1990). Children with learning disabilities: The role of achievement in their social, personal, and behavioral functioning. In H. L. Swanson & B. Keogh (Eds.), *Learning disabilities: Theoretical and research issues* (pp. 333–352). Hillsdale, NJ: Erlbaum.

Leahy, R. L. (Ed.). (1985). *The development of the self.* Orlando, FL: Academic Press.

Leary, M. (1999). Making sense of self-esteem. *Current Directions in Psychological Science, 8,* 32–35.

Lefrancois, G. R. (1990). *The lifespan* (3rd ed.). Belmont, CA: Wadsworth.

Lewandowski, L., & Arcangelo, K. (1994). The social adjustment and self-concept of adults with learning disabilities. *Journal of Learning Disabilities, 27*(9), 598–605.

Li, A. K. F. (1985). Early rejected status and later social adjustments: A 3-year follow-up. *Journal of Abnormal Child Psychology, 13,* 567–577.

Marsh, H. W. (1988). *Self-Description Questionnaire, I.* San Antonio, TX: Psychological Corporation.

Marsh, H. W. (1989). Age and sex effects in multiple dimensions of self-concept: Preadolescence to adulthood. *Journal of Educational Psychology, 81,* 417–430.

Marsh, H. W. (1990a). The influence of internal and external frames of reference on the formation of math and English self-concepts. *Journal of Educational Psychology, 82,* 107–116.

Marsh, H. W. (1990b). *Self-Description Questionnaire, II.* San Antonio, TX: Psychological Corporation.

Marsh, H. W., & Yeung, A. S. (1997a). Causal effects of academic self-concept on academic achievement: Structural equation models of longitudinal data. *Journal of Educational Psychology, 89*(1), 41–54.

Marsh, H. W., & Yeung, A. S. (1997b). Coursework selection: Relations to academic self-concept and achievement. *American Educational Research Journal, 34*(4), 691–720.

McInerney, D. M., Roche, L. A., McInerney, V., & Marsh, H. W. (1997). Cultural perspectives on school motivation: The relevance and application of goal theory. *American Educational Research Journal, 34*(1), 207–236.

McIntosh, R., Vaughn, S., Schumm, J., Haager, D., & Lee, O. (1993). Observations of students with learning disabilities in general education classrooms. *Exceptional Children, 60*(3), 249–261.

Merrell, K. W. (1991). Teacher ratings of social competence and behavioral adjustment: Differences between learning-disabled, low-achieving, and typical students. *Journal of School Psychology, 29*(3), 207–217.

Montgomery, M. S. (1994). Self-concept and children with learning disabilities: Observer-child concordance across six context-dependent domains. *Journal of Learning Disabilities, 27*(4), 254–262.

Palombo, J. (2001). *Learning disorders and disorders of the self in children and adolescents.* New York: Norton.

Parker, J. G., & Asher, S. R. (1987). Peer relations and later personal adjustment: Are low-accepted children at risk? *Psychological Bulletin, 102,* 357–389.

Piers, E. V. (1984). *The Piers-Harris Children's Self-Concept Scale.* Nashville, TN: Counselor Recordings and Tests.

Prout, H. T., Marcal, S. D., & Marcal, D. C. (1992). A meta-analysis of self-reported personality characteristics of children and adolescents with learning disabilities. *Journal of Psychoeducational Assessment, 10*(1), 59–64.

Purkey, W. W., & Novak, J. M. (1996). *Inviting school success: A self-concept approach to teaching, learning, and democratic practice* (3rd ed.). Belmont, CA: Wadsworth.

Renick, M. J., & Harter, S. (1988). *Self-Perception Profile for Learning Disabled Students.* Denver, CO: University of Denver Press.

Renick, M. J., & Harter, S. (1989). Impact of social comparisons on the developing self-perceptions of learning disabled students. *Journal of Educational Psychology, 81,* 631–638.

Shavelson, R. J., Hubner, J. J., & Stanton, G. C. (1976). Self-concept: Validation of construct interpretations. *Review of Educational Research, 46,* 407–441.

Swann, W. B. (1996). *Self-traps: The elusive quest for higher self-esteem.* New York: Freeman.

Twain, M. (1929). *What is man? and other essays.* New York: Harper & Brothers.

Vaughn, S., & Elbaum, B. E. (1999). The self-concept and friendships of students with learning disabilities: A developmental perspective. In R. Gallimore, L. Bernheimer, D. L. MacMillan, D. L. Speece, & S. Vaughn (Eds.), *Developmental perspectives on children with high incidence disabilities* (pp. 81–110). Mahwah, NJ: Erlbaum.

Vaughn, S., Elbaum, B., & Boardman, A. G. (2001). The social functioning of students with learning disabilities: Implications for inclusion. *Exceptionality, 9*(1), 49–67.

Vaughn, S., & Haager, D. (1994). Social competence as a multifaceted construct: How do students with learning disabilities fare? *Learning Disability Quarterly, 17*(4), 253–266.

Vaughn, S., Haager, D., Hogan, A., & Kouzekanani, K. (1992). Self-concept and peer acceptance in students with learning disabilities: A four- to five-year prospective study. *Journal of Educational Psychology, 84*(1), 43–50.

Vaughn, S., Hogan, A. Kouzekanani, K., & Shapiro, S. (1990). Peer acceptance, self-perceptions, and social skills of learning disabled students prior to identification. *Journal of Educational Psychology, 82*(1), 101–106.

Vaughn, S., McIntosh, R., & Spencer-Rowe, J. (1991). Peer rejection is a stubborn thing: Increasing peer acceptance of rejected students with learning disabilities. *Learning Disabilities Research and Practice, 6*(2), 65–132.

Wentzel, K. R., & Erdley, C. A. (1993). Strategies for making friends: Relations to social behavior and peer acceptance in early adolescence. *Developmental Psychology, 29*(5), 819–826.

Wiest, D., Wong, E. H., & Kreil, D. A. (1998). Predictors of global self-worth and academic performance among regular education, learning disabled, and continuation high school students. *Adolescence, 33*(131), 601–618.

15

Neurological Correlates of Reading Disabilities

Carlin J. Miller
Juliana Sanchez
George W. Hynd

Learning disabilities are a heterogeneous group of behaviorally diagnosed disorders thought to have a negative impact on the learning of an estimated 3–6% of all school-age children (Kibby & Hynd, 2001). Diagnosis assumes adequate intelligence, intact sensory systems, and the absence of a handicapping condition or environment that would cause a person to have significant difficulty learning (American Psychiatric Association, 2000). Although learning disabilities exist in many domains, it is the area of severe reading disabilities, also known as developmental dyslexia, that has been the focus of the majority of research and in which the neurobiological basis of the disorder is best understood.

The neurobiological basis of learning problems has been the subject of research for over a century. In the late 19th century, the lateralization of language to the left hemisphere and the localization of the language areas in the brain were beginning to be explored by Broca and Wernicke, among others (Kral, Nielson, & Hynd, 1998). Hinshelwood (1900), among others, first proposed the idea that damage to or variation in brain development of these cortical language areas might lead to difficulties in

learning to read (Kibby & Hynd, 2001). Hinshelwood suggested that an abnormality of or damage to the angular and supramarginal gyri on the left side of the brain might manifest itself by difficulty in learning to read. Incredibly, these same areas of the brain are the focus of research on the biological basis of reading disabilities today.

Reading disabilities are primarily characterized by difficulties with reading and spelling, but also include difficulties with phonemic segmentation (Hynd, Semrud-Clikeman, Lorys, Novey, & Eliopulos, 1990), rapid and automatic recognition and decoding of single words (Lyon, 1996), articulation (Huettner, 1994), sensorimotor coordination (Zeffiro & Eden, 2001), and anomia (Temple, 1997). Although there is a high comorbidity with attention-deficit/hyperactivity disorder (ADHD; Barkley, 1997), the two appear to be unique disorders that often co-occur each with a potentially different etiology (Barkley, 1997; Hynd et al., 1990).

In the last decade, a consensus has been reached among most researchers in the field that the core deficit in reading disabilities is difficulty with phonological processing

(Huettner, 1994; Hynd et al., 1995; Lyon, 1996; Shaywitz & Shaywitz, 1999; Siegel, 1993). Although most researchers agree that phonological processing is a core deficit of this disorder, evidence remains that visual deficits also exist in some people with reading disabilities (Eden, Van Meter, Rumsey, & Zeffiro, 1996). There has been some debate in the literature as to whether or not orthographic processing is another core deficit of developmental dyslexia. The work of Eden and others has shown that individuals with developmental dyslexia are impaired on a number of tasks that involve early sensory mechanisms, including visual motion, visuomotor, and visuospatial processing (Zeffiro & Eden, 2001). Thus, although the most common and accurately identified type of reading disability is phonological dyslexia (Stanovich, 1999), an orthographic or "surface" subtype might exist in conjunction with or independent of phonological dyslexia.

Reading disabilities and associated difficulties reflect a persistent deficit manifest persist throughout the lifespan (Lyon, 1996; Shaywitz & Shaywitz, 1999). For example, of children who are reading disabled in the third grade, 74% remain disabled in the ninth grade (Temple, 1997). This persistence throughout development is concordant with the evidence that there is a strong genetic component in the development of these disorders, with 35% to 45% familial risk rates consistently reported in the literature (Hynd et al., 1995). Neurobiological evidence as to the etiology of reading disabilities is supported by postmortem, electrophysiological, family, genetic, and brain-imaging studies (Galaburda, 1993; Hynd et al., 1995; Hynd & Semrud-Clikeman, 1989; Kinsbourne, 1989; Lyon, 1996; Temple, 1997; Zeffiro & Eden, 2001).

Evidence from these studies suggests disruption of the neurological system for language in individuals with dyslexia. Most of the structures which have been implicated in the neurobiological basis of reading disabilities are known to process language and/or visual information; thus it is not surprising that abnormalities in these structures are linked with the language and/or visual deficits seen in reading disabilities. These structures include, but are not limited to, Broca's area, the angular gyrus, the planum temporale, and the perisylvian cortex, all of which are thought to be involved in the processing of language (Galaburda, 1993; Hynd, Hynd, Sullivan, & Kingsbury, 1987; Hynd et al., 1990; Hynd & Semrud-Clikeman, 1989; Leonard et al., 1993; Riccio & Hynd, 1996; Temple, 1997; Zeffiro & Eden, 2001). The magnocellular pathway of the visual system (including the lateral geniculate nucleus of the thalamus), the occipital cortex, and the corpus callosum, all of which process visual information or are involved in the transfer of visual information to the language centers, have also been implicated (Hynd et al., 1995; Zeffiro & Eden, 2001). The remainder of this chapter provides an overview of the literature on the neurobiological basis of reading disabilities.

Review of the Research Literature on Reading Disabilities

The Double-Deficit Hypothesis

The double-deficit theory of dyslexia is currently receiving considerable attention in the neuropsychological literature. According to Wolf and Bowers (1999), the double-deficit hypothesis of dyslexia posits "phonological deficits and processes underlying naming speed represent two separable sources for reading dysfunction" (p. 415), such that there are separate types of reading disabilities characterized by single deficits in phonological processing or rapid naming as well as a more pervasive and severe form of dyslexia characterized by deficits in both phonological processing and rapid naming. Phonological processing is a skill that allows an individual to hear and manipulate individual sounds in spoken language (Cutting & Denckla, 2001). It is a part of the larger skill units of auditory perception and discrimination, but it is involved only in sounds that correspond to speech. Rapid naming is a skill that allows an individual to access concept names from their store of highly automatized information using visual prompts (Denckla & Rudel, 1974).

Many studies have examined the role phonological processing and rapid naming ability play in the acquisition of reading skills. Several studies have documented that these skills contribute uniquely to the variance in reading ability (e.g., Cronin &

Carver, 1998; Wagner et al., 1997). It also appears that the relationship between phonological processing and reading ability is bidirectional; thus, as phonological processing develops so does reading ability which in turn allows phonological processing to develop further (e.g., Wagner, Torgesen, & Rashotte, 1994). In addition, early phonological processing skills predict later reading achievement (e.g., Torgesen, Wagner, & Rashotte, 1994).

Most of the studies testing the double deficit hypothesis of dyslexia have focused on using phonological processing and rapid naming skills to differentiate good readers from children with reading disabilities. These studies suggest that children with impaired phonological processing and rapid naming deficits are at most significant risk for reading disabilities and also represent the most impaired readers, confirming the double-deficit hypothesis (e.g., Manis, Doi, & Bhadha, 2000). Attempts are being made to connect research on the double-deficit hypothesis to neurological characteristics associated with dyslexia in our research and by others.

The double-deficit theory of dyslexia has also been used to differentiate children with dyslexia from children who are garden-variety poor readers. The latter group is made up of children who fail to exhibit a discrepancy between reading achievement and cognitive ability due to low-cognitive-ability scores. These children are often not eligible for special education support services because their cognitive ability is too low for them to meet the criteria for a learning disability in reading. Conversely, their cognitive ability is too high to meet the criteria for mental retardation. The double-deficit model has been used to justify, amid significant controversy, providing special education intervention to children who display weaknesses in phonological processing and rapid naming, regardless of cognitive ability (Vellutino et al., 1996). The research in this area suggests that a redefinition of what constitutes a reading disability may be in order. Traditionally, learning disabilities have been diagnosed on the basis of a discrepancy between intellectual ability and reading achievement. These diagnostic criteria, which have been used in research and clinical settings, are based on the assumption

that an individual with a reading disability has a specific deficit in reading, but not in other domains of achievement, that is "unexplained" by intellectual ability (Stanovich, 1999).

These challenges in the appropriate diagnosis of reading disability have been under debate. Stanovich and Siegel have proposed that the aptitude–achievement discrepancy model be abandoned for reading disability diagnosis (Siegel, 1988, 1999; Stanovich, 1991, 1999; Stanovich & Siegel, 1994). They cite as basis for their proposal that fact that the neurolinguistic deficits of poor readers are the same regardless of intellectual ability (Fletcher, Francis, Rourke, Shaywitz, & Shaywitz, 1994; Stanovich, 1999; Stanovich & Siegel, 1994) and there is no evidence that low-IQ and high-IQ poor readers respond differently to intervention (Stanovich, 1999).

As an alternative to the aptitude–achievement discrepancy model, Siegel (1999) proposed a cutoff model of reading disability diagnosis. In this model, poor performance on a single test of psuedo-word reading is the primary indicator of a reading disability. Performance below a standard score of 85 on this task, a measure of phonological processing, with intellectual ability at or above a standard score of 85, would indicate a reading disability according to the Siegel criteria. Stanovich (1999) suggested that reading disabilities be indicated by performance below the 15th percentile on either a measure of pseudo-word reading or a test of word recognition, with intellectual ability playing no role in the diagnosis. But, this model may serve to simply sample the lower end of the distribution for reading achievement, rather than assessing students who experience what some would refer to as dyslexia, a more severe form of reading disability, always thought to have a neurobiological etiology.

The Planum Temporale

Brain-based research of dyslexia has focused a great deal of attention on a structure referred to as the planum temporale. In a seminal study, Geschwind and Levitsky (1968) reported their findings on the asymmetry of the planum temporale, an area that contains the bilateral auditory association cortices. This area is thought to be important in language. Of 100 normative postmortem brains, 65% showed a larger left planum temporale, 11% showed a larger right planum temporale, and the remaining 24% were of equal size. These findings are highly significant and have led other researchers to examine the role of the planum temporale in language-based deficits, including reading disabilities.

Galaburda and Kemper (1979) described results from a postmortem examination of a young man diagnosed with dyslexia during his childhood. They documented symmetrical plana with polymicrogyri. Polymicrogyria, a collection of many unusually small gyria, are considered an anomaly of neurological ontogeny. In a follow-up study, symmetrical plana were noted in three other dyslexic males on postmortem examination (Galaburda, Sherman, Rosen, Aboitiz, & Geschwind, 1985). In 1990, Humphreys, Kaufman, and Galaburda reported on postmortem results for three female dyslexics, all of whom had symmetrical plana. The theoretical interpretation was that some factor had an impact on pruning the normal process of neuronal elimination during development of the right plana, thus allowing for inefficient processing auditory–linguistic stimuli. Although these results provided additional information about the nature of the dyslexic brain, a more specific protocol for measurement of the planum temporale was needed as well as a method for measuring the planum temporale in a living person. Magnetic resonance imaging (MRI) and functional magnetic resonance imaging (fMRI) has provided the means to achieve this goal.

In 1990, a pattern of smaller left plana when compared to the right plana (reversed asymmetry) and symmetry was noted in children with dyslexia (Hynd et al., 1990). These measures were calculated from MRI scans using clinically identified children. Using a somewhat similar methodology, Larsen, Hoien, Lundberg, & Odegaard (1990) found that individuals with dyslexia were more likely to have a larger right plana and this rightward asymmetry was associated with phonological processing problems. Different measurement techniques were used which may have accounted for these slightly different findings. Regardless, both

of these studies documented deviations from normal patterns of plana asymmetry.

In an attempt to further elucidate the relationship between length of the planum temporal and reading deficits, a study the following year used the same measurement technique used by Hynd and colleagues to measure the plana from MRI scans. Results indicated that individuals with leftward asymmetry were significantly better on measures of total reading achievement, word attack, reading comprehension, confrontational naming, and rapid naming ability (Semrud-Clikeman, Hynd, Novey, & Eliopulos, 1991). The relationship held when the contrast groups had rightward asymmetry and symmetrical plana. To some degree, the literature then began to shift from measuring the length of the plana toward developing typologies of the morphology of the perisylvian region.

Gyral Morphology of the Perisylvian Region

Theory and research into the biological basis of dyslexia have traditionally focused on the left perisylvian region, which includes the planum temporale. The left hemisphere has been the focus of the majority of the research because it is the dominant hemisphere for language in most individuals. In recent years, some researchers have begun to investigate the gyral and sulcal morphology of the region and its possible relation to learning disabilities.

In a postmortem and MRI study of 120 left and right hemispheres of presumably non-learning disabled individuals, Steinmetz, Ebeling, Huang, and Kahn (1990) classified four main types of gyral morphology patterns. Figure 15.1 illustrates these typologies. Figure 15.2 contains examples of the typologies from MRI scans of children. The typologies were classified on the basis of the relative size and position of the posterior ascending ramus (PAR) of the Sylvian fissure and the inferior postcentral sulcus (POCS). The Type I, or "textbook," pattern according to Steinmetz and colleagues, the PAR of the Sylvian fissure ascends posterior to the POCS. This morphology was the most common as it was found in 67% and 65% of left hemispheres and 82% and 85% of right hemispheres in the postmortem and MRI samples. Type II is characterized by the

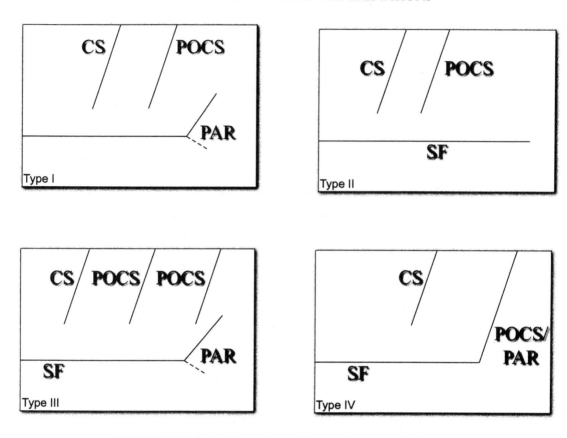

FIGURE 15.1. Perisylvian region subtypes (Steinmetz et al., 1990).

absence of a PAR of the Sylvian fissure and was found only in 10% of the postmortem sample and 25% the MRI sample and only in left hemispheres. In the Type III morphology, which was found only in 5% of right hemispheres and only in the postmortem sample, a second POCS exists, creating an extra gyrus. Type IV gyral morphology is characterized by the continuation of the PAR into the POCS. This type was found in the left hemisphere in 2% and 5% of the postmortem and MRI samples, respectively, and 13% and 15% of the right hemispheres.

Both Leonard and colleagues (1993) and Heimenz and Hynd (2000) have attempted to link the Steinmetz classification system to reading disabilities by comparing the gyral morphology of individuals with dyslexia and controls. Leonard and colleagues found an increase of Type III gyral morphology and a smaller incidence of Type I morpholo-

gy in the left hemisphere of dyslexics compared to controls and suggested that the increase in Type III morphology could be related to learning disabilities. This conjecture was strengthened by the finding that the first-degree relatives, or individuals who share 50% of their genetic material, such as parents and children or full siblings, of individuals with dyslexia, also had increased incidence of Type III morphology in the left hemisphere, which Leonard suggested could be evidence for genetic transmission of gyral morphology. Heimenz and Hynd found that although the Steinmetz typologies were not useful in the differentiated diagnosis of dyslexia, gyral morphology did relate to performance on neurolinguistic measures of receptive language. Specifically, left-hemisphere Type I morphology was associated with better performance on the Peabody Picture Vocabulary Test—Revised (PPVT-R) when compared to Type II and III mor-

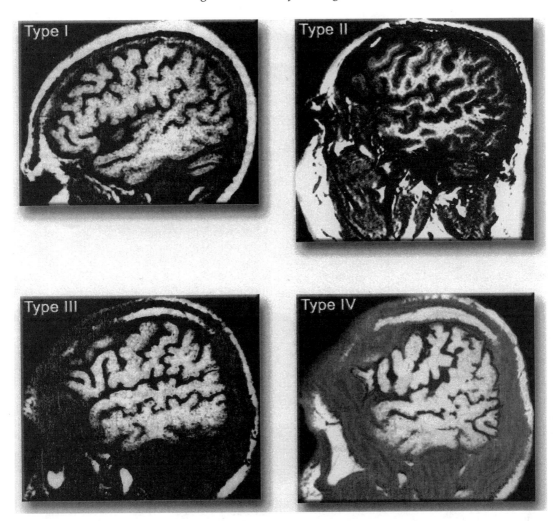

FIGURE 15.2. Perisylvian region subtype examples from MRI scans of human brains.

phologies, causing the authors to conclude that the absence of an extra gyrus in the left hemisphere may confer an advantage in receptive language. Interestingly, Heimenz and Hynd found that Type II occurred only in four male subjects who were diagnosed with both dyslexia and ADHD, suggesting the possibility of a unique and rare dyslexia syndrome.

The Corpus Callosum

Galaburda has theorized that development dyslexia is due, in part, to a larger right planum temporale, and evidence for this anatomical difference in dyslexics and normal readers is substantial (Galaburda, 1995; Geschwind & Galaburda, 1985). Galaburda goes on to suggest that the larger right planum temporale is interfering in the normal dominance of the left planum temporale for language processing. As noted previously, the right planum temporale is thought to be larger due to insufficient pruning in early ontogeny, and Galaburda, Rosen, and Sherman (1990) also suggest that increased callosal connections might be related to insufficient pruning. In this conceptualization, the interference of the right planum temporale on the left planum temporale's dominance for language may manifest itself through the morphological variation in the corpus callosum.

Although there has been conflicting evidence regarding the size of the corpus callosum in developmental dyslexia (Duara et al., 1991; Hynd et al., 1995, Preis, Steinmetz, Knorr, and Jancke, 2000), most studies have found significant differences in size. These differences are thought to be related to reduced cortical asymmetry. Hynd and colleagues (1995) found that the genu of the corpus callosum (most anterior part) was smaller in dyslexics. Other researchers (Larsen et al., 1992), however, have found a larger corpus callosum in developmental dyslexia. Preis and colleagues (2000) points out that the current results in studies examining this issue are split evenly, leaving us no closer to a conclusion about the potential role of the corpus callosum on language and language disorders. These discrepancies in research findings are likely due methodological differences which remain to be resolved in this line of research, including criteria for inclusion in the clinical and control groups, the method of measuring the corpus callosum and other relevant brain structures, and variability varieties in the imaging technology.

Cortical Abnormalities of the Temporal–Parietal Region

In addition to the structures with measurable differences in size and morphology already described, the literature suggests that there may be differences at the level of microneuropathology in the brains of individuals with dyslexia. Although these differences are difficult to image and are best described from the standpoint of histology upon postmortem examination, it appears that differences caused by focal dysplasias or heterotopias and polymicrogyria may contribute to the performance of individuals with dyslexia (Hynd, Morgan, & Vaughn, 1997).

Focal dysplasias or heterotopias are "ectopic gray matter in the cerebral hemispheres" (Hynd et al., 1997, p. 49). There are two types of focal dysplasias: laminar heterotopias and nodular heterotopias. Laminar heterotopias are gray matter in symmetrical ribbons in the centrum semiovale (Friede, 1989). Laminar heterotopias are not associated with deficits in performance when limited in scope. When dysplasias are present to a significant degree

throughout the cortex, laminar heterotopias are often associated with mental retardation and epilepsy (Palmini et al., 1991).

Nodular heterotopias are clustered masses of gray matter in irregularly formed nodules separated by thin myelinated fibers located near lateral ventricles (Friede, 1989; Hynd & Willis, 1988). Typically, nodular heterotopias are asymptomatic when they occur in small numbers (Aicardi, 1992). When there are more migrational deficits, nodular heterotopias have been associated with agenesis of the corpus callosum and micrencephaly (Friede, 1989). Important to this discussion, however, nodular heterotopias have been found in brains of individuals with dyslexia upon postmortem examination (Galaburda, et al., 1985). The distribution and severity of the dysplasias may determine the degree of impact upon learning (Hynd & Willis, 1988). Focal dysplasias are typically the result of migration errors during the second gestational trimester where only a limited number of migrational waves of neurons are affected (Palmini et al., 1991). According to Palmini and colleagues (1993), the extent of the migration deficits and the clinical manifestations may be related such that more migration deficits may be associated with a greater degree of clinical impairment.

As previously indicated, polymicrogyria are atypical gyri that are crowded and small; convolutional patterns are also atypical in polymicrogyria (Aicardi, 1992). Polymicrogyria can cover the entire cortical surface of either one or both hemispheres but are typically localized to a limited area of the cortex (Aicardi, 1992; Friede, 1989). Polymicrogyria can be asymptomatic, but it has also been associated with the incidence of learning disabilities (Galaburda & Kemper, 1979; Galaburda et al., 1985). Generally, polymicrogyria are associated with dyslexia when the affected area is in the perisylvian region (Galaburda & Kemper, 1979; Hynd & Willis, 1988). Polymicrogyria is the result of disturbances in cortical gyration that takes place during the fifth to sixth gestational month following neuronal migration (Aicardi, 1992; Friede, 1989). It is not clear what causes these disturbances, but maternal influenza, severe trauma, secondary fetal asphyxia, and genetic transmission have been implicated in polymicrogyria (Hynd et al., 1997).

Neuronal Pruning Hypothesis

Noting clinical observations of the high incidence of autoimmune disorders and left-handedness among dyslexics, Geschwind (and later in collaboration with Galaburda) hypothesized that autoimmune function, left-handedness, and dyslexia might be related to androgen secretion during development (Geschwind & Behan, 1982; Geschwind & Galaburda, 1985). Geschwind assumed as the basis of his theory that dyslexia is associated with symmetry or reversed asymmetry of the planum temporale (Galaburda et al., 1985; Geschwind & Levitsky, 1968; Humphreys et al., 1990) and noted that the symmetrical plana of dyslexics were bilaterally larger than that of controls (Galaburda et al., 1985).

Researchers theorized that the symmetry or reversed asymmetry of the plana is due to decreased rates of ontogenetic cell death in the left planum temporale during the period of corticogenesis that occurs between the fifth and seventh month of human fetal development (Geschwind & Behan, 1982; Hynd & Semrud-Clikeman, 1989). Galaburda and colleagues (1985) suggested that this decreased rate of cell death during corticogenesis may be associated with a familial tendency toward autoimmune and allergic disorders, while Geschwind's hypothesis (Geschwind & Behan, 1982) pointed to a high level of prenatal testosterone as the a potential cause of dyslexia, left-handedness, and autoimmune disorders. In fact, testosterone can decrease ontogenetic cell death (Kelley, 1993) and has been thought to affect the development of the immune system (Geschwind & Galaburda, 1985).

The important role of testosterone in the development of these two disorders is strengthened by studies which show a higher prevalence rate of developmental dyslexia in boys (Geschwind & Galaburda, 1985). Later studies, however, have attributed this difference in prevalence rates on selection bias (Shaywitz, Shaywitz, Fletcher, & Escobar, 1990). Furthermore, evidence associating left-handedness, immune disorders, and dyslexia has not consistently supported the Geschwind hypothesis (Pennington, Lefly,

Van Orden, Bookman, & Smith, 1987). Galaburda (1990) stated that in addition to the impact of testosterone on fetal brain development, a genetic predisposition toward developing bilateral plana is likely involved.

Genetics

The recent national interest in the human genome has increased the emphasis on genetic research in all fields. Not surprisingly, research on dyslexia has followed this trend, but the investigation of dyslexia's genetic basis is not new. Since the early 1970s, research has indicated a dramatic increase in risk for a childhood reading disability to occur when a parent also had a reading disability. In considering genetic research on dyslexia, it is important to remember that reading is a complex cognitive task that involves attention, memory, phonological processing, and rapid naming, among other abilities. As a result, any findings related to individual chromosomal linkage might actually identify a chromosomal difference associated with aspects of cognition or linguistic abilities associated with the clinical manifestation of dyslexia.

However, it is important to emphasize that research suggests particular chromosomal loci associated with reading and language disabilities. Several studies implicate chromosomes 6 and 15 in reading disabilities (Grigorenko et al., 1997). Previous research suggests that dyslexia is the result an autosomal dominant transmission with variable expression and incomplete penetrance (Elbert & Seale, 1988). This means that each child of a parent with the genes hypothesized to cause dyslexia has a 25% probability of inheriting those genes. These genes are not sex linked, and in children who inherit the genes, the expression of dyslexia can range from being nonapparent to causing severe impairment. Profiles of impairment may vary across family members.

Research also suggests that both genetic and environmental etiological factors have an impact on developmental dyslexia. Specifically, children with dyslexia demonstrate skill profiles that are similar to those of their nonimpaired siblings (DeFries, Singer, Foch, & Lewitter, 1978) and their parents (Foch, DeFries, McClearn, & Singer, 1977). Using behavioral genetic techniques, research using nuclear families has identified an allele for dyslexia that explains 54% of the phenotypical variance in reading performance (Gilger, Pennington, & DeFries, 1991).

Data collected in studies of twins suggest that 50% of the variance in reading problems experienced by children with dyslexia is due to heritable influences, but there is also a significant environmental component as well (Wadsworth, Olson, Pennington, & DeFries, 1992). Another study found that what is inherited is reading performance, rather than reading disabilities per se, with data to demonstrate that parent reading performance predicts child reading performance regardless of whether or not dyslexia is present (Alarcon, DeFries, & Gillis, 1994).

Summary of Consistent Findings

Developmental dyslexia is a complex behaviorally diagnosed disorders that reflects underlying cognitive deficits that are believed to be related to neurobiological abnormalities. The primary behavioral deficit is an inability to rapidly decode words (word attack), which results in poor and dysfluent reading. The primary underlying cognitive deficit is theorized to be related to phonological processing and rapid naming speed (Wolf & Bowers, 1999), although evidence also exists that there is an orthographic or visual component in some individuals (Eden et al., 1996; Pennington et al., 1987), which might constitute a separate subtype.

The neurobiological correlates believed to underlie these cognitive deficits are centered around the left temporal–parietal region. Differences in the asymmetry of the planum temporale have consistently been found in association with reading disabilities (Galaburda & Kemper, 1979; Galaburda et al., 1985; Hynd & Semrud-Clikeman, 1989). Specifically, symmetry of the planum temporale (Galaburda et al., 1985; Humphreys et al., 1990) due to a larger right plana or a reversal of the normal pattern of left greater than right asymmetry (Hynd et al., 1990) has been found in individuals with developmental dyslexia. Although the research finding have been inconsistent, most studies have found differences in the size of the cor-

pus callosum in individuals with developmental dyslexia (Preis et al., 2000). Furthermore, in the first reported postmortem cases of a dyslexic's brain, cortical abnormalities including polymicrogyri were found in the temporal–parietal region (Galaburda, LeMay, & Kemper, 1978). Recently, research has begun to focus on the relationship between reading difficulties, verbal ability, and gyral morphology of the perisylvian region (Heimenz & Hynd, 2000; Leonard et al., 1993), which could be associated with the relative size and position of receptive language areas such as the planum temporale.

The morphology of these areas of the brain is likely related to genetic factors as well as to variability in fetal development. In fact, there is consistent evidence that reading disabilities tend to run in families, with 50% of the variance in reading problems explained by genetics (Wadsworth et al., 1992). Several studies have implicated chromosomes 6 and 15 (Grigorenko et al., 1997). Perinatal environment has also been implicated in the development of reading disabilities. The Geschwind hypothesis theorized that higher levels of testosterone *in utero* could decrease pruning that normally occurs during corticogenesis and could affect immune functioning, leading to developmental dyslexia, left-handedness, and autoimmune disorders (Geschwind & Behan, 1982; Geschwind & Galaburda, 1985). It must be remembered, however, that aspects of the postuterine environment, such as exposure to language and reading, certainly play an important role in the development of reading problems.

Whereas the neurobiological evidence seems to support the notion that neurodevelopmental variation during fetal ontogeny is associated with deficient language and reading skills found in dyslexics, it is not exactly clear what cognitive abilities are most affected. In this context, it is helpful to examine models of cognitive processes most representative of the dyslexic syndrome.

Competing Models

The models described in this section are not necessarily contradictory to those previously described. In fact, all three models provide complementary information that enhances the predominant research focus in dyslexia studies. These models include descriptions of dyslexia from the perspectives of deficits in the visual processing system, a nondiscrepancy-based model, and one that focuses on the role of orthographic processing in the presentation of the reading deficits associated with dyslexia.

The Visual Processing Model

The model proposed by Eden and colleagues (1996) focuses on the visual processing of rapidly presented information. Although this paradigm for the investigation of dyslexia appears opposed to the more linguistic models, it represents a perspective that posits global temporal-processing deficits, both auditory and visual, as the underlying factors in dyslexia. As a result, this model is complementary to the neurolinguistic model of dyslexia. According to this model, these deficits are related to magnocellular processing in the visual pathway system. According to Livingstone and Hubel (1988), the magnocellular system is responsive to stimulus onset and offset, rather than motion or color sensitivity. Research by Felmingham and Jakobson (1995) suggests evidence for magnocellular deficits and deficient flicker/motion detection abilities in individuals with dyslexia. Furthermore, Eden and colleagues present evidence that the extrastriate area of the cortex receives mostly magnocellular projects fails to show normal activation patterns in adults with dyslexia.

As an additional component in the visual-processing model, poor eye movement may also be implicated in dyslexia. There is evidence to suggest that poor eye movement stability or fixation may also be deficient in individuals with dyslexia, although these deficits may be better understood as a result of linguistic deficits (Eden, Stein, Wood, & Wood, 1994). This evidence confirmed earlier work by Pirozzolo and Rayner (1979).

Orthographic processing

Orthographic processing is more closely related to the visual aspects of reading, described by Eden and others, than to the phonological components. Orthographic processing is the interpretation of abstract representations (series of letters that form words) during the process of reading. Orthographic processing is most closely related to sight word reading where the individual does not use decoding strategies to read words but, rather, knows the entire word "on sight." Research on orthographic coding suggests that it contributes significantly to word-reading ability (Olson, Forsberg, & Wise, 1994). Furthermore, this contribution appears to be beyond that of the contributions of phonological processing to the reading process (Cunningham, Perry, & Stanovich, 2001).

Although there is evidence to suggest that phonological processing is influenced by genetic factors, there is little evidence to suggest the same for orthographic coding. In fact, Stanovich and colleagues have noted in multiple articles that orthographic processing is linked to exposure to print and other environmental indicators of reading (e.g., Cunningham & Stanovich, 1993; Olson, Wise, Conners, Rack, & Fulker, 1989). This may explain, in part, why genetic factors only account for 50% of the variance in reading performance.

Conclusions and Future Directions

An abundance of evidence supports a neurobiological basis for developmental dyslexia. Persistent differences in the patterns of normal symmetry and/or morphology have consistently been noted in the temporal–parietal region of the left hemisphere, specifically the planum temporale (Galaburda & Kemper, 1979; Galaburda et al., 1985; Hynd & Semrud-Clikeman, 1989). Cortical abnormalities have also been documented (Galaburda, LeMay, & Kemper, 1978). Research is now turning toward examining the pattern of gyral morphology in this region and its relation to performance on neurolinguistic measures and diagnosis (Heimenz & Hynd, 2000; Leonard et al., 1993).

There is evidence that the origin of the neurological abnormalities found in dyslexia is a genetic one, as reading disabilities tend to run in families (Wadsworth et al., 1992). Controversial theories have also implicated high perinatal levels of testosterone as a possible causal factor of abnormal brain development in the language cortex (Geschwind & Galaburda, 1985).

Though many researchers have concluded that the core deficit in dyslexia is phonological processing (Huettner, 1994; Hynd et al., 1995; Lyon, 1996; Shaywitz & Shaywitz, 1999; Siegel, 1993), competing models exist. They include the visual processing model, which implicates the magnocellular pathway of the visual system as dysfunctional, and the orthographic processing model, which implicates difficulties with accurate perception and processing of visual symbols. Both models have been described by Eden and colleagues (1996) and propose visual deficits in reading as opposed to the auditory deficits proposed in the phonological model and double-deficit model. These theories are by no means mutually exclusive, and it is likely that neurolinguistic deficits occur in both auditory and visual processing in individuals with reading disabilities, and that these deficits have a neurological basis. It is clear that research should continue to examine the relationship between and prevalence of both auditory and visual processing difficulties.

It should also be pointed out that variability in pattern of plana symmetry or asymmetry is not a sufficient cause of severe reading disability or dyslexia. This is because symmetry and reversed asymmetry of the plana appear in the normative population (Geschwind & Levitsky, 1968; Hynd et al., 1990). As Galaburda and colleagues (1985) suggest, it may be that cortical or subcortical dysplasias must also be present in the brain to such a degree that they seriously disrupt normal language processes so essential to the development of fluent reading ability. Unfortunately for research purposes, these cortical abnormalities cannot be imaged using MRI as the spatial resolution is not yet sufficient to reveal abnormalities in the microstructure of the brain.

An additional area that merits further investigation is the link between the brain-based deficits in dyslexia and intervention. Although recent studies of dyslexia have used fMRI technology to further describe the involved brain–behavior relationships, this technology has yet to be applied to the efficacy of intervention strategies. Although there is no way to intervene in childhood to change planum temporale asymmetry or perisylvian morphology, research using fMRI may facilitate targeting intervention strategies to specific deficits observed in the metabolic functioning in brain regions in the future. If fMRI becomes part of the technologies used by to monitor progress in the remediation of specific reading deficits, this may lead to the identification of more effective intervention efforts. Furthermore, if intervention can be demonstrated to be effective in changing how a child reads, it may further the knowledge about the nature of dyslexia.

A final area warranting mention as a future area of study on dyslexia is further research about the nature of the genetics involved in dyslexia. Although the reviewed research suggests a strong heritable component for reading processes, there are many unknowns yet to be explored. For example, although certain genes have been targeted as being involved in dyslexia, it is not known how these chromosomes cause the manifestation of reading deficits. Furthermore, the nature of the relationship between these chromosomal differences and the visual processes involved in reading has yet to be explored. In addition, there has been little investigation on the genetic contributions to dyslexia in minority populations. Without additional study, there may be more unanswered questions about the nature of dyslexia than questions with answers.

Acknowledgment

Preparation of this chapter was supported in part by a grant to the third author (GWH) from the National Institute for Child Health and Human Developmental, National Institutes of Health (No. 26890-06).

References

Aicardi, J. (1992). *Diseases of the nervous system in childhood*. New York: MacKeith Press.

Alarcon, M., DeFries, J. C., & Gillis, J. J. (1994). Familial resemblance for measures of reading performance in families of reading-disabled and control twins. *Reading and Writing, 6,* 93–101.

American Psychiatric Association. (2000). *Diagnostic and statistical manual of mental disorders* (4th ed., text revision). Washington, DC: Author.

Barkley, R. A. (1997). Behavioral inhibition, sustained attention, and executive functions: Constructing a unifying theory of ADHD. *Psychological Bulletin, 121,* 65–94.

Cronin, V., & Carver, P. (1998). Phonological sensitivity, rapid naming, and beginning reading. *Applied Psycholinguistics, 19,* 441–460.

Cunningham, A. E., Perry, K. E., & Stanovich, K. E. (2001). Converging evidence for the concept of orthographic processing. *Reading and Writing, 14,* 549–568.

Cunningham, A. E., & Stanovich, K. E. (1993). Children's early literacy environments and early word recognition subskills. *Reading and Writing, 5,* 193–204.

Cutting, L. E., & Denckla, M. B. (2001). The relationship of rapid serial naming and word reading in normally developing readers: An exploratory model. *Reading and Writing, 14,* 673–705.

DeFries, J. C., Singer, S. M., Foch, T. T., & Lewitter, F. I. (1978). Familial nature of reading disability. *British Journal of Psychiatry, 132,* 361–367.

Denckla, M. B., & Rudel, R. G. (1976). Rapid "automatized" naming of pictured objects, colors, letters, and numbers by normal children. *Cortex, 10,* 186–202.

Duara, R., Kushch, A., Gross-Glenn, K, Barker, W., Jallad, B., Pascal, S., Loewenstein, D. A., Sheldon, J., Rabin, M., Levin, B., & Lubs, H. (1991). Neuroanatomic differences between dyslexia and normal readers on magnetic resonance imaging scans. *Archives of Neurology, 48,* 410–416.

Eden, G. F., Van Meter, J. W., Rumsey, J. M., & Zeffiro, T. A. (1996). The visual deficit theory of developmental dyslexia. *Neuroimage, 4,* S108–S117.

Eden, G. F., Stein, J. F., Wood, H. M., & Wood, F. B. (1994). Differences in eye movements and reading problems in dyslexic and normal children. *Vision Research, 34,* 1345–1358.

Elbert, I. C., & Seale, T. W. (1988). Complexity of the cognitive phenotype of an inherited form of a learning disability. *Developmental Medicine and Child Neurology, 30,* 181–189.

Felmingham, K. L., & Jakobson, L. S. (1995). Visual and visuomotor performance in dyslexic children. *Experimental Brain Research, 106,* 467–474.

Fletcher, J. M., Francis, D. J., Rourke, B. P., Shaywitz, S. E., & Shaywitz, B. A. (1994). The validity of discrepancy-based definitions of reading disabilities. *Journal of Learning Disabilities, 25,* 555–561.

Foch, T. T., DeFries, J. C., MacClearn, G. E., & Singer, S. M. (1977). Familial patterns of impairment in reading disability. *Journal of Educational Psychology, 69,* 316–329.

Friede, R. L. (1989). *Developmental neuropathology* (2nd ed.). Berlin, Germany: Springer-Verlag.

Galaburda, A. M. (1990). The testosterone hypothesis: Assessment since Geschwind & Behan, 1982. *Annals of Dyslexia, 40,* 18–38.

Galaburda, A. M. (1993). The planum temporale. *Archives of Neurology, 50,* 457.

Galaburda, A. M. (1995). Anatomic basis of cerebral dominance. In R. J. Davidson & K. Hugdahl (Eds.), *Brain asymmetry* (pp. 51–74). Cambridge, MA: MIT Press.

Galaburda, A. M., & Kemper, T. L. (1979). Cytoarchitectonic abnormalities in developmental dyslexia: A case study. *Annals of Neurology, 6,* 94–100.

Galaburda, A. M., LeMay, M., & Kemper, T. L. (1978). Right–left asymmetries in the brain: Structural differences between hemispheres may underlie differences. *Science, 199,* 852–856.

Galaburda, A. M., Rosen, G. D., & Sherman, G. F. (1990). Individual variability in cortical organization: Its relationship to brain laterality and implications to function. *Neuropsychologia, 28,* 529–546.

Galaburda, A. M., Sherman, G. F., Rosen, G. D., Aboitiz, F., & Geschwind, N. (1985). Developmental dyslexia: Four consecutive patients with cortical abnormalities. *Annals of Neurology, 18,* 222–233.

Geschwind, N., & Behan, P. (1982). Left-handedness: Association with immune disease, migraine, and developmental learning disorder. *Proceedings of the National Academy of Sciences of the United States of America, 79,* 5097–5100.

Geschwind, N., & Galaburda, A. (1985). Cerebral lateralization: Biological mechanisms, associations, and pathology: I. A hypothesis and program for research. *Archives of Neurology, 42,* 428–459.

Geschwind, N., & Levitsky, W. (1968). Human brain: Left–right asymmetries in temporal speech region. *Science, 161,* 186–187.

Gilger, J. W., Pennington, B. F., & DeFries, J. C. (1991) Risk for reading disability as a function of parental history in three family studies. *Reading and Writing, 3,* 205–217.

Grigorenko, E. L., Wood, F. B., Meyer, M. S., Hart, L. A., Speed, W. C., Shuster, A., & Pauls, D. L. (1997). Susceptibility loci for distinct components of developmental dyslexia on chromosomes 6 and 15. *American Journal of Genetics, 60,* 27–39.

Heimenz, J. R., & Hynd, G. W. (2000). Sulcal/gyral pattern morphology of the perisylvian language region in developmental dyslexia. *Brain and Language, 74,* 113–133.

Hinshelwood, J. (1900). Congenital word-blindness. *Lancet, 1,* 1506–1508.

Huettner, M. I. S. (1994). Neuropsychology of language and reading development. In P. A. Vernon (Ed.), *The neuropsychology of individual differences* (pp. 9–34). San Diego, CA: Academic Press.

Humphreys, P., Kaufman, W. E., & Galaburda, A. (1990). Developmental dyslexia in women: Evidence for a subgroup with a reversal of cerebral asymmetry. *Annals of Neurology, 28,* 727–738.

Hynd, G. W., Hall, J., Novey, E. S., Eliopulos, D., Black, K., Gonzalez, J. J., Edmonds, J. E., Riccio, C., & Cohen, M. (1995). Dyslexia and corpus callosum morphology. *Archives of Neurology, 52,* 32–38.

Hynd, G. W., Hynd, C. R., Sullivan, H. G., & Kingsbury, T. B. (1987). Regional cerebral blood flow (rCBF) in developmental dyslexia: Activation during reading in a surface and deep dyslexic. *Journal of Learning Disabilities, 20,* 294–300.

Hynd, G. W., Morgan, A. E., & Vaughn, M. (1997). Neurodevelopmental anomalies and malformations. In C. R. Reynolds & E. Fletcher-Janzen (Eds.), *Handbook of clinical child neuropsychology: Critical issues in neuropsychology* (pp. 42–62). New York: Plenum Press.

Hynd, G. W., & Semrud-Clikeman, M. (1989). Dyslexia and brain morphology. *Psychological Bulletin, 106,* 447–482.

Hynd, G. W., Semrud-Clikeman, M., Lorys, A., Novey, E., & Eliopulos, D. (1990). Brain morphology in developmental dyslexia and attention deficit hyperactivity disorder. *Archives of Neurology, 47,* 919–926.

Hynd, G. W., & Willis, W. G. (1988). *Pediatric neuropsychology.* Needham Heights, MA: Allyn & Bacon.

Kelley, D. B. (1993). Androgens and brain development: Possible contributions to developmental dyslexia. In A. M. Galaburda (Ed.), *Dyslexia and development: Neurobiological aspects of extraordinary brains* (pp. 21–41). Cambridge, MA: Harvard University Press.

Kibby, M. Y., & Hynd, G. W. (2001). Neurobiological basis of learning disabilities. In D. P. Hallahan & B. K. Keogh (Eds.), *Research and global perspectives in learning disabilities: Essays in honor of William M. Cruickshank* (pp. 25–42) Mahwah, NJ: Erlbaum.

Kinsbourne, M. (1989). Mechanisms and development of hemisphere specialization in children. In C. R. Reynolds & E. Fletcher-Janzen (Eds.), *Handbook of clinical child neuropsychology. Critical issues in neuropsychology* (2nd ed., pp. 69–85). New York: Plenum Press.

Kral, M., Nielson, K., & Hynd, G. W. (1998). Historical conceptualization of developmental dyslexia: Neurolinguistic contributions from the 19th and early 20th centuries. In R. Licht, A. Bouma, W. Slot, & W. Koops (Eds.), *Child neuropsychology* (pp. 1–16). Delft, The Netherlands: Eburon.

Larsen, J. P., Hoien, T., Lundberg, I., & Odegaard, H. (1990). MRI evaluation of the size and symmetry of the planum temporale in adolescents with developmental dyslexia. *Brain and Language, 39,* 289–301.

Larsen, J. P., Hoien, T., & Odegaard, H. (1992). Magnetic resonance imaging of the corpus callosum in developmental dyslexia, *Cognitive Neuropsychology, 9,* 123–134.

Leonard, C., Voeller, K. K. S, Lombardino, L., Morris, M., Hynd, G. W., Alexander, A., Andersen, H., Garofalakis, M, Honeyman, J., Mao, J., Agee, H., & Staab, E. (1993). Anomalous cerebral structure in dyslexia revealed with magnetic resonance imaging. *Archives of Neurology, 50,* 461–469.

Livingstone, M. S., & Hubel, D. (1988). Segregation of form, color, movement, and depth: Anatomy, physiology, and perception. *Science, 240,* 740–749.

Lyon, G. R. (1996). Learning disabilities. In E. J. Mash & R. A. Barkley (Eds.), *Child psychopathology* (pp. 390–435). New York: Guilford Press.

Manis, F. R., Doi, L. M., & Bhadha, B. (2000). Naming speed, phonological awareness, and orthographic knowledge in second graders. *Journal of Learning Disabilities, 33,* 325–333.

Olson, R. K., Forsberg, H., & Wise, B. (1994). Genes, environment, and the development of orthographic skills. In V. W. Berninger (Ed.), *The varieties of orthographic knowledge, 1: Theoretical and developmental issues. Neuropsychology and cognition* (Vol. 8, pp. 27–71). Norwell, MA: Kluwer Academic.

Olson, R., Wise, B., Conners, F., Rack, J., & Fulker, D. (1989). Specific deficits in component reading and language skills: Genetic and environmental influences. *Journal of Learning Disabilities, 25,* 562–573.

Palmini, A., Andermann, F., Aicardi, J, Dulac, O., Chaves, F., Ponsot, G., Pinard, J. M., Goutieres, F., Livingston, J., Tampieri, D., Andermann, E., & Robitaille, Y. (1991). Diffuse cortical dysplasia, or the "double cortex" syndrome: The clinical and epileptic spectrum in 10 patients. *Neurology, 41,* 1656–1662.

Palmini, A., Andermann, F., de Grissac, H., Tampieri, D., Robitaille, Y., Langevin, P., Desbiens, R., & Andermann, E. (1993). Stages and patterns of centrifugal arrest of diffuse neuronal migration disorders. *Developmental Medicine and Child Neurology, 35,* 331–339.

Pennington, B. F., Lefly, D. L., Van Orden, G. C., Bookman, M. O., & Smith, S. D. (1987). In phonology bypassed in normal or dyslexic development. *Annals of Dyslexia, 37,* 62–89.

Pirozzolo, F. J., & Rayner, K. (1979). Cerebral organization and reading disability. *Neuropsychologia, 17,* 485–491.

Preis, S., Steinmetz, H., Knorr, U., & Jancke, L. (2000). Corpus callosum size in children with developmental language disorder. *Cognitive Brain Research, 10,* 37–44.

Riccio, C. A., & Hynd, G. W. (1996). Neuroanatomical and neurophysiological aspects of dyslexia. *Topics in Language Disorders, 16,* 1–13.

Semrud-Clikeman, M., Hynd, G. W., Novey, E. S., & Eliopulos, D. (1991). Dyslexia and brain morphology: Relationships between neuroanatomical variation and neurolinguistic tasks. *Learning and Individual Differences, 3,* 225–242.

Shaywitz, S. E., & Shaywitz, B. A. (1999). Cognitive and neurobiologic influences in reading and in dyslexia. *Developmental Neuropsychology, 16,* 383–384.

Shaywitz, S. E., Shaywitz, B. A., Fletcher, J. M., & Escobar, M. D. (1990). Prevalence of reading disability in boys and girls: Results of the Connecticut Longitudinal Study. *Journal of the American Medical Association, 264,* 998–1002.

Siegel, L. S. (1988). Evidence that IQ scores are irrelevant to the definition and analysis of reading disability. *Canadian Journal of Psychology, 42,* 201–215.

Siegel, L. S. (1993). Phonological processing deficits

as the basis of a reading disability. *Developmental Review, 13,* 246–257.

Siegel, L. S. (1999). Issues in the definition and diagnosis of learning disabilities: A perspective on *Guckenberger v. Boston University. Journal of Learning Disabilities, 32,* 304–320.

Stanovich, K. E. (1991). Conceptual and empirical problems with discrepancy definitions of reading disability. *Learning Disabilities Quarterly, 14,* 269–280.

Stanovich, K. E. (1999). *Who is rational?: Studies of individual differences in reasoning.* Mahwah, NJ: Erlbaum.

Stanovich, K. E., & Siegel, L. S. (1994). Phenotypic performance profile of children with reading disabilities: A regression-based test of the phonological core variable-difference model. *Journal of Educational Psychology, 86,* 24–53.

Steinmetz, H., Ebeling, U., Huang, Y., & Kahn, T. (1990). Sulcus topography in the parietal opercular region: An anatomic and MR study. *Brain and Language, 38,* 515–533.

Temple, C. M. (1997). Reading disorders. In C. M. Temple (Ed.). *Developmental cognitive neuropsychology* (pp. 163–223). Hove, East Sussex, UK: Psychology Press.

Torgesen, J. K., Wagner, R. K., & Rashotte, C. A. (1994). Longitudinal studies in phonological processing and reading. *Journal of Learning Disabilities, 27,* 276–286.

Vellutino, F. R., Scanlon, D. M., Sipay, E. R., Small, S. G., Pratt, A., Chen, R., & Denckla, M. B. (1996). Cognitive profiles of difficult-to-remediate and easily remediated poor readers: Early intervention as a vehicle for distinguishing between cognitive and experiential deficits as basic causes of specific reading disability. *Journal of Educational Psychology, 88,* 601–638.

Wadsworth, S. J., Olson, R. K., Pennington, B. F., & DeFries, J. C. (1992). Differential genetic etiology of reading disability as a function of IQ. *Journal of Learning Disabilities, 33,* 192–199.

Wagner, R. K., Torgesen, J. K., & Rashotte, C. A. (1994). Development of reading related-phonological processing abilities: New evidence of bidirectional causality from a latent variable longitudinal study. *Developmental Psychology, 30,* 73–87.

Wagner, R. K., Torgesen, J. K., Rashotte, C. A., Hecht, S. A., Barker, T. A., Burgess, S. R., Donahue, J., & Garon, T. (1997). Changing relations between phonological processing abilityies and word-level reading as children develop from beginning to skilled readers: A five-year longitudinal study. *Developmental Psychology, 33,* 468–479.

Wolf, M., & Bowers, P. G. (1999). The double-deficit hypothesis for developmental dyslexias. *Journal of Educational Psychology, 91,* 415–438.

Zeffiro, T., & Eden, G. (2001). The cerebellum and dyslexia. Perpetrator or innocent bystander?: Comment from Thomas Zeffiro and Guinevere Eden to Nicholson et al. *Trends in Neurosciences, 24,* 512–513.

16

Genetic Influences on Reading and Writing Disabilities

Jennifer B. Thomson
Wendy H. Raskind

Dyslexia and dysgraphia are common complex disorders characterized by difficulty learning to read and/or write, not attributable to general cognitive delay, psychiatric or neurological disorder, sensory impairment, or inadequate instruction. There is now considerable evidence that genetic factors contribute to the development of dyslexia and dysgraphia (Raskind, 2001), although given the complex interactions between genetic background and environmental factors, genetic information is not likely to be the definitive diagnostic test for dyslexia/dysgraphia. The phenotype (behavioral expression) for dyslexia and dysgraphia is complex and is different for each affected individual, and the occurrence and manifestations of the disorder in an individual may depend on the interaction of genetic factors (genes), environmental factors (e.g., amount and quality of educational exposure), and stochastic processes (i.e., chance events). Nevertheless, delineating these genetic influences will not only lead to a better understanding of the biological mechanisms of the disorder but will also be valuable for assessment and intervention purposes.

For example, knowledge of the genes involved in these disorders might facilitate earlier intervention for children at higher risk. Because the optimal developmental window for acquisition of reading and writing skills is narrow, a delay in triaging struggling children for the special education services they need may have an adverse effect on their eventual learning outcome. Educators may be reluctant to label younger children as potentially "learning disabled" when they may merely be at the lower end of the normal range of developing readers or writers. A suggestive family history of learning disability and a "high risk" genotype might spur earlier remediation for a child who demonstrates a slow trajectory of acquisition of basic reading skills.

In addition, genetic information could have clinical applicability in the choice of a specific instructional plan and prognosis for the intensity and duration of early intervention required. For example, our research showing that phonological short-term memory has a genetic etiology (Wijsman et al., 2000) led to an instructional program in which word reading begins with creating a precise representation of syllables and phonemes in spoken polysyllabic words rather than beginning with written words (Berninger, 2000). Our research showing that the efficiency (rate) of phonological decoding has a genetic etiology (Raskind, Hsu, Berninger, Thomson, & Wijsman, 2000) led to treatment aimed at automatizing phonological decoding (Berninger, 2000). Thus, a knowledge of genetic influences on dyslexia and dysgraphia may also contribute to development of effective instructional interventions tailored to genetically constrained processes in reading and writing.

Terms

Every discipline has a vocabulary that is peculiar to itself. Although this vocabulary facilitates communication between experts within the field, it may bar others from a full understanding of the area. Appendix 16.1 provides a short list of frequently used terms in human genetics. This list will help readers understand this chapter and publications about other genetic investigations. For many of these terms, the reader may need to refer to other words in the glossary for additional definitions.

Familial Aggregation

The concept that reading disabilities may have a hereditary basis is not new. Since the first descriptions of dyslexia, researchers have noted that reading disability clustered in families (e.g., Fisher, 1905; Hinshelwood, 1907; Stephenson, 1907; Thomas, 1905). Later, it was observed that there is a greater prevalence of reading difficulties in first-degree relatives of individuals with dyslexia as compared to controls (e.g., Decker & De-Fries, 1981; DeFries, Singer, Foch, & Lewitter, 1978; Finucci, Guthrie, Childs, Abbey, & Childs, 1976; Foch, DeFries, McClearn, & Singer, 1977; Owen, Adams, Forrest, Stolz, & Fisher, 1971; Wolff & Melngailis, 1994). Familial aggregation is necessary but not sufficient to prove a genetic etiology because families tend to experience the same environmental as well as genetic influences. Diseases such as lead poisoning or asbestosis and behaviors such as speaking French or eating tropical fruits are examples of familial traits that do not have a genetic etiology.

Estimates of the Heritability of Reading/Writing Disabilities

Research strategies involving twins have long been used to explore the relative contributions of genetic and environmental factors. In the traditional twin design, differences between identical, or monozygotic (MZ), and fraternal, or dizygotic (DZ), co-twins are studied. Both types of twins share their home and school environments to a substantial degree, but they differ in their genetic similarity. Because MZ twins arise from the splitting of one early embryo, their genetic constitution is the same. DZ twins, on the other hand, arise from two ova separately fertilized by two sperm; they have the same genetic relationship as other siblings and have in common, on average, one-half of their genes. For a dichotomous trait that is entirely genetically determined, MZ twins should be fully concordant, whereas DZ twins should be less often concordant.

Based on a categorical definition of dyslexia, the majority of early twin studies found greater concordance among MZ than DZ co-twins. In the first reported study of reading disability in five sets of twins, two were concordant MZ pairs, one was a concordant opposite-sex DZ pair, and two were discordant opposite-sex DZ pairs (Hallgren, 1950). Hermann and Norrie (1958) reported that 4 of 19 same-sex and 6 of 11 opposite-sex DZ twin pairs were concordant for reading disability, whereas all 9 MZ twin pairs were concordant. A weakness of this report is the lack of information regarding ascertainment or diagnostic procedures. Bakwin (1973) later reported that 26 of 31 MZ twin pairs ascertained on the basis of history of reading problems in the proband twin and only 9 of 31 same-sex DZ co-twins were concordant for reading disability. The differences in concordance rates were significant. Significant differences between DZ and MZ concordance rates in the larger of the studies and in aggregate provide evidence for a genetic etiology of reading/writing disabilities. However, the observation that concordance among MZ twins is less than complete reflects the existence of nongenetic factors in the development of reading and writing disabilities.

Given the evidence that reading and writing skills are normally distributed in the population and that the threshold between categorically defined affected and nonaffected status is somewhat arbitrary, it is more precise to use quantitative data. For a genetically determined continuous trait phenotype, the scores of DZ co-twins of probands selected for scoring in one tail of the normal distribution should regress halfway to the population mean, whereas those of MZ co-twins should not. On the other hand, for a continuous trait that is entirely determined by environmental influence, the scores of co-twins in both MZ and DZ types of twin sets should regress equally to the population mean. In twin studies, an estimate of heritability can therefore be derived by comparing the average regressions to the population mean for MZ and DZ co-twins of probands (DeFries & Fulker, 1985).

This method was first applied to a subject set of 64 MZ and 55 DZ twin pairs ascertained as part of a longitudinal study of reading and writing skills in children attending elementary schools in Colorado (DeFries, Fulker, & LaBuda, 1987). Probands were selected on the basis of low achievement on a composite measure based on the Reading Recognition, Reading Comprehension, and Spelling subtests of the Peabody Individual Achievement test (Dunn & Markwardt, 1970), verbal intelligence of no more than two-thirds standard deviations below the mean (Wechsler, 1974), and no evidence of neurological, sensory, or emotional deficit. Average regressions of 1.16 and 0.77 standard deviation units toward the mean were found for DZ co-twins and MZ co-twins, respectively, yielding an estimated heritability for reading/writing disability of 0.29 (p = .003). A much higher heritability estimate of 0.58 was obtained in a more recent analysis of a larger twin sample from the same project—223 pairs of MZ twins and 169 pairs of same-sex DZ twins (Wadsworth, Olson, Pennington, & DeFries, 2000).

Reading and writing disabilities are heterogeneous disorders with multiple subtypes, and it is possible that some subtypes may have an appreciable genetic etiology and others may not. Therefore, the heritability of the underlying processes thought to contribute to reading and writing ability has also been evaluated. Both phonological coding (ability to analyze sound patterns in spoken words) and orthographic coding (ability to distinguish between written real and pseudo-word homonyms) have been reported to be significantly heritable (approximately 31–60%) (Castles, Datta, Gayan, & Olson, 1999; Olson, Forsberg, & Wise, 1994; Olson, Wise, Connors, Rack, & Fulker, 1989).

Although twin studies have provided information regarding the heritability of a variety of phenotypes, there are some inherent limitations. For research on learning disabilities, a major assumption has been that environmental influences on MZ and DZ co-twins' reading/writing development are equivalent. It may be the case, however, that MZ twins share a more similar environment than do DZ twins (Grayson, 1989; Joseph, 2001; Kendler, Neale, Kessler, Heath, & Eaves, 1993). The genetic etiology of comorbid behaviors that modify the reading and writing phenotype may confound the interpretation of studies on learning disabilities in twins. For example, a substantial genetic contribution to attention/concentration skills has recently been reported (e.g., Faraone & Doyle, 2001; Willcutt, Pennington, & DeFries, 2000). If MZ co-twins are more similar with regard to their ability to attend to written material, this may result in more similarity with regard to their attention to reading and writing tasks. Another potential limitation in twin research lies in the generalization of these data to the population at large. Are there etiological factors that are unique to the twinning situation for the variables under study? Does the greater likelihood of participation in studies by MZ than DZ twin pairs and by females than males contribute to a systematic bias? Overall, however, twin research supports the heritability of reading disability and of the phonological and orthographic processing abilities underlying it.

Modes of Inheritance of Reading/Writing Disabilities

The observation that dyslexia is highly familial and moderately heritable does not necessarily imply that it is the result of a single gene. There are several possible modes of transmission of a genetically influenced trait. The phenotype can be caused by one or more independent, single major genes (Mendelian), by several genes acting in combination (oligogenic), or by many genes each of which contributes a small amount of variation (polygenic) (Smith & Goldgar, 1986). This distinction is of more than theoretical interest because it may be difficult to identify the multiple genes involved in a polygenic trait when none has a big enough effect to be distinguished on its own. On the other hand, if an allele of one of the genes has a more pronounced (major) effect on the phenotype than do the other genes, the gene may be identified even if the overall heritability of the trait is not high.

Traits with Mendelian inheritance may be autosomal or sex linked and dominant, codominant, or recessive. Although some observational family studies suggested a simple autosomal dominant mode of transmission of reading disability (e.g., Drew, 1956; Hallgren, 1950) and a genetic linkage study in a single large family found evidence for involvement of a gene with autosomal dominant effect (Fagerheim et al., 1999), the growing consensus is that the most prevalent pattern of dyslexia in pedigrees does not fit a simple Mendelian mode of inheritance (e.g., Finucci et al., 1976; Hohnen & Stevenson, 1999; Omenn & Weber, 1978). In contrast to a simple Mendelian trait in which one gene's alleles determine a phenotype, in complex disorders the genotypes of a set of genes act in concert with environmental factors to affect the probability that an individual will manifest the phenotype; alterations of a single gene are not sufficient to cause the disorder. In addition, for most complex disorders, the population cannot simply be categorized as "affected" or "unaffected" because there is a range of manifestations. In fact, when the genes are cloned and studied in detail, even many "simple" disorders are found to be much more complex than previously thought. Their phenotypic effects can be quite varied, even without the involvement of independent modifying genes and environmental factors (e.g., Cohn, Bornstein, & Jowell, 2000; Gayther et al., 1997; Quinzii & Castellani, 2000).

Although data from the Colorado Reading Project twin study supported the existence of a major gene effect on reading disability (e.g., Alarcón & DeFries, 1995), twin studies do not provide precise information about the mode of inheritance. To answer this question, a variety of mathematical approaches have been developed to model the inheritance patterns of a trait in families. Detailed descriptions of the methods are beyond the scope of this chapter, but summaries of the major findings in reading and writing disabilities are provided herein.

Segregation Analysis

One way to evaluate the mode of inheritance of a trait in families is through segregation analysis. The method of ascertainment of families for these studies is of paramount importance because systematic bias can lead to a model of inheritance that does not reflect the actual transmission pattern of the trait in the larger, unselected, population (see Smith & Goldgar, 1986, for a discussion regarding ascertainment correction). In essence, segregation analysis evaluates a variety of possible modes of inheritance for their ability to explain the observed familial pattern of the trait. In its simplest form, the proportion of affected children of probands (the segregation ratio) is computed and tested to evaluate whether the observed ratio fits the expected one (Smith & Goldgar, 1986). For example, in the classic transmission of an autosomal dominant trait with no environmental influence and 100% penetrance, the expected segregation ratio is .50 because it is expected that half the offspring of matings in which one parent is affected and the other is not affected would be affected if enough families are studied.

In complex segregation analysis (CSA), a mathematical equation describing a more complete model of the inheritance pattern of a single gene is generated. In this method the potential contributions of other genes are combined into one polygenic term, terms for both shared and unshared environment effects can also be included, and a single model is chosen that best fits the data (Bonney, 1986; Morton & MacLean, 1974). An estimate of the number of genes that are involved can be obtained using a newly devised sophisticated Bayesian Monte-Carlo Markov-Chain stochastic method (MCMC) that models several Mendelian loci simultaneously but does not include a polygenic component (e.g., Daw, Heath, & Wijsman, 1999; Heath, 1997; Wijsman et al., 2000).

Hallgren (1950) was the first to use segregation analysis in his sample of 116 reading disabled children and their families, finding no evidence for a sex-linked mode of inheritance but good agreement with an autosomal dominant mode of transmission. Finucci and colleagues (1976) studied 20 families and found that the mode of transmission did not fit any one mode of single gene inheritance. Lewitter, DeFries, and Elston (1980) found that although there was no evidence for a single gene mode of transmission in a set of 133 families, plausible models could explain several subsets of these families. For example, the data were compatible with a major recessive gene for reading disability in families with female probands. In a study of four independently ascertained samples, Pennington and colleagues (1991) obtained results consistent with a sex-influenced, dominant, or major gene effect in three of four samples and with polygenic transmission in the fourth. The latter two studies highlight the importance of careful phenotyping of families because the identification of reliable subtypes could help in the identification of distinct genetic etiologies.

Because reading ability is normally distributed in the population (Shaywitz, Escobar, Shaywitz, Fletcher, & Makuch, 1992), the boundary between abnormal and normal reading is indistinct and analyses using quantitative data may be more appropriate. In a population of 125 nuclear families ascertained through a reader without disabilities, Gilger, Borecki, DeFries, and Pennington (1984) reported evidence that low penetrant common alleles of one or more dominant genes contributed a significant proportion of the variance to a continuous measure of reading ability based on the Reading Recognition, Reading Comprehension, and Spelling subtests of the Peabody Individual Achievement Test (Dunn & Markwardt, 1970). In addition, Wijsman and colleagues (2000) reported evidence for the presence of one or more genes contributing to performance on a continuous measure of phonological nonword memory using both complex and MCMC segregation analysis methods.

Linkage Analyses

If there is a gene of major effect that contributes to a phenotype, it is possible to locate its position in the genome by a process called linkage analysis. When the mode of transmission of the phenotype is known, powerful model-based linkage methods can be employed. Parameters estimated in segregation analyses, such as gene frequency, the relative effects of genetic and nongenetic influences, and potential heterogeneity, can be incorporated into these linkage analyses. On the other hand, when the mode of transmission of a phenotype is not known, nonparametric methods, such as sib- and other affected relative-pair analyses, which are relatively model free, must be used. Regardless of the analysis method, the question asked during each step in a linkage study is whether two loci segregate independently in meiosis.

During meiosis, chromosomal segments derived from the individual's parents are exchanged in a process, "crossing over," which recombines the DNA that had been inherited from the individual's parents. The ovum thus contains DNA from both parents of the mother and the sperm contains DNA from both parents of the father. Therefore, an individual in the next generation inherits some alleles from each of the four grandparents. What makes linkage analyses feasible is the existence of DNA sequence differences between individuals. In essence, the locus responsible for the phenotype of interest (affected or unaffected, in the case of a categorical phenotype) whose place in the genome is unknown is evaluated with a series of polymorphic loci (markers) whose places in the genome are known. When two loci are far apart, for instance, on different chromosomes, their alleles segregate independently from each other. Assume, for example, that a phenotype being studied results from a mutation (–) in a gene on one chromosome pair and there is a marker locus on another chromosome pair with alleles A and a (the genotype of the affected parent is +/– at the gene and A/a at the marker). Only one chromosome of each pair is transmitted to each offspring. The possible outcomes of independent segregation of the phenotype and the marker locus are –/A and –/a and each is equally likely to be observed. In contrast, alleles at loci that are close to each other on the same chromosome will stay together much more often than would be predicted by chance. For example, if the allele causing the phenotype is on the same chromosome as allele A of the linked marker locus, offspring with the phenotype will more often inherit allele A than allele a. If cosegregation of alleles of the known locus and the phenotype of the unknown locus is observed more frequently than 50% of the time, the chromosomal position of the unknown gene relative to the known locus can be estimated. The distance between two locations in the genome is often expressed as the fraction of gametes in which there has been a recombination (i.e., the recombination fraction, θ).

In the affected relative pair method, usually done on sib pairs, constraints are not placed on the model of transmission. It is assumed that if the trait locus and the marker are linked, the sib pair will be concordant for both the trait and an allele at the marker. If the phenotype is linked to the marker, there should be a correspondence between the phenotypical and genotypical similarities between the relatives regardless of the mode of inheritance.

Model-based methods are more powerful than sib-pair methods, at least in part because information about all members of the family, affected and not affected, can be used. A ratio of the probability of linkage to the probability of nonlinkage, under the proposed model of transmission, is computed at several recombination frequencies for each family. The log of the ratios, called the LOD score (log of the odds of likelihood of linkage), are calculated so that LOD scores at various θ levels can be summed across families. Given the large number of genes and markers in the genome, the a priori likelihood of linkage of any two locations is extremely low. Therefore, the hypothesis of linkage is accepted (at the $p < .05$ level) when a LOD score greater than 3.0 is obtained (1,000:1 odds in favor of linkage). For a simple Mendelian trait, an LOD score of less than –2.0 (100:1 odds against linkage) is conventionally used to reject the

linkage hypothesis (Morton, 1955). It has been suggested that more stringent significance levels be required to reach the same conclusions for a complex trait (Lander & Kruglyak, 1995; Thomson, 1994). Linkage studies also have the capacity to detect genetic heterogeneity in the sample and to estimate the proportion of families in which the trait locus appears to be linked to a specific location. The linkage analysis can then be repeated in the subset of unlinked families to map another locus.

Association Studies and Linkage Disequilibrium Mapping

For the linkage analysis just described, the specific marker alleles are not relevant to the phenotype. They merely allow the transmission of the phenotype to be analyzed concurrently with the segregation of a locus in the genome in each family. Another category of analytic methods relies on the phenomenon of linkage disequilibrium—that is, the association of the phenotype with a specific allele at a marker. Such an association will occur when the allele has an effect on the phenotype or when there has not been sufficient time for the specific genetic change responsible for the phenotype and an allele at a closely linked marker to reach equilibrium. It takes time (in the form of generations) for a new allele that arises by mutation at one site to be separated by the process of recombination from the specific alleles at a nearby site on the same chromosome. For a while, these alleles will be transmitted together in a unit called a haplotype. A state of equilibrium exists when the alleles at both loci are distributed in the population as is predicted for the distance between the two loci. Because the frequencies of alleles at a locus may vary considerably between different ethnic populations, the analysis must control for ethnicity (Schaid et al., 1999; Terwilliger & Ott, 1992).

Genetic Mapping and Association Studies in Reading and Writing Disabilities

Given the phenotypical heterogeneity of reading and writing disorders, it is not surprising that linkage results have also been diverse. Potential locations for genes influencing reading and spelling disorders have been reported on chromosomes 1, 2, 6, 15, and 18, as reviewed later and partially summarized previously in a table (Raskind, 2001). It is important to note that because of differences in ascertainment procedures, measures used to define reading/spelling disorders, and analytic methods, these studies are not directly comparable.

Smith, Kimberling, Pennington, and Lubs (1983) were the first to report a significant linkage finding for reading disability. In this initial study of eight families chosen for apparent autosomal dominant transmission of dyslexia, a dichotomous classification of reading disability was used based on oral reading and written spelling at least 2 years below expected grade level (determined by mathematics and general information tests) for children and history for adults. Using a cytogenetically observable polymorphism at the proximal portion of the long arm of chromosome 15 as the marker, a LOD score of 3.241 at a recombination fraction of 0.13 was found. The putative dyslexia locus was assigned the name DYX1. However, when additional families were included and DNA markers were used, the overall LOD score decreased and there was evidence of significant genetic heterogeneity, with about 20% of the families showing linkage to chromosome 15 but the remainder not demonstrating linkage (Smith, Pennington, Kimberling, & Ing, 1990). A single large family provided most of the evidence for linkage. There was some evidence for a chromosome 15 localization when nonparametric multiple regression techniques were applied to the quantitative scores in a subset of the most severely affected sibships (Fulker et al., 1991).

The chromosome 15 locus was subsequently evaluated by other groups for linkage to a variety of reading and writing phenotypes. Significant evidence for linkage was found by parametric methods for a dichotomous phenotype based on deficits in single word reading in a sample of six extended families containing at least four affected members (Grigorenko et al., 1997). Results for a phenotype based on spelling deficits, categorically defined, were consistent with linkage to chromosome 15, but the LOD scores were too low to provide independent confirmation of this localization (Schulte-Körne et al., 1998). Markers in this region have also been significantly associat-

ed with deficits in oral prose reading in a recent study of parent–proband trios (Morris et al., 2000). In addition, there is suggestive evidence for the localization to chromosome 15 of a gene that modifies the expression of dyslexia in a family whose dyslexia appears to be linked to chromosome 2 (Fagerheim et al., 2000). Finally, in one family, three of four individuals carrying a balanced translocation involving chromosome band 15q21 had dyslexia (Nopola-Hemmi et al., 2000). However, in a second family, only one of four carriers of a translocation involving the same region of chromosome 15q was affected by dyslexia. Not all researchers have been able to replicate the chromosome 15 linkage findings (Bisgaard, Eiberg, Moller, Niebuhr, & Mohr, 1987; Sawyer et al., 1998), even when the original families were included in the sample studied (Cardon et al., 1994; Lubs et al., 1991; Rabin et al., 1993).

One of these groups reported suggestive evidence for linkage to the distal portion of the short arm of chromosome 1 (1p34–36) in nine of the extended families with a three-generation history of reading disability, including the one that had previously provided much of the evidence for linkage to chromosome 15 (Lubs et al., 1991; Rabin et al., 1993). Supporting evidence for a dyslexia locus on the short arm of chromosome 1 was found in another set of extended families with deficits in single word reading, phonological decoding, and rapid automatized naming (Grigorenko et al., 2001). However, no study has obtained significant evidence for linkage to chromosome 1p, and at least one study reported no evidence for linkage to this region (Cardon et al., 1994).

Evidence for a dyslexia locus on the short arm of chromosome 6, DYX2, has also been reported. This region had been targeted for analysis because of earlier reports of an increased prevalence of autoimmunity in families of children with learning disabilities (Geschwind & Behan, 1982; Pennington, Smith, Kimberling, Green, & Haith, 1987), although subsequent research has not supported this association (Gilger et al., 1998). The first suggestion of linkage here was reported by Smith, Kimberling, and Pennington (1991) in a study of a subset of families whose linkage to chromosome 15 (as reported previously) was questioned. Using the sib-pair analysis method specialized for DZ twins (DeFries & Fulker, 1985), Cardon and colleagues (1994, 1995) found evidence for linkage to 6p for a continuous scale discriminant score derived from performance on measures of reading recognition, reading comprehension, and spelling. In a new sample of sibs, modest supporting evidence was obtained for a quantitative trait locus on 6p for an orthographic task involving discrimination of a real word and a nonword homophone (orthographic choice) and for phonological decoding (Gayán et al., 1999). In targeted studies, this localization was replicated by two other groups. The phenotypes providing the evidence included categorically defined phonological segmentation (Grigorenko et al., 1997), real word reading, and spelling/vocabulary (Grigorenko et al., 2001) subtypes and continuous measures of ability to read irregular real words (orthographic processing) and phonological decoding of nonwords (Fisher et al., 1999). However, several other groups found no evidence for linkage to 6p for a measure of phonological decoding (Field & Kaplan, 1998), for spelling disabilities (Schulte-Körne et al., 1998), or for measures of phonological awareness, phonological decoding, spelling, and rapid automatized naming (Petryshen, Kaplan, Liu, & Field, 2000).

In the first genome-wide scan for a dyslexia locus, using a qualitative affectation status, significant evidence for linkage to a locus on chromosome 2q was found in a single large Norwegian family with an apparent autosomal dominant mild to moderate reading and spelling disability (Fagerheim et al., 1999). This locus has been assigned the name DYX3. Although mildly positive linkage results were obtained to the pericentromeric region of chromosome 15, where the DYX1 locus was originally specified, linkage to DYX2 was excluded in this family (Fagerheim et al., 1999, 2000).

A second genome-wide scan investigated several quantitative reading-related phenotypes in two samples from the United States and the United Kingdom, using two nonparametric methods (Fisher et al., 2001). Genotypes of parents and their children were included in the analyses, but quantitative data were available only for the siblings. Both samples provided strong evi-

dence for a locus on the short arm of chromosome 18 (18p11.2) for single-word reading ability. Weaker evidence for linkage to the same site was found for measures of orthographic (irregular word reading and orthographic choice) and phonological (phonological awareness and phonological decoding) processing. This localization was confirmed in an independent sample of families from the United Kingdom for the phenotype of phonological awareness. The U.S. sample provided suggestive evidence for a second locus on the long arm of chromosome 18. It is also interesting that some evidence for a locus on chromosome 2p15-p16 emerged in both the U.K. and U.S. samples, suggesting that DYX3 may be involved in the broader population of dyslexia than just the rare family with a monogenic form of reading disability (Fagerheim et al., 1999).

This increasing list of genomic locations for genes involved in reading and spelling disabilities is not unexpected given the complex nature of the phenotype. The relative contribution of each of these putative genes to reading and spelling disabilities is not known, nor is it clear how they interact to produce the variation in the phenotype that is seen within as well as between families. To answer these questions, it will be necessary to identify the genes. The genetics of learning disabilities might be more tractable if the phenotypes studied could be reduced to simpler or more phenotypically precise subphenotypes. If genetic models can be constructed for these subphenotypes, it would be possible to use model-based gene-mapping methods that are inherently more powerful than model-free methods and that can be used to refine the localizations of the suggested dyslexia gene sites (Wijsman & Amos, 1997). The University of Washington Multidisciplinary Learning Disabilities Center (UWMLDC) was established in 1995 and began ascertaining and phenotyping multigenerational families to address these considerations.

Genetic Research at the University of Washington Multidisciplinary Learning Disabilities Center

Probands were ascertained without regard to family size or family history of reading and/or writing problems. These potential probands were administered an approximately 4-hour battery of 23 tests that spanned the following domains:

1. *Verbal comprehension.* The Verbal Comprehension factor of the Wechsler scales of intelligence (1981, 1992) was administered to provide an overall indication of verbal ability. Although there is controversy regarding the use of verbal intelligence to qualify children for special education services within the school system, the use of verbal intelligence was warranted for genetic research for two reasons. First, the exclusion of children with verbal intelligence of less than 90 made it less likely that a sizable portion of the probands might have more global impairment in cognition due to neurological, neurogenetic, or psychiatric disorders, rather than a specific disability in the area of reading or writing. Second, previous genetic research has provided evidence that reading disabilities defined by a discrepancy criterion may be more heritable than reading disabilities as defined by low performance alone (Olson, Datta, Gayan, & DeFries, 1999), and reading disability in groups of children with higher intelligence may be more heritable than reading disability in groups of children with lower intelligence (Wadsworth et al., 2000).

2. *Academic achievement.* Several measures of reading accuracy, reading rate, reading comprehension, handwriting, spelling, written composition, mathematics calculation, and mathematical problem solving were also administered. If a child demonstrated verbal comprehension skills of at least SS = 90 and academic achievement of one standard deviation below verbal ability, in addition to academic performance below the mean, the child was included in our study as a proband and their family was invited to be tested (see Berninger, Abbott, Thomson, & Raskind, 2001, for complete details regarding tests administered and ascertainment procedures).

3. *Language processing.* In addition to verbal ability and academic achievement, a large battery of language-processing measures was also administered to gain information regarding the underlying processes involved in reading or writing disability. In-

formation regarding these basic language processes (phonological processing, orthographic coding, and rapid automatized naming) was deemed necessary to understand the various subphenotypes that may exist within and between families.

Careful characterization of the phenotype was initially performed on 102 nuclear families containing 409 individuals (Berninger et al., 2001). Structural equation modeling was used to validate that four different language processes—Verbal Comprehension, Orthographic Coding, Rapid Automatized Naming, and Phonological Processing—contribute to the expression of the phenotype but that different patterns of covariance across processes and different patterns of paths from these language processes to the academic achievement measures were found within child probands and between child probands and their affected parents. It was found that the phonological processing factor had significant paths to all reading and writing skills except reading rate and handwriting in both probands and adults, but in adults only if the effect of verbal IQ was removed. For the orthographic coding factor, significant paths to all reading and writing factors with the exception of reading comprehension were found in both probands and adults. Rapid naming had a significant path only to reading rate in probands and adults. Verbal IQ had significant paths to reading comprehension in probands and adults, and to reading accuracy, reading rate, spelling, and composition in adults but not probands. These data demonstrate that the same set of language processing skills are used differently across academic tasks and across ages.

Additional phenotyping studies have also been carried out with the data from these original 102 families. In a study of the comorbidity of calculation and reading disabilities, it was found that children with both disabilities were more likely to have a rapid automatized naming deficit than were other children in the study, but they did not differ on measures of verbal IQ or phonological processing (Busse, Thomson, Abbott, & Berninger, 1999). This observation suggests that a deficit in phonological processing may lead to a reading disability but that deficits in automaticity may lead to dual disability with calculation and reading. In a further analysis, it was found that those children with the dual reading and calculation disability actually had a triple deficit in reading, calculation, and written expression and were more severely affected in all three domains (as well as language processing markers) than those with a reading disability alone (Busse et al., 1999).

To evaluate the familial patterns of each measure in the battery, aggregation analyses of the quantitative data were performed (Raskind et al., 2000). Using a generalized estimating equation (GEE)-based approach that can handle correlated data, such as various measurements on the same subject or on related subjects, and that is not influenced by the different size of pedigrees (Liang & Zeger, 1986; Zhao, Grove, & Quaioit, 1992), correlations between nuclear family members were computed for all measures to identify patterns consistent with a genetic basis. If there is a genetic basis for a trait, the correlations between relatives should reflect the degree of genetic relatedness. Therefore, the correlation between siblings should exceed the correlation between parents and their children, and both correlations should be positive. In contrast, unless there is assortative mating or inbreeding, the trait should show no correlation between the parents. Two measures were identified that met these criteria with a statistical significance at $p < 0.05$ for both sibling and parent–offspring correlations: rate or automaticity of phonological decoding and phonological memory for nonwords. Three measures had slightly weaker patterns with one correlation significant at $p < 0.05$ and the other significant at $p < 0.1$: accuracy of phonological decoding, short-term memory for digits, and one measure of written spelling from dictation. Five additional measures showed at least suggestive evidence for an appropriate aggregation pattern with only one of the two correlations significant at $p < 0.1$: another measure of written spelling from dictation, accuracy, fluency and comprehension of oral reading, and one measure of rapid automatized naming.

Aggregation analyses were then performed on pairs of related measures in order to gain information regarding their interdependence. We reasoned that some measures may be accounting for the observed aggregation patterns of others. If a promising aggregation pattern disappeared when another measure was included as a covariate, perhaps the covariate measure was accounting for the promising aggregation pattern in the first measure. Using covariate analyses, we found that there may be a genetic contribution to phonological decoding rate in addition to the genetic contribution it shares with phonological decoding accuracy, a genetic contribution to phonological nonword memory in addition to the genetic contribution it shares with written spelling from dictation, a genetic contribution to written spelling from dictation in addition to the genetic contribution it shares with phonological decoding accuracy, and a genetic contribution to self-regulation of cognition (inattention ratings) in addition to the genetic contribution it shares with rapid automatized naming or oral reading rate (Hsu, Wijsman, Berninger, Thomson, & Raskind, 2002).

Although the familial patterns were consistent with an underlying genetic component, aggregation analyses do not provide information about the mode of inheritance or the number of genes involved. To investigate these questions, two candidate phenotypes, phonological nonword memory and digit span, were chosen for further investigation in more labor-intensive segregation analyses (Wijsman et al., 2000). This research diverged from other segregation studies in that we evaluated only one component process of reading/writing disability rather than attempting to analyze the genetic contribution of reading or writing skills as a whole. In single-measure analyses, we found evidence supporting a major-gene mode of inheritance for both the nonword memory task and digit-span task. Results obtained by reciprocal adjustment of the measures suggested that the genes contributing to the nonword memory score completely account for the genetic basis of the digit-span score but that there is an additional genetic contribution to the nonword memory task that is not accounted for by the digit-span measure.

Unraveling the genetics of complex phenotypes such as reading and writing disabilities will require large data sets. Mapping broad genomic locations for contributing genes is an important first step. Subsequent steps include refinement of the locations, candidate gene analysis or positional cloning, mutational analysis, genotype/phenotype/environment correlations, and searches for modifying genes. Therefore, continued ascertainment and assessment of study subjects is a priority. The study sample currently consists of 183 families containing 1,093 first-degree and more distant relatives. Additional phenotypes, such as morphology (especially derivational suffixes that convey grammatical information) and syntax, are being analyzed for the possibility of a genetic etiology, and segregation and linkage analyses are being performed for promising subtypes.

Conclusion

Research on the genetic contribution to reading and writing disabilities has progressed substantially over the years, from early observational studies of its familial aggregation to sophisticated linkage analyses made feasible through advances in the Human Genome Project and development of powerful genetic statistical methods. Several possible sites on five different chromosomes (1, 2, 6, 15, and 18) have been implicated in the expression of reading/writing disorders in a number of families, but no etiological genes have yet been identified. The next decade promises to be an exciting time in the history of dyslexia research when continued enlargement of the study populations and development of even more powerful analytic methods culminate in the cloning of these genes. This milestone will usher in a new phase of research into genotype/phenotype correlations, biological consequences of specific genetic changes, and potential intervention strategies guided by genetic profiles.

Appendix 16.1. Glossary

Allele: One of the alternative versions of a gene or marker.

Ascertainment: The method of selection of individuals for inclusion in a study.

Association: In human genetics, this describes the situation in which a particular allele is found more or less often in a group of affected indivuals than would be expected by chance in the general population.

Autosome: Any nuclear chromosome other than the sex chromosomes. There are 22 pairs of autosomes.

Chromosome: A threadlike structure in the cell's nucleus that contains DNA. There are normally 46 chromosomes in each cell organized into 23 pairs.

Complex trait inheritance: A pattern of inheritance that is not Mendelian and usually reflects involvement of alleles at more than one locus interacting with environmental factors.

Concordance: The presence of the same trait in a set of individuals, such as a pair of twins.

Dichotomous trait: A phenotype that is either present or absent.

Discordance: The presence of a trait in only one member of a set of individuals.

DNA (deoxyribonucleic acid): The molecule composed of four different elements (bases) that encode genetic information for the individual and that allows transmission of this genetic information from one generation to another.

Dominant: One copy of the trait-causing form of the gene is sufficient for the phenotype.

Epigenetic: A factor that can affect the phenotype without any change in the genotype.

Epistasis: Technically means that an allele of one gene can block the phenotypical expression of all alleles of another gene. Often used to imply a gene that has an effect on the expression of the alleles at another gene.

Expressivity: The degree to which a heritable trait is exhibited in an individual. When different phenotypes or severity of the phenotype may result from the action of a gene, the gene is said to manifest "variable expressivity."

Gene: A sequence of DNA that contains all the information necessary for synthesis of an RNA molecule, which, in turn, contains the information to produce a protein product.

Genetic heterogeneity: More than one genetic mechanism can produce the same phenotype.

Genetic statistical modeling: A process that seeks to describe in mathematical terms the inheritance pattern of an observed phenotype.

Genome: All the DNA of a cell or individual.

Genotype: The alleles at a specific locus or portion of the genome.

Haplotype: A set of closely linked loci that tend to be inherited toegether as a unit.

Heritability: The proportion of the variation in a trait that is attributable to genetic (or inherited) factors.

Linkage analysis/Gene mapping: A statistical method in which the chromosomal location of a gene responsible for a trait is identified by tracking the inheritance of a gene or phenotypical trait and a DNA marker in a family or group of families. The closer together two loci are (the marker and the trait gene), the more often they will stay together during meiosis. When two loci are unlinked they will be transmitted independently.

Locus: A position in the DNA sequence.

Major gene: A gene that is responsible for a detectable portion of the variation in a phenotype.

Marker: A site in the genome that has a known location and more than one form (allele). It may be a gene or a DNA sequence that is not part of a gene.

Mendelian inheritance: The pattern of a phenotype in a family that can be explained by transmission of a locus that follows Mendel's first law of independent segregation; that is, at a single locus, the alleles that were inherited from the two parents are independently segregated during transmission to the offspring. The phenotype may be autosomal (the locus for the gene is on an autosome) or sex linked (the locus for the gene is on the X or Y chromosome) and dominant, codominant, or recessive.

Oligogenic inheritance: The effects of several genes combine to cause the phenotype.

p: The short arm of a chromosome.

Penetrance: The proportion of individuals who have the trait-associated genotype who exhibit the trait phenotype. This number is expressed as a percent and may differ with age of the individuals.

Phenotype: The phenotype is what is observed. It can be a physical attribute, such as eye color, or a measurable attribute, such as performance on a test. It can be defined categorically (blue eyes or brown eyes, affected or unaffected) or quantitatively (blood pressure, verbal IQ).

Proband: The affected person through whom the other family members are ascertained.

Polygenic inheritance: The phenotype is determined by many genes at different loci, each with small additive effects.

Polymorphism: A common variation in the sequence of DNA at the same site among individuals.

q: The long arm of a chromosome.

Qualitative trait: A trait that is categorical, often dichotomous. The individual either has the trait or does not have it.

Quantitative trait: A trait that shows a continuous and quantitative distribution in the population.

Quantitative trait locus: A chromosomal region that contains a gene that contributes part of the variance of an oligogenic trait.

Recessive: All copies of the gene must have the trait-causing form for the phenotype to be expressed.

Recurrence risk: The probability that a genetic disorder present in a member of a family will recur in another member of the same family or a later generation.

Sex chromosomes: The X and Y chromosomes.

Segregation analysis: A statistical genetic method that assesses the pattern of a trait in families to determine the most likely mode of inheritance.

Acknowledgment

Both authors are supported by NIH Grant No. P50 HD33812.

References

Alarcón, M., & DeFries, J. C. (1995) Quantitative trait locus for reading disability: An alternative test. *Behavior Genetics, 25,* 253.

Bakwin, H. (1973). Reading disability in twins. *Developmental Medicine and Child Neurology, 15,* 184–187.

Berninger, V. (2000). Dyslexia, the invisible, treatable disorder: The story of Einstein's Ninja Turtles. *Learning Disability Quarterly, 23,* 175–195.

Berninger, V. W., Abbott, R. D., Thomson, J. B., & Raskind, W. H. (2001). Language phenotype for reading and writing disability: A family approach. *Scientific Studies of Reading, 5,* 59–106.

Bisgaard, M. L., Eiberg, H., Moller, N., Niebuhr, E., & Mohr, J. (1987). Dyslexia and chromosome 15 heteromorphism: negative LOD score in a Danish material. *Clinical Genetics, 32,* 118–119.

Bonney, G. (1986). Regressive logistic models for familial disease and other binary traits. *Biometrics, 42,* 611–625.

Busse, J., Thomson, J., Abbott, R., & Berninger, V. (1999, August). *Cognitive processes related to dual disability in reading and calculation.* Paper presented at the annual meeting of the American Psychological Association, Boston.

Cardon, L. R., Smith, S. D., Fulker, D. W., Kimberling, W. J., Pennington, B. F., & DeFries, J. C. (1994). Quantitative trait locus for reading disability on chromosome 6. *Science, 266,* 276–279.

Cardon, L. R., Smith, S. D., Fulker, D. W., Kimberling, W. J., Pennington, B. F., & DeFries, J. C. (1995). Quantitative trait locus for reading disability: correction [Letter]. *Science, 268,* 1553.

Castles, A., Datta, H., Gayan, J., & Olson, R. K. (1999). Varieties of developmental reading disorder: Genetic and environmental influences. *Journal of Experimental Child Psychology, 72,* 73–94.

Cohn, J. A., Bornstein, J. D., & Jowell, P. S. (2000). Cystic fibrosis mutations and genetic predisposition to idiopathic chronic pancreatitis. *Medical Clinics of North America, 3,* 621–631, ix.

Daw, E. W., Heath, S. C., & Wijsman, E. M. (1999). Multipoint oligogenic analysis of age-at-onset data with applications to Alzheimer's disease pedigrees. *American Journal of Human Genetics, 64,* 839–851.

Decker, S. N., & DeFries, J. C. (1981). Cognitive abilities in families with reading disabled children. *Developmental Medicine and Child Neurology, 23,* 217–227.

DeFries, J. C., & Fulker, D. W. (1985). Multiple regression analysis of twin data. *Behavior Genetics, 15,* 467–473.

DeFries, J. C., Fulker, D. W., & LaBuda, M. C. (1987). Evidence for a genetic aetiology in reading disability of twins. *Nature, 329,* 538–539.

DeFries, J. C., Singer, S. M., Foch, T. T., & Lewitter, F. I. (1978). Familial nature of reading disability. *British Journal of Psychiatry, 132,* 361–367.

Drew, A. L. (1956). A neurological appraisal of familial congenital word-blindness. *Brain, 79,* 440–460.

Dunn, L. M., & Markwardt, F. C. (1970). *Peabody Individual Achievement Test.* Circle Pines, MN: American Guidance Service.

Fagerheim, T., Raeymaekers, P., Tonnessen, F. E., Pedersen, M., Tranebjaerg, L., & Lubs, H. A. (1999). A new gene (DYX3) for dyslexia is located on chromosome 2. *Journal of Medical Genetics 36,* 664–669.

Fagerheim, T., Raeymaekers, P., Tonnessen, F. E., Sandkuijl, L. A., Lubs, H. A., & Tranebjaerg, L. (2000). A genome wide search for dyslexia loci in a large Norwegian family. *American Journal of Human Genetics, 67*(Suppl.), A1712.

Faraone, S. V., & Doyle, A. E. (2001). The nature and heritability of attention-deficit/hyperactivity disorder. *Child and Adolescent Psychiatric Clinics of North America, 10,* 299–316, viii–ix.

Field, L. L., & Kaplan, B. J. (1998). Absence of linkage of phonological coding dyslexia to chromosome 6p23-p21.3 in a large family data set. *American Journal of Human Genetics, 63,* 1448–1456.

Finucci, J. M., Guthrie, J. T., Childs, A. L., Abbey, H., & Childs, B. (1976). The genetics of specific reading disability. *Annals of Human Genetics, 40,* 1–20.

Fisher, J. H. (1905). Case of congenital word blindness (inability to learn to read). *Ophthalmological Review, 24,* 315–318.

Fisher, S. E., Francks, C., Marlow, A. J., MacPhie, I. L., Newbury, D. F., Cardon, L. R., Ishikawa-Brush, Y., Richardson, A. J., Talcott, J. B., Gayan, J., Olson, R. K., Pennington, B. F., Smith, S. D., DeFries, J. C., Stein, J. F., & Monaco, A. P. (2001). Independent genome-wide scans identify a chromosome 18 quantitative-trait locus influencing dyslexia. *Nature Genetics, 30,* 86–91

Fisher, S. E., Marlow, A. J., Lamb, J., Maestrini, E., Williams, D. F., Richardson, A. J., Weeks, D. E., Stein, J. F., & Monaco, A. P. (1999). A quantitative-trait locus on chromosome 6p influences different aspects of developmental dyslexia. *American Journal of Human Genetics, 64,* 146–156.

Foch, T. T., DeFries, J. C., McClearn, G. E., & Singer, S. M. (1977). Familial patterns of impairment in reading disability. *Journal of Educational Psychology, 69,* 316–329.

Fulker, D. W., Cardon, L. R., DeFries, J. C., Kimberling, W. J., Pennington, B. F., & Smith, S. D. (1991). Multiple regression analysis of sib-pair data on reading to detect quantitative trait loci. *Reading and Writing: An Interdisciplinary Journal, 3,* 299–313.

Gayán, J., Smith, S. D., Cherny, S. S., Cardon, L. R., Fulker, D. W., Brower, A. M., Olson, R. K., Pennington, B. F., & DeFries, J. C. (1999). Quantitative-trait locus for specific language and reading deficits on chromosome 6p. *American Journal of Human Genetics, 64,* 157–164.

Gayther, S. A., Mangion, J., Russell, P., Seal, S., Barfoot, R., Ponder, B. A., Stratton, M. R., & Easton, D. (1997). Variation of risks of breast and ovarian cancer associated with different germline mutations of the BRCA2 gene. *Nature Genetics, 15,* 103–105.

Geschwind, N., & Behan, P. (1982). Left-handedness: association with immune disease, migraine, and developmental learning disorder. *Proceedings of the National Academy of Sciences USA, 79,* 5097–5100.

Gilger, J. W., Borecki, I. B., DeFries, J. C., & Pennington, B. F. (1994). Commingling and segregation analysis of reading performance in families of normal reading probands. *Behavior Genetics, 24,* 345–355.

Gilger, J. W., Pennington, B. F., Harbeck, R. J., DeFries, J. C., Kotzin, B., Green, P., & Smith, S. (1998). A twin and family study of the association between immune system dysfunction and dyslexia using blood serum immunoassay and survey data. *Brain and Cognition, 36,* 310–333.

Grayson, D. A. (1989) Twins reared together: Minimizing shared environmental effects. *Behavior Genetics, 19,* 593–604.

Grigorenko, E. L., Wood, F. B., Meyer, M. S., Hart, L. A., Speed, W. C., Shuster, A., & Pauls, D. L. (1997). Susceptibility loci for distinct components of developmental dyslexia on chromosomes 6 and 15. *American Journal of Human Genetics, 60,* 27–39.

Grigorenko, E. L., Wood, F. B., Meyer, M. S., Pauls, J. E. D., Hart, L. A., & Pauls, D. L. (2001). Linkage studies suggest a possible locus for developmental dyslexia on chromosome 1p. *American Journal of Medical Genetics, 105,* 120–129.

Hallgren, B. (1950). Specific dyslexia (congenital word blindness): A clinical and genetic study. *Acta Psychiatrica et Neurologica, 65*(Suppl.), 1–287.

Heath, S. C. (1997). Markov chain Monte Carlo segregation and linkage anlysis for oligogenic models. *American Journal of Medical Genetics, 61,* 748–760.

Hermann, K., & Norrie, E. (1958). Is congenital word blindness a hereditary type of Gerstmann's syndrome? *Psyciatria et Neurologia, 136,* 59–73.

Hinshelwood, J. (1907). Four cases of congenital word-blindness occurring in the same family. *British Medical Journal, 2,* 1229–1232.

Hohnen, B., & Stevenson, J. (1999). The structure of genetic influences on general cognitive, language, phonological and reading abilities. *Developmental Psychology, 35,* 590–603.

Hsu, L., Wijsman, E. M., Berninger, V. W., Thomson, J. B., & Raskind, W. H. (2002). Familial aggregation of dyslexia phenotypes: Paired correlated measures. *American Journal of Medical Genetics (Neuropsychiatric Genetics Section), 114,* 471–478.

Joseph, J. (2001). Separated twins and the genetics of personality differences: A critique. *American Journal of Psychology, 114,* 1–30.

Kendler, K. S., Neale, M., Kessler, R., Heath, A., & Eaves, L. (1993). A twin study of recent life events and difficulties. *Archives of General Psychiatry, 50,* 789–796.

Lander, E., & Kruglyak, L. (1995). Genetic dissection of complex traits: Guidelines for interpreting and reporting linkage results. *Nature Genetics, 11*, 241–247.

Lewitter, F. I., DeFries, J. C., & Elston, R. C. (1980). Genetic models of reading disability. *Behavior Genetics, 10*, 9–30.

Liang, K. Y., & Zeger, S. L. (1986). Longitudinal data analysis using generalized linear models. *Biometrika, 73*, 13–22.

Lubs, H. A., Duara, R., Levin, B., Jallad, B., Lubs, M.L., Rabin, M., et al. (1991). Dyslexia subtypes—Genetics, behavior, and brain imaging. In D.D. Duane & D.B. Gray (Eds.), *The reading brain: The biological basis of dyslexia* (pp. 89–117). Parkton, MD: York Press.

Morris, D. W., Robinson, L., Turic, D., Duke, M., Webb, V., Milham, C., Hopkin, E., Pound, K., Fernando, S., Easton, M., Hamshere, M., Williams, N., McGuffin, P., Stevenson, J., Krawczak, M., Owen, M. J., O'Donovan, M. C., & Williams, J. (2000). Family-based association mapping provides evidence for a gene for reading disability on chromosome 15q. *Human Molecular Genetics, 9*, 843–848.

Morton, N. (1955). Sequential tests for the detection of linkage. *American Journal of Human Genetics, 7*, 277–318.

Morton, N., & MacLean, C. (1974). Analysis of family resemblance. III. Complex segregation analysis of quantitative traits. *American Journal of Human Genetics, 26*, 489–503.

Nopola-Hemmi, J., Taipale, M., Haltia, T., Lehesjoki, A. E., Voutilainen, A., & Kere, J. (2000). Two translocations of chromosome 15q associated with dyslexia. *Journal of Medical Genetics, 37*, 771–775.

Olson, R. K., Datta, H., Gayan, J., & DeFries, J. (1999). A behavioral-genetic analysis of reading disabilities and component processes. In R. M. Klein & P. A. McMullen (Eds.), *Converging methods for understanding reading and dyslexia* (pp. 133–151). Cambridge, MA: MIT Press.

Olson, R., Forsberg, H., & Wise, B. (1994). Genes, environment, and the development of orthographic skills. In V. W. Berninger (Ed.), *The varieties of orthographic knowledge I: Theoretical and developmental issues* (pp. 27–71). Dordrecht, The Netherlands: Kluwer Academic.

Olson, R., Wise, B., Conners, F., Rack, J., & Fulker, D. (1989). Specific deficits in component reading and language skills: Genetic and environmental influences. *Journal of Learning Disabilities, 22*, 339–348.

Omenn, G. S., & Weber, B. A. (1978). Dyslexia: Search for phenotypic and genetic heterogeneity. *American Journal of Medical Genetics, 1*, 333–342.

Owen, F. W., Adams, P. A., Forrest, T., Stolz, L. M., & Fisher, S. (1971). Learning disorders in children: sibling studies. *Monographs of the Society for Research in Child Development, 36*, 1–77.

Pennington, B. F., Gilger, J. W., Pauls, D., Smith, S. A., Smith, S. D., & DeFries, J. C. (1991). Evidence for major gene transmission of developmental dyslexia. *Journal of the American Medical Association, 266*, 1527–1534.

Pennington, B. F., Smith, S. D., Kimberling, W. J., Green, P. A., & Haith, M. M. (1987). Left-handedness and immune disorders in familial dyslexics. *Archives of Neurology, 44*, 634–639.

Petryshen, T. L., Kaplan, B. J., Liu, M. F., & Field, L. L. (2000). Absence of significant linkage between phonological coding dyslexia and chromosome 6p23–21.3, as determined by use of quantitative-trait methods: Confirmation of qualitative analyses. *American Journal of Human Genetics, 66*, 708–714.

Quinzii, C., & Castellani, C. (2000). The cystic fibrosis transmembrane regulator gene and male infertility. *Journal of Endocrinological Investigation, 10*, 684–689.

Rabin, M., Wen, X. L., Hepburn, M., Lubs, H. A., Feldman, E., & Duara, R. (1993). Suggestive linkage of developmental dyslexia to chromosome 1p34-p36. *Lancet, 342*, 178.

Raskind, W. H. (2001). Current understanding of the genetic basis of reading and spelling disability. *Learning Disability Quarterly, 24*, 141–157.

Raskind, W., Hsu, L., Berninger, V., Thomson, J., & Wijsman, E. (2000). Familial aggregation of phenotypic subtypes in dyslexia. *Behavior Genetics, 30*, 385–399.

Sawyer, D. L., Krishnamani, M. R. S., Hannig, V. L., Garcia, M., Kim, J. K., Haines, J. L., & Phillips, J. A. (1998). Genetic analysis of phonological core deficit dyslexia (PCDD). *American Journal of Human Genetics, 63*, A1776.

Schaid, D. J., Buetow, K., Weeks, D. E., Wijsman, E., Guo, S. W., Ott, J., & Dahl, C. (1999). Discovery of cancer susceptibility genes: Study designs, analytic approaches, and trends in technology. *Journal of the National Cancer Institute Monograph, 26*, 1–16.

Schulte-Körne, G., Grimm, T., Nothen, M. M., Muller-Myhsok, B., Cichon, S., Vogt, I. R., Propping, & Remschmidt, H. (1998). Evidence for linkage of spelling disability to chromosome 15. *American Journal of Human Genetics, 63*, 279–282.

Shaywitz, S. E., Escobar, M. D., Shaywitz, B. A., Fletcher, J. M., & Makuch, R. (1992). Evidence that dyslexia may represent the lower tail of a normal distribution of reading ability. *New England Journal of Medicine, 326*, 145–150.

Smith, S. D., & Goldgar, D. E. (1986). Single gene analyses and their application to learning disabilities. In S. D. Smith (Ed.), *Genetics and learning disabilities* (pp. 47–65). San Diego, CA: College-Hill Press.

Smith, S. D., Kimberling, W. J., & Pennington, B. F. (1991). Screening for multiple genes influencing dyslexia. *Reading and Writing, 3*, 285–298.

Smith, S. D., Kimberling, W. J., Pennington, B. F., &

Lubs, H. A. (1983). Specific reading disability: Identification of an inherited form through linkage analysis. *Science, 219,* 1345–1347.

Smith, S. D., Pennington, B. F., Kimberling, W. J., & Ing, P. S. (1990). Familial dyslexia: Use of genetic linkage data to define subtypes. *Journal of the American Academy of Child and Adolescent Psychiatry, 29,* 204–213.

Stephenson, S. (1907). Six cases of congenital word-blindness affecting three generations of one family. *Ophthalmoscope, 5,* 482–484.

Terwilliger, J. D., & Ott, J. (1992). A haplotype-based "haplotype relative risk" approach to detecting allelic associations. *Human Heredity, 42,* 337–346.

Thomas, C. J. (1905). Congenital "word-blindness" and its treatment. *Ophthalmoscope, 3,* 380–385.

Thomson, G. (1994). Identifying complex disease genes: Progress and paradigms. *Nature Genetics, 8,* 108–110.

Wadsworth, S. J., Olson, R. K., Pennington, B. F., & DeFries, J. C. (2000). Differential genetic etiology of reading disability as a function of IQ. *Journal of Learning Disabilities, 33,* 192–199.

Wechsler, D. I. (1981). *Wechsler Adult Intelligence Scale—Revised.* San Antonio, TX: Psychological Corporation.

Wechsler, D. I. (1992). *Wechsler Intelligence Scale for Children—Third edition.* San Antonio, TX: Psychological Corporation.

Wijsman, E. M., & Amos, C. I. (1997). Genetic analysis of simulated oligogenic traits in nuclear and extended pedigrees: summary of GAW10 contributions. *Genetic Epidemiology, 14,* 719–735.

Wijsman, E. M., Peterson, D., Leutenegger, A. L., Thomson, J. B., Goddard, K. A., Hsu, L., Berninger, V. W., & Raskind, W. H. (2000). Segregation analysis of phenotypic components of learning disabilities: Nonword memory and digit span. *American Journal of Human Genetics, 67,* 631–646.

Willcutt, E. G., Pennington, B. F., & DeFries, J. C. (2000). Twin study of the etiology of comorbidity between reading disability and attention-deficit/hyperactivity disorder. *American Journal of Medical Genetics, 96,* 293–301.

Wolff, P. H., & Melngailis, I. (1994). Family patterns of developmental dyslexia: Clinical findings. *American Journal of Medical Genetics, 54,* 122–131.

Zhao, L. P., Grove, J., & Quiaoit, F. (1992). A method for assessing patterns of familial resemblance in complex complex human pedigrees, with as application to the nevus-count data in Utah kindreds. *American Journal of Human Genetics, 51,* 178–190.

III
EFFECTIVE INSTRUCTION

17

Effective Remediation of Word Identification and Decoding Difficulties in School-Age Children with Reading Disabilities

Maureen W. Lovett
Roderick W. Barron
Nancy J. Benson

I don't have any trouble with the sentences; it's the words that get in my way.
—A 9-YEAR-OLD STRUGGLING READER (2000)

The cognitive psychology of reading and its contributing processes enjoys a long and honorable scientific history spanning more than 100 years, from the pioneering interests of Cattell (1886) and Huey (1908) to current research in the cognitive neuroscience of reading and its disorders (e.g., Pugh, Mencl, Jenner, Katz, Lee, et al., 2000; Pugh, Mencl, Jenner, Katz, Frost, et al., 2001; Simos et al., 2002) and molecular genetic studies of the transmission of reading ability and disability across generations (Grigorenko, 2001). As Pennington (1997) phrased it, reading can be considered "a cognitive science success story" (p. 13).

Similarly, it has been recognized for more than a century that a sizable minority of otherwise intelligent, healthy, and well-developing children experience unexpected failures in learning to read (Hinshelwood, 1917; Morgan, 1896). Surprisingly, it has only been in the last two decades that there has been a scientific literature worth citing with respect to what constitutes effective in-

struction for these children in their struggle to learn to read. In this chapter, we review the literature on reading acquisition difficulties in children, evidence on the most persistent underlying learning deficits that appear central to reading disabilities, and what is known to date of what constitutes effective remediation.

Although the existence of developmental reading disabilities has been acknowledged for the past century, it is only within the past 10–15 years that reliable evidence from controlled evaluations has been reported on its remediation. In the mid–1980s, there was almost no scientifically credible evidence to indicate that reading disabilities were amenable to intervention or that any one remedial approach was better than any other (Gittelman, 1983; Hewison, 1982; Lovett, 1992). This dearth of evidence regarding the effectiveness of remediation over so many decades led to inevitable questions about the amenability of the disorder to treatment (Lovett, 1997, 1999).

Methodological and Design Limitations of Past Intervention Research on Reading Disabilities

Few studies were reported in the mid to late 1980s that evaluated the efficacy of interventions in a controlled research design in which alternative intervention approaches were systematically compared. Failures to include a control group and to compare two or more interventions rendered reported evidence as little more than anecdotal in import (Lovett & Barron, 2002). Only when alternative approaches are evaluated in controlled designs is there an opportunity to separate treatment-specific effects from general treatment effects (e.g., halo effects due to inclusion in a special program, individualized attention, access to a teacher/therapist with specialized reading disabilities expertise) and change due to maturation and experience.

Until relatively recently, the intervention literature on reading disorders has been characterized by serious measurement and methodological problems. There has been limited recognition of the fact that outcome is necessarily a multidimensional and multivariate construct, and its measurement is complex. Even in recent years, measurement issues continue to plague otherwise successful intervention protocols yielding positive and specific intervention effects: It is extremely difficult, for example, to adequately measure reading comprehension skills in a child with word identification problems and to evaluate whether word identification gains have yielded improved text reading and comprehension abilities (Berninger & Abbott, 1994; Levy, Abello, & Lysynchuk, 1997). The efficacy of an intervention requires assessment with respect to the transfer, generalization, and maintenance of its effects, yet basic questions remain regarding their reliable and valid measurement (Lyon, 1996; Lyon & Moats, 1997; Shanahan & Barr, 1995).

It is also a concern that the outcome measures that have been used in many studies have varied enormously in their power and sensitivity to treatment-related change. Many standardized measures with steep item gradients, for example, allow relatively few chances for an improving reader with disabilities to demonstrate newly acquired reading skills before item difficulty levels rise and ceilings are quickly reached (Lovett, Hinchley, & Benson, 1997). As can be expected, experimental measures with more trials per level of difficulty result in more visible gains and better opportunities to demonstrate treatment-related change over the short term. At present, many questions remain open regarding the best measurement models for evaluating the success or failure of a given intervention (Lyon & Moats, 1997). The lack of power inherent to traditional measurement choices has perhaps masked the effects of some potentially promising remedial approaches.

Characterizing the Core Deficits Contributing to Reading Acquisition Failure and Assessing Children's Response to Remediation

Despite these challenges, the contributions of intervention researchers in the past 15 years have been scientifically sophisticated at a level unprecedented in the field only two decades ago. With an ambitious research funding program announced by the National Institute of Child Health and Human Development (NICHD) in the United States in the early 1990s, clear incentives to conduct rigorous research on remedial interventions for phonologically based reading disorders became available (Lyon, 1995; Lyon & Moats, 1997; Moats & Foorman, 1997); and large-scale scientific research on what constitutes effective remediation for childhood reading disabilities started in earnest. Advances in our understanding of the neurobiological and genetic substrates of reading disability and other developmental learning disorders in the mid-1990s and beyond (Filipek, 1995, 1999; Grigorenko, 2001; Grigorenko et al., 1997; Pennington, 1997, 1999; Shaywitz et al., 1998) have focused increased research attention on the nature and underlying causes of these developmental learning disorders and the extent to which the underlying cognitive processing deficits can be ameliorated with effective intervention methods.

Many children who experience serious difficulty learning to read have precursor problems in highly specific aspects of speech and language development. Prospective research studies have confirmed the relationship between early specific speech and language difficulties and later reading disabilities in childhood (Bishop & Adams, 1990; Gathercole & Baddeley, 1987; Scarborough, 1990, 1998). There has been remarkable consensus in the learning disabilities literature in the past two decades that a core language-related deficit associated with and predictive of reading acquisition failure involves a domain of linguistic competence known as "phonological awareness." Children with significant reading difficulties typically exhibit a range of signature deficits in their explicit awareness of and ability to manipulate the sound structure of spoken words (Brady, 1997; Snowling & Hulme, 1993). Whether reading disorders are defined on the basis of a significant discrepancy between measured IQ and actual reading achievement or simply on the basis of significant underachievement in reading based on age or grade-level expectations, the deficits identified as potentially causal to this class of learning disorders appear to be concentrated within the word identification and phonological processing domains (Fletcher et al., 1994; Francis, Shaywitz, Stuebing, Shaywitz & Fletcher, 1996; Stanovich & Siegel, 1994).

Disabled readers have been characterized as having a dysfunction "in the phonological component of their natural capacity for language" (Liberman, Shankweiler, & Liberman, 1989, p. 1). Phonological awareness represents a multifaceted and complex set of processing and metalinguisitic capabilities recognized to have different developmental trajectories (Barron, 1998; Goswami & Bryant, 1990). Reading disabled individuals often experience significant difficulty segmenting and differentiating individual speech sounds in spoken words, blending individual speech sounds to form a spoken word, and effectively using phonological codes to aid working memory performance (Liberman & Mattingly, 1985; Mann, 1986; Stanovich, 1991, 1994; Wagner & Torgesen, 1987). It is thought that all these difficulties may stem from a more basic problem in the ability to form phonological representations and to encode phonological information accurately (Brady, 1997; Elbro, Borstrom, & Petersen, 1998).

This basic dysfunction in phonological processing is thought to underlie the struggling reader's defining deficits in acquiring alphabetic and phonologically based reading skills (Brady, 1997; Lovett, 1997, 1999; Lovett & Barron, 2003; Torgesen, Wagner, & Rashotte, 1997). The significance of these deficits in phonological processing has been emphasized by findings of different profiles of brain activation while doing phonologically demanding tasks—a distinct "neurobiological signature" for individuals with reading disorders revealed in functional neuroimaging studies (Shaywitz et al., 1998) which compare disabled and able readers of similar age and background. Behaviorally and neurobiologically, the weight of evidence identifies phonological processing deficits, disruptions in word identification learning, and difficulty acquiring the alphabetic principle as defining features of developmental reading disabilities.

Deficits in these areas of speech and language development have been characterized as an "arrest in development" (Bruck, 1992); and they are known to persist into adulthood for individuals with childhood histories of reading disability (Bruck, 1992, 1998; Felton & Brown, 1990; Scarborough, 1984; Shaywitz et al., 1999). In one study, even the highest-functioning adults with dyslexia exhibited lower levels of phonemic awareness than did third-grade children with lower reading and spelling achievement (Bruck, 1992). Recognition of the depth and longevity of these phonological processing deficits in individuals with developmental reading disorders led to concerns about whether phonologically based reading disabilities were amenable to remediation (e.g., Wagner, Torgesen, & Rashotte, 1994). New incentives and funding opportunities from the NICHD encouraged scientists to conduct rigorous research evaluating remedial interventions for phonologically based reading disabilities (Lyon, 1995; Lyon & Moats, 1997; Moats & Foorman, 1997) and early intervention programs for young children constitutionally and environmentally at-risk for reading acquisition failure.

Early Intervention Studies

Because of these incentives, in the past decade, several controlled and comparative research studies have been reported assessing the efficacy of different approaches to the remediation and/or prevention of reading acquisition problems in the early elementary grades (Foorman, Francis, Fletcher, Schatschneider, & Mehta, 1998; Foorman et al., 1997; Scanlon & Vellutino, 1997; Torgesen et al., 1997, 1999; Vellutino, Scanlon, Sipay, et al., 1996). Foorman and colleagues (1998) conducted an important and influential study assessing the reading development of 285 children in first and second grades across 66 classrooms in several Title 1 schools in Texas. These investigators sought to understand how the nature and type of letter–sound instruction in early reading programs would interact with individual differences in the children's entry-level skills in phonological awareness. Subjects were children who scored in the bottom 18% on an early literacy assessment conducted by the school district.

Three types of experimental classroom programs were compared with the standard curriculum in the district. The three experimental instruction programs differed in the type of phonics instruction offered: One provided direct instruction in letter–sound correspondences and practice with decodable text (direct code); another offered less direct instruction in letter–sound correspondences embedded in authentic literature samples (embedded code); and a third provided implicit instruction in the alphabetic code while children read authentic text (implicit code). All teachers received ongoing training experiences specific to their program. Children from the direct code instructional condition demonstrated better word identification skills and steeper learning curves in word reading than did those receiving implicit code instruction. This advantage was greater for those children who entered the programs with the lowest levels of phonological awareness. Although the direct code instruction did not normalize the reading achievement of all instructed children, Torgesen (2000) derived a population-based failure rate from this study computed at 6%. As Fletcher and Lyon (1998) discuss, however, a failure rate of 6% for any instructional method represents a significant reduction in the 15–20% of students with reading difficulty in the United States currently. The findings of Foorman and colleagues (1998) provide important evidence that explicit instruction in letter–sound correspondences can prevent reading underachievement in children at risk for reading failure because of poor phonological awareness at school entry or a lack of literacy experiences in the home environment (see also Juel & Minden-Cupp, 2000; Torgesen et al., 1999; Vellutino et al., 1996).

Torgesen and colleagues (1999) also reported a landmark early intervention study. At-risk children entering kindergarten were included in the study, and the participants were children who scored in the bottom 12th percentile on kindergarten measures of letter knowledge and phonological awareness. Children were randomly assigned to one of four instructional conditions. The first condition provided phonological awareness and synthetic phonics training (the Lindamood Auditory Discrimination in Depth program) including explicit instruction in articulatory-based phonological awareness and much practice in phonetic decoding and word identification (ADD). The second condition also provided explicit phonics instruction but allocated far more instructional time on application to the reading and writing of connected text materials and the acquisition of a sight vocabulary (embedded phonics, or EP). A third condition provided regular classroom support (i.e., tutorial group), and the fourth was a no-treatment control group. Children in the experimental conditions received one-to-one instruction in 20-minute sessions 4 days a week over 2½ years. At the end of this 2½-year instructional period, children who had received the ADD instruction were the strongest readers when average scores were assessed. Both their nonword reading (Word Attack) and word reading (Word Identification) skills fell overall within the average range. Their advantage relative to the other groups was not consistently established, however, on word identification and reading comprehension measures at the end of second grade. Torgesen and his colleagues note, in addition, that there was substantial variability in response to the instruction, with 38% and 39% of the ADD group scoring less than the 30th percentile on the word attack and word identification subtests, respectively. Similar to calculations for the Foorman and colleagues (1998) study, population-based estimates suggest that if the strongest condition were to be applied more broadly, approximately 4% of children would remain relatively weak in decoding ability and 5% in sight word reading at the end of second grade (Torgesen, 2000). These investigators concluded that despite enormous advances in our understanding of the nature and etiology of reading disabilities, there remained limited knowledge about how to effectively remediate the more *severe* forms of developmental reading disability and help these children to become independent and fluent readers (Torgesen et al., 1997, 1999; Torgesen, Alexander, et al., 2001).

Can the Deficits of Older Reading Disabled Children Be Remediated?

Given the persistence of reading disorders and the negative sequelae of cumulative reading experience deficits and more widespread academic difficulties in the later grades (Shaywitz et al., 1999; Stanovich, 1986), it might be expected that it would be easier to prevent reading acquisition failure in at-risk children than to remediate it in older children diagnosed with reading disability. There is evidence, for example, that first-grade reading achievement is a remarkably strong predictor of high school reading achievement (Cunningham & Stanovich, 1997), reinforcing the conclusion that the gap between able and less able readers widens rather than decreases with time and development (Rayner, Foorman, Perfetti, Pesetsky, & Seidenberg, 2001). Research on adolescent and adult outcomes of children with developmental reading disorders indicates that reading ability *does* improve with age and intervention for most individuals with reading disabilities, but that the signature deficits of reading disorder typically persist into adulthood, particularly in more severe cases. Phonological deficits persist, even in cases with relatively good literacy outcomes (Bruck 1992, 1998; Scarborough, 1984; Shaywitz et al., 1999). Problems also frequently persist with spelling accuracy, word recognition speed, and reading rate.

Prospective longitudinal data from the Connecticut Longitudinal Study reveals that the natural course of reading disorder follows a deficit rather than a developmental lag model over time (Francis et al., 1996; Shaywitz et al., 1999). When children who met criteria for reading disability in grades 2 through 6 were compared with normally developing children with average and above-average reading skills in those grades, the persistently poor readers continued to demonstrate deficits in phonological coding in adolescence and to experience continuing problems in reading, spelling, and reading rate (Shaywitz et al., 1999). These results were considered "sobering" by the authors, particularly as children in the persistent poor reader group all had received special education services. There was no evidence that children in the persistent RD group had caught up in their reading skills by high school. In fact, another study has revealed that typical special education placements in grades 4 and 5 accelerate students' reading development only by .04 standard deviations over the rate of growth achieved by these children in their regular classroom placements (Hanushek, Kain, & Rivkin, 1998). *Can* the deficits of older disabled readers be effectively remediated?

Remediation Studies with Older Children

Results from remediation studies focusing on the phonological reading deficits of older children with reading disabilities have also been reported in recent years (Olson, Wise, Ring, & Johnson, 1997; Torgesen, Alexander, et al., 2001; Wise & Olson, 1995; Wise, Ring, Sessions, & Olson, 1997). Solid converging evidence is now available demonstrating that significant improvement *can* be attained on speech-based and phonological reading measures for both older children with reading disabilities *and* young children at significant risk for reading disability (Foorman et al., 1998; Lovett et al., 1994; Lovett, Lacerenza, Borden, Frijters, et al., 2000; Olson et al., 1997; Torgesen et al., 1997, 1999; Torgesen, Alexander, et al., 2001; Vellutino et al., 1996); these results confirm that phonologically based decoding and beginning reading skills are "teachable aspects of reading for most children" (Moats & Foorman, 1997, p. 188). Additional evidence from controlled comparative intervention studies has demonstrated that, with focused and systematic intervention, measurable progress in phonological reading skills *can* be achieved throughout the elementary school years even with the most severely disabled readers of a clinical sample (Lovett & Steinbach, 1997; Lovett, Steinbach, & Frijters, 2000).

Significant questions remain, particularly regarding the normalization of phonologically based and fluent reading skills in reading disabled individuals (Foorman & Torgesen, 2001; Torgesen, Rashotte, & Alexander, 2001; Wolf & Katzir-Cohen, 2001). Progress has been made, however, in identifying some of the ingredients of effective remediation. A recent empirical review concludes that effective reading interventions with struggling readers must include "(a) phonological awareness training, (b) systematic phonics instruction that is linked to spelling, and (c) oral reading practice with decodable texts (i.e., texts that include only words using the accumulating set of letter–sound correspondences that have been taught" (Rayner et al., 2001, p. 45). These conclusions emphasize the necessity of direct remediation of phonological awareness deficits, systematic and explicit instruction in letter- and letter cluster–sound mappings, and reinforcement of word identification learning through ample text reading practice using controlled decodable reading vocabulary.

Within the past decade, there have been mixed results and a range of outcomes from remediation studies with readers who are more severely disabled and with older children. Foorman and colleagues (1997) compared the relative efficacy of three remediation programs for second- and third-graders with identified reading disorders; the programs differed in instructional approach and in the size of the print-to-sound unit emphasized in reading instruction. In analytic phonics, words were segmented into onset and rime units, in synthetic phonics into letter–sound units, and in sight word approaches instructed as whole words. After the instruction, the synthetic phonics group appeared superior to the other two groups on testing, but their treatment advantage was not confirmed when the influences of

demographic and verbal IQ differences were statistically controlled. This constitutes a particularly important qualification to this study because random assignment to instructional condition was not feasible. The synthetic phonics subjects did demonstrate greater gains in phonological analysis ability relative to the other two groups, but this advantage did not generalize to superior performance on measures of word identification skill.

Reports by other researchers have also focused on deficient phonological processing and the phonologically based reading deficits of older reading disabled children. Olson, Wise, and their colleagues (Olson et al., 1997; Wise & Olson, 1995; Wise, Ring, & Olson, 2000; Wise et al., 1997) conducted an intervention study in which they combined features of an oral–motor program for training phonological awareness, reading, and spelling skills (the Lindamood ADD Program; Lindamood & Lindamood, 1975, cited in Torgesen et al., 1999) with their own computer-based reading training program (Reading with Orthographic and Speech Support, or ROSS). Two groups of children with reading disabilities from grades 2 through 5 received phonological decoding and digitized speech support to help them read unknown words in story reading on the computer; with this training experience, one group received additional phonological awareness training using the ADD oral–motor methods and the other group received extra training in reading comprehension strategies. There was no control group in this study. The group that received extra phonological awareness (PA or ADD) training was superior in phonological awareness and phonological decoding skill both right after training and at 1-year follow-up testing. The PA group's superiority on phonological measures did not, however, result in superior word recognition performance at 1- or 2-year follow-up assessments. These negative findings 1 and 2 years after remediation were contrary to the expectation that the PA group's advantage in phonological awareness and nonword decoding skills would be associated with greater word recognition development over time (Olson et al., 1997; Share, 1995). Wise and colleagues (2000) concluded that "this amount of this type of (PA) training has not been sufficient for children to transfer the improved phonological skills to independent accurate reading compared to less intensive phonologically supported instruction" (p. 202). Individual differences were apparent however: Younger, lower-performing readers were found to gain more from intervention and to benefit more from phonological training instruction than were older, higher-performing children (Wise et al., 2000).

Generalization of phonological processing gains and improvements in nonword decoding skills to other aspects of reading skill development has posed a hurdle for which relatively few remediation programs have proved effective. Despite the gains observed in children's phonologically based word attack and decoding skills, many investigators have found that these often sizable gains do not reliably generalize to other dimensions of reading development. Children who, after intervention, could "sound out" new words or nonwords were not always improved relative to other instructional groups in their word recognition, text reading, or reading comprehension skills. Generalization failures have been reported for many intervention methods evaluated in the literature (e.g., Olson et al., 1997; Torgesen et al., 1997) and for interventions that we assessed in our early remediation studies at The Hospital for Sick Children in Toronto (Lovett, Ransby, Hardwick, Johns, & Donaldson, 1989; Lovett, Warren-Chaplin, Ransby, & Borden, 1990). As Moats and Foorman (1997) note in their summary of several notable intervention studies with positive findings,

> These gains are to be celebrated although . . . generalization and transfer of decoding proficiency to fluent word recognition and better reading comprehension was not automatic and constitutes a next phase of remediation that needs . . . additional study. (p. 188)

Wise and colleagues (2000, p. 231) conclude their report with a parallel observation:

> Researchers must try to specify how best to achieve transfer from improved phonological skills to greater long-term growth in read-

ing. . . . We believe that future research should include longer training times and investigate supplementary methods to increase automaticity and application, to help children to transfer improved phonological skills to similarly improved reading even after training has ceased.

Generalization in Disabled Readers' Response to Remediation: Components of Effective Instruction for Children with Reading Disabilities

Torgesen and colleagues (1997) have suggested that the generalization problem in these intervention studies may reflect in part the complexity of the processing deficits seen in readers with more severe disabilities. In fact, it is now acknowledged that the core processing impairments of many children with reading disabilities extend beyond the realm of phonological awareness to other domains of function. Wolf and Bowers have identified the deficit in naming speed as potentially causal to developmental reading disability (Bowers & Wolf, 1993; Wolf, 1991; Wolf & Bowers, 1999, 2000). Both phonological awareness and naming speed deficits impede reading acquisition at the lexical level and the existence of both deficits in combination are known to constitute a risk factor for more severe forms of reading disability than demonstration of either deficit separately (Lovett, Steinbach, & Frijters, 2000; Wolf, Bowers, & Biddle, 2000).

Many of the generalization failures experienced by children with reading disabilities could also be attributed to a more general difficulty with acquiring effective, flexible word identification strategies and with monitoring and evaluating the effectiveness of their strategic efforts. Difficulties with specific aspects of executive functioning and strategy learning appear to exist in readers with learning disabilities independent of their phonological processing difficulties (Levin, 1990; Swanson, 1999a; Swanson & Alexander, 1997). Recent research has also highlighted the specificity of the transfer-of-learning deficit, however: Transfer-of-learning problems for children with reading disabilities appear specific to printed language learning and are not evident on other learning tasks with similar cognitive demands but no phonological processing requirements (Benson, 2000; Benson, Lovett, & Kroeber, 1997).

Our clinical research program at The Hospital for Sick Children in Toronto has a long history of specific interest in generalization and transfer-of-learning questions. Difficulties in achieving generalization of intervention gains have motivated much of our recent remediation research with severely reading disabled children referred to our laboratory classrooms. We have described research in which children were randomly assigned to one of two remedial reading programs or to an active control treatment that worked on helping them acquire better study, organizational, and problem-solving skills (CSS for Classroom Survival Skills Program; Lovett et al., 1994; Lovett & Steinbach, 1997; Lovett, Steinbach, & Frijters, 2000). Both of the reading interventions targeted the problem of generalization of instructional gains in word identification learning, but they addressed this problem with quite different remedial approaches and at different levels of print-to-sound segmentation.

The PHAB/DI (Phonological Analysis and Blending/Direct Instruction) Program consisted of lessons from the direct instruction decoding programs developed by Engelmann and his colleagues at the University of Oregon; these programs train phonological analysis, phonological blending, and letter–sound association skills in the context of intensive systematic word recognition and decoding instruction (see Reading Mastery I/II Fast Cycle, and Corrective Reading Program: Engelmann & Bruner, 1988; Engelmann, Carnine, & Johnson, 1988; Engelmann et al., 1988). The other remedial reading program was called WIST (Word Identification Strategy Training). WIST has a strong metacognitive focus, instructs through a teacher-led dialogue, and teaches the children how to use and monitor the application of four metacognitive decoding strategies. The WIST program was developed in our laboratory classrooms at The Hospital for Sick Children and is based in part on the original Benchmark School Word Identification/Vocabulary Development Program developed by Irene Gaskins and her colleagues (Gaskins, Downer, & Gaskins,

1986). WIST adapts the Benchmark Program's dialogue structure for strategy instruction, their keywords, and their Compare/Contrast strategy (a strategy of "Word Identification by Analogy"). WIST differs from the Benchmark Program in its inclusion of three additional word identification strategies ("Vowel Variation"—trying variant vowel pronunciations in order of the frequency with which they occur in spoken English; "Peeling Off" prefixes and suffixes in a multisyllabic word; and "Spy"—spying the part(s) of a word you already know), its direct training focus on the subskills necessary for strategy implementation, and its provision of a metacognitive "Game Plan" to train flexibility in strategy choice and evaluation of the success of those choices.

Both PHAB/DI and WIST recognize the need for subsyllabic segmentation during word identification learning and its importance to attaining transfer of learning to uninstructed words (Lovett, 1991; Lovett et al., 1990). The PHAB/DI and WIST programs, however, work on subsyllabic segmentation using subword units of different size: PHAB/DI emphasizes the smallest spelling-to-sound units (letter–sound) and WIST focuses on recognition of larger subsyllabic units, particularly the rime. Both remedial programs attempt to promote generalization of word identification skills in different ways—PHAB/DI through intensive remediation of core sound analysis and blending deficits in the context of systematic decoding training, WIST by teaching a set of flexible and effective word identification strategies and the specific skills and content required to implement them successfully. Every lesson of the PHAB/DI and WIST programs includes practice using new word identification skills in context—by reading connected text with controlled vocabulary and at carefully selected levels of difficulty.

In a controlled research design, both the PHAB/DI and the WIST programs proved far more effective than our previous intervention programs (Lovett, Ransby, & Barron, 1988; Lovett et al., 1989, 1990) from the perspective of achieving generalization of remedial gains: PHAB/DI- and WIST-trained children were reliably improved on several standardized and experimental test measures and demonstrated significant generalization on word reading measures including transfer probes varying in their distance from instructed target words included in the PHAB/DI and WIST lessons (Lovett et al., 1994; Lovett & Steinbach, 1997; Lovett, Steinbach, & Frijters, 2000). Although both programs were associated with large positive effects, different patterns of transfer were observed following the two programs on some measures, confirming the existence of some treatment-specific effects. The phonological program, PHAB/DI, was associated with broader-based and deeper generalization specifically within the phonological skill domain (speech- and print-based), and the WIST program, with its strategy training focus, resulted in broader-based generalization for real English words (i.e., generalization was observed on regular *and* exception words).

Three findings from this line of research were particularly encouraging: (1) the demonstration of generalization within the domain of word identification learning, (2) the finding that the phonological skills and decoding performance of children with severe reading disabilities could be improved with focused intensive remediation of this type, and (3) that positive effects were achieved even with later (e.g., grades 5–6) intervention (Lovett & Steinbach, 1997) and even for the most disabled children of a very reading disabled sample (Lovett, Steinbach, & Frijters, 2000). The phonological processing and reading deficits of these children were not ameliorated after this short-term intervention, but both print- and speech-based phonological skills were reliably improved and moved closer to age-appropriate expectations. After only 35 hours of instruction, PHAB/DI and WIST graduates typically were not reading at grade level; however, they demonstrated markedly improved letter–sound knowledge, better decoding abilities, and more accurate word identification skills. Before their remedial interventions, these children with severe reading disabilities were incorrectly identifying one-syllable words such as *way, left,* and *put*: After PHAB/DI or WIST instruction, many of these children were able to decode accurately (although often slowly) challenging multisyllabic words such as *unintelligible, mistakenly,* and *disengaged.* (These examples are taken from the test protocols of a 10-year-old girl with a reading disability.)

In a subsequent study, we used a sequential crossover design to address the question of whether phonologically based remediation is sufficient to achieve the best remedial outcomes for children with severe reading disabilities, or whether a combination of phonological and strategy training approaches would produce superior outcomes (Lovett, Lacerenza, Borden, et al., 2000). The efficacy of a combination of the PHAB/DI and WIST programs was compared to that of longer-term intervention with each approach separately. Eighty-five children, 7–13 years of age and severely reading disabled, were randomly assigned to 70 hours of remedial instruction in one of five program sequences: PHAB/DI → WIST; WIST → PHAB/DI; PHAB/DI × 2; WIST × 2; or CSS → MATH (Classroom Survival Skills → Mathematics, a control treatment offering study skills and then math instruction). Each child's skills were assessed at five time points: before, at three points during, and following 70 hours of intervention; this testing schedule allowed a closer examination of the *time course* of remedial gains and their generalization within the different instructional conditions. Generalized treatment effects were demonstrated on standardized measures of word recognition, passage comprehension, and nonword reading, confirming the effectiveness of the present instructional programs on multiple indices of reading skill acquisition.

The most critical findings of this research were the demonstration of superior outcomes and steeper learning curves for those children who had received a sequential combination of the phonological and strategy-based instruction. A combination of PHAB/DI and WIST proved superior to either intervention alone on measures of phonological reading skill (nonword reading), tests of letter–sound and keyword knowledge, and three word identification measures (two of near and far transfer words and the third of uninstructed multisyllabic challenge words). These results provide evidence of the separate instructional contributions of both the phonological and the strategy-based methods. More important, these findings demonstrate that generalization from nonword decoding to other reading measures can be best achieved with a *combination* of effective remedial compo-

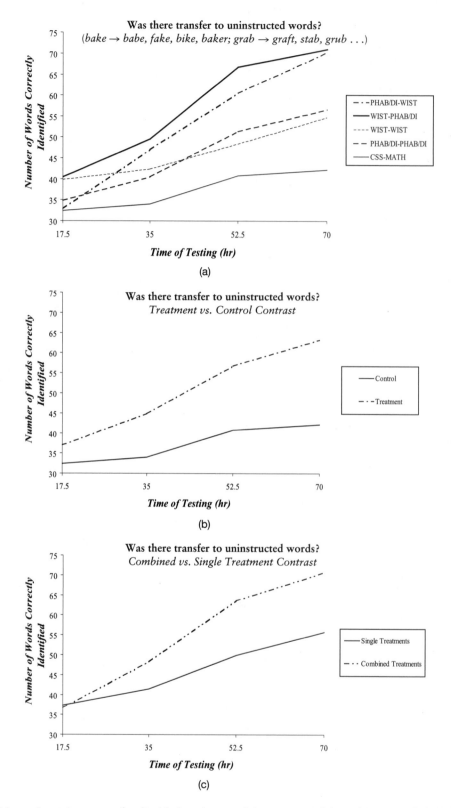

FIGURE 17.1a–c. Learning curves for disabled readers receiving a sequential combination of phonological and strategy-based instruction (PHAB/DI → WIST; WIST → PHAB/DI); phonological (PHAB/DI) or strategy-based instruction alone (WIST); or a control treatment program (CSS → MATH). From Lovett, Lacerenza, Borden, Frijters, et al. (2000). Copyright 2000 by the American Psychological Association. Reprinted by permission.

nents. Figure 17.1 summarizes representative learning curves and average group outcomes on a transfer test of word identification skill.

The results of this intervention research suggest that phonologically based approaches alone are *not* sufficient for achieving optimal remedial outcomes with individuals with reading disabilities. While systematic phonologically based, deficit-directed interventions appear necessary to achieve gains, generalization of those gains is more probable if a *multidimensional* approach to core reading-related deficits is used. Our findings indicate that faster learning and superior outcomes are attained when a broader-based intervention approach is adopted—particularly one combining direct and dialogue-based instruction, explicitly teaching children different levels of subsyllabic segmentation, and training them in the acquisition and effective use of multiple decoding strategies. The central importance of strategy instruction and the promotion of a flexible approach to word identification and text reading tasks cannot be overemphasized when it comes to achieving generalization of remedial gains.

Conclusions from this research are compatible with recent findings from a meta-analysis of the treatment outcome literature on learning disabilities: Swanson and Hoskyn (1998) conducted a rigorous review of 180 intervention studies; they concluded that the optimal approach in instructing children with learning disabilities was a combined intervention model that included both direct instruction and strategy instruction methods. Additional work by Swanson (1999b) has focused specifically on meta-analytic analyses of remedial reading interventions. Again, Swanson has demonstrated in this report that a combined direct instruction/strategy training approach is particularly important when outcomes in the domain of reading comprehension and text reading are considered.

The PHAST Track Reading Program

Based on the results previously summarized, our research team at The Hospital for Sick Children worked to integrate these two approaches into a single intervention program for struggling readers. Called the PHAST Track Reading Program (PHAST for Phonological *and* Strategy Training), this new program begins with PHAB/DI's program of phonological and letter–sound training and uses it as a framework on which each of the four WIST strategies are introduced and scaffolded. A detailed description of the instructional design of the PHAST Track Reading Program, of its component instructional parts (PHAB/DI and WIST), of the dialogue structure used for the acquisition and monitoring of each word identification strategy, and of sample lesson materials developed for each program section has been published (Lovett, Lacerenza, & Borden, 2000).

This part of the PHAST program covers lessons 1–70 and focuses on the development of the five PHAST word identification strategies and acquisition of the prerequisite skills and knowledge needed to implement them successfully. The five PHAST word identification strategies are sounding out (the left-to-right letter–sound decoding strategy of PHAB/DI), rhyming (word identification by analogy, using a bank of known keywords to decode an unknown word with the same spelling pattern), peeling off (stripping prefixes and suffixes from a multisyllabic word to get a smaller root word which can then be decoded using one of the other strategies), vowel alert (trying variable vowel sounds in the order in which they occur in spoken English to see which pronunciation gives a word the child knows), and I spy (seeking smaller parts of a word that the child already knows). Every lesson includes some instructional time acquiring the skills and knowledge to execute the strategies successfully. For sounding out, the child learns the constituent letter–sounds of words in an order specified by the Reading Mastery I/II Fast Cycle or the Corrective Reading programs. To use the rhyming strategy, the child learns a corpus of keywords, which represent 120 high-frequency spelling patterns in the English language (adapted from the original Benchmark School Word Identification/Vocabulary Development Program [Gaskins et al., 1986]). Figure 17.2 lists the PHAST keywords. Peeling off requires the recognition of affixes whch are taught in a specific order dictated by frequency of occurrence (e.g.,

a	**e**	**i**	**o**	**u**
grab	he	hi	go	club
place	speak	nice	boat	luck
pack	scream	kick	job	glue
dad	ear	did	rock	bug
made	eat	slide	dog	drum
rag	red	wife	oil	jump
page	see	pig	broke	fun
nail	need	right	fold	skunk
rain	queen	like	on	up
take	keep	file	phone	bus
talk	sweet	will	long	use
all	tell	him	zoo	nut
am	them	time	food	
name	ten	in	good	
champ	end	find	look	
man	tent	vine	fool	**y**
and	her	king	cop	
nap	yes	sink	for	cry
car	test	ship	more	baby
shark	let	squirt	corn	gym
smart	flew	this	nose	
has		wish	not	
smash		it	could	
mask		white	round	
cat		dive	out	
ate		give	cow	
gave			glow	
paw			down	
pay			boy	

FIGURE 17.2. The PHAST Keyword Bank: A physical organization of keyword spelling patterns by vowel and rime units. From the Benchmark School Word Identification/Vocabulary Development Program by Gaskins, Downer, and Gaskins (1986). Copyright 1986 by Benchmark School. Adapted by permission. Figure from Lovett, Lacerenza, and Borden (2000). Copyright 2000 by PRO-ED, Inc. Reprinted by permission.

pre-, re-, un-, -ing, -ly, and -ment). Vowel alert requires the learning of short and long pronunciations for single vowels and instruction in vowel combinations and other variants (ea, oo, ie, ow).

PHAST is designed to teach the child context-free word identification skills and strategies and to promote their immediate and effective application to the desired goal—reading connected text for meaning. The 70 daily PHAST lessons include many opportunities for the children to practice applying a metacognitive Game Plan in regular story reading and in various challenge word games. In the Game Plan, children choose, use, check, and score their application of the five PHAST strategies. The Game Plan dialogue both guides their implementation of the different strategies they have selected for a particular unknown word and monitors the effectiveness of strategy application in decoding the word sucessfully. The game Pyramid Challenge provides an attractive gameboard on which readers navigate a pyramid's different levels and tunnels by correctly decoding difficult challenge words. The challenge games present the readers—now equipped with a treasure chest of several effective decoding strategies—a playing field on which to practice various decoding plans and further refine their skills and strategies. Figure 17.3 summarizes the PHAST Game Plan and Table 17.1 presents sample dialogue for application of the Game Plan in decoding an unknown word.

The PHAST Track Reading Program is intended to be situated as part of a linguistically enriched and literature-based balanced

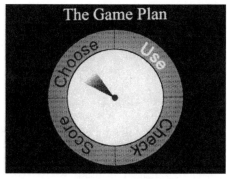

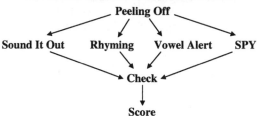

FIGURE 17.3. The Game Plan: A formula for strategy selection, application, monitoring, and evaluation. Lovett, Lacerenza, and Borden (2000). Copyright 2000 by PRO-ED, Inc. Reprinted by permission.

literacy program. PHAST is an intensive program to teach word identification and word attack skills and to promote the development of the basic skills necessary to permit independent decoding and reading for meaning, information, or pleasure. The metacognitive instructional focus and the dialogue structure of the PHAST Track Reading Program are compatible with dialogue-based approaches to text comprehension and writing training. Ideally, full implementation of the PHAST Program in a classroom setting would place it as part of a highly integrated approach to reading, spelling, and writing instruction—an approach that allows intense instruction in spelling-to-sound and sound-to-spelling analysis at the subsyllabic, lexical, and connected text levels. Our goal is to foster the development of reading, spelling, comprehension, and literacy skills in a manner that would equip the child for a world where the demands for fluent, effective, multifaceted literacy capabilities are ever increasing.

The PHAST Track Reading Program was developed for struggling readers in our own laboratory classrooms, but it is adaptable to the needs of precocious and average readers in the early elementary years. Current developments and extensions of the PHAST Program include a PHAST Reading Comprehension Track (Lessons 71–140) that builds on and follows the word identification lessons in Lessons 1–70. Supplementary spelling and writing tracks are also being piloted to accompany the decoding and text comprehension segments of the PHAST Track Reading Program. Finally, a new adaptation of PHAST for older individuals with reading disorders is in development

TABLE 17.1. A Sample of Strategy Execution Using the Metacognitive Dialogue "GAME Plan" from the PHAST Track Reading Program

The following is an example of the prompts and the dialogue of Game Plan as it is used to decode the word *unstacking*:

Step 1. CHOOSE:
"My Game Plan is to first use Peeling Off. Then I am going to use the Rhyming Strategy and look for the spelling patterns I know."

Step 2. USE:
"I am Peeling Off *un* and *ing*. My next Game Plan is Rhyming. I see the spelling pattern *a-c-k*. The key word is *pack*. If I know *pack,* then I know *stack*."

Step 3. CHECK:
"I have to *stop and think* about whether I'm using the strategy(ies) properly. Is it working? Yes, I'll keep on going. I will put all the parts together—*un-stack-ing*."

Step 4. SCORE/RE-CHOOSE:
"The word is *unstacking*. I scored! I used Peeling Off and Rhyming to help me figure out this word and they worked." (If the strategy did not result in a real word, the child begins again at Step 1, and *chooses* another strategy to try.)

Note. From Lovett, Lacerenza, and Borden (2000). Copyright 2000 by PRO-ED, Inc. Reprinted by permission.

(the PHAST PACES Program for struggling high school readers and young adults).

The PHAST Track Reading Program (Lessons 1–70) has been evaluated in a large multisite intervention study funded by NICHD: In this project, Robin Morris, Maryanne Wolf, and the first author are evaluating the effectiveness of two different dual-focus, deficit-directed intervention programs for young children with reading disabilities (PHAST Lessons 1–70 [Lovett, Lacerenza, & Borden, 2000] and PHAB/DI + RAVE-O [Wolf, Miller, & Donnelly, 2000]) against both an alternative treatment control program (Classroom Survival Skills + Math [see Lovett, Lacerenza, Borden, Frijters, et al., 2000]) and a phonological treatment control program (PHAB/DI + CSS). A second NICHD grant to our multisite group is supporting evaluation of longer multifocus intervention programs based on the original aforementioned 70-hour programs. A 125-hour PHAST Track Reading Program is being evaluated as part of this design and includes both integrated Decoding and Reading Comprehension tracks. The reader is referred to the published papers for more detailed descriptions of the interventions described in these pages.

Beyond the Acquisition of Basic Reading Skills: The Attainment of Reading Fluency in Individuals with Developmental Reading Disorders

In a recent study assessing two intensive and individualized remediation programs for 8–10-year-old children with reading disabilities, Torgesen, Alexander, and colleagues (2001) found significant improvement in generalized reading skills that were maintained over a 2-year follow-up period but little impact in terms of their subjects' continued impairment in reading rate. Extended individual instruction in both remedial programs (each 67½ hours and differing in the pedagogical focus of the phonological training) was associated with good growth in these children's reading skills, and graduates of the two programs scored on average within the age-appropriate range of reading achievement 2 years after intervention. These improvements were demonstrated for measures of word identification and passage comprehension only, however. The subjects remained 2 full standard deviations below age-level expectations on measures of reading rate at follow-up; this deficit persisted despite an overall increase in the number of words per minute read at follow-up and substantial improvement in the children's basic reading skills. Torgesen and his colleagues speculate that to "close the gap" for older children with reading disorders, they would have to add sight words (words that can be recognized immediately, without phonologically mediated decoding) to their lexicons at a rate that exceeded that of their agemates without disabilities. These investigators also acknowledge that some of the older children with reading disabilities may have severe constraints upon levels of processing speed, a deficit perhaps indexed by their slowed naming speeds on rapid automatized naming tasks (Wolf, Bally, & Morris, 1986; Wolf & Bowers, 1999).

There has been recent recognition that extended models of remedial intervention need to be developed if children with reading disabilities are to make gains in phonological processing skills, word identification and text reading accuracy *and* in word identification speed and text reading fluency with intervention. In fact, there remains little consensus in definitions of reading fluency (Meyer & Felton, 1999; Wolf & Katzir-Cohen, 2001). Meyer and Felton (1999) describe fluency as "the ability to read connected text rapidly, smoothly, effortlessly, and automatically with little conscious attention to the mechanics of reading such as decoding" (p. 284), a definition similar to LaBerge and Samuels' (1974) early model of reading fluency. LaBerge and Samuels suggested that fluency results from the automatization of component processes which allows attentional resources to be reallocated to other levels of processing. Berninger, Abbott, Billingsley, and Nagy (2001) propose a "systems" conceptualization of reading fluency, based on their research investigating components of reading, spelling, and written language development in children. Berninger and her colleagues suggest that fluency depends on three main sources of influence: characteristics of the informational input (visual or speech), the efficiency and automaticity of component language processing systems, and coordination by an executive function (management) system.

Wolf and Katzir-Cohen (2001) propose a developmental and component-based framework for understanding and promoting the acquisition of reading fluency. They define reading fluency as

> the product of the initial development of accuracy and the subsequent development of automaticity in underlying sublexical processes, lexical processes, and their integration in single-word reading and connected text. These include perceptual, phonological, orthographic, and morphological processes at the letter, letter-pattern, and word level, as well as semantic and syntactic processes at the word level and connected text level. After it is fully developed, reading fluency refers to a level of accuracy and rate where decoding is relatively effortless; where oral reading is smooth and accurate with correct prosody; and where attention can be allocated to comprehension. (p. 219)

It should be recognized, however, that much remains unknown about the nature and reciprocity of the relationships between reading fluency and text comprehension. It has long been assumed that increased efficiency and automatization of word recognition and decoding processes result in a freeing up of attentional resources for text comprehension processes; however, whether direct reciprocal relationships between fluency and comprehension exist has not been established (Meyer & Felton, 1999; Wolf & Katzir-Cohen, 2001).

From their developmental model of reading fluency, Wolf and her colleagues at Tufts University have developed an experimental reading intervention program called RAVE-O to facilitate its development (Wolf, Miller, & Donnelly, 2000). RAVE-O is taught in combination with a systematic phonologically based intervention program that teaches letter–sound knowledge, decoding, and word identification skills while remediating the speech-based phonological processes of children with reading disabilities. In combination with this decoding program, RAVE-O (for Retrieval, Automaticity, Vocabulary elaboration, Engagement with language, and Orthography) is designed (1) to promote accuracy and automaticity in reading subskills and compo-

nent processes; (2) to facilitate the development of fluency in word identification, word attack, and text reading and comprehension processes; and (3) to retrain the attitudes and affect of disabled readers in their approach to words and written language. RAVE-O encourages the children to learn to play with the English language through animated computer games (e.g., Speed Wizards; Wolf & Goodman, 1996), the building of imaginative word webs, instruction in systematic yet playful word-retrieval strategies, and the reading of minute mystery stories.

Like the PHAST Track Reading Program described earlier, the RAVE-O program in combination with the previously described PHAB/DI Program (Engelmann et al., 1988; Lovett et al., 1994) is being evaluated in the same multisite intervention study funded by NICHD. In this 5-year, three-city project, Morris, Wolf, and the first author have been investigating the effectiveness of different multicomponent intervention programs for young children with reading disabilites (PHAB/DI + RAVE-O; and PHAB/DI + WIST—i.e., the PHAST Track Reading Program [Lovett, Lacerenza, & Borden, 2000]) against both an alternative treatment control program (Classroom Survival Skills + Math [see Lovett et al., 2000]) and a phonological treatment control program (PHAB/DI + CSS). Again, the reader is referred to the published papers for a more complete description of the PHAST and RAVE-O interventions described in these pages. In a second 5-year intervention study by the same investigators and funded by NICHD, we are extending the intervention period and focus to evaluate the effectiveness of extended PHAST and RAVE-O Programs (125 hours) and to develop and evaluate a triple-focus program that integrates the PHAST Track Reading (Decoding and Reading Comprehension Tracks) Program and RAVE-O.

Final Comments

New conceptualizations of developmental reading disabilities, the core underlying learning impairments, and their effective remediation place us in a better position to undertake rigorous and productive research on reading disorders, their prevention in at-risk populations, their optimal remediation, and long-term outcome. Recent developments will allow us to refine our methodologies for the measurement of change, its evaluation and analysis, and now place us in a position to study individual and developmental variation within a richer and more coherent theoretical context and with significantly improved research tools. Questions about what mediates, moderates, and predicts change for children with developmental reading disorders and what treatment or treatment combinations will best serve them can now be productively addressed. Advances in the cognitive neuroscience of reading and in functional neuroimaging techniques allow additional evaluation of whether the functional and neurobiological substrates of reading in the brain change with effective remediation of reading problems (Simos et al., 2002).

Within the past 5 years, there has been growing recognition of the need to study the remedial response of individuals with reading disabilities along a continuum of skill development—addressing accuracy and rate criteria of skill acquisition in each reading-related domain (Lovett, 1984; 1987). With recognition of the multidimensional nature of the learning involved, we will be better able to assess not only what components of effective intervention allow children with reading disabilities to acquire basic decoding and word identification skills but also what types of training allow them to consolidate and automatize newly acquired skills to the point that word identification and decoding processes are relatively automatized and that different types of text are read fluently and with good comprehension (Foorman & Torgesen, 2001; Torgesen, Alexander, et al., 2001; Torgesen, Rashotte, & Alexander, 2001; Wolf & Katzir-Cohen, 2001). Foorman and Torgesen (2001) claim that if current research findings on effective classroom reading instruction were implemented, meeting the additional needs of the at-risk child for effective, intense, and explicit individual or small-group instruction, the literacy needs of *all* children could be met. This is a case in which advances in the science of reading disorders and intervention research, if brought to the front line of educational practice, could change the life circumstances of millions of at-risk children.

Acknowledgments

Preparation of this chapter was supported by a National Institute of Child Health and Human Development Grant (HD30970-01A1) to Georgia State University, Tufts University, and The Hospital for Sick Children/University of Toronto. The remediation research reported here was supported, in addition, by operating grants to the authors from the Ontario Mental Health Foundation, the Velleman Foundation, and the Social Sciences and Humanities Research Council of Canada.

We gratefully acknowledge the conceptual contributions of our collaborators and colleagues over the years, particularly those of Robin Morris and Maryanne Wolf. We also gratefully acknowledge the intellectual contributions of senior members of the Learning Disabilities Research Program (LDRP) at The Hospital for Sick Children—Karen A. Steinbach, Maria De Palma, Jan C. Frijters, Meredith Temple, Léa Lacerenza, Denis Murphy, Gail Markson, Jody Chong, and the whole LDRP staff who have contributed so much to past and current intervention studies.

Correspondence regarding this paper may be directed to the authors at The Hospital for Sick Children, 555 University Avenue, Toronto, Ontario, CANADA M5G 1X8 or via e-mail at mwl@sickkids.ca. Inquires about the Learning Disabilities Research Program may be directed to ldrp@sickkids.ca.

References

Barron, R. W. (1998). Proto-literate knowledge: Antecedents and influences on phonological awareness and literacy. In C. Hulme & R. M. Joshi (Eds.), *Reading and spelling: Development and disorders* (pp. 153–173). Mahwah, NJ: Erlbaum.

Benson, N. J. (2000). Analysis of specific deficits: Evidence of transfer in disabled and normal readers following oral–motor awareness training. *Journal of Educational Psychology, 92*(4), 646–658.

Benson, N. J., Lovett, M. W., & Kroeber, C. L. (1997). Training and transfer-of-learning effects in disabled and normal readers: Evidence of specific deficits. *Journal of Experimental Child Psychology, 64*(3), 343–366.

Berninger, V. W., & Abbott, R. D. (1994). Redefining learning disabilities: Moving beyond aptitude–achievement discrepancies to failure to respond to validated treatment protocols. In G. R. Lyon (Ed.), *Frames of reference for the assessment of learning disabilities: New views on measurement issues* (pp. 163–183). Baltimore: Brookes.

Berninger, V. W., Abbott, R. D., Billingsley, F., &

Nagy, W. (2001). Processes underlying timing and fluency of reading: Efficiency, automaticity, coordination, and morphological awareness. In M. Wolf (Ed.), *Dyslexia, fluency, and the brain* (pp. 383–413). Timonium, MD: York Press.

Bishop, D. V., & Adams, C. (1990). A prospective study of the relationship between specific language impairment, phonological disorders and reading disabilities. *Journal of Child Psychology and Psychiatry, 31*(7), 1027–1050.

Bowers, P. G., & Wolf, M. (1993). Theoretical links between naming speed, precise mechanisms, and orthographic skill in dyslexia. *Reading and Writing: An Interdisciplinary Journal, 5*, 69–85.

Brady, S. A. (1997). Ability to encode phonological representations: An underlying difficulty of poor readers. In B. A. Blachman (Ed.), *Foundations of reading acquisition and dyslexia* (pp. 21–47). Hillsdale, NJ: Erlbaum.

Bruck, M. (1992). Persistence of dyslexics' phonological awareness deficits. *Developmental Psychology, 28*, 874–886.

Bruck, M. (1998). Outcomes of adults with childhood histories of dyslexia. In C. Hulme & R. M. Joshi (Eds.), *Reading and spelling: Development and disorders* (pp. 179–200). Mahwah, NJ: Erlbaum.

Cattell, M. (1886). The time it takes to see and name objects. *Mind, 2*, 63–85.

Cunningham, A. E., & Stanovich, K. (1997). Early reading acquisition and its relation to reading experience and ability. *Developmental Psychology, 33*, 934–945.

Elbro, C., Borstrom, I., & Petersen, D. K. (1998). Predicting dyslexia from kindergarten: The importance of distinctness of phonological representations of lexical items. *Reading Research Quarterly, 33*(1), 36–60.

Engelmann, S., & Bruner, E. C. (1988). *Reading Mastery I/II Fast Cycle: Teacher's guide.* Chicago: Science Research Associates.

Engelmann, S., Carnine, L., & Johnson, G. (1988). *Corrective reading: Word attack basics, decoding A.* Chicago: Science Research Associates.

Engelmann, S., Johnson, G., Carnine, L., Meyer, L., Becker, W., & Eisele, J. (1988). *Corrective reading: Decoding strategies, decoding B1.* Chicago: Science Research Associates.

Felton, R. H., & Brown, I. S. (1990). Phonological processes as predictors of specific reading skills in children at risk for reading failure. *Reading and Writing: An Interdisciplinary Journal, 2*, 39–59.

Filipek, P. A. (1995). Neurobiological correlates of developmental dyslexia: What do we know of how dyslexics' brains differ from those of normal readers? *Journal of Child Neurology, 10*(Suppl.), S62–S69.

Filipek, P. A. (1999). Neuroimaging in the developmental disorders: The state of the science. *Journal of Child Psychology and Psychiatry, 40*(1), 113–128.

Fletcher, J. M., & Lyon, G. R. (1998). Reading: A research-based approach. In W. M. Evers (Ed.), *What's gone wrong in America's classrooms* (pp. 49–90). Stanford, CA: Hoover Institution Press.

Fletcher, J. M., Shaywitz, S. E., Shankweiler, D. P., Katz, L., Liberman, I. Y., Stuebing, K. K., Francis, D. J., Fowler, A. E., & Shaywitz, B. A. (1994). Cognitive profiles of reading disability: Comparisons of discrepancy and low achievement definitions. *Journal of Educational Psychology, 86*(1), 6–23.

Foorman, B. R., Francis, D. J., Fletcher, J. M., Schatschneider, C., & Mehta, P. (1998). The role of instruction in learning to read: Preventing reading failure in at-risk children. *Journal of Educational Psychology, 90*(1), 37–55.

Foorman, B. R., Francis, D. J., Winikates, D., Mehta, P., Schatschneider, C., & Fletcher, J. M. (1997). Early interventions for children with reading disabilities. *Scientific Studies of Reading, 1*(3), 255–276.

Foorman, B. R., & Torgesen, J. (2001). Critical elements of classroom and small-group instruction promote reading success in all children. *Learning Disabilities Research and Practice, 16*(4), 203–212.

Francis, D. J., Shaywitz, S. E., Stuebing, K. K., Shaywitz, B. A., & Fletcher, J. M. (1996). Developmental lag versus deficit models of reading disability: A longitudinal, individual growth curves analysis. *Journal of Educational Psychology, 88*(1), 3–17.

Gaskins, I. W., Downer, M. A., & Gaskins, R. W. (1986). *Introduction to the Benchmark School Word Identification/Vocabulary Development program.* Media, PA: Benchmark School.

Gathercole, S. E., & Baddeley, A. D. (1987). The processes underlying segmental analysis. *European Bulletin of Cognitive Psychology, 7*, 462–464.

Gittelman, R. (1983). Treatment of reading disorders. In M. Rutter (Ed.), *Developmental Neuropsychiatry* (pp. 520–541). New York: Guilford Press.

Goswami, U., & Bryant, P. E. (1990). *Phonological skills and learning to read.* Hove, East Sussex, UK: Erlbaum.

Grigorenko, E. L. (2001). Developmental dyslexia: An update on genes, brains, and environments. *Journal of Child Psychology and Psychiatry, 42*(1), 91–125.

Grigorenko, E. L., Wood, F. B., Meyer, M. S., Hart, L. A., Speed, W. C., Shuster, A., & Pauls, D. L. (1997). Susceptibility loci for distinct components of developmental dyslexia on chromosomes 6 and 15. *American Journal of Human Genetics, 60*, 27–39.

Hanushek, E. A., Kain, J. F., & Rivkin, S. G. (1998). *Does special education raise academic achievement for students with disabilities?* National Bureau of Economic Research, Working Paper No. 6690, Cambridge, MA.

Hewison, J. (1982). The current status of remedial intervention for children with reading problems. *Developmental Medicine and Child Neurology, 24*, 183–186.

Hinshelwood, J. (1917). *Congenital word blindness.* London: H. K. Lewis.

Huey, E. B. (1908). *The psychology and pedagogy.* New York: MacMillan.

Juel, C., & Minden-Cupp, C. (2000). Learning to read words: Linguistic units and instructional strategies. *Reading Research Quarterly, 35*(4), 458–492.

LaBerge, D., & Samuels, S. J. (1974). Toward a theory of automatic information processing in reading. *Cognitive Psychology, 6,* 293–323.

Levin, B. E. (1990). Organizational deficits in dyslexia: Possible frontal lobe dysfunction. *Developmental Neuropsychology, 6,* 95–110.

Levy, B. A., Abello, B., & Lysynchuk, L. (1997). Transfer from word training to reading in context: Gains in reading fluency and comprehension. *Learning Disability Quarterly, 20*(3), 173–188.

Liberman, A., & Mattingly, I. G. (1985). The motor theory of speech perception revised. *Cognition, 21,* 1–36.

Liberman, I. Y., Shankweiler, D., & Liberman, A. M. (1989). The alphabetic principle and learning to read. In D. Shankweiler & I. Y. Liberman (Eds.), *Phonology and reading disability: Solving the reading puzzle* (pp. 1–33). Ann Arbor: University of Michigan Press.

Lindamood, C. H., & Lindamood, P. C. (1975). *Auditory discrimination in depth.* Allen, TX: DLM Teaching Resources.

Lovett, M. W. (1984). A developmental perspective on reading dysfunction: Accuracy and rate criteria in the subtyping of dyslexic children. *Brain and Language, 22,* 67–91.

Lovett, M. W. (1987). A developmental approach to reading disability: Accuracy and speed criteria of normal and deficient reading skill. *Child Development, 58,* 234–260.

Lovett, M. (1991). Reading, writing, and remediation: Perspectives on the dyslexic learning disability from remedial outcome data. *Learning and Individual Differences, 3,* 295–305.

Lovett, M. W. (1992). Developmental dyslexia. In I. Rapin & S. J. Segalowitz (Eds.), *Handbook of neuropsychology, Vol. 7: Child neuropsychology* (pp. 163–185). Amsterdam: Elsevier Science.

Lovett, M. W. (1997). Developmental reading disorders. In T. E. Feinberg & M. J. Farah (Eds.), *Behavioral neurology and neuropsychology* (pp. 773–787). New York: McGraw-Hill.

Lovett, M. W. (1999). Defining and remediating the core deficits of developmental dyslexia: Lessons from remedial outcome research with reading disabled children. In R. Klein & P. McMullen (Eds.), *Converging methods for understanding reading and dyslexia. Language, speech, and communication* (pp. 111–132). Cambridge, MA: MIT Press.

Lovett, M. W., & Barron, R. W. (2003). Neuropsychological perspectives on reading development and developmental reading disorders. In S. J. Segalowitz & I. Rapin (Eds.), *Handbook of neuropsychology. Child neuropsychology* (2nd ed., Vol. 8, Part II, pp. 255–300). Amsterdam: Elsevier Science.

Lovett, M. W., & Barron, R. W. (2002). The search for individual and subtype differences in reading disabled children's response to remediation. In D. L. Molfese & V. J. Molfese (Eds.), *developmental variations in learning: Applications to social, executive function, language, and reading skills* (pp. 309–337). Mahwah, NJ: Erlbaum.

Lovett, M. W., Borden, S. L., DeLuca, T., Lacerenza, L., Benson, N. J., & Brackstone, D. (1994). Treating the core deficits of developmental dyslexia: Evidence of transfer-of-learning following phonologically- and strategy-based reading training programs. *Developmental Psychology, 30*(6), 805–822.

Lovett, M. W., Hinchley, J., & Benson, N. J. (1997). *Assessing the remedial gains of disabled learners: Conceptual, measurement, and statistical considerations in the evaluation of remedial outcome.* Unpublished manuscript.

Lovett, M. W., Lacerenza, L., & Borden, S. L. (2000). Putting struggling readers on the PHAST track: A program to integrate phonological and strategy-based remedial reading instruction and maximize outcomes. *Journal of Learning Disabilities, 33*(5), 458–476.

Lovett, M. W., Lacerenza, L., Borden, S. L., Frijters, J. C., Steinbach, K. A., & De Palma, M. (2000). Components of effective remediation for developmental reading disabilities: Combining phonological and strategy-based instruction to improve outcomes. *Journal of Educational Psychology, 92*(2), 263–283.

Lovett, M. W., Ransby, M. J., & Barron, R. W. (1988). Treatment, subtype, and word type effects in dyslexic children's response to remediation. *Brain and Language, 34,* 328–349.

Lovett, M. W., Ransby, M. J., Hardwick, N., Johns, M. S., & Donaldson, S. A. (1989). Can dyslexia be treated? Treatment-specific and generalized treatment effects in dyslexic children's response to remediation. *Brain and Language, 37,* 90–121.

Lovett, M. W., & Steinbach, K. A. (1997). The effectiveness of remedial programs for reading disabled children of different ages: Is there decreased benefit for older children? *Learning Disability Quarterly, 20*(3), 189–210.

Lovett, M. W., Steinbach, K. A., & Frijters, J. C. (2000). Remediating the core deficits of developmental reading disability: A double deficit perspective. *Journal of Learning Disabilities, 33*(4), 334–358.

Lovett, M. W., Warren-Chaplin, P. M., Ransby, M. J., & Borden, S. L. (1990). Training the word recognition skills of reading disabled children: Treatment and transfer effects. *Journal of Educational Psychology, 82,* 769–780.

Lyon, G. R. (1995). Research initiatives in learning disabilities: Contributions from scientists supported by the National Institute of Child Health and Human Development. *Journal of Child Neurology, 10*(1), S120–S126.

Lyon, G. R. (1996). Learning disabilities. In E. J.

Marsh & R. A. Barkley (Eds.), *Child psychopathology* (pp. 390–435). New York: Guilford Press.

Lyon, G. R., & Moats, L. C. (1997). Critical conceptual and methodological considerations in reading intervention research. *Journal of Learning Disabilities, 30*(6), 578–588.

Mann, V. (1986). Why some children encounter reading problems. In J. Torgesen & B. Wong (Eds.), *Psychological and educational perspectives on learning disabilities* (pp. 133–159). New York: Academic Press.

Meyer, M. M., & Felton, R. H. (1999). Repeated reading to enhance fluency: Old approaches and new direction. *Annals of Dyslexia, 49,* 283–306.

Moats, L. C., & Foorman, B. R. (1997). Introduction to special issue of SSR: Components of effective reading instruction. *Scientific Studies of Reading, 1*(3), 187–189.

Morgan, W. P. (1896). A case of congenital word-blindness. *British Medical Journal, 2,* 1378.

Olson, R. K., Wise, B., Ring, J., & Johnson, M. (1997). Computer-based remedial training in phoneme awareness and phonological decoding: Effects on the posttraining development of word recognition. *Scientific Studies of Reading, 1*(3), 235–254.

Pennington, B. F. (1997). Using genetics to dissect cognition. *American Journal of Human Genetics, 60,* 13–16.

Pennington, B. F. (1999). Toward an integrated understanding of dyslexia: Genetic, neurological, and cognitive mechanisms. *Development and Psychopathology, 11,* 629–654.

Pugh, K. R., Mencl, W. E., Jenner, A. R., Katz, L., Frost, S. J., Lee, J. R., Shaywitz, S. E., & Shaywitz, B. A. (2001). Neurobiological studies of reading and reading disability. *Journal of Communication Disorders, 34*(6), 479–492.

Pugh, K. R., Mencl, W. E., Jenner, A. J., Katz, L., Lee, J. R., Shaywitz, S. E., & Shaywitz, B. A. (2000). Functional neuroimaging studies of reading and reading disability (developmental dyslexia). *Mental Retardation and Developmental Disabilities Review, 6,* 207–213.

Rayner, K., Foorman, B. R., Perfetti, C. A., Pesetsky, D., & Seidenberg, M. S. (2001). How psychological science informs the teaching of reading. *Psychology in the Public Interest, 2,* 31–74.

Scanlon, D. M., & Vellutino, F. R. (1997). A comparison of the instructional backgrounds and cognitive profiles of poor, average, and good readers who were initially identified as at risk for reading failure. *Scientific Studies of Reading, 1*(3), 191–216.

Scarborough, H. S. (1984). Continuity between childhood dyslexia and adult reading. *British Journal of Psychology, 75*(3), 329–348.

Scarborough, H. S. (1990). Very early language deficits in dyslexic children. *Child Development, 61,* 1728–1743.

Scarborough, H. S. (1998). Early identification of children at risk for reading disabilities. In B. K. Shapiro, P. J. Accardo, & A. J. Capute (Eds.), *Specific reading disability: A view of the spectrum* (pp. 75–119). Timonium, MD: York Press.

Shanahan, T., & Barr, R. (1995). Reading Recovery: An independent evaluation of the effects of an early instructional intervention for at-risk learners. *Reading Research Quarterly, 30*(4), 958–996.

Share, D. L. (1995). Phonological recoding and self-teaching. Sine qua non of reading acquisition. *Cognition, 55,* 151–218.

Shaywitz, S. E., Fletcher, J. M., Holahan, J. M., Schneider, A. E., Marchione, K. E., Stuebing, K. K., Francis, D. J., Pugh, K. R., & Shaywitz, B. A. (1999). Persistence of dyslexia: The Connecticut Longitudinal Study at adolescence. *Pediatrics, 104*(6), 1351–1359.

Shaywitz, S. E., Shaywitz, B. A., Pugh, K. R., Fulbright, R. K., Constable, R. T., Mencl, W. E., Shankweiler, D. P., Liberman, A. M., Skudlarski, P., Fletcher, J. M., Katz, L., Marchione, K. E., Lacadie, C., Gatenby, C., & Gore, J. C. (1998, March). Functional disruption in the organization of the brain for reading in dyslexia. *Proceedings of the National Academy of Sciences of the United States of America, 95,* 2636–2641.

Simos, P. G., Fletcher, J. M., Bergman, E., Breier, J. I., Foorman, B. R., Castillo, E. M., Davis, R. N., Fitzgerald, M., & Papanicolaou, A. C. (2002). Dyslexia-specific brain activation profile becomes normal following successful remedial training. *Neurology, 58,* 1203–1213.

Snowling, M., & Hulme, C. (1993). Developmental dyslexia and language disorders. In G. Blanken, J. Dittmann, H. Grimm, J. C. Marshall, & C.-W. Wallesch (Eds.), *Linguistic disorders and pathologies: An international handbook* (pp. 724–732). New York: Walter de Gruyter.

Stanovich, K. E. (1986). Matthew effects in reading: Some consequences of individual differences in the acquisition of literacy. *Reading Research Quarterly, 21,* 360–407.

Stanovich, K. E. (1991). Changing models of reading and reading acquisition. In L. Rieben & C. A. Perfetti (Eds.), *Learning to read: Basic research and Its implications* (pp. 19–31). Hillsdale, NJ: Erlbaum.

Stanovich, K. E. (1994). Annotation: Does dyslexia exist? *Journal of Child Psychology and Psychiatry, 55*(4), 579–595.

Stanovich, K. E., & Siegel, L. S. (1994). Phenotypic performance profile of children with reading disabilities: A regression-based test of the phonological-core variable-difference model. *Journal of Educational Psychology, 86*(1), 24–53.

Swanson, H. L. (1999a). Reading comprehension and working memory in learning-disabled readers: Is the phonological loop more important than the executive system? *Journal of Experimental Child Psychology, 72,* 1–31.

Swanson, H. L. (1999b). Reading research for students with learning disabilities: A meta-analysis of intervention outcomes. *Journal of Learning Disabilities, 32*(6), 504–532.

Swanson, H. L., & Alexander, J. E. (1997). Cognitive processes as predictors of word recognition and reading comprehension in learning-disabled and skilled readers: Revisiting the specificity hypothesis. *Journal of Educational Psychology, 89*(1), 128–158.

Swanson, H. L., & Hoskyn, M. (1998). Experimental intervention research on students with learning disabilities: A meta-analysis of treatment outcomes. *Review of Educational Research, 68*(3), 277–321.

Torgesen, J. K. (2000). Individual differences in response to early interventions in reading: The lingering problem of treatment resisters. *Learning Disabilities Research and Practice, 15*(1), 55–64.

Torgesen, J. K., Alexander, A. W., Wagner, R. K., Rashotte, C. A., Voeller, K. K. S., & Conway, T. (2001). Intensive remedial instruction for children with severe reading disabilities: Immediate and long-term outcomes from two instructional approaches. *Journal of Learning Disabilities, 34*(1), 33–58.

Torgesen, J. K., Rashotte, C. A., & Alexander, A. W. (2001). Principles of fluency instruction in reading: Relationships with established empirical outcomes. In M. Wolf (Ed.), *Dyslexia, fluency, and the brain* (pp. 333–355). Timonium, MD: York Press.

Torgesen, J. K., Wagner, R. K., & Rashotte, C. A. (1997). Approaches to the prevention and remediation of phonologically-based reading disabilities. In B. A. Blachman (Ed.), *Foundations of reading acquisition and dyslexia: Implications for early intervention* (pp. 287–304). Mahwah, NJ: Erlbaum.

Torgesen, J., Wagner, R., Rashotte, C., Lindamood, P., Rose, E., Conway, T., & Garvan, C. (1999). Preventing reading failure in young children with phonological processing disabilities: Group and individual responses to instruction. *Journal of Educational Psychology, 91*(4), 579–593.

Vellutino, F. R., Scanlon, D. M., Sipay, E. R., Small, S. G., Pratt, A., Chen, R., & Denckla, M. B. (1996). Cognitive profiles of difficult-to-remediate and readily remediated poor readers: Early intervention as a vehicle for distinguishing between cognitive and experiential deficits as basic causes of specific reading disability. *Journal of Educational Psychology, 88*(4), 601–638.

Wagner, R. K., & Torgesen, J. K. (1987). The nature of phonological processing and its causal role in the acquisition of reading skills. *Psychological Bulletin, 101,* 192–212.

Wagner, R. K., Torgesen, J. K., & Rashotte, C. A. (1994). Development of reading-related phonological processing abilities: New evidence of bidirectional causality from a latent variable longitudinal study. *Developmental Psychology, 30*(1), 73–87.

Wise, B. W., & Olson, R. K. (1995). Computer-based phonological awareness and reading instruction. *Annals of Dyslexia, 45,* 99–122.

Wise, B. W., Ring, J., & Olson, R. K. (2000). Individual differences in gains from computer-assisted remedial reading. *Journal of Experimental Child Psychology, 77,* 197–235.

Wise, B. W., Ring, J., Sessions, L., & Olson, R. K. (1997). Phonological awareness with and without articulation: A preliminary study. *Learning Disability Quarterly, 20*(3), 211–225.

Wolf, M. (1991). Naming speed and reading: The contribution of the cognitive neurosciences. *Reading Research Quarterly, 26,* 123–141.

Wolf, M., Bally, H., & Morris, R. (1986). Automaticity, retrieval processes, and reading: A longitudinal study in average and impaired readers. *Child Development, 57*(4), 988–1000.

Wolf, M., & Bowers, P. G. (1999). The double-deficit hypothesis for the developmental dyslexias. *Journal of Educational Psychology, 91*(3), 415–438.

Wolf, M., & Bowers, P. G. (2000). Naming-speed processes and developmental reading disabilities: An introduction to the special issue on the double-deficit hypothesis. *Journal of Learning Disabilities, 33*(4), 322–324.

Wolf, M., Bowers, P. G., & Biddle, K. (2000). Naming-speed processes, timing, and reading: A conceptual review. *Journal of Learning Disabilities, 33*(4), 387–407.

Wolf, M., & Goodman, G. (1996). *Speed wizards* [Computer software], Tufts University, Boston and Rochester Institute of Technology, Rochester, NY.

Wolf, M., & Katzir-Cohen, T. (2001). Reading fluency and its intervention. *Scientific Studies of Reading, 5*(3), 211–239.

Wolf, M., Miller, L., & Donnelly, K. (2000). Retrieval, automaticity, vocabulary elaboration, orthography (RAVE-O): A comprehensive, fluency-based reading intervention program. *Journal of Learning Disabilities, 33*(4), 375–386.

18

Teaching Text Structure to Improve Reading Comprehension

Joanna P. Williams

Comprehending what is read presents a genuine challenge for many students with learning disabilities. Sometimes the difficulty stems from a lack of fluency in word recognition. However, in many cases children who read fluently do not understand what they read because of cognitive processing problems such as working memory limitations, lexical processing difficulties, poor inference making, and ineffective comprehension monitoring (Gersten, Fuchs, Williams, & Baker, 2001). In other cases their knowledge, either of word meanings or of a particular domain, may be minimal (Perfetti, Marron, & Foltz, 1996). Of course, many of these same problems are sometimes seen in students who do not have learning disabilities; these students, too, have trouble understanding what they read.

About 30 years ago, researchers began to investigate the nature of reading comprehension by analyzing the strategies used by proficient readers. Today a focus on teaching such strategies has become the main approach to comprehension instruction (Pressley, 2000). Most strategy instruction involves a strong emphasis on metacognition; that is, instruction is geared toward an awareness of one's cognitive processes and

how to deploy them (Swanson & Hoskyn, 1998). Students are directed to stop occasionally during their reading to monitor their understanding by asking themselves questions or by trying to summarize. They are taught to take steps to ensure their understanding by rereading, by trying to connect the material to be learned with what they already know, and by using other general study skills (Swanson & Hoskyn, 1998). These strategies can be thought of as ways to put oneself in a position to comprehend. They might be considered remedial in the sense that good readers seem to use them without specific instruction and indeed often without even being aware that they are using them.

Some strategies involve more than becoming aware of, manipulating, and monitoring one's cognitive processing. Well-structured text enhances recall and comprehension, for those who have acquired sensitivity to structure (Pearson & Dole, 1987), and instruction designed to teach students to recognize the underlying structure of the text that they are reading improves comprehension. This instruction typically involves teaching students to identify the important structural elements of a particular type of text and then to memorize a list of generic questions that cue a search for those important elements. This instruction involves new knowledge about text structure and how to use this knowledge in a strategy.

Different types of text are organized in different ways. Narrative text can be described as following a single general structural pattern (often called story grammar; Mandler & Johnson, 1977), and informational text comes in a variety of patterns (e.g., description, sequence, compare–contrast, cause–effect, and problem–solution). Children develop sensitivity to narrative structure early, and they use it to comprehend simple stories before they enter school. But informational text, because it comprises a variety of structures and also because it more often deals with unfamiliar content, is more difficult to comprehend (Kucan & Beck, 1997). It has been considered so challenging for young children that until recently, one rarely saw any informational text in elementary school classrooms.

There was a considerable amount of research on text structure in the 1980s. But in the 1990s, under the influence of a constructivist philosophy (Bean, 2000; Rosenblatt, 1978), the focus of research efforts shifted. Attention turned away from the effects of features of text to issues such as the characteristics of the reader and the social nature of comprehension. Unfortunately, this change in research focus occurred long before the implications of the findings on text structure had been thoroughly investigated and effective instructional programs developed.

One of the hallmarks of the new constructivist approach that has strongly influenced the selection of instructional materials is its emphasis on using only authentic texts. Arguments have been made that because only a small proportion of authentic text actually follows any single specific structure (and yet proficient readers, of course, do understand the more complicated text that they usually encounter), there is little reason to spend much instructional time on text structure. However, one could argue that to base early instruction on what proficient readers do, as many recommend, is not necessarily the best approach to take. For example, proficient readers do not sound out individual letters in words; they

process larger units (Perfetti, 1985). Yet synthetic phonics is an effective way to teach beginning reading (National Reading Panel, 2000). Similarly, it is reasonable to suggest that early comprehension instruction might be more effective when it is not based strictly on a model of proficient reading. Texts that are well structured (even if "contrived" for specific instructional purposes) may prove to be useful materials for the classrooms.

It should be kept in mind that the specific structures that we are talking about are not limited to text; they are rhetorical structures that reflect universal cognitive processes. The thinking of young children exhibits forms of all these structures. By the time children enter school, they tell stories, compare and contrast objects, order events in a temporal sequence, and may even impute causality in rudimentary ways. But children have not had sufficient practice to be able to use these structures easily, and sometimes they do not even recognize opportunities for using them to enhance their comprehension. Helping students recognize the structure inherent in text—and match it to their own cognitive structures—will help them understand and produce not only text but also spoken discourse. And when they encounter text whose structure is complex or text that is poorly organized, they will be able to simplify or reorganize it in order to better comprehend it.

The Student with Learning Disabilities

The field of learning disabilities has been plagued since its inception by difficulties of definition (Hammill, 1990). When I first began to work on reading instruction for children with learning disabilities, I was perplexed by the question of what "learning disabilities" really meant. I realized that many people had the same question. My own main interest was in reading and in instructional design, and so after considerable reflection, I decided that I could work with children with reading difficulties whom someone else had labeled as having a learning disability. My rationale was that what I was trying to do was develop materials and techniques for poor readers in general, a more inclusive category. If I succeeded, then surely those who had specific learning disabilities would be helped.

I still hold that point of view, and I believe that the evidence is bearing me out. That is, regardless of the important controversies about the nature and extent of learning disabilities, instructional techniques that are found to be effective and are recommended for students with learning disabilities who have reading problems are not qualitatively different from those recommended for other poor readers (Williams, 1992). For each of the studies I describe here, I provide a description of the population drawn from. In all cases the students who have been designated as having learning disabilities have difficulty with reading; I refer to them either as students with learning disabilities or with reading disabilities.

Finding the Main Idea

"Comprehension" is a general term, encompassing a wide variety of skills and performances. The core of reading comprehension is the ability to get from a text its gist or its point. Traditionally, this ability is called finding the main idea (Pearson & Johnston, 1978). Without being able to understand the point of a text, one cannot draw appropriate inferences from it; nor can one compare texts without understanding the main points of each. This ability is fundamental to basic comprehension, to effective studying, and to critical thinking. The fact that instruction in how to find main ideas has always been one of the most common elements of the elementary-school curriculum underscores its importance.

"Main idea" is rather a challenge to teach. Children often have difficulty in identifying main ideas of even rather simple texts (Baumann, 1984). Available instructional materials have been evaluated and found wanting. It is often suggested that teachers give children explanations that go like this: "To find the main idea, pick out the most important point," or "If you have picked out the most important sentence, you have probably found the main idea." Such statements communicate the importance of finding main ideas, but they do not tell or show how to find one. In fact, there is nothing you can tell children directly that

will tell them what to do. That is the real challenge of much comprehension instruction . . . and the reason why so much emphasis is placed on general metacognitive strategies.

Our initial focus was on normally achieving children in the fourth to sixth grades. In a series of studies (William, Taylor, & Ganger, 1981), my students and I asked children to read short paragraphs and to select an appropriate title from an array of choices and write a summary sentence for the paragraph. These are typical tasks that one might see in a classroom. All of our paragraphs were written on a low readability level, so that difficulties with decoding would not confound our findings.

Consider the following paragraph:

Cowboys had to protect the herd from cattle robbers. Cowboys had to brand cattle to show who owned them. They had to ride around the ranch to keep cattle from straying too far. Sometimes cowboys had to separate the cattle that were to be sent to market.

In this paragraph, each sentence instantiates a global topic ("cowboys"), and the reader can construct a proposition that at a higher level subsumes the three sentences (van Dijk, 1980, p. 46): "Cowboys had jobs to do."

We found that there was a clear developmental progression in ability across school grades, and that performance was better when readers had merely to select the main idea from an array than when they had to formulate it as a summary sentence. Also, children performed better on paragraphs with topic sentences than on those without (although only when the topic sentences were highlighted). We replicated these findings with children with learning disabilities (Taylor & Williams, 1983); we compared them with normally achieving children who were matched in terms of IQ and word knowledge scores. All children were reading at the fourth- or fifth-grade level. Across all our experimental tasks, the children with learning disabilities did just as well as the younger children without disabilities. This finding suggested to us that the two groups were not qualitatively different with respect to the ability to generate macrostructure, and that instruction that focuses on the development of main idea skills should not necessarily be different for children with disabilities than for children without disabilities—a conclusion that is consonant with the general point of view that instructional development for the reading disabled should focus on whatever strategies and techniques are effective for the general category of slow readers.

There was, however, one finding that differentiated the two groups. We included what we called parenthetical information in some of the paragraphs, information that was either unrelated to or else only tangentially related to the propositional hierarchy of the text. We did this on the grounds that natural text does not always consist of well-structured paragraphs, and so it is important for readers to be able to disregard anomalous information when reading for gist.

We asked the children to identify the inappropriate sentence in the paragraph. For example, in the cowboy paragraph, that sentence might read, "Cowboys often wear leather jackets and fancy boots." The position of the anomalous sentence was varied across paragraphs, appearing as either the second, third, or fourth (last) sentence. Children without disabilities were able to identify a sentence as anomalous the closer it was to the end of the paragraph, but the children with learning disabilities showed no such effect, suggesting that the latter were not as good at building up a representation gradually as the information in each succeeding sentence was processed. They were just as willing to accept the anomalous sentence even when it appeared late in the paragraph: They did not edit.

I do not believe that this difficulty is the same as saying that children with learning disabilities do not monitor their comprehension; that is, when they are faced with the task of saying whether a sentence belongs in the paragraph, they probably do compare what the sentence says with their current representation of the paragraph, as, presumably, good readers do. Rather, I think that their representation of the paragraph develops less adequately than that of the child without disabilities; thus when the child with disabilities *does* compare sentence with paragraph representation, the outcome of the comparison is not likely to be on target.

We went on, in this main idea work, to develop an instructional sequence (Williams, Taylor, Jarin, & Milligan, 1983). We used the same sort of simple, highly structured paragraphs as we had in our experimental studies and designed a program that emphasized clear definition of main idea, clear description of the task, and an explanation of why it was important.

In addition, we incorporated general principles of instruction into the design: (1) the use of well-structured examples of the prototypical task, (2) consistent modeling of the strategies being taught, (3) a sequence of tasks, (4) a sequence of response demands that reflected a progression from easier to more difficult material, (5) gradual removal of the teacher from the task, and (6) provision for extensive practice and feedback. We also chose to externalize some of the steps in the comprehension process that are, in actuality, implicit, that is, to externalize their thinking. We did this by having the students highlight some of the textual cues, that is, circle the most frequent word or idea, to help figure out the general category that encompassed each sentence.

Another aspect of our training was our use of anomalous sentences and the systematic introduction of different types of anomaly: first, sentences totally unrelated to the topic of the paragraph, then sentences that were tangentially related and therefore rather confusing. Children were taught to identify the deviant sentence, to cross it out, as part of this "externalization" of the thought process, and then to formulate a main idea on the marked-up paragraph.

In evaluating the program (Williams et al., 1983), we worked with 11-year-old children with learning disabilities, about two grade levels below average reading level for their age. Children given 10 lessons were better able than children who did not receive the lessons to identify anomalous sentences and to write sentences on both materials that had been used in training and similar materials that had not.

One of the major concerns in this sort of work is to determine whether our instructional efforts lead to transfer, that is, that students will learn to work with new material: It is their ability to comprehend in general that we are concerned about. In this case, we can say that there was transfer, albeit only to similarly structured materials. We did not do any posttesting on other types of material. However, although the texts used in this study were structurally simple, we are convinced that work with materials such as these is an appropriate beginning step in the development of a sophisticated understanding of main idea and in using this comprehension skill in a variety of more complex materials.

It turns out that starting out by trying to teach students to get the main idea was not the simplest choice we might have made. What we were able to do, we decided, was to provide the students with a model or template. We could not tell students directly how to find the main idea, but we could provide a clear and simple pattern that could be used later as a standard for comparison. What main idea comprehension amounts to, on this level, is categorization (Williams, 1984). And categorization depends strongly on domain knowledge. The textual cues that we identified were content dependent. That is, in our sample paragraph, readers could be directed to circle the most frequent words ("cowboys") as an aid to determining what the paragraph was about. However, unless they knew the concept of "job" and could identify the activity listed in each sentence as a job, they would not get the main idea. This is a simple illustration of how content and structure interact in comprehension. A complete instructional model must provide students with domain knowledge as well as explicit instruction about text structure.

Comprehension of Narrative Text

What corresponds to finding the "main idea" in narrative text? The most analogous task is finding a theme of a story. A theme is sometimes expressed in terms of a concept such as "friendship," that is, as a relationship among story components in a form that is abstracted from the specific story context. Our definition adds another element: A theme is expressed as the concept along with a commentary, either evaluative or not, for example, "Some people steal"; or "People who are upset sometimes get distracted" (Williams, Brown, Silverstein, & deCani, 1994).

Although by the time they start school most children have a good grasp of narrative structure on the level of the plot, they often have difficulty identifying the theme of a story (Lehr, 1988). We found that this is true especially of children with learning disabilities. In one study, we worked with children who had been classified as reading disabled by the private school for children with learning disabilities that they were attending (Williams, 1993). Their test scores fell within the normal range of intelligence, and their reading levels were at least 2 years below what was expected for their age. Their mean age was 13½ years. A group of students without disabilities drawn from the fourth, fifth, and sixth grades of a regular private school was matched with the group with reading disabilities on reading level (middle of the sixth grade). Their mean age was 10½ years. Another group of students without disabilities was drawn from the seventh and eighth grades, matched on age to the group with reading disabilities. Their reading comprehension was substantially higher than that of the other two groups. Students listened to a story (West, 1953), summarized it, and answered questions about its theme in a structured interview (they listened so that any difficulties with lower-order reading skills would not confound our findings about comprehension). The students with learning disabilities were comparable to the reading-level-matched younger students without disabilities on summarizing, predicting, and answering questions. A close analysis of the students' protocols suggested that there was one difference between the groups: In their summaries, the students with learning disabilities imported more irrelevant and implausible information into their summaries than did the students without disabilities. This suggests that they did not build up an accurate representation of the story. The inaccurate representation interfered with their getting the point. The fact that students with reading disabilities seem to have a more difficult time in identifying themes than do the students without disabilities does not mean that no students without disabilities have difficulty with this task; indeed, our data indicated that students without disabilities demonstrated a wide range of performance.

Teaching Theme Identification

Theme is usually found to be the most difficult story component to teach (Dimino, Gersten, Carnine, & Blake, 1990; Gurney, Gersten, Dimino, & Carnine, 1990), even to students without disabilities (Singer & Donlan, 1982). We decided to develop an instructional program that would focus specifically on this aspect of narrative understanding. We began by considering current reading comprehension instruction. Most of today's instruction is constructivist; in this view, each reader brings a unique knowledge base to the reading of a text and ends up with a unique interpretation of the text. The instruction that follows from this type of approach is typically organized around discussion in which students contribute their individual interpretations so that all can expand and refine their own meaning construction (Allington, Guice, Michelson, Baker, & Li, 1996). Teachers serve as facilitators who contribute their own interpretations, without imposing them on the group. This constructivist paradigm has been found to be successful for many students (Allington et al., 1996).

However, this is relatively unstructured instruction. In addition, it presumes that all students have stable knowledge bases and interpretations to begin with, so that the class discussions can effectively modify and refine the interpretations and understanding of individual students. We decided that this constructivist approach would not fully meet the needs of students with learning disabilities, who have been shown to respond well to structured, direct instruction (Simmons, Fuchs, Fuchs, Mathes, & Hodge, 1995). Thus we designed our Theme Identification program to incorporate constructivist *goals* of comprehension instruction with an instructional approach that is effective for students with learning disabilities and others at risk for academic failure. That is, our program emphasized the holistic and constructive nature of the comprehensive process and the importance of integrating text meaning with concepts and experiences that are personally meaningful, but it also acknowledged the demonstrated value of structured, direct instruction for poor readers.

There is one important difference between teaching main idea and teaching theme. As pointed out earlier, it is difficult to provide any explicit strategic routine for determining a main idea. However, a theme is derived from the basic plot components of a story, which can be taught, and a series of generic questions that apply generally (starting with plot questions and going beyond those) can be taught as a strategy to guide theme identification. Dorfman and Brewer (1994), who worked with fables, proposed that in order to identify a theme, one must attend to two of the basic plot elements: the central event and the outcome. Given the event, one evaluates the outcome in terms of one's moral understanding; this evaluation is essentially a moral judgment. The combination of the plot components and the evaluation results in the theme. Our definition of theme is more encompassing than this, but we believe that the Dorfman and Brewer model applies even in stories whose themes are not evaluative. In any event, we decided to focus on evaluative themes in our research because of their simplicity and their ubiquity in children's literature.

The purpose of our instructional program is to help students learn about the concept of theme, identify theme in stories, and apply themes to real life. The instruction follows the tried-and-true paradigm of teacher explanation and modeling, guided practice, and independent practice. It focuses on teaching plot-level components via organizing (schema) questions, as previous studies have done. Then it teaches teaching theme identification via additional questions. A final set of questions helps students generalize the theme to relevant life situations. We call our set of questions the Theme Scheme. We use simple stories with single, clear and accessible themes. Some of the theme concepts we have used include perseverance, cooperation, greed, and honesty. All our themes are of the evaluative commentary type and are expressed in a simple, common format: "We should cooperate," "We should not be greedy."

The original version of the program consisted of a series of 12 40-minute sessions, each organized around a single story and comprising five parts as outlined herein. The 12 stories were taken from four basal reader series. In most cases, the stories originally appeared in trade books. Five of the stories exemplified a single theme, "We should persevere." Each of the other seven stories exemplified a different theme concept, such as cooperation, responsibility, and respect for others, all expressed in the theme format (We should . . .), described earlier.

1. *Prereading discussion about lesson purpose and story topic.* In the first part of each lesson, theme is defined as a lesson you can learn from a story, the value of understanding themes is discussed, and background for the specific story for that lesson is introduced, including its relevance to personal experiences. This instruction is heavily scaffolded, with teachers initially modeling each step and students gradually taking on more responsibility. In the first three lessons, teachers define theme and lead the discussion on the importance of theme and the story topic, making associations between the story and personal experiences. Starting in lesson 4, the students offer definitions of theme and lead the discussions themselves. As is the case throughout the lessons, only a general outline is given to the teachers, who use their own expertise in developing discussions and guiding the instruction.

2. *Reading the story.* Next, the teacher reads the story aloud while students follow along with their texts (so that decoding difficulties do not interfere with comprehension). At various points during the reading, the teacher imposes questions. These questions are designed to encourage students to process the text actively (to make associations between their own knowledge and the text information and to clarify the text information). The teacher asks the students to make predictions about what would happen next in the story and to explain major story events. Student responses are discussed, and students are encouraged to ask their own questions.

After reading the story, the class discusses the main points and reads a summary highlighting the main events and outcome. This is done because students with learning disabilities are particularly likely to have trouble identifying the important story components (Wong, 1984), and their story comprehension is often idiosyncratic (Williams, 1993).

3. *Discussion of important story information using organizing (schema) questions.* Teacher and students discuss five questions designed to help organize the im-portant story components and derive the thematic material. Over the course the lesson series, the teacher provides opportunities to practice these questions so that students can recall them on their own.

The first three organizing questions focus on the important story components from which a theme concept will be derived: main character, central event, and outcome. The questions are:

- Who is the main character?
- What did he or she do?
- What happened?

These questions direct students to focus on the important information and enable them to extract and organize important story components independently. Again, instruction is scaffolded.

The final two organizing questions are designed to encourage the students to make the judgments that, when combined with the theme concept, lead to theme identification. These questions are:

- Was this good or bad?
- Why was this good or bad?

Although teachers model their responses to the first four questions for four lessons, the final question—Why was this good or bad?—requires teacher modeling through lesson 7. Also through lesson 7, teachers model the way in which the answers to the five questions lead to a theme, and they state the theme. After lesson 7, responsibility for identifying and stating the theme is gradually transferred to the students. Teachers provide feedback to help the students in this process.

4. *Identification of the theme in standard format.* Students next learn to state the theme in a standard format defined as a "should" statement. Teachers model two generic statement frames:

- (Main character) should have (should not have)
  _____.

- We should (should not)
  _____.

The first frame puts the theme into the should format. The second theme applies the theme to situations and people in general rather than just to those in the story. Students practice stating the theme in this format.

5. *Application of theme to real-life experiences.* The last two questions help extend the theme to specific and often personal real-life scenarios:

- To whom would this theme apply?
- When would it apply? (In what situation?)

In this step, too, instruction proceeds by means of scaffolding. For each story, more explicit forms of the questions are also included in the lesson, elaborating on "who" and "in what situation," to be used as prompts when necessary.

Evaluation of the Program

First Evaluation

Our first evaluation involved fifth- and sixth-grade students in eight New York City classrooms that included both normally achieving students and those with learning disabilities that were mild enough to permit mainstreaming (Williams et al., 1994). This evaluation allowed us to assess the effectiveness of the Theme Identification program initially with children who were making satisfactory progress. Our assumption was that any difficulties we found would not be attributable to the children's learning problems but, rather, would lie in the program. In this study, students were taught by their own teachers, in classrooms that had been randomly assigned either to receive the instructional program or to serve in a control condition receiving no special instruction.

This initial study provided positive evidence for the effectiveness of our instructional program. Specifically, the students in the Theme Identification classrooms understood the concepts of theme and the concept of perseverance better, both of which represented content that they had been explicitly taught. They also did better on application of the perseverance theme (i.e., generating a story with that theme), which also had been explicitly taught. And, they were better at identifying the theme of a previously unheard perseverance story,

which can be considered a near transfer task (Brown & Palincsar, 1989). Finally, they were better at identifying the theme of a novel story whose theme had not appeared at all during the instruction, a task we considered to qualify as far transfer. Both the students with mild disabilities and the students without disabilities performed at similar levels.

Encouraged by these results but recognizing the preliminary nature of the findings (they were based on a no-treatment control), we turned to the evaluation of our comprehension instruction for students with more severe learning disabilities. It was for those students, who do not respond well to normal classroom instruction, that our program was really designed.

Second Evaluation

Here we compared the performance of students who were given our Theme Identification program with students who were given more traditional instruction that emphasized vocabulary acquisition and plot-level comprehension (the Story Comprehension program) (Williams et al., 1994). Twelve seventh- and eighth-grade special education classrooms in a small city near New York were randomly assigned to each treatment. All students received all their instruction in their own classrooms; they were not mainstreamed. All had been certified by the school as having learning disabilities, although many of them had IQ scores below 85, the usual minimum for a classification as having learning disabilities. As is our custom, we did not impose any further criteria on this school-identified group because we feel that instructional studies are most useful if conducted in ecologically valid settings (i.e., in actual classroom situations as they exist in schools).

The students in the Theme Identification classrooms performed significantly better than the students in the traditional-instruction classrooms. First, they understood the concept of theme and the concept of perseverance better, and they were also better at identifying the theme of a previously unheard perseverance story. Thus, the Theme Identification program aided students in their comprehension and promoted near transfer. But they were not superior at applying the perseverance theme. And when we asked the students to identify the theme of a previously unheard story that had a novel theme, one that was not represented at all during the instruction, the two instructional treatments did not differ. Thus, these students with severe learning disabilities, unlike the students in the first study, did not demonstrate any transfer to stories with novel themes.

However, it should be pointed out that while it might seem that we achieved only a modest degree of generalization, the results actually demonstrated a level of transfer that represents substantial achievement for students with severe learning disabilities (Pressley & McCormick, 1995). We concluded that the students with learning disabilities were able to respond positively to an integrated, well-structured approach to comprehension.

Third Evaluation

We decided to work further on our program because it appeared as if it could be modified so that it would lead to even greater transfer. To accomplish this goal, we made one major change in the program (Wilder & Williams, 2001). In its original version, almost half of the instruction focused on a single theme and the rest included one instance each of several other themes. Traditional recommendations concerning training for transfer propose that transfer be built into the original instruction by using multiple instances in a variety of contexts (Pressley et al., 1990). Following these recommendations, we included three themes in the instruction, each one exemplified in four stories. These themes were "We should not prejudge," "We should be ourselves," and "We should keep trying." We presented these themes in a sequence that made it impossible to predict what the theme of the next story would be.

We also made some other changes in the program. We added three questions to the Theme Scheme (making it a 12-step program). We added one question at the plot level ("What was his/her problem?", and two redundant, reinforcing questions, "The theme of this story is . . ." and "In what situation will . . . (not) help?" We also included additional activities that we thought

would engage the students, such as drawing, role playing, and song writing.

This evaluation involved 10 classrooms for students with learning disabilities in three junior high schools in New York City. The classrooms were randomly assigned to the Theme Identification program or to the Story Comprehension program.

Our efforts proved successful. In this study, the students in the Theme Identification classes were significantly better than the others, not only on the posttest measures on which there had been differences in the previous study, but also on application of the instructed themes and on identification of the theme of a new story whose theme had not been part of the instruction ("We should be honest"). Thus students with severe learning disabilities did demonstrate far transfer. The effect sizes for the comparisons that were significant ranged from 1.18 (Theme Identification of a novel theme) to 5.93 (Theme Identification of an instructed theme). We believe that it was the combination of the sequencing of the lessons as recommended in the literature on transfer plus the explicit and highly structured instruction, including the Theme Scheme, that were the effective elements of our instruction.

Fourth Evaluation

We conducted one final study, to determine whether our program could be adapted successfully for use with elementary school students in inclusion classrooms (Williams et al., 2002). In this study, 10 intact inclusion second- and third-grade classrooms in Harlem were assigned randomly to the Theme Identification Program or the Story Comprehension program. The only substantive modification we made was in the materials—we selected stories that we thought would be especially appealing to younger children. The three theme concepts we worked with were perseverance, greed, and honesty. In this study the classrooms whose students had been given the Theme Identification program showed superiority on measures of explicit teaching; they scored higher on the concept of theme and on theme concepts. They also showed evidence of near transfer, that is, they were better at identifying the three instructed themes in the (novel) posttest stories. Effect sizes for the comparisons that were significant ranged from 0.68 (Theme Concepts) to 2.71 (Concept of "Theme"). However, these students showed no evidence of far transfer in that they were not superior on questions dealing with theme identification or applications when dealing with a story whose theme concept (cooperation) had not come up during instruction. In this respect they were different from the middle school students with severe learning disabilities that we had studied (Wilder & Williams, 2001). This discrepancy in outcomes indicates the difficulty that abstract thinking poses for younger children (Williams, 1998).

Responsiveness to Instruction

We posed an additional question in this last study. Was the Theme Identification program effective for all students? This question is especially important in school settings in which there is a wide range of ability levels (including children who have been identified as having a learning disability or who have been referred for evaluation for special education). Full inclusion intensifies the demand for a diversity of effective instructional treatments. We found that the program was effective for students at high-, average-, and low-achievement levels, including those with learning disabilities or who had been referred for special education evaluation. The program was effective at both second and third grade. Given that on the pretest the basic theme comprehension scores were essentially 0 at both grade levels, the significant grade effects on the posttest indicate that the program was more effective for third-graders. However, there was no indication that the second-graders had reached a performance asymptote; it is likely that they could have attained a higher level of performance, perhaps as high as the third-graders, if they had had additional instructional time.

There were, as there usually are, a few children who were not responsive to the program. It is instructive to examine individual differences in responsiveness with an eye toward improving the program or deciding when to use it. Of course, the program is short and circumscribed in nature.

Also, there is no consensus in the field of comprehension instruction as to what constitutes an acceptable level of performance, as there may be in decoding instruction (Al Otaiba & Fuchs, in press). With these caveats in mind, we determined criteria for designating nonresponders that included low performance on either explicit teaching or transfer. We identified 10 nonresponders in grade 2 and four in grade 3. We found that the only student characteristics that were associated with nonresponding were scores on reading and listening tests. There was no significant relationship between nonresponders and special education status in either grade. That is, the probability that students who had learning disabilities or who had been referred for evaluation for special education were nonresponders was no different from the probability that students without disabilities were nonresponders.

Students also gained from the instruction presented in the comparison program, which also featured carefully selected stories, well-organized lessons, and substantial discussion. Substantial differences between the two instructional programs appeared on transfer measures, suggesting that to promote generalization, more direct and structured instruction is valuable. We believe that current recommendations to focus comprehension instruction on discussion should be supplemented with further recommendations concerning choice of content and its organization, as well as direct instruction.

In summary, our Theme Identification program helped students learn the fundamental aspects of theme comprehension and to generalize what they had learned. The program was effective for students at all achievement levels, and also for students with learning disabilities. It was effective, with appropriate adaptations, from second grade through junior high school. Across the studies, effect sizes for significant effects were almost always substantial.

Informational Text

Most recently my students and I have returned to a consideration of informational text. Most children do not encounter much of this type of text until the third or even the fourth grade, at a time when they are expected to use reading as a tool for learning new content. In the last several years the field has recognized the need for students to be exposed to informational text in the early elementary grades (Caswell & Duke, 1998) and has called for research in this area (Pearson & Duke, 2002). Fortunately, instruction does not have to start from scratch. As part of our research program, Kristen Lauer has found in her dissertation study that as early as the second grade, students are sensitive to informational text structure; structure makes an independent contribution to comprehension, along with content familiarity and reading ability.

Certain types of informational text lend themselves to an instructional approach similar to the one we took in our Theme Identification program, in that, in contrast to main idea, there are specific structures that can be taught. Our work involves the development of instruction that focuses solely and intensively on a single structure, *compare–contrast,* and that provides elementary school students with direct instruction on how to understand that structure. As content to teach, we have chosen the classification of animals into the five classes of vertebrates (which aligns with the New York City Core Science Curriculum Standards for the elementary grades).

Kendra Hall, in her dissertation study, has examined a nine-lesson (15-session) program in second-grade inclusion classrooms that include students with learning disabilities and students who have been referred for evaluation for special education. The instruction includes the teaching of several strategies, such as the use of clue words (e.g., "alike" and "but"), graphic organizers, and questions that outline the text structure (What two things is this paragraph about? How are they the same? How are they different?) Each lesson includes reading and discussing the content of informational trade books, analysis of short, well-structured, compare–contrast paragraphs, work on content vocabulary (e.g., oxygen and warm-blooded), and writing as well as reading practice.

The study compares this program with more traditional instruction that involves the same materials (trade books and paragraphs) but focuses on content and not on text structure and also with a no-treatment control group. Preliminary data analysis indicates that the compare–contrast program is successful in teaching the strategies and in helping students acquire proficiency in constructing, orally and in writing, well-structured comparative statements in their summary of text. Moreover, there is indication of transfer, in that the effects are seen both on text that involves animals and on text whose content is unrelated to animals. We believe that our very direct and structured approach aids children in acquiring proficiency in reading informational text in the same way as it has been shown to be successful for narrative text.

Summary

Our evaluation studies have clearly indicated that our instructional programs are effective with respect to achievement. They have been successful in helping children with learning disabilities, even severe disabilities, to acquire higher-order comprehension skills. Students also can generalize what they have learned to other similar texts. On the basis of these findings, it appears certain that direct instruction that provides children with knowledge about text structure, and how to use that knowledge strategically, is an effective way to improve their comprehension. Simply providing opportunities for exposure to particular types of text is important but far from the whole story. Explicit instruction is valuable.

We have had positive and enthusiastic responses from both teachers and students. Informal feedback from students indicates that they enjoy the lessons. Teachers' responses on evaluation questionnaires indicate that they deem the programs educationally beneficial and enjoyable. They like the explicitness, repetition, and organization of the programs (Williams, 2002).

In conclusion, with appropriate materials and methods, students with learning disabilities who have reading problems can achieve competence in higher-order comprehension. The materials and methods that are effective for these students are also effective with other low-functioning students—indeed, they are effective with all levels of students in the classrooms that we have worked in. It is encouraging to see that students with learning disabilities respond well when a well-structured and integrated approach to comprehension is used and to realize that there is no need to limit instruction for these students to low-level tasks.

References

Allington, R., Guice, S., Michelson, N., Baker, K., & Li, S. (1996). Literature-based curricula in high poverty schools. In M. F. Graves, P. van den Broek, & B. M. Taylor (Eds.), *The first R: Every child's right to read* (pp. 141–162). New York: Teachers College Press.

Al Otaiba, S., & Fuchs, D. (In press). Characteristics of children who are unresponsive to early literacy intervention. *Remedial and Special Education.*

Baumann, J. F. (1984). The effectiveness of a direct instruction paradigm for teaching main idea comprehension. *Reading Research Quarterly, 20,* 93–115.

Bean, T. (2000). Reading in the content areas: Social constructivist dimensions. In M. L. Kamil, P. B. Mosenthal, P. David Pearson, & R. Barr (Eds.), *Handbook of reading research* (Vol. 3, pp. 629–644). Mahwah, NJ: Erlbaum.

Brown, A. L., & Palincsar, A. M. (1989). Guided, co-operative learning and individual knowledge acquisition. In L. B. Resnick (Ed.), *Knowing and learning: Essays in honor of Robert Glaser* (pp. 393–451). Hillsdale, NJ: Erlbaum.

Caswell, L. J., & Duke, N. K. (1998). Non-narrative as a catalyst for literacy development. *Language Arts, 75,* 108–117.

Dimino, J., Gersten, R., Carnine, D., & Blake, G. (1990). Story grammar: An approach for promoting at-risk secondary students' comprehension of literature. *Elementary School Journal, 91,* 19–32.

Dorfman, M. H., & Brewer, W. F. (1994). Understanding the points of fables. *Discourse Processes, 17,* 105–129.

Gersten, R., Fuchs, L. S., Williams, J. P., & Baker, S. (2001). Teaching reading comprehension strategies to students with learning disabilities: A review of research. *Review of Educational Research 71,* 279–320.

Gurney, D., Gersten, R., Dimino, J., & Carnine, D. (1990). Story grammar: Effective literature instruction for high school students with learning disabilities. *Journal of Learning Disabilities 23,* 335–348.

Hammill, D. D. (1990). On defining learning disabilities: An emerging consensus. *Journal of Learning Disabilities, 23,* 120–124.

Kucan, L., & Beck, I. L. (1997). Thinking aloud and reading comprehension research: Inquiry, in-struction, and social interaction. *Review of Educational Research, 67,* 271–299.

Lehr, S. (1988). The child's developing sense of theme as a response to literature. *Reading Research Quarterly, 23,* 337–357.

Mandler, J. M., & Johnson, N. S. (1977). Remembrance of things parsed: Story structure and recall. *Cognitive Psychology, 9,* 11–151.

National Reading Panel. (2000). *Teaching children to read: An evidence-based assessment of the scientific research literature on reading and its implications for reading instruction.* Washington, DC: National Institute of Child Health and Human Development and U.S. Department of Education.

Pearson, P. D., & Dole, J. A. (1987). Explicit comprehension instruction: A review of research and a new conceptualization of instruction. *The Elementary School Journal, 88,* 151–165.

Pearson, P. D., & Duke, N. K. (2002). Comprehension instruction in the primary grades. In C. C. Block & M. Pressley (Eds.), *Comprehension instruction: Research-based best practices* (pp. 247–258). New York: Guilford Press.

Perfetti, C. A. (1985). *Reading ability.* New York: Oxford University Press.

Perfetti, C. A., Marron, M. A., & Foltz, P. W. (1996). Sources of comprehension failure: Theoretical perspectives and case studies. In C. Cornoldi & J. Oakhill (Eds.), *Reading comprehension difficulties: Processes and interventions* (pp. 137–165). Mahwah, NJ: Erlbaum.

Pressley, M. (2000). What should comprehension instruction be the instruction of? In M. L. Kamil, P. B. Mosenthal, P. David Pearson, & R. Barr (Eds.), *Handbook of reading research* (Vol. 3, pp. 545–562). Mahwah, NJ: Erlbaum.

Pressley, M., & McCormick, C. (1995). *Advanced educational psychology.* New York: Harcourt Brace.

Pressley, M., Woloshyn, V., Lysynchuk, L. M., Martin, V., Wood, E., & Willoughby, T. (1990). A primer of research on cognitive strategy instruction: The important issues and how to address them. *Educational Psychology Review, 2,* 1–33.

Rosenblatt, L. M. (1978). *The reader, the text, and the poem.* Carbondale: Southern Illinois University Press.

Simmons, D. C., Fuchs, L. S., Fuchs, D., Mathes, P. G., & Hodge, J. P. (1995). Effects of explicit teaching and peer tutoring on the reading achievement of learning-disabled and low-performing students in regular classrooms. *Elementary School Journal, 95,* 387–408.

Singer, H., & Donlan, D. (1982). Active comprehension: Problem-solving schema with question generation for comprehension of complex short stories. *Reading Research Quarterly, 17,* 166–186.

Swanson, H. L, & Hoskyn, M. (1998). Experimental intervention research on students with learning disabilities: A meta-analysis of treatment outcomes. *Review of Educational Research, 68,* 277–321.

Taylor, M. B., & Williams, J. P. (1983). Comprehension of LD readers: Task and text variations. *Journal of Educational Psychology, 75,* 743–751.

van Dijk, T. A. (1980). *Macrostructures.* Hillsdale, NJ: Erlbaum.

West, J. (1953). *Cress Delahanty.* New York: Harcourt Brace.

Wilder, A. A., & Williams, J. P. (2001). Students with severe learning disabilities can learn higher-order comprehension skills. *Journal of Educational Psychology, 93,* 268–278.

Williams, J. P. (1984). Categorization, macrostructure, and finding the main idea. *Journal of Educational Psychology 76,* 874–879.

Williams, J. P. (1992). Reading instruction and learning disabled students. In M. J. Dreher & W. H. Slater (Eds.), *Elementary school literacy: Critical issues* (pp. 157–181). Norwood, MA: Christopher-Gordon.

Williams, J. P. (1993). Comprehension of students with and without disabilities: Identification of narrative themes and idiosyncratic text representations. *Journal of Educational Psychology, 85,* 631–641.

Williams, J. P. (1998). Improving the comprehension of disabled readers. *Annals of Dyslexia, 48,* 213–238.

Williams, J. P. (2002). Using the Theme Scheme to improve story comprehension. In C. C. Block & M. Pressley (Eds.), *Comprehension instruction: Research-based best practices* (pp. 126–139). New York: Guilford Press.

Williams, J. P., Brown, L. G., Silverman, A. K., & deCani, J. S. (1994). An instructional program for adolescents with learning disabilities in the comprehension of narrative themes. *Learning Disabilities Quarterly, 17,* 205–221.

Williams, J. P., Lauer, K. D., Hall, K. M., Lord, K. M., Gugga, S. S., Bak, S. J., Jacobs, P. R., & deCani, J. S. (2002). Teaching elementary school students to identify story themes. *Journal of Educational Psychology, 94,* 235–248.

Williams, J. P., Taylor, M. B., & Ganger, S. (1981). Text variations at the level of the individual sentence and the comprehension of simple expository paragraphs. *Journal of Educational Psychology, 73,* 851–865.

Williams, J. P., Taylor, M. B., Jarin, D. C., & Milligan, E. S. (1983). *Determining the main idea of expository paragraphs: An instructional program for the learning-disabled and its evaluation* (Tech. Rep. #25). Research Institute for the Study of Learning Disabilities, Teachers College, Columbia University.

Wong, B. Y. L. (1984). Metacognition and learning disabilities. In T. Waller, D. Forrest, & E. MacKinnon (Eds.), *Metacognition, cognition and human performance* (pp. 137–180). New York: Academic Press.

19

Enhancing the Mathematical Problem Solving of Students with Mathematics Disabilities

Lynn S. Fuchs
Douglas Fuchs

Converging evidence (Badian, 1983; Gross-Tsur, Manor, & Shalev, 1996; Kosc, 1974) reveals that 6–7% of the school-age population suffers from mathematics disability (MD). Despite its prevalence, MD has been the focus of less systematic study than has reading disability (RD) (cf. Rasanen & Ahonen, 1995). This relative neglect is unfortunate. In school, mathematics skill is important for success; after school, mathematics competence accounts for employment, income, and work productivity even after intelligence and reading have been explained (Rivera-Batiz, 1992).

Despite this relative neglect, important work on MD has been accomplished over the past two decades. The literature describes functional arithmetic difficulties of students with MD and demonstrates how cognitive deficits are associated with the development of arithmetic cognition (see Geary, 1993, for review). This literature has, nevertheless, focused disproportionately on acquisition of basic facts, with relatively few studies on algorithmic competence. And, when problem solving has been studied (e.g., Jordan & Hanich, 2000), it has been confined largely to linguistically presented one-step problems involving addition and subtraction number facts.

Although straightforward to measure and study, these arithmetic story problems fail to represent the kind of tasks that increasingly are incorporated in school curricula beyond the earliest grades. In fact, mathematics education reform over the past 15 years has prompted schools to emphasize the development of more complex problem-solving capacity (e.g., Resnick & Resnick, 1992; Rothman, 1995), with a measurement focus on performance assessments that pose real-world problem-solving dilemmas and require students to develop solutions involving the application of multiple skills. Therefore, generalizations from the MD literature to MD as it occurs in schools and generalizations to the kinds of mathematical competence required in the real world are tenuous. So, a focus on mathematical competence beyond arithmetic and arithmetic story problems is required to understand, prevent, and remediate MD in its many forms, as it develops in schools and as it pertains to the real world.

Our research on mathematics serves to illustrate an expanding focus that corresponds roughly to how mathematics curriculum has evolved over time within schools. Our early studies, illustrated by Fuchs, Fuchs, Hamlett, and Stecker (1990), were dedicated to mathematics operations (addition, subtraction, multiplication, and division of whole number, fractions, and decimals). As schools, however, broadened their mathematics domain, we adapted by focusing on mathematics concepts and applications (see, e.g., Fuchs et al., 1997). Of course, these measurement methods and this instructional content were confined largely to discrete skills and artificially structured word problems. Thus, beginning in 1995, we reoriented our research program to mathematics problem solving, more broadly conceptualized and as increasingly reflected in the schools.

In this chapter, we summarize our research program on mathematical problem solving. We begin by describing our conceptualization of problem solving and the corresponding measurement work we necessarily conducted to make the study of mathematics problem solving possible. Next, we describe a series of studies conducted with normally developing students to gain insight into how we might effect better learning on challenging mathematical problem-solving tasks for students with MD. Then, we discuss recent studies in which we applied those findings to students with MD. In these studies, to qualify as having a MD, students had to score at least 90 on an intelligence test and at least 1.5 standard deviations below the mean on a mathematics achievement test.

Conceptualizing and Identifying Tasks to Study Mathematical Problem Solving

Mathematical Problem Solving

We conceptualized mathematical problem solving as a transfer challenge, which requires students to apply knowledge, skills, and strategies to novel problems (cf. Bransford & Schwartz, 1999; Mayer, Quilici, & Moreno, 1999). Effecting this form of transfer can be especially difficult for primary-grade children (Durnin, Perrone, & MacKay, 1997) and for students with disabilities, who have demonstrated generalization problems (White, 1984).

As conceptualized by Cooper and Sweller

(1987), three variables contribute to problem-solving transfer. Students must (1) master the rules for problem solution, (2) develop categories for sorting problems that require similar solutions, and (3) be aware that novel problems are related to previously solved problems. Research has substantiated the importance of the first variable, mastering rules for problem solution (e.g., Mawer & Sweller, 1982; Sweller & Cooper, 1985). As students master problem-solution rules, they allocate less working memory to the details of the solution and instead devote cognitive resources to identify connections between novel and familiar problems and to plan their work.

Cooper and Sweller's (1987) second variable suggests that schemas play a role in transfer. As defined by Gick and Holyoak (1983), a *schema* is a generalized description of two or more problems, which individuals use to sort problems into groups requiring similar solutions. The broader the schema, the greater the probability that individuals will recognize the connections between familiar and novel problems and that transfer, therefore, will occur. To gain insight into the role schemas play in transfer, Cooper and Sweller questioned eighth-graders as they worked novel algebra problems. The researchers coded responses in terms of whether statements reflected schemas (e.g., when faced with a new problem, students reported thinking about how an earlier problem had been solved) and demonstrated that schemas strongly influence performance on problems that fall within the boundaries of those schemas. They also noted, however, that participants' schemas were disappointingly narrow. The challenge in effecting transfer, of course, is to help learners develop broad schemas.

At the same time, it remains unclear how to address Cooper and Sweller's (1987) third transfer-inducing variable: triggering awareness of the connections between training and transfer tasks. Prior work does, however, reveal the importance of such awareness. For example, using two sets of paired associates, Asch (1969) demonstrated that many students enjoyed no savings in learning one pair that was identical across the lists; only participants who recognized the pair as familiar realized the savings, but once students were told that an old pair might be on the new list, all students demonstrated the expected savings. In this and related studies (e.g., Catrambone & Holyoak, 1989; Gick & Holyoak, 1983; Ross, 1989), performance increased when participants were cued to anticipate similarities across tasks. This finding demonstrates how awareness of the potential connections across novel and familiar tasks is a key ingredient for transfer. Of course, to achieve mathematical problem-solving transfer, it is necessary to go beyond cuing by an external agent. Instead, students must independently activate searches for connections between novel and familiar tasks.

To broaden schemas and evoke independent searches for connections between transfer and familiar tasks without the need for external cueing. Salomon and Perkins (1989) provided the following theoretical framework. They distinguished between two forms of transfer. Low-road transfer is accomplished via extensive, varied practice; it occurs as a function of the automatic triggering of well-learned, stimulus-controlled behavior in a new situation; using math facts to solve multi-step computation problems is an example of low-road transfer. Mathematical problem solving, by contrast, is a form of high-road transfer, which involves the deliberate abstraction of principles that apply across contexts or tasks. High-road transfer requires individuals to formulate and search for these abstract connections between transfer and familiar tasks. As Salomon and Perkins suggested, the hallmark of high-road transfer is *mindful abstraction*. (For *mindfulness*, we substitute the more familiar, educationally relevant term "metacognition.")

To *abstract* a principle is to identify a generic quality or pattern across instances of the principle. In formulating an abstraction, an individual deletes details across examplars, which are irrelevant to the abstract category (e.g., ignoring that an airplane is metal and or that a bird has feathers to formulate the abstraction of "flying things"). These abstractions are represented in symbolic form and avoid contextual specificity so they can be applied to other instances or across situations. Because abstractions, or schemas, subsume related cases, they promote transfer. With *metacognition*, an individual withholds an initial response and, instead, deliberately examines the task at hand and generates alternative solutions by considering ways in which the novel task shares connections with familiar tasks. So, with high-road transfer, abstraction provides the bridge from one context to the other; metacognition is the conscious recognition and effortful application of that abstraction across contexts.

Salomon and Perkins (1989) further described two forms of high-road transfer. With forward-reaching high-road transfer, the abstraction is generated in the initial learning context; as learners engage in the initial task, they consider other situations in which the abstraction might apply. By contrast, with backward-reaching high-road transfer, abstraction occurs in the transfer situation, where the learner thinks back to previous tasks to search for relevant connections and abstractions. As discussed by Salomon and Perkins, both forms of high-road transfer provide a theoretical basis for teaching explicity for transfer. For example, as teachers formulate the scientific factors relevant to electricity, they highlight how these principles apply to other domains of science. This promotes forward-reaching transfer. Furthermore, when addressing subsequent topics, teachers capitalize on the potential for backward-reaching transfer. Here, teachers encourage students to search their knowledge of scientific principles gleaned from electricity for relevant analogies. Salomon and Perkins asserted that helping students (a) anticipate how abstractions may facilitate success with novel learning tasks (as in forward-reaching tansfer) and (b) conduct independent searches for relevant abstractions that apply across tasks (as in backward-reaching transfer) represents an untapped instructional opportunity to explicitly teach students to transfer. We used this framework to study and enhance mathematical problem solving.

Tasks to Study Mathematical Problem Solving

To identify tasks with which to study mathematical problem solving, we relied on this conceptual framework. So, we developed measures of mathematical problem solving along a continuum of contextual realism. We predicted that as problems achieved greater verisimiltude, the challenge of identifying familiar problem solutions would increase. Essentially, we hypothesized that contextual realism is achieved as the variety of possible solutions needed to answer problems increases, the nature of the required operations becomes more varied, the amount of information described in the problem situation increases, and the location of that information is removed from the problem questions. Herein, we briefly summarize our work in developing technically viable measurement at a point toward the difficult end of this continuum: The Mathematics Performance Assessment (Fuchs, Fuchs, Karns, et al., 2000).

This measure, which incorporates six alternate forms at each level (grades 2–6), requires students to apply 10 essential grade-level skills to a contextually realistic situation. The assessment presents an introductory narrative that includes nonessential details and irrelevant numbers, with multiple related questions removed from the narrative. At each grade, we developed parallel forms by first creating one preliminary fourth-grade assessment for illustrative purposes. Next, we held a focus group meeting at which teachers individually completed the illustrative assessment, learned to use the scoring rubric, and divided into grade-level teams to score five sample protocols and to make suggestions for modifying the scoring rubric and the basic structure of the illustrative assessment. Then, in grade-level teams, teachers identified 10 core skills to incorporate into the assessment at their grade level. They began by reviewing the statewide mathematics curriculum to select the 10 skills most essential for successful entry to the next grade and the 10 skills most essential for successful entry into the grade they teach. Then, in one large group, the teachers compared (a) the skills they specified as important for entering the next higher grade with (b) the skills identified by teachers in that next higher grade as critical for successful entry. With this input, teachers returned to grade-level teams to finalize lists of core grade-level skills. Finally, in grade-level teams, teachers identified and rank-ordered 20 themes that represented real-life situations students might face now or in the next few years, were interesting, could incorporate the 10 core skills, and were age appropriate.

Working with this input, we collectively developed one assessment at each grade. We piloted each test with three students who were entering and three who were exiting the target grade. Based on the range of performances and the students' input about what they liked, disliked, and found confusing, we modified these initial tests. We next developed a framework for creating the remaining five parallel forms at each grade level and then developed those remaining tests. The following sequence then recurred three times. At each grade level, five experienced teachers completed each of the six assessments. These adults, who were unfamiliar with the development process, identified every skill they applied in answering the questions; described inconsistencies in difficulty level and required skill applications across parallel forms; and noted potential sources of confusion within the narrative and questions. Based on this input, we revised the tests. Finally, at each grade, four students (two exiting and two entering the target grade level) completed all six tests. Based on their responses and input, we made a final set of revisions.

Each two- to three-page test begins with a multiparagraph narrative describing the problem situation. Each dilemma also presents students with tabular and graphic information for potential application. The problem includes questions that provided students with opportunities to (1) apply the core set of skills, (2) discriminate relevant from irrelevant information in the narrative, (3) generate information not contained in the narrative, (4) explain their mathematical work, and (5) generate written communication related to the mathematics.

These tests initially were scored according to the rubric shown adapted from the Kansas Quality Performance Assessment (Kansas State Board of Education, 1991). This rubric structured scoring along four dimensions (conceptual underpinnings, computational applications, problem-solving strategies, and communicative value). Each dimension was scored on a 6-point holistic scale. In later work, we enhanced reliability by converting this scoring system to award points on a fine-grained basis ranging from 1 to 70. As shown by Fuchs and colleagues (in press-a) ($n = 412$), alpha coefficient was .94; concurrent validity with the TerraNova (CTB/McGraw-Hill, 1997) was .67.

Because Fuchs, Fuchs, Karns, and colleagues (2000) illustrated the deleterious effects of unfamiliarity with performance assessments, we administer the task in the following way. Prior to measurement, testers deliver a 45-min lesson on how performance assessments are structured, strategies for approaching performance assessments, and scoring procedures. This lesson first provides students an opportunity to work on a performance assessment below their grade level; then, using that assessment, presents examples of student work to illustrate the topics. In all assessment situations, text is read and reread aloud as requested.

We had hypothesized that the variety of possible problem solutions and the amount and location of the information needed to set up the problem all contribute to contextual realism. This, in turn, increases the difficulty students experience in recognizing a novel problem as belonging to a familiar problem type, for which they know a solution method. In fact, we (Fuchs & Fuchs, 2002) contrasted features of our performance assessments with Jordan and Hanich's (2000) arithmetic story problems task (i.e., linguistically presented one-step number fact problems). All indices of problem difficulty (i.e., number of words, sentences, words per sentence, verbs, numbers, and math steps) were lower for arithmetic story problems than for the real-world problem-solving measure. Each feature increases the difficulty of mathematics problem-solving tasks. In addition, we compared student performance as a function of task (Fuchs & Fuchs, 2002). Among students with MD without comorbid RD, accuracy fell from 75% for arithmetic story problems to 12% for real-world problem solving; for students with comorbid MD and RD, percentages were 55 and 5. Thus, performance differentials were dramatic when comparing arithmetic story problems to our performance assessments.

It is also interesting to consider the source of the dramatic performance drop for students with MD between arithmetic and real-world problem solving, where increasing complexity was derived from greater text-based demands, the need to apply more varied math operations, and the inclusion of nonessential details. Previous work demonstrates the deleterious effects of longer text with more words and more verbs per sentence (Cohen & Stover, 1981; Cook, 1973; Helwig, Rosek-Toedesco, Tindal, Heath, & Almond, 1999; Jerman & Mirman, 1974) as well as multiple operational steps and irrelevant information. The challenge, of course, is to separate the effects of these potential sources of difficulty. We attempted to provide some insight on this matter by reporting separate scores for operations and problem solving, so that problem-solving capacity was not confounded with operational competence. In fact, the magnitude of drop on both performance dimensions was comparable, suggesting that operational demands as well as informational richness contribute to difficulty. Multidetermined difficulty provides some support for conceptualizing contextual realism (determined by variety of possible problem solutions, operational demands, and amount and location of information in the problem) as the source of challenge in mathematical problem solving. It is also consistent with the notion that transfer is the essential feature of mathematical problem solving, whereby contextual realism increases the difficulty of classifying problems as belonging to categories for which solutions are known. This measurement work provided the groundwork for studying methods to enhance mathematical problem solving.

Enhancing Mathematical Problem Solving among Nondisabled Students with Varying Histories of Mathematics Achievement

Using this conceptual framework and relying on this measurement task, we conducted a series of three studies to identify methods for enhancing mathematical problem solving among students without disabilities with varying mathematics achievement histories. The first study described instruction and student learning in mathematical problem solving when teacher planning was informed by ongoing performance assessment feedback. The second study examined the effects of explicitly teaching students to transfer, and the third study extended those findings by investigating the added contribution of self regulation. In this chapter, we focus on the first two studies and refer briefly to the third.

Teacher Planning and Student Learning with Ongoing Performance Assessment Feedback

We (Fuchs, Fuchs, Karns, Hamlett, & Karzaroff, 1999) were interested in exploring how teachers designed instruction to enhance their students' mathematical problem-solving performance. Because teachers were relatively unfamiliar with a problem-solving curriculum and with the performance assessments that measure performance on that curriculum, we supported teacher efforts—but in a relatively unobtrusive way. We familiarized them with the concept of performance assessment; we helped them administer, score, interpret, and provide student feedback on performance assessments every 3 weeks; and we released them to consult with fellow teachers every 3 weeks about how to improve their students' problem-solving performance. The design of this study was experimental. We identified 16 teachers at grades 2–4, then, stratifying by grade level, we randomly assigned teachers to "experimental" and contrast groups. At the beginning of the school year, we identified students in each class as above, at, or below grade level in math and examined effects on student learning as a function of these achievement designations and as a function of teachers' study condition. We used teacher as the unit of analysis.

Results indicated that the modest level of support we provided did increase teachers' understanding of what mathematics problem-solving performance assessment is and how feedback on students' performance assessment might be used to improve problem-solving performance. When asked to develop a performance assessment, experimental teachers constructed problems that incorporated more features associated with performance assessment. When asked how performance assessment might be used to formulate instructional decisions, experimental teachers cited more strategies. Results were statistically significant and large, with effect sizes (ESs) exceeding 1 standard deviation. Of course, this is not surprising.

One might expect knowledge about performance assessment to increase as teachers, over the course of several months, scored performance assessments, provided students feedback on those problem-solving assessments, and consulted with fellow teachers to design instruction to enhance student performance.

More noteworthy is the finding that as a function of participating in the experimental condition, teachers' curricular focus expanded to incorporate a greater emphasis on mathematical problem solving. Compared to the contrast group, experimental teachers decreased emphasis on math facts and computation and increased focus on problem solving, with ESs ranging from 0.62 for math facts to 1.51 for problem solving. Thus, in response to a relatively modest intervention, teachers' thinking about mathematics curriculum changed. This echoes previous work on the effects of statewide accountability programs incorporating performance assessment (e.g., Koretz, Barron, Mitchell, & Stecher, 1996; Koretz, Mitchell, Barron, & Keith, 1996).

Importantly, however, our study extended previous work by showing how teachers' actual instructional plans reflect changing curricular emphasis. As experimental teachers, over three planning cycles, brainstormed collaboratively with colleagues to identify methods for increasing student performance, they each committed themselves to many (i.e., 9–17) instructional ideas, which represented three important instructional strategies. First, approximately one of every four ideas that teachers incorporated into their plans was designed to expand mathematical problem-solving performance. And, importantly, some of these activities, such as peer-mediated learning (e.g., King, 1991) and problem demonstrations (e.g., Cooper & Sweller, 1987), resemble research-based practices with demonstrated efficacy for promoting mathematical problem solving. Second, as represented by their use of test-like practice, teachers incorporated extended mathematical problem-solving activities. This is noteworthy because extended problem-solving activities offer students opportunity to discover the relations among knowledge elements and problem features, which are important to the development of problem solving, and because prior work (Stigler & Hiebert, 1997) suggests that teachers typically avoid extended mathematics activities, allocating as much as 96% of students' time to practice on routine problems. The third strategy represented in the teachers' instructional plans was helping students demonstrate and communicate about the mathematical competence they already possessed: One of every four instructional ideas was designed to improve students' labels and explanations. Of course, some may construe two of these instructional procedure, clarifying methods for showing/explaining work and providing test-like practice, as "teaching to the test" and view these activities as cause for concern. After all, these two foci collectively represented half the teachers' instructional plans—or double the teachers' use of more guided methods for extending students' mathematical problem solving (e.g., peer-mediated learning or problem demonstrations). Moreover, as shown in previous work on the effects of statewide accountability programs, teachers can structure these activities in ways that constitute "coaching" (Firestone, Mayrowetz, & Fairman, 1998), which can lead to rapid, initial gains that do not represent true learning (Hambleton et al., 1995).

It is not surprising, therefore, that effects on student learning were not entirely supportive of the teachers' methods and differed as a function of students' achievement histories. Superior problem solving was demonstrated by *above-grade-level students* (ESs = 0.93–1.47). *At-grade-level students* also demonstrated impressive learning—at least on the two measures most similar to the performance assessments administered over the course of the study (ESs = 0.76–1.15). Yet, on the most novel measure (a commercial performance assessment) where transfer demands were greatest, effects were not statistically significant, with a correspondingly modest ES of 0.30. For the two measures in which we observed effects, format and scoring were identical to the classroom performance assessments, whereas the format and scoring of the novel measure differed dramatically. This provides the basis for supposing that students may have suffered from inadequate awareness of how the knowledge and strategies they had in fact garnered from the classroom activities

(as evidenced by their superior performance on the two similarly formatted and scored measures) might apply to the novel measure. Essentially, superficial differences in the novel measure may have interfered in prompting metacognitive awareness of relations across problem situations (Brown, Campione, Webber, & McGilly, 1992). This argument also seems plausible in light of experimental teachers' failure to incorporate instructional activities designed to help students analyze and articulate similarities and differences among problem contexts. Such pattern-finding activities, in which students analyze contrasting cases, have been shown to enhance problem solving (Schwartz & Bransford, 1998). Thus, we hypothesize that metacognitive awareness of the relations across problem-solving situations may have mediated at-grade-level students' problem-solving capacity. This hypothesis provided the basis for future research described later.

Meanwhile, results for *below-grade-level students* were disappointing. We found one statistically significant effect on one problem-solving measure for the communicative value scoring dimension—the dimension most sensitive to the experimental teachers' guidance about how to label and explain work. Moreover, below-grade-level experimental students actually performed somewhat lower than contrast counterparts on the most novel transfer problem, which differed in format and scoring (ES = −0.28). These findings echo previous work showing the challenges associated with effecting mathematical problem solving among low-achieving students. For example, Cooper and Sweller (1987) found that students with previously low achievement required longer periods and more worked examples to acquire mathematical problem solving. Mayer (1998) demonstrated that when teachers used an approach consistent with the National Council of Teachers of Mathematics's (NCTM's) standards, students with higher incoming achievement levels benefited more. In a similar way, Woodward and Baxter (1997) showed that students with learning disabilities or those who scored below the 34th percentile on a standardized achievement test profited less from a problem-solving mathematics curriculum than did average achievers. Clearly, for below-grade-level students, results were discouraging, and they augured poorly for students with MD.

Explicitly Teaching Students to Transfer

One major conclusion from Fuchs and colleagues (1999) was that teachers required greater structure and guidance to address mathematical problem solving effectively. Although teachers' instructional plans reflected impressive attempts to incorporate innovative activities, some promising approaches for guiding students in the development of problem-solving capacity were noticeably absent. And, for low-achieving and for some average-achieving students, more explicit forms of instruction may be required to develop problem-solving schema and metacognitive awareness.

We therefore designed a treatment to teach explicitly for transfer (Fuchs et al., in press-a). Relying on the conceptual work of Cooper and Sweller (1987) and Salomon and Perkins (1989), the treatment attempted to increase awareness of the connections between novel and familiar problems by (1) broadening the categories by which students group problems requiring the same solution methods (i.e., promoting a higher level of abstraction) and (2) explicitly prompting students to search novel problems for these broad categories (i.e., increasing metacognition). We combined this explicit transfer treatment with explicit instruction designed to teach solution methods for different types of problems. We contrasted the effectiveness of a combined treatment (transfer + solution instruction) to solution instruction alone and to teacher-designed.

Solution instruction addressed Cooper and Sweller's (1987) first variable, teaching rules for problem solution. Our explicit transfer treatment, by contrast, was designed to effect abstraction and metacognition in the service of mathematical problem solving. With respect to *abstraction,* our explicit transfer treatment attempted to broaden students' schemas for sorting problems that require similar solutions. Toward that end, we taught four types of superficial problem features, which change problems without altering the problems' structure or solution (Ross, 1989). Our four types of superficial problem features were format, key-

word vocabulary, additional question posed, and placement in a larger problem-solving context. In the Appendix, we illustrate how each type of superficial feature changes a sample problem. As shown, the manipulation of superficial problem features affects neither the structure of the problem nor the required solution. We provided students with practice in sorting novel problems according to which superficial problem feature had changed and in solving those novel problems. In this way, we promoted the development of broader schemas, which permitted students to recognize that a broader range of problems belonged to a unifying problem structure and thereby required the known solution. In terms of *metacognition,* we explicitly taught students the concept of transfer. Moreover, we cautioned students that, when faced with novel problems, they should search for connections to familiar problem structures and for the superficial problem features they knew could change a problem without altering the required solution. By broadening schemas and triggering awareness of the connections between familiar and novel problems, this explicit transfer treatment addressed Cooper and Sweller's second and third transfer-inducing varibles. The combination of problem solution instruction with transfer instruction addressed all three transfer-inducing variables.

The study included four conditions, all of which received the school district's mathematics program from which the four problem structures had been selected and received comparable amounts of math instruction time. Teacher-designed (i.e., control) instruction incorporated the district's curriculum, which addressed the four problem structures. The other three conditions were experimental, designed to incorporate explicit instruction (Carnine, 1997), heavy use of worked examples (Cooper & Sweller, 1987), and peer-mediated practice (Fuchs et al., 1997). In one experimental condition, students received only solution instruction. The other two experimental groups combined solution with transfer treatment. Because the solution treatment required 20 sessions and the transfer treatment entailed another 10 sessions, combining treatments posed a dilemma about how to control the amount of experimenter-designed instructional time. So, we combined treatments in two ways. In one combined condition, the number of experimental sessions were equal for the solution and for the combined condition; to accomplish this, we cut the number of solution sessions in half. The other combined treatment permitted the full set problem solution sessions. Intervention lasted 16 weeks.

Not surprisingly, we found evidence to support the utility of the problem solution instruction. On the acquisition test, which required students to solve the four problem structures when fresh cover stories constituted the only source of novelty, the two groups that received more of the solution treatment grew significantly and substantially more than the combined group that received less of the solution treatment (ES = 1.49–2.08). This provides evidence for the importance of Cooper and Sweller's (1987) first transfer-inducing, as operationalized by our solution treatment. Of course, the extent of transfer required on the acquisition task was minimal because problems varied from the content of the solution treatment only in terms of cover stories. Thus, the effectiveness of the solution treatment is illustrated better with findings the near transfer measure, which not only varied cover stories but also manipulated, for each problem, one additional superficial problem feature addressed in the transfer treatment. Results indicated that although this near transfer measure was aligned more closely with the transfer than the solution treatment, all three experimental conditions, including the experimental group that did not receive the transfer treatment, again improved significantly and substantially more than the control group (ESs = 2.11–2.25). Moreover, the combined condition with the full set of solution sessions persuasively outgrew the combined condition with only half the solution sessions (ES = 1.29).

In addition to lending support for the effectiveness of the solution treatment, the near-transfer results also provided evidence for the utility of the explicit transfer treatment, which was designed to broaden the categories by which students group problems requiring the same solution methods (i.e., promoting a higher level of abstraction) and to prompt students to search novel problems for these broad categories (i.e.,

increasing metacognition). Support for this transfer treatment was found on the near-transfer measure, in the dramatically superior growth of the combined treatment (transfer + the full set of solution lessons) versus the solution condition alone without transfer instruction (ES = 1.45). Both conditions had received all the solution lessons; the key difference was the provision of the transfer treatment. Although the simple addition of experimenter-controlled instructional time in the full solution + transfer condition might explaining this effect, this explanation is unpersuasive in light of improvement on the acquisition measure, where the contrast between these two conditions was not statistically significant (ES = 0.19).

Of course, the most convincing measure of learning in this study was the far-transfer test—our real-world problem-solving measure, which posed questions with the greatest degree of novelty: an unfamiliar cover story, simultaneous manipulation of all four superficial problem features taught in the transfer treatment, and inclusion of irrelevant information as well as additional problem structures and content taught in the district's curriculum. Also, we minimized extraneous cuing by formatting the far transfer measure to resemble commercial achievement tests and using unfamiliar testers. Results on this far-transfer measure further substantiated the additive effect of the transfer treatment: Both groups that received the transfer treatment impressively outgrew the control group (ES = 1.01–1.16). Moreover, the solution condition, which did not receive the transfer treatment, did not outgrow the control group (ES = 0.39).

On the improvement score for each measure, we also examined interactions between study condition and the mathematics grade-level status with which students began the study. We found no significant interaction. Therefore, effects were not mediated by students' prior achievement histories. This is notable in light of previous work indicating that transfer is more difficult to effect among low-achieving students (Cooper & Sweller, 1987; Fuchs et al., 1999; Mayer, 1998; Woodward & Baxter, 1997). Effects may have accrued for below-grade students because our treatments were more explicit and longer in duration than most previous experimental interventions.

Consequently, results strengthened previous work (e.g., Cooper & Sweller, 1987) showing the importance of instruction designed to teach rules for problem solution. At the same time, the study's major contribution was the demonstration that explicitly teaching for transfer, by broadening the categories by which students group problems requiring the same solution methods (i.e., promoting a higher level of abstraction) and prompting students to search novel problems for these broad categories (i.e., increasing metacognition), facilitates mathematical problem solving. In subsequent work (Fuchs et al., in press-b), we also documented how self-regulation enhances the effectiveness of the combined solution/transfer treatment.

Applying Findings to Students with MD

Our work also provides the basis for examining related effects on students with MD. In this chapter, we focus on two databases. First, our study examining effects of explicitly teaching for transfer on nondisabled students (as just described; Fuchs et al., in press-a) also incorporated a small sample of students with MD. This database permits an estimate of the efficacy of the treatments when that instruction is delivered in whole-class arrangement. Second, we recently conducted an experiment (Fuchs, Fuchs, Hamlett, & Appleton, 2002) examining the effects of the combined solution and transfer treatments specifically on students with MD when that instruction is provided in small groups. Below, we summarize these findings.

Effects of Explicitly Teaching for Transfer in Whole-Class Arrangement

As just noted, our experiment examining the effects of solution and transfer instruction (Fuchs et al., in press-a) on students without disabilities also included a small group of students with MD. Among these children, effects were least supportive for the combined condition that incorporated only the partial set of solution lessons. In that condition, 60% to 80% of students with MD (depending on outcome measure) failed to progress more than the control group of students with MD. This unacceptable rate of nonresponsiveness reveals the need to develop a strong foundation in problem solutions before instruction designed to promote transfer can contribute to learning.

For the other treatments, which incorporated the full set of lessons designed to teach solution methods, some findings were encouraging. Specifically, on the acquisition measure, effects, although smaller in magnitude than for students without disabilities (where ESs ranged between 1.49 and 2.08), were in fact respectably strong (ESs = .66–1.78). Thus, it appeared that the explicit instruction, with strong reliance on worked examples and peer mediation, was effective in helping students with MD master the rules for problem solution, when novel word problems (i.e., new cover stories and quantities) were presented in the exact same format in which they had been taught.

Unfortunately, as problems became increasingly novel from those practiced during instruction, the discrepancy of effects between students with and without MD grew. For near transfer, ESs for students without disabilities who received transfer instruction ranged between 2.11 and 2.25; for students with MD, the effect, while moderate, was dramatically lower (0.45 in the transfer condition with the full set of solution lessons). And, on the far-transfer measure where the problem situation approximated real-world problem solving, there was essentially no effect for students with MD (ES = 0.07) whereas students without disabilities clearly transferred their knowledge to the novel problem-solving situation (ES = 1.01–1.16). From this database, we concluded that we needed to examine the efficacy of our mathematical problem-solving treatment using a service delivery mechanism that permitted greater intensity.

Effects of Explicit Instruction on Solutions and Transfer in Small-Group Arrangement

Consequently, in the following year, we conducted an experiment to examine the effectiveness of problem-solving tutoring, conducted in small groups of two to four, with fourth-grade students with MD. The lessons, which were identical to those used in the larger whole-class study, integrated explicit instruction on problem solution rules and transfer. To create a stringest test of efficacy, we assessed the contribution of this treatment to computer-assisted practice on real-world problem-solving tasks, where students actually had intensive, guided, direct practice on the alternate forms of the study's far-transfer task. Students were randomly assigned to problem-solving tutoring (or not) and to computer-assisted practice (or not), creating four conditions: problem-solving tutoring, computer-assisted practice, problem-solving tutoring plus computer-assisted practice, and control, all of which received the same mathematics curriculum from which the four problem structures were selected and the same base unit on problem solving. As with Fuchs and colleagues (in press-a), tutoring incorporated explicit instruction (Carnine, 1997), heavy use of worked examples (Cooper & Sweller, 1987), and peer-mediated practice (Fuchs et al., 1997). Computer-assisted practice included incorporated guided feedback with motivational scoring.

Six special education teachers agreed to have their fourth-grade students with MD participate. Teachers nominated 62 students who met two criteria: (1) According to cumulative records, their standard scores on an individually administered intelligence test were 90 or above, and (2) their special education teachers reported that they had MD. To these 62 students, we administered the Test of Computational Fluency (Fuchs, Fuchs, Eaton, Hamlett, & Karns, 2000), to identify students ($n = 40$) who scored at least 1.5 standard deviations below a regional normative sample.

Stratifying so that each condition was represented approximately equally for each teacher, we randomly assigned students so that 10 students were in each of four conditions: problem-solving tutoring with computer-assisted practice, computer-assisted practice, problem-solving tutoring, and control. Inferential statistics indicated group comparability on students' sex, free/reduced lunch status, race, and problematic classroom behavior. We also documented comparable mathematics pretreatment performance across the treatment groups on tests of computational fluency, mathematics ap-

plications, and arithmetic story problems (Jordan & Hanich, 2000).

Results showed that problem-solving tutoring, which provided students with explicit instruction on rules for problem solution and explicit instruction on transfer in small groups, did promote mathematical problem-solving growth among students with MD. Importantly, this growth was manifested on the full range of measures, although with smaller effects on the real-world problem-solving, far-transfer measure.

On the acquisition and near-transfer measures, tutoring produced statistically significant improvement compared to a control condition, in which students had received a 3-week instructional unit on word problems. On the acquisition measure, effect sizes comparing the tutoring condition with this control group exceeded 2 standard deviations and clearly were in the same range as those documented in the earlier study for students without disabilities (2.11–2.25). On the near-transfer measure, effects were reliable and large (0.88)—nearly double those revealed for students with MD when lessons were delivered in whole-class arrangement (0.45).

In addition, although results for the real-world problem-solving, far-transfer measure were not statistically significant, the corresponding effect size exceeded a half standard deviation. This figure approximated the effect size (0.63) associated with the computer-assisted practice condition, even though the computer-assisted group spent all its experimental time practicing problems analogous to the real-world problem-solving task. Moreover, the effect size of 0.61 for students with MD when lessons were delivered in small groups was substantially larger than the figure of 0.07 for students with MD when lessons were delivered in whole-class arrangement. Across the three tasks, therefore, results support the value of small-group instruction (Elbaum, Vaughn, Hughes, & Moody, 2000), where opportunities to respond, to seek clarification, and to obtain guided feedback are substantially greater than in whole-class instruction. Of course, this effect size of 0.61 for students with MD, when lessons were provided in *small* groups, still pales in comparison to effect sizes exceeding 1 standard deviation for students without disabilities when lessons were delivered in *large* groups.

Thus, this study provided the basis for some optimism and some caution. On the one hand, results documented the efficacy of explicit instruction on problem solutions and transfer delivered within the context of small groups and paralleled findings for students without disabilities, at 3 points on the achievement continuum, when the problem-solving program was delivered in large-class format (Fuchs et al., in press-a). As documented by Fuchs and colleagues (in press-a), the effectiveness of the problem-solving program resides in both components: Instruction on rules for problem solution explains growth on the acquisition measure; the explicit transfer component explains growth on the near- and far-transfer measures. Of course, tutoring across both the problem solution rules and the transfer components was explicit (Carnine, 1997), with heavy use of worked examples (Cooper & Sweller, 1987), peer mediation (Fuchs et al., 1997), and small-group arrangements (Elbaum et al., 2000)—instructional features with proven efficacy for promoting reading. The study extends previous work by documenting effects on mathematical problem solving, a curricular area that has received relatively little attention, especially for students with MD, and where previous work indicates that outcomes are difficult to effect among low-achieving students (Cooper & Sweller, 1987; Fuchs et al., 1999; Mayer, 1998; Woodward & Baxter, 1997). Clearly, findings provide the basis for an important message to practitioners: Teachers can improve the mathematical problem-solving performance of students with MD. On the other hand, effects on far transfer, although respectable, were lower than for students without disabilities. Thus, clearly, additional work is warranted to identify how to enhance outcomes for students with MD.

It is also interesting to consider the effects of computer-assisted practice, as operationalized in this study. Our software provided intensive, instructional feedback with motivational scoring. Results on real-world problem solving, although not achieving statistical significance, did produce scores that exceeded the control group by a notable 0.63 standard deviation. This might have been expected given that computer-assisted practice was conducted on tasks directly paralleling the real-world problem-solving measure. More notable was a similar ES of 0.60 on the acquisition measure along with a small ES of 0.31 on near transfer, suggesting that some "downward" transfer occurred. Together, these ESs provide the basis for additional research on computer-assisted practice designed to guide students toward enhanced problem solving. Future research should incorporate greater power, not only with larger samples but also with software that enhances the instructional value of the practice provided. We currently are undertaking this effort because of the strong appeal of improved mathematical problem solving without the need for expensive adult guidance.

It is, nevertheless, interesting to note that with the explicit, small-group, peer-mediated instruction on rules for problem solution and transfer in place, our computer-assisted practice condition provided no added value. On acquisition and near transfer, the comparison between the tutoring treatments with and without computer-assisted practice revealed small effect sizes favoring the tutoring with*out* computer-assisted practice. On far transfer, which paralleled the very tasks students practiced via computer, the ES favoring tutoring plus computer-assisted practice was a disappointingly low 0.14. From a research design perspective, this lends credence to the value of the tutoring treatment because the combined treatment, which failed to effect better growth, incorporated twice the amount of problem-solving worktime. Substantively, results are bolstered by the fact that, on acquisition and near transfer, direct contrasts between the computer and the tutoring treatments reliably favored tutoring: ESs comparing tutoring plus computer-assisted practice versus computer-assisted practice alone were 1.27 and 0.93; for tutoring without computer-assisted versus computer-assisted practice alone, 1.50 and 1.02. As revealed with the software used in this study, computer-guided practice failed to provide a meaningful substitute for or addition to carefully formulated adult tutoring. Perhaps software designed to provide better elaborated instruction would effect better outcomes—or might be used in conjunction with problem-solving tutoring to reduce the amount of teacher time (an expensive resource) required to enhance mathematical problem solving.

Conclusions

On the basis of this program of research, we draw some tentative conclusions about how to enhance mathematical problem solving among students with MD. We first offer some specific recommendations based on our work; then, we provide a general comment about the state of knowledge about "effective instruction" within special education. We conclude by offering some directions for future study within the area of mathematical problem solving for students with MD.

Specific Recommendations

Our program of research reveals that to promote mathematical problem solving for students with MD, a strong foundation in the rules for problem solution is necessary. This means that children must master solution methods on problems with low transfer demands (i.e., identically worded problems that only vary cover stories and quantities). This is necessary before we should expect to see mathematical problem solving, which necessarily requires transfer to problems presented with superficial differences that make recognition of known problem solutions difficult. The need for mastery of problem solutions has been substantiated in earlier research (e.g., Mawer & Sweller, 1982; Sweller & Cooper, 1985), showing that as students master problem-solution rules, they allocate less working memory to the details of the solution and instead devote cognitive resources to identify connections between novel and familiar problems and to plan their work (Kotovsky et al., 1985).

A second conclusion about enhancing mathematical problem solving, based on our research, is more novel. It involves the need for explicit instruction on transfer, designed to increase awareness of the connections between novel and familiar problems by (1) broadening the categories by which students group problems requiring the same solution methods (i.e., promoting a higher level of abstraction) and (2) explicitly prompting students to search novel problems for these broad categories (i.e., increasing metacognition). Our experiments illustrate the contribution of such explicit instruction on transfer for students without disabilities; effect sizes were substantial on the range of transfer measures examined. Moreover, as shown by Fuchs and colleagues (in press-a), this approach also promotes important improvement for students with MD. Of course, among students with MD, results are more impressive and reliable for near- than for far-transfer problem-solving measures. Additional work is required to identify strategies for increasing the magnitude and range of problem-solving effects.

A General Observation about the Nature of "Effective Instruction"

With respect to the state of knowledge about "effective instruction," we offer the following observation. Within special education, research on instructional practices is strong on process variables that provide the foundation for instruction. These variables (e.g., Englert, 1984; Gersten, Woodward, & Darch, 1986; Haynes & Jenkins, 1986) include, but are not limited to, modeling, quick pace, frequent responding and high proportion of engaged time, overrehearsal, and guided feedback. Our work on mathematical problem solving has incorporated these principles by, for example, relying on modeling via worked examples; encouraging quick pace via scripted lessons; requiring frequent response via choral responding; providing a high proportion of engaged time, overrehearsal, and guided feedback via small-group teacher-led instruction and peer-mediated practice; and encouraging task-focused goals via accountability of individual performance and self-regulation procedures that include goal setting, self-scoring, self-charting of progress, and reporting transfer opportunities and events.

As important as these variables are, however, it is important for the field to acknowledge that they simply provide a foundation over which substantive explanations must be superimposed. And special education research has allocated relatively little attention to principles for designing those explanations, beyond the notion of explicitness (e.g., Carnine, 1987). In our research on mathematical problem solving, we have attempted to optimize the quality of explanations by incorporating concrete algorithms that make visible the conceptual underpinnings behind operations (e.g., drawing items into "bags" to concretize step-up functions before relying on repeated addition or division to derive answers) and using everyday examples that are accessible to a wide range of children's experiences to illustrate principles (e.g., exemplifying *transfer* with babies learning to drink from a toddler cup, then a glass, then a soda pop bottle). The challenges associated with constructing effective explanations cannot, however, be overestimated. Given the constraints imposed on teachers' time to plan, the need to provide clearly articulated explanations for teachers to borrow is great. We believe that the field needs to dedicate effort not only to studying principles of strong explanations but also to build those explanations within specific academic domains.

Some Future Directions for Research

Extension to the literature on enhancing mathematical problem solving is required; we identify four areas for additional work. First, as already stated, work is needed to identify principles of effective explanations and to build effective explanations that promote mathematical problem solving. Second, continued research is required to strenghthen performance on far-transfer, real-world problem-solving tasks. In our studies, we have documented effects of six-tenths of a standard deviation among students with MD; methods are required to boost these effect sizes so that they better approximate effects of 1 or more standard deviation observed for students without disabilities. Intensifying instruction by, for example relying on one-to-one tutoring or configuring computer-delivered practice in effective ways represents one potential strategy for accomplishing this goal. Better developed explanations represent another possible method.

A third direction for future study addresses the fact that relatively little is known about the cognitive correlates associated with responsiveness to instruction within the domain of mathematical problem solving. In terms of number fact retrival and arithmetic story problems, Jordan and Montani (1997) examined performance on spoken number facts, spoken one- and two-step arithmetic story problems, and nonverbal number facts as a function of the children's language and visuospatial profiles. The researchers showed that these tasks were differentially sensitive to variation in cognitive ability. The language-impaired group (receptive vocabulary and grammatic closure < 30th percentile) performed significantly lower than nonimpaired peers on story problems, but not on either number fact task. By contrast, the visuospatial-impaired group performed comparably to the nonimpaired group across tasks. Unfortunately, consensus on this performance pattern is lacking in the literature. For example, Rourke (1993) identified two similar groups of children with MD: those with verbal deficits (who had MD with reading and spelling deficits) and those with tactual-perceptual, visuoperceptual, motor, and reasoning difficulties (whose functional difficulties were limited to math). In contrast to Jordan et al.'s findings, however, Rourke's visuospatial-deficit group manifested a more pervasive pattern of mathematics difficulties, which involved a larger number and wider range of procedural errors than did the verbal-deficit group. Based on the literature, a wide set of cognitive correlates provide the basis for productive study. From arithmetic research, these include articulatory speed, short-term memory, speed of retrieving information from long-term memory, and general speed of processing From arithmetic problem solving as well as our own work on more extended problem solving, relevant cognitive correlates are metacognition, language-related variables associated with reading and listening comprehension difficulties, motivation and perseverance, visuospatial ability, generalization deficits/inference-making difficulties, and semantics.

Finally (and in a related way), the effects of mathematical problem-solving treatment for subgroups of students with MD, who do and do not present comorbid RD, is required. MD research typically fails to account for reading competence in the study of mathematical problem solving. This is unfortunate because research suggests that unique patterns of functional competence (e.g., Hanich, Jordan, Kaplan, & Dick, 2001; Jordan & Hanich, 2000; Jordan & Mondani, 1997) as well as unique patterns of verbal strength and visual-perceptual organizational weakness (e.g., Fletcher, 1985; Fuchs & Fuchs, 2002; McLean & Hitch, 1999; Rourke & Finlayson, 1978; Siegel & Linder, 1994; Siegel & Ryan, 1989) underlie MD and MD + RD. In light of the semantic challenges associated with mathematics problem solving, regardless of whether problems are accessed through reading or listening, the verbal performance deficits of comorbid students along with their more pervasive disruptions of language (Rourke, 1993) may render mathematical problem solving a more difficult outcome to effect for students with comorbidity. Future research should identify effective practices for effecting this outcome for students with serious problems in reading and math.

Acknowledgments

The research described in this chapter was supported by Grants No. H324V980001 and No. H327A000035 from the U.S. Department of Education, Office of Special Education Programs, and Core Grant NHD15052 from the National Institute of Child Health and Human Development to Vanderbilt University. Statemens do not reflect the position or policy of these agencies, and no official endorsement by them should be inferred.

References

Asch, S. E. (1969). A reformulation of the problem of associations. *American Psychologist, 24,* 92–102.

Badian, N. A. (1983). Dyscalculia and nonverbal disorders of learning. In H. R. Myklebust (Ed.), *Progress* (pp. 235–264). New York: Grune & Stratton.

Bransford, J. D., & Schwartz, D. L. (1999). Rethinking transfer: A simple proposal with multiple implications. In A. Iran-Nejad & P. D. Pearson (Eds.), *Review of research in education* (pp. 61–100). Washington, DC: American Educational Research Association.

Brown, A. L., Campione, J. C., Webber, L. S., & McGilly, K. (1992). Interactive learning environments: A new look at assessment and instruction. In B. R. Gifford & M. C. O'Connor (Eds.), *Changing assessments: Alternative view of aptitude, achievement, and instruction* (pp. 37–75). Boston: Kluwer Academic.

Carnine, D. (1997). Instructional design in mathematics for students with learning disabilities. *Journal of Learning Disabilities, 30,* 130–141.

Catrambone, R., & Holyoak, K. J. (1989). Overcoming contextual limitations on problem-solving transfer. *Journal of Experimental Psychology: Learning, Memory, and Cognition, 15,* 1127–1156.

Cohen, S. A., & Stover, G. (1981). Effects of teaching sixth-grade students to modify format variables of math word problems. *Reading Research Quarterly, 16,* 175–199.

Cook, B. (1973, February). *An analysis of arithmetic, linguistic , and algebraic structural variables that contribute to problem solving difficulty in algebra word problems.* Paper presented at the annual meeting of the American Educational Research Association, New Orleans. (ERIC Document Reproduction Service No. ED 076 433)

Cooper, G., & Sweller, J. (1987). Effects of schema acquisition and rule automation on mathematical problem-solving transfer. *Journal of Educational Psychology, 79,* 347–362.

CTB/McGraw-Hill. (1997). *TerraNova technical manual.* Monterey, CA: Author.

Durnin, J. H., Perrone, A. E., & MacKay, L. (1997). Teaching problem solving in elementary school mathematics. *Journal of Structural Learning and Intelligent Systems, 13,* 53–69.

Elbaum, B., Vaughn, S., Hughes, M. T., & Moody, S. W. (2000). How effective are one-to-one tutoring programs in reading for elementary students at risk for reading failure? A meta-analysis of the intervention research. *Journal of Educational Psychology, 92,* 605–619.

Englert, C. S. (1984). Effective direct instruction practices in special education settings. *Remedial and Special Education, 5,* 38–47.

Fletcher, J. M. (1985). Memory for verbal and nonverbal stimuli in learning disabilities subgroups: Analysis by selective reminding. *Journal of Experimental Child Psychology, 40,* 244–259.

Firestone, W. A., Mayrowetz, D., & Fairman, J. (1998). Performance-based assessment and instructional change: The effects of testing in Maine and Maryland. *Educational Evaluation and Policy Analysis, 20,* 95–113.

Fuchs, L. S., & Fuchs, D. (2002). Mathematical problem-solving profiles of students with mathematics disabilities with and without comorbid reading disabilities. *Journal of Learning Disabilites, 35,* 563–573.

Fuchs, L. S., Fuchs, D., Eaton, S., Hamlett, C. L., & Karns, K. (2000). Supplementing teacher judgments of mathematics test accommodations with objective data sources. *School Psychology Review, 20,* 65–85.

Fuchs, L. S., Fuchs, D., Hamlett, C. L., & Appleton, A. K. (2002). Explicitly teaching for transfer: Effects on the mathematical problem-solving performance of students with nathematics disabilities. *Learning Disabilities Research and Practice, 17,* 90–106.

Fuchs, L. S., Fuchs, D., Hamlett, C. L., Phillips, N. B., Karns, K., & Dutka, S. (1997). Enhancing students' helping behavior during peer-mediated instruction with conceptual mathematical explanations. *Elementary School Journal, 97,* 223–250.

Fuchs, L. S., Fuchs, D., Karns, K., Hamlett, C. L., Dutka, S., & Karzaroff, M. (2000). The importance of providing background information on the structure and scoring of performance assessments. *Applied Measurement in Education, 11,* 1–34.

Fuchs, L. S., Fuchs, D., Karns, K., Hamlett, C. L., & Karzaroff, M. (1999). Mathematics performance assessment in the classroom: Effects on teacher planning and student problem solving. *American Educational Research Journal, 36,* 609–646.

Fuchs, L. S., Fuchs, D., Prentice, K., Burch, M., Hamlett, C. L., Owen, R., Hosp, M., & Jancek, D. (in press-a). Explicitly teacher for transfer: Effects on third-grade students' mathematical problem solving. *Journal of Educational Psychology.*

Fuchs, L. S., Fuchs, D., Prentice, K., Burch, M., Owen, R., Hamlett, C. L., & Schroeter, K. (in press-b). Enhancing third-grade students' mathematical problem solving with self-regulated learning strategies. *Journal of Educational Psychology*

Geary, D. C. (1993). Mathematical disabilities: Cognitive, neuropsychological, and genetic components. *Psychological Bulletin, 114,* 345–362.

Gersten, R., Woodward, J., & Darch, C. (1986). Direct instruction: A research-based approach to curriculum design and teaching. *Exceptional Children, 53,* 17–31.

Gick, M. L., & Holyoak, K. J. (1983). Analogical problem solving. *Cognitive Psychologist, 12,* 306–355.

Gross-Tsur, V., Manor, O., & Shalev, R. S. (1996). Developmental dyscalculalia: Prevalence and demographic features. *Developmental Medicine and Child Neurology, 38,* 25–33.

Hambleton, R. K., Jaeger, R. M., Koretz, D., Linn, R. L., Millman, J., & Phillips, S. (1995). *Review of the measurement quality of the Kentucky Instructional Results Information System, 1991–1994.* Frankfort: Office of Education Accountability, Kentucky General Assembly.

Hanich, L. B., Jordan, N. C., Kaplan, D., & Dick, J. (2001). Performance across different areas of mathematical cognition in children with learning disabilities. *Journal of Educational Psychology, 93,* 615–626.

Haynes, M., & Jenkins, J. R. (1986). Reading instruction in special education resource rooms. *American Educational Research Journal, 23,* 161–190.

Helwig,R., Rosek-Toedesco, M. A., Tindal, G., Heath, B., & Almond, P. J. (1999). Reading as an access to mathematics problem solving on multiple-choice tests for sixth-grade students. *Journal of Educational Research, 91,* 113–125.

Jerman, M. E., & Mirman, S. (1974). Linguistic and compuational variables in problem solving in elementary mathematics. *Educational Studies in Mathematics, 5,* 317–362.

Jordan, N. C., & Hanich, L. B. (2000). Mathematical thinking in second-grade children with different forms of LD. *Journal of Learning Disabilites, 33,* 567–578.

Jordan, N. C., & Montani, T. O. (1997). Cognitive arithmetic and problem solving: A comparison of children with specific and general mathematics difficulties. *Journal of Learning Disabilities, 30,* 624–634.

Kansas State Board of Education. (1991). *Kansas Quality Performance Accreditation.* Topeka, KS: Author.

Koretz, D., Barron, S., Mitchell, K., & Stecher, B. (1996). *Perceived effects of the Kentucky Instructional Results Information System (KIRIS).* National Center for Research on Evaluation, Standards, and Student Testing (CRESST). Santa Monica, CA: Rand.

Koretz, D., Mitchell, K., Barron, S., & Keith, S. (1996). *Final Report: Perceived effects of the Maryland School Performance Assessment Program.* National Center for Research on Evaluation, Standards, and Student Testing (CRESST). Los Angeles: University of California.

Kosc, L. (1974). Developmental dyscalculalia. *Journal of Learning Disabilities, 7,* 164–177.

Mawrer, R., & Sweller, J. (1985). What do students learn while solving mathematics problems? *Journal of Educational Psychology, 77,* 272–284.

Mayer, D. P. (1998). Do new teaching standards undermine performance on an old test? *Educational Evaluation and Policy Analysis, 15,* 1–16.

Mayer, R. E., Quilici, J. L., & Moreno, R. (1999). What is learned in an after-school computer club? *Journal of Educational Computing Research , 20,* 223–235.

McLean, J. F., & Hitch, G. J. (1999). Working memory impairments in children with specific arithmetic learning difficulties. *Journal of Experimental Child Psychology, 74,* 240–260.

Rasanen, P., & Ahonen, T. (1995). Arithmetic disabilities with and without reading difficulties: A comparison of arithmetic errors. *Developmental Neuropsychology, 11,* 275–295.

Resnick, L. B., & Resnick, D. P. (1992). Assessing the thinking curriculum: New tools for educational reform. In B. R Gifford & M. C. O'Connor (Eds.), *Changing assessments: Alternative views of aptitude, achievement, and instruction* (pp. 37–75). Boston: Kluwer Academic.

Rivera-Batiz, F. L. (1992). Quantitative literacy and the likelihood of employment among young adults in the United States. *Journal of Human Resources, 27,* 313–328.

Ross, B. H. (1989). Distinguishing types of superficial similarities: Different effects on the access and use of earlier problems. *Journal of Experi-*

mental Psychology: Learning, Memory, and Cognition, 15, 456–468.

Rothman, R. (1995). *Measuring up: Standards, assessments, and school reform.* San Francisco: Jossey-Bass.

Rourke, B. P. (1993). Arithmetic disabilities specific and otherwise: A neuropsychological perspective. *Journal of Learning Disabilities, 26,* 214–226.

Rourke, B. P., & Finlayson, M. A. I. (1978). Neuropsychological significance of variations in patterns of academic performance: Verbal and visual-spatial abilities. *Journal of Abnormal Child Psychology, 6,* 121–133.

Salomon, G., & Perkins, D. N. (1989). Rocky roads to transfer: Rethinking mechanisms of a neglected phenomenon. *Educational Psychologist, 24,* 113–142.

Schwartz, D. L., & Bransford, J. D. (1998). A time for telling. *Cognition and Instruction, 16,* 475–522.

Siegel, L. S., & Linder, B. (1984). Short-term memory process in children with reading and arithmetic disabilities. *Developmental Psychology, 20,* 200–207.

Siegel, L. S., & Ryan, E. B. (1989). The development of working memory in normally achieving and subtypes of learning disabled children. *Child Development, 60,* 973–980.

Stigler, J. W., & Hiebert, J. (1997). Understanding and improving classroom mathematics instruction. *Phi Delta Kappan, 79*(1), 14–21.

Sweller, J., & Cooper, G. A. (1985). The use of worked examples as a substitute for problem solving in algebra. *Cognition and Instruction, 2,* 59–89.

White, O. R. (1984). Descriptive analysis of extant research literature concerning skill generalization and the handicapped. In M. Boer (Ed.), *Investigating the problem of skill generalization: Literature review* (pp. 1–19). Seattle: University of Washington, Washington Research Organization.

Woodward, J., & Baxter, J. (1997). The effects of an innovative approach to mathematics on academically low-achieving students in inclusive settings. *Exceptional Children, 63,* 373–388.

20

Students with Learning Disabilities and the Process of Writing: A Meta-Analysis of SRSD Studies

Steve Graham
Karen R. Harris

A few years ago, we overheard two children swapping jokes. Most of their jokes were pretty corny and not especially funny (at least to an adult), but one caught our attention because it was about writing.

TEACHER: Why is it, Johnny, that everyone else had a five-page report and your paper is only one page long?
JOHNNY: I was writing about condensed milk.

The joke yielded no more than a tiny grin from the listening child. For the two eavesdropping adults, however, the joke provided a useful metaphor for describing how most students with learning disabilities write. Not only is what they write condensed, but so is how they write.

Recent models of skilled writing (e.g., Hayes, 1996; Hayes & Flower, 1980; Zimmerman & Risemberg, 1997) emphasize that composing is a complex cognitive activity, involving the activation of a variety of processes (Graham & Harris, in press). Hayes and Flower (1980), for example, indicate that writing involves three basic processes: planning what to say and how to say it, translating plans into written text, and reviewing to improve existing text.

Planning, in turn, is composed of three ingredients—setting goals, generating ideas, and organizing ideas into a writing plan—whereas reviewing includes reading and editing text. Skilled writers deftly orchestrate and monitor the use of these processes in order to accomplish their goals and complete writing tasks.

In contrast, most students with learning disabilities (LD) use a "condensed" or simplified version of this model. They mostly rely on the generating ideas component of the Hayes and Flower (1980) model, which involves converting writing tasks into tasks of simply telling what one knows about a topic, or writing as remembering (Scardamalia & Bereiter, 1986). With this approach, little attention is directed at rhetorical goals, whole-text organization, the needs of the reader, or the constraints imposed by the topic (Graham & Harris, 1994).

An important goal in writing instruction for students with LD, therefore, is to help them develop a more sophisticated approach to composing—one that draws on the same types of composing processes and strategies employed by more skilled writers. In this chapter, we examine how we have tackled this problem head on, by explicitly and directly teaching planning, revising, and other self-regulation procedures for writing to students with LD. However, we first set the stage for this examination by reviewing what is currently known about these children's planning and revising behavior.

How Do Students with LD Write?

A One-Trick Pony: Composing as Content Generation

The idea that children create multiple drafts of their compositions, planning and revising them, is so common today that some of the terminology surrounding these processes have worked their way into more mundane everyday tasks. One parent disclosed (Loranger, 2000) that his 8-year-old daughter responded, "No Dad, it's only a rough draft," when he commented, "You call that a made bed?"

Though the idea of planning, writing, and reworking a composition may be commonplace for some children, students with LD often minimize their use of these processes. In contrast to skilled writers who typically devote considerable effort to planning and thinking about their compositions before they write an initial draft (Graham & Harris, 2000), students with LD generally do little or no planning before starting to write. This is the case even when they are asked to plan in advance. For example, when we prompted fifth- and sixth-grade students with LD to plan before writing, they averaged less than 1 minute of advanced planning time (MacArthur & Graham, 1987), whether they were writing papers by hand, typing their compositions on a word processor, or dictating them to an adult.

The approach to writing that students with LD most often employ involves little in the way of planning, monitoring, evaluating, and so forth (Graham, 1990; Thomas, Englert, & Gregg, 1987). Instead, it relies heavily on a single composing process: the generation of writing content (Scardamalia & Bereiter, 1986). With this approach, students compose by creating or drawing from memory a relevant idea, writing it down, and using each preceding phrase or sentence to stimulate the next idea. Little effort is made to evaluate or rework these ideas or to consider the constraints imposed by the top-

ic, the needs of the audience, or the organization of text. The resulting composition is generally a list of topic-related ideas rather than a coherent discussion or examination of the topic. According to McCutchen (1988), this approach to writing functions much like an automated and forward-moving content-generation program. Although this approach may be useful for writing a note to a friend or describing a personal experience, it is not particularly effective for many school-related writing tasks, such as writing an essay, a report, or even a story. A good story, for example, includes a plot, is organized in a logical manner, and is sensitive to the needs and interests of the audience. This process requires more than generating or retrieving ideas on the fly.

Although content generation dominates the planning and composing process for most students with LD, it is a relatively unproductive approach. One of the most striking characteristics of these students' writing is that there is so little of it. Their papers are inordinately short, containing little elaboration or detail (Graham, Harris, MacArthur, & Schwartz, 1991).

One reason why these children's writing is so impoverished is that they have difficulty sustaining the writing effort. In one study involving fourth- and sixth-grade students with LD (Graham, 1990), the average amount of time that students spent writing an opinion essay was 6 minutes. They only composed for 1 minute when they were asked to dictate an essay. Moreover, their essays typically began with a positive or negative statement indicating either agreement or disagreement with the essay topic (e.g., Should boys and girls play sports together?), followed by one or two briefly stated reasons, abruptly ending without a resolution or a concluding statement. Other researchers (Thomas et al., 1987) have noted that students with LD experience problems sustaining their thinking about writing topics, as they have difficulty producing multiple statements about familiar subjects.

A second reason why students with LD produce so little content is that they fail to gain access to the knowledge they possess. We found that the output of fourth- and sixth-grade students with LD could be doubled or even tripled by repeatedly prompting them to write more about an assigned topic (Graham, 1990). This was true for both writing by hand and composing via dictation.

A third reason for their meager output is that difficulties with the mechanics of writing interfere the process of generating content. The writing of students with LD is replete with mechanical miscues, including malformed letters, misspelled words, and errors in punctuation and capitalization (Graham et al., 1991). Having to attend to mechanical concerns, such as how to spell a word or write a letter, can presumably interfere with the execution of other writing processes (Graham, Harris, & Fink, 2000, in press). For example, having to figure out how to spell a word while composing may lead a child to forget writing plans or ideas being held in working memory. Likewise, students may lose ideas or plans because their handwriting is not fast enough to keep up with their thoughts.

The theoretical effect of mechanical difficulties on writing output are supported by three sources of information:

1. Handwriting fluency and spelling account for 66% and 41% of the variability in writing output of primary and intermediate grade students, respectively (Graham, Berninger, Abbott, Abbott, & Whitaker, 1997).
2. Removal of mechanical demands through dictation usually results in a corresponding increase in written output (De La Paz & Graham, 1995). For instance, the length of stories produced by fifth- and sixth-grade students with LD tripled when they were asked to dictate rather than write or type their compositions (MacArthur & Graham, 1987).
3. Providing extra handwriting instruction for poor writers has a positive impact on their writing output (Berninger et al., 1997, 1998).

I Don't Do Substance, But I Do Correct Errors

The following revision exemplifies the general approach of students with LD.

> Please Correct: "The bull and the cow is in the field."
>
> Subsequent Revision: "The cow and the bull is in the field."

Students with LD employ a "thesaurus" approach, focusing most of their efforts on making word substitutions, correcting mechanical errors, and producing a neater product (MacArthur & Graham, 1987: MacArthur, Graham, & Schwartz, 1991). In contrast to skilled writers who modify their text extensively, less than 20% of the revisions made by students with LD appreciably change what they write. The majority of their revisions involve minor changes in the surface-level features of text (MacArthur & Graham, 1987: MacArthur et al., 1991). More than 70% of these changes are attempts to correct capitalization, punctuation, spelling, format, and other mechanical errors. The changes made are generally ineffective, as the only thing that typically improves across drafts is the legibility of handwriting (MacArthur et al., 1991).

SELF-REGULATION

One reason students with LD revise in such a limited manner is that they have difficulty managing the processes involved in revising (Graham & Harris, 2000). In two separate experiments (De La Paz, Swanson, & Graham, 1998; Graham, 1997), we found that students' revising improved when they received procedural support designed to ensure that the separate elements of the revising process were coordinated and occurred in a regular way. In the first study (Graham, 1997), fifth- and sixth-grade students with LD executed a revising routine where they evaluated each sentence written, explained their evaluation, selected a tactic for revising the sentence (if one was needed), and executed the revision.

Revising one sentence at a time, the child first selected one of seven possible evaluations (each was written on a separate index card). Three of the evaluations were written from the writer's perspective (i.e., "this doesn't sound right," "this is not what I wanted to say," and "this is not useful to my paper") and three from the reader's perspective (i.e., "people may not understand this part," "people won't be interested in this part," and "people won't buy this part"). The seventh evaluative statement was "This is good." Once they selected an evaluation, they then explained how it applied. Next, they selected a tactic for revising the sentence, drawing on five possible directives (again each was written on a separate index card). The directives were "Leave it the same," "say more," "leave this part out," "change the wording," and "cross out and say it a different way." After selecting a directive, they executed the intended change. This routine reduced the executive burden involved in revising by signaling movement from one element of revising to the next and limiting the number of evaluative and tactical decisions made by students.

The participating students indicated that the procedure made the process of revising easier by helping them carry out part or all of the revising process. There was also an improvement in the quality of their revisions and the type of text that they changed. In comparison to their typical approach to revising, the procedure resulted in more revisions involving larger units of text, such as phrases or t-units (i.e., independent plus any accompanying dependent clauses).

Even more impressive results were obtained in the second study (De La Paz et al., 1998), where eighth-grade students with LD used a somewhat similar routine that involved making two passes through their composition. The first pass focused on more global concerns (e.g., "two few ideas" or "part of the essay is not in the right order"), whereas the second pass concentrated on local concerns primarily situated at the sentence-level (e.g., "this one doesn't sound right" or "this is an incomplete idea"). Again students indicated that the executive routine made revising easier. It also prompted more, better, and larger revisions. The changes that students made were substantive enough to improve the overall quality of their text.

OTHER PROBLEMS

Although the studies by Graham and his colleagues (De La Paz et al., 1998; Graham, 1997) showed that students with LD experience difficulty coordinating and managing the elements of revision, other factors hamper their revising as well. First, the evaluation criteria that students used in both studies generally focused children's attention on substantive concerns. Even with this focus,

60% of the revisions made by students in the first study (Graham, 1997) involved the mechanics of writing or minor word changes.

It is possible that inexperienced writers may not be able to turn off or turn down their attention to issues of form easily or at will (Scardamalia & Bereiter, 1986). This proposition was tested in the second study (De La Paz et al., 1998) by telling students not to worry about errors that involved spelling, punctuation, and capitalization, as these would be corrected by the examiner. When given such instructions, students were able to adjust how much attention they paid to mechanics; just 19% of their changes involved usage and form.

The most obvious reason why these students focus so much of their attention on form, unless otherwise directed, is that their papers contain an inordinate number of mechanical errors. For instance, MacArthur and Graham (1987) reported that fifth- and sixth-grade students with LD misspelled one-eighth of the words in their papers and one-third of their sentences lacked initial capitalization or final punctuation. But this is not the only reason. Many of these students view revising as proofreading. They are more likely than their normally achieving counterparts to emphasize mechanical issues when asked to talk about writing and revising (Graham, Schwartz, & MacArthur, 1993; Wong, Wong, & Blenkinsop, 1989). For example, when asked how they would revise a paper to make it better, 61% of their responses focused on the mechanical attributes of text, such as "make it neater" or "spell words correctly" (Graham et al., 1993).

A second limitation in the revising of students with LD is that they are often indifferent to reader-based concerns. In the revising/self-regulation study by Graham (1997) reviewed previously, three of the evaluation cards were written from the writer's perspective (e.g., "this is not what I wanted to say") and three from the reader's perspective (e.g., "people may not understand this part"). The participating students appeared to have difficulty taking the perspective of an absent reader, as only 6% of their evaluations focused on the possible reaction of an audience to their text. Furthermore, when they did select a reader-based evaluation card, only 25% of the resulting revisions were rated as improving text. In contrast, 60% of revisions cued by a writer-based evaluation resulted in an improvement.

A third limitation involves students competence with the individual elements underlying the revising process. In both of the revising/self-regulation studies (De La Paz et al., 1998; Graham, 1997), there were many instances in which students failed to make a constructive evaluation. For example, one child told us that he changed "he *loved* farmwork" to "he *liked* farmwork" (a neutral change) because the reader probably would not understand why the main character "loves farmwork." Another child indicated that he deleted three sentences that were central to understanding his story (a negative change), because "people won't care about that part."

There were also a number of instances in which revisions were ineffective because of difficulties in executing the intended change. For instance, one child correctly identified that the sentence "But sometimes you need a girl's more than you do a boy's" was not a complete idea and decided that she needed to add information. Instead of adding the word *advice* after the word *girl* (the preceding sentence made it clear that this was what she meant), she added an additional sentence: "And sometimes you don't have advice to give." This did not correct the problem but further clouded what she was trying to say, as it did not support the claim that she was trying to establish, namely, that boys and girls should be educated together because they can give each other advice.

"A Theme Is a Thing" and Other Tales of Incomplete Knowledge

When asked to define a theme, one young man indicated that it is "a thing that runs down the side of your trousers" (Abbington, 1952). For many students with LD, their knowledge about writing—its genres, devices, and conventions—is quite limited. Even with a relatively familiar genre such as story writing, they are often unfamiliar with the basic attributes or parts of a story. In a recent interview with a third-grade child with LD, for example, he started off on the right track but quickly veered into questionable territory. When asked to tell a friend what kinds of things are included in a story, he indicated: "I would tell him main character, a subject, predicate, and main idea." These students' incomplete knowledge is further noticeable in their stories where they often omit basic elements such as the location, problem, ending, or moral (Graham & Harris, 1989a; Sawyer, Graham, & Harris, 1992).

Gaps in the writing knowledge of students with LD are not just limited to lore about genres and other aspects of the written product but also extend to knowledge about how to write. When compared with their regularly achieving peers, for instance, students with LD are less knowledgeable about the processes involved in organizing and categorizing writing ideas as well as evaluating and revising text (Englert, Raphael, Anderson, Gregg, & Anthony, 1989).

Unshakable Confidence: At Least on the Surface

Students with LD often remind us of a child who told Art Linkletter, the host of *House Party,* "I am the best they is in English." When interviewed by others, these children are generally overconfident about their capabilities. When we assessed the self-efficacy of 10- to 14-year-old students with LD, for example, they were just as positive about their writing capabilities as their peers who were better writers (Graham et al., 1993). Both groups of students favorably rated their ability to write reports, stories, and book reports. They were also positive about their abilities to get and organize ideas for writing, transcribe ideas into sentences, sustain their writing effort, and correct mistakes in their paper. Although a positive judgment about one's capabilities may promote persistence in spite of a history of poor performance (Sawyer et al., 1992), there is a downside as well. Children who overestimate their capabilities may fail to allocate needed resources and effort, believing that this is unnecessary.

Surprisingly little is known about these children's attitudes toward writing. When the students in the aforementioned study were asked to indicate their agreement or disagreement with six attitude questions (e.g., "Writing is a waste of time."), the students with LD were generally positive about writing. Their responses stand in contrast to anecdotal and clinical reports where such children frequently indicate that they avoid writing if they can (Berninger et al., 1997).

How Can We Help Students with LD Become More Strategic Writers?

When we asked a fourth-grade child with LD to tell us what good writers do, he hesitated only for a moment before declaring, "Write large!" Though this is clearly a strategic response, it is not one that we want to support. How then do we help students with LD set aside the low-effort approach that they so often employ and take up a more thoughtful and insistence course to composing?

One means for doing this is to tackle the problem head on by teaching students with LD to use the same types of strategies employed by more skilled writers. This is the primary tactic we have used in our research program.

A second approach involves constructing an environment that nourishes the development of self-regulation (Graham & Harris, 1994, 1997). This environment includes assigning writing topics that serve real purposes and promote strategic behavior; allowing students to work on topics of their own choosing; encouraging them to share their writing with others; establishing predictable classroom routines where planning and revising are expected and reinforced; letting students arrange their writing environment and work at their own pace; and creating a classroom milieu that is supportive, pleasant, and nonthreatening.

Clearly, these two approaches are not incompatible, and we (e.g., Danoff, Harris, & Graham, 1993; MacArthur, Graham, Schwartz, & Schafer, 1995; MacArthur, Schwartz, & Graham; 1991; MacArthur, Schwartz, Graham, Molloy, & Harris, 1996) and other researchers (Englert et al., 1991) have used both in tandem. Nevertheless, it should be noted that the second approach by itself may not be powerful enough for many children with LD who struggle with writing. For example, Troia and Graham (in press) found that the writing of students with LD who were asked to plan and write compositions in an environment that included many of the features described previously actually declined over time. In contrast, Danoff, Harris, and Graham (1993) reported that the writing performance of students with LD in a similarly supportive environment improved once they were taught a strategy for planning and writing their papers.

Self-Regulated Strategy Development

Alexander and her colleagues (Alexander, Graham, & Harris, 1998) have argued that the development of competence is closely tied to changes in strategic knowledge, subject-matter knowledge, and motivation. To help students form a more sophisticated approach to composing then, it is important to design instructional procedures that shape the development of each of these abilities. This is especially important for students with LD, as many of these children experience problems in each of these areas (see Harris, Graham, Deshler, 1998). They often use inefficient and ineffective strategies, experience difficulty activating and regulating strategic behavior, possess incomplete and poorly integrated knowledge, hold maladaptive beliefs and self-doubts, and exhibit low levels of engagement.

Consequently, we developed an approach to strategy instruction, referred to as self-regulated strategy development (SRSD), designed to enhance students' strategic behaviors, self-regulation skills, content knowledge, and motivational dispositions (Harris & Graham, 1996, 1999). Strategic knowledge is elevated by teaching students more sophisticated strategies for accomplishing an academic task or problem (e.g., report writing). Self-regulation is advanced by teaching them how to use goal setting, self-monitoring, self-instructions, and/or self-reinforcement to regulate their use of the target strategies, the task, and their behaviors. Content knowledge is increased by teaching any information (or skills) students need to use the selected strategies or self-regulation procedures. Motivation is boosted by a variety of procedures, including emphasizing the role of effort in learning, making the positive effects of instruction concrete and visible, and promoting an "I can do" attitude.

A writing study by Sexton, Harris, and Graham (1998) illustrates how SRSD can be used to address each of these areas. Teachers identified fifth- and sixth-grade students with LD who had difficulty with writing and exhibited low levels of motivation as well as maladaptive beliefs about the causes of writing success and failure. These students were explicitly taught a strategy for planning and writing an opinion essay. The strategy involved a series of steps designed to help them establish a goal for writing, generate an initial outline for their paper, and continue the process of planning while writing. The strategy was designed to upgrade their approach to composing, as they typically did little planning in advance of writing.

In developing an outline for their paper, students were taught to generate ideas in response to the basic components of an opinion essay (i.e., a thesis, supporting reasons, and a conclusion). To do so required that they become familiar with the elements of such an essay. As a result, this content knowledge was taught by introducing and defining these elements, identifying them in essays written by others, and generating ideas for each element when using different essay topics.

To help students learn to regulate their use of the strategy, the teacher modeled how to use it, while thinking out loud. While modeling aloud, she used a variety of self-statements to direct the use of the strategy and the writing process. This included self-statements involving problem definition (e.g., "What do I need to do?"), self-evaluation (e.g., "Did I say what I really believe?"), error correction (e.g., "Whoops, I forgot to do this; I need to do all of the strategy steps."), and self-reinforcement (e.g., "Great, this is a good reason."). Students and teacher discussed the importance of such statements, identified the things the teacher said that helped her work better, generated self-statements that they would use, and were encouraged and reinforced for using their statements while learning the strategy. Students further regulated their writing behavior by setting goals to include all the basic parts in their compositions, emphasizing that this could be accomplished by using the strategy.

To increase students' motivation, the teacher made it clear how learning the strategy would improve their writing, stressed students' role as collaborators in the learning process, taught students how to monitor the effects of the strategy, and encouraged students to support each other during instruction. Students' maladaptive beliefs about the causes of writing success and failure were addressed by emphasizing the role of effort in learning and writing. For example, students were encouraged during writing to use personal self-statements that attributed success to the use of effort ("Work hard," "Write better.").

Characteristics of SRSD Instruction

There are five critical characteristics of SRSD instruction:

1. Strategies, accompanying self-regulation procedures, and needed knowledge are explicitly taught, as children with LD typically require more extensive and direct instruction to master processes and knowledge that other students acquire more easily (Reeve & Brown, 1985).
2. The SRSD model stresses interactive learning between teacher and students, consistent with the dialectical constructivist viewpoint (Pressley, Harris, & Marks, 1992). Children are viewed as active collaborators who work with the teacher and each other during instruction.
3. Instruction is individualized so that the processes, skills, and knowledge targeted for instruction are tailored to children's needs and capabilities For instance, in a class where students were taught the content outline from the Sexton and colleagues (1998) study described above, the strategy would be modified for students who already included the basic parts (i.e., thesis, supporting reasons, and conclusion) in their persuasive writing. An appropriate modification might include generating one or more possible examples for each supporting reason. Instruction is further individualized through the use of individually tailored feedback and support.
4. Instruction is criterion rather than time based, as students move through each in-

structional process at their own pace and do not proceed to later stages of instruction until they have met the criteria for doing so. Just as importantly, instruction does not end until the student can use the strategy and self-regulation procedures efficiently and effectively.

5. SRSD is an ongoing process in which new strategies are introduced and previously taught strategies are upgraded. For example, the content outline from the Sexton and colleagues (1998) study could be upgraded by adding an additional essay element, namely, refuting reasons that run counter to the writer's thesis.

Stages of Instruction

Six instructional stages provide the structural framework for SRSD (Harris & Graham, 1996). These stages represent a "meta-script," providing a general guideline for instruction, but stages can be reordered, combined, or modified to meet student and teacher needs. Example lesson plans can be found at www.vanderbilt.edu/CASL/.

1. *Develop background knowledge.* The teacher helps students develop the knowledge and skills needed to understand, acquire, and execute target strategies and self-regulation procedures.

2. *Discuss it.* Teacher and students examine and discuss current performance and the strategies used to accomplish specific assignments or tasks. The target strategies, their purpose and benefits, and how and when to use them are then examined. Students are asked to make a commitment to learn the strategies and act as a collaborative partner in this endeavor. Negative or ineffective self-statements or beliefs that students currently use may also be addressed at this time. Teachers may further introduce the concept of progress monitoring, teaching students how to monitor the impact of learning the strategies.

3. *Model it.* The teacher models aloud how to use the strategies, employing appropriate self-instructions. The self-instructions include a combination of problem definition, planning, strategy use, self-evaluation, error correction, coping, and self-reinforce-

ment statements. After analyzing the model's performance, teacher and students may collaborate on how to change the strategies to make them more effective or efficient. Each student develops and records personal self-statements they plan to use. These self-statements may be designed to regulate strategy use, the task, or interfering student behavior. Teachers may model how to use the strategy more than once, depending on how quickly students' grasp the concepts illustrated by the teacher.

4. *Memorize it.* The steps of the strategies, any accompanying mnemonic for remembering them, and students' personalized self-statements are memorized; paraphrasing is allowed as long as the original meaning is maintained. Practice memorizing the strategies, mnemonics, and personalized self-statements may begin during the "discuss it" stage. This stage is included for students with severe learning and memory problems and is not needed by all students.

5. *Support it.* Students practice using the strategies, self-statements, and any other self-regulation processes (e.g., self-assessment and goals setting) introduced here or earlier, receiving help from the teacher, their peers, or both until they can use these procedures independently. Teacher help ranges from direct assistance in applying the strategies (i.e., collaborative practice) to remodeling part or all of the strategies to corrective feedback and praise. Students may also support each other by working together as they initially learn to use the strategies. Both teacher and peer help as well as instructional facilitators, such as self-statement lists and strategy reminder charts, are faded as quickly as possible, and students are encouraged to begin using their self-statements covertly (i.e., in their head).

6. *Independent performance.* Students use the strategies independently. If goal setting and self-assessment procedures are still in use, the teacher may decide to fade them at this time.

Procedures for promoting maintenance and generalization are integrated throughout the SRSD model. This includes discussing opportunities to use, and results of using, the strategies and self-regulation procedures with other tasks and in other settings; asking parents and other teachers to comment on the student's success in using the strategies; and working with other teachers to prompt the use of the strategies in their classrooms.

Impact of SRSD Instruction in Writing

SRSD Studies in Writing

To date, 26 studies have examined the use of SRSD. Most of this research has involved students' writing (see Harris & Graham, 1999), but reading and math have been investigated as well (Bednarczyk, 1991; Case, Harris, & Graham, 1992; Johnson, Graham, & Harris, 1997). This chapter only examines SRSD writing intervention studies. Tables 20.1 through 20.4 presents effect sizes for these 18 studies. Studies by Harris and colleagues (2002) and Sawyer and colleagues (1992) involved component analysis of the SRSD model, so only effect sizes for the full treatment were computed.

Not included in Tables 20.1 through 20.4 are a qualitative study of SRSD implementation (MacArthur et al., 1996), an evaluation of SRSD using a one-group pretest–posttest design (Collins, 1993), a component analysis of SRSD that did not include a control group (Graham & Harris, 1989a), and the study of a writing program that included SRSD as one of several instructional components (MacArthur et al., 1995). A study by Troia and Graham (in press) that was partially modeled after SRSD was also not included, because interactive learning between teacher and students, a hallmark of the SRSD model, was purposefully limited. In addition, a study by Tanhouser (1994) was not included because the investigator included only 3 days of instruction, limiting the amount of practice and time students were given to master the target strategy. This violates a basic characteristic of the SRSD model, namely, the use of criterion, not time-based, learning.

For SRSD writing studies that involved group comparisons, effect sizes were computed by subtracting the posttest mean of the control group from the posttest mean of the SRSD group and dividing by the standard deviation for the control group. An ef-

fect size of 0.20 is considered small, 0.50 medium, and 0.80 large. For single-participant design studies, effect sizes were calculated using the percentage of nonoverlapping data (PND) points recommended by Scruggs and Mastropieri (2001). The PND is "the proportion of data points in a given treatment condition that exceeds the extreme value in a baseline condition" (p. 230). PND scores above 90% represent very effective treatments, scores between 70% and 90% represent effective treatments, scores between 50% and 70% are of questionable effectiveness, and scores below 50% are ineffective. Because the PND metric was used, it was not possible to calculate effect size for all the variables collected in the single-participant design studies. PND can only be calculated when the data for each assessment point are provided. When multiple measures are collected in single-participant studies, such data is usually provided for only the most critical variables (usually in the form of one or more graphs). This was the case for many of the single-participant studies reviewed here.

Thirteen of the 18 studies (72%) presented in Tables 20.1 through 20.4 involved students with LD. The students with LD were in fourth to eighth grade. In addition to being identified as LD by the schools, they typically met the following additional criteria: a score between 80 and 120 on an intelligence test, achievement 2 years or more below grade level on a standardized achievement test, and problems with writing. Students who were poor writers or low achievers were included in three studies (De La Paz, 2001; Harris et al., 2002; Saddler, Moran, Graham, & Harris, 2002), average writers in three studies (Danoff, Harris, & Graham, 1993; De La Paz, 1999; De La Paz & Graham, in press), and good writers or gifted students in two studies (Albertson & Billingsley, 1997; De La Paz, 1999). Finally, a mixture of students with special needs (LD, attention-deficit/hyperactivity disorder, etc.) were included in three studies (De La Paz, 2001; De La Paz & Graham, 1997b; Harris et al., 2002). Thus, the effectiveness of SRSD has been tested with a variety of different types of children. Moreover, SRSD has been experimentally tested with children as early as second grade (Saddler et al.,

TABLE 20.1. Effect Sizes for Self-Regulated Strategy Development Planning Studies Involving Story Writing

Study	Design	Grades	Students	Teacher	Posttests	ES	Maintenance tests	ES	Generalization tests	ES
Harris, Graham, & Mason (2002)	Group design	3	Poor writers	GAs	(Quiet room) Length	2.21	(8–10 weeks) Length	0.49	(Narratives) Length	0.27
					Elements	1.76	Elements	1.16	Elements	1.23
					Quality	1.90	Quality	0.82	Quality	0.56
Sawyer, Graham, & Harris (1992)	Group design	5–6	LD	GAs	(Quiet room) Story grammar	3.52				
					Quality	1.47				
Saddler, Moran, Graham, & Harris (2002)	SP	2	Poor writers	GAs	(Quiet room) Elements	100%	(2–4 weeks) Elements	86%	(Narratives) Elements	83%
Troia, Graham, & Harris (1999)	SP	5	LD	Researchers	(Quiet room) Story grammar	100%	(3 weeks) Story grammar	67%	(Essays) Elements	75%
Albertson & Billingsley (1997)	SP	6	Gifted	Researcher	(Home setting) Length	71%				
					Story grammar	100%				
					Sentences	100%				
Danoff, Harris, & Graham (1993)	SP	4–5	LD	Teacher	(Regular class) Elements	100%	(2–4 weeks) Elements	100%	(Different teacher) Elements	100%
					Story grammar	100%	Story grammar	100%	Story grammar	100%
		4–5	Normal writers	Teacher	Elements	100%	Elements	100%	Elements	100%
					Story grammar	100%	Story grammar	100%	Story grammar	100%
Harris, & Graham (1985)	SP	6	LD	GAs	(Quiet room) Action verbs	100%	(2–14 weeks) Action verbs	100%	(Classroom) Action verbs	100%
				Adjectives	Adjectives 100%	Adjectives 100%	Adjectives 100%	Adjectives 50%	Adjectives 100%	Adjectives 75%
					Adverbs	88%	Adverbs	75%	Adverbs	100%

Note. Effect sizes for group studies were calculated by subtracting the posttest mean of the control condition from the posttest mean of the SRSD condition and dividing by the standard deviation for the control condition; effect size for single-participant design studies was the percentage of nonoverlapping data points. Quiet room, a quiet room in the school where instruction was delivered; SP, single-participant design; LD, learning disability; GAs, graduate assistants.

TABLE 20.2. Effect Sizes for Self-Regulated Strategy Development Planning Studies Involving Opinion Essays

Study	Design	Grades	Students	Teacher	Posttests	ES	Maintenance tests	ES	Generalization tests	ES
Harris, Graham, & Mason (2002)	Group design	3	Poor writers	GAs	(Quiet room) Length Elements Quality	1.83 1.07 2.14			(Informative) Length Quality	1.58 1.15
De La Paz & Graham (1997a)	Group design	7–8	LD	GAs	(Quiet room) (Task—writing) Length Elements Coherence Quality (Task—dictation) Length Elements Coherence Quality	.32 .55 1.10 .48 5.18 3.74 .44 1.43	(2 weeks) (Task—writing) Length Elements Coherence Quality (Task—dictation) Length Elements Coherence Quality	.58 1.53 1.19 .48 1.38 2.11 .40 .90		
Sexton, Harris, & Graham (1998)	SP	5–6	LD	Researcher	(Regular class) Elements	70%	(3–8 weeks) Elements	33%	(Different teacher) Elements	100%
De La Paz & Graham (1997b)	SP	5	LD/Gifted LD/MMR, LD	Researcher	(Quiet room) Elements	100%	(6–8 weeks) Elements	100%		
Graham, MacArthur, Schwartz, & Page-Voth (1992)	SP	5	LD	GAs	(Quiet room) (Word processing) Elements	100%	(4–15 weeks) (Word processing) Elements	100%	(Stories) (Word processing) Elements	88%
Graham & Harris (1989b)	SP	6	LD	GAs	(Quiet room) Elements	100%	(3–12 weeks) Elements	75%	(Class) Elements (Stories) Elements	100% 88%

Note. Effect sizes for group studies were calculated by subtracting the posttest mean of the control condition from the posttest mean of the SRSD condition and dividing by the standard deviation for the control condition; effect size for single-participant design studies was the percentage of nonoverlapping data points. SP, single-participant design; LD, learning disability; MMR, mild mental retardation; GAs, graduate assistants.

333

TABLE 20.3. Effect Sizes for Self-Regulated Strategy Development Planning Studies Involving Essays Involving Explanation

Study	Design	Grades	Students	Teacher	Posttests	ES	Maintenance tests	ES
De La Paz & Graham (in press)	Group design	7–8	Normal writers	Teachers	(Class) Length Vocabulary Quality	0.82 1.13 1.71	(4 weeks) Length Vocabulary Quality	1.07 0.94 0.74
De La Paz (1999)	SP	7–8	LD	Teachers	(Class) Length Elements Quality	89% 89% 89%	(4 weeks) Length Elements Quality	100% 100% 100%
			Poor writers		Length Elements Quality	100% 100% 100%	Length Elements Quality	100% 100% 100%
			Average writers		Length Elements Quality	100% 67% 100%	Length Elements Quality	100% 100% 100%
			Good Writers		Length Elements Quality	50% 83% 100%	Length Elements Quality	100% 100% 100%
De La Paz (2001)	SP	7–8	ADHD and speech/lang	Teachers	(Class) Elements	100%	(4 weeks) Elements	100%

Note. Effect sizes for group studies were calculated by subtracting the posttest mean of the control condition (SRSD) from the posttest mean of the SRSD condition and dividing by the standard deviation for the control condition; effect size for single-participant design studies was the percentage of nonoverlapping data points. SP, single-participant design; LD, learning disability; ADHD, attention-deficit/hyperactivity disorder; speech/lang, speech and language disorders.

2002) and as late as eighth grade (e.g., De La Paz, 1999).

Does SRSD Improve Students' Writing Performance?

To answer this question, we first looked at the impact of SRSD on students in general and then examined its impact on specific kinds of students, including those with and without LD. To examine overall and differential effects of SRSD writing instruction, average effect sizes (ESs) were calculated for the four variables that appeared most frequently in the SRSD studies summarized in Tables 20.1 though 20.4. These were quality (11 ESs), elements (15 ESs), story grammar scale (5 ESs), and length (10 ESs). Quality measured the overall impact or value of a student's composition. Elements assessed the inclusion of basic genre elements or parts in a composition. With a story, for example, papers were analyzed by the re-

searcher to determine whether they included a main character(s), a location, time frame, goals for the characters, actions, expressed emotions, and an ending. Elements tabulated in opinion essays included the writer's premise, counter premise, supporting reasons, refutation of counterreasons, elaborations, and ending. The story grammar scale examined the inclusion and quality of story elements or parts. Finally, length was the number of words in a composition.

Table 20.5 summarizes the average effect size for these four variables across all studies (i.e., overall) and by specific type of students (i.e., LD, poor writers, and average students). The number in the parentheses following each average effect size specifies the *n*, or number of effect sizes used to compute that average. *n* ranged from 11 to 1. Effect sizes for good writers (i.e., good writers or gifted students) were not included in Table 20.5 because *n* was never greater than 1 on any of the four target variables. For

TABLE 20.4. Effect Sizes for Self-Regulated Strategy Development Revising Studies Where Students Wrote Using Word Processing

Study	Design	Grades	Students	Teacher	Posttests	ES	Maintenance tests	ES	Generalization tests	ES
MacArthur, Schwartz, & Graham (1991)	Group Design	4–6	LD	Teachers	(Class) (Narratives)					
					Total revisions	1.29				
					S—revisions	1.41				
					NS—revisions	0.64				
					Spelling	0.54				
					Punctuation	0.33				
					Capitalization	0.14				
					Quality	1.19				
Albertson & Billingsley (1997)	SP	6	Gifted	Researcher	(Home setting) (Stories)					
					Revising time	100%				
Stoddard & MacArthur (1993)	SP	7–8	LD	Researcher	(Quiet room) (Narratives)		(4–9 weeks) (Narratives)		(Paper and pencil) (Narratives)	
					NS—revisions	100%	NS—revisions	100%	NS—revisions	100%
					MNS—revisions	100%	MNS—revisions	100%	MNS—revisions	83%
					S—revisions	75%	S—revisions	83%	S—revisions	67%
Graham & MacArthur (1988)	SP	5–6	LD	GAs	(Quiet room) (Opinion essays)		(4–9 weeks) (Opinion essays)		(Paper and pencil) (Opinion essays)	
					Total revisions	60%	Total revisions	75%	Total revisions	67%
					MC—revisions	100%	MC—revisions	100%	MC—revisions	100%
					MP—revisions	30%	MP—revisions	50%	MP—revisions	33%

Note. Effect sizes for group studies were calculated by subtracting the posttest mean of the control condition from the posttest mean of the SRSD condition and dividing by the standard deviation for the control condition; effect size for single-participant design studies was the percentage of nonoverlapping data points. Quiet room, a quiet room in the school where instruction was delivered; SP, single-participant design; LD, learning disability; GA, graduate assistants; NS, surface-level revisions; NS—revisions, non-surface-level revisions; MNS—revisions, meaning changing non-surface level revisions; MC—revisions, meaning-changing revisions; MP—revisions, meaning-preserving revisions.

335

TABLE 20.5. Summary of Average Effect Sizes for Quality, Elements, Story Grammar, and Length for Self-Regulated Strategy Development Studies

Measures	Overall				LD				Poor writers				Average students		
	Post.	Maint.	General. genre	General. P & P	Post.	Maint.	General. genre	General. P & P	Post.	Maint.	General. genre	General. P & P	Post.	Maint.	General. P & P
Quality															
Group	1.47 (7)	0.74 (4)	0.86 (2)	—	1.14 (4)	0.69 (2)	—	—	1.67 (2)	0.82 (2)	0.86 (2)	—	1.71 (1)	0.74 (1)	—
SP	97% (4)	100% (4)	—	—	89% (1)	100% (1)	—	—	100% (1)	100% (1)	—	—	100% (1)	100% (1)	—
Elements															
Group	1.87 (4)	1.60 (3)	1.23 (1)	—	2.15 (2)	1.82 (2)	—	—	1.42 (2)	1.16 (1)	1.23 (1)	—	—	—	—
SP	92% (11)	90% (11)	84% (4)	100% (4)	93% (6)	85% (6)	84% (3)	100% (3)	100% (2)	93% (2)	83% (1)	—	84% (2)	100% (2)	100% (1)
Story grammar															
Group	3.52 (1)	—	—	—	3.52 (1)	—	—	—	—	—	—	—	—	—	—
SP	100% (4)	89% (3)	75% (1)	100% (2)	100% (2)	84% (2)	—	100% (1)	—	—	—	—	100% (1)	100% (1)	100% (1)
Length															
Group	2.07 (5)	.88 (4)	.93 (2)	—	1.86 (2)	0.98 (2)	—	—	2.02 (2)	.49 (1)	0.93 (2)	—	.82 (1)	1.07 (1)	—
SP	82% (5)	100% (4)	—	—	89% (1)	100% (1)	—	—	100% (2)	100% (1)	—	—	100% (1)	100% (1)	—

Note. Post., posttest; Maint., maintenance; General. genre, generalization to different genre; General. P & P, generalization to different person or place; LD, learning disabilities; Group, Group design; SP, single-participant studies; the number in parentheses following the effect size is the number of effect sizes the average effect size was computed from; effect sizes for good writers/high-achieving students were not included in this table because there was no more than one effect size for any test (posttest, maintenance, etc.).

each variable, the average effect size, when available, was provided for both group design and single-participant studies. Whenever possible, these average effect sizes were calculated for posttest (immediately following instruction), maintenance (2 to 15 weeks following instruction), generalization to a different genre (e.g., story writing to opinion essay writing), and generalization to a different person or place (e.g., from a special setting to the regular classroom).

OVERALL

As can be seen in Table 20.5, SRSD writing instruction produced large effects for students in general. When all studies were considered together, average effect sizes at posttest for group design investigations ranged from 1.47 for quality, 1.78 for elements, and 2.0 and above for length and story grammar scores. Likewise, average PNDs for quality, elements, and story grammar were all above 90%, indicating that SRSD writing instruction is an effective treatment in single-participant design studies as well. Thus, SRSD had a strong and positive effect on the quality, structure, and length of students' writing.

STUDENTS WITH LD

Of particular importance to this review is the impact of SRSD on the writing of students with LD. Average effect sizes at posttest for group and single-participant design studies show that this is a powerful treatment for these students (see Table 20.5). Average effect sizes for group studies ranged from 1.14 for quality, 1.86 for length, and above 2.0 for elements and story grammar. All the average PNDs were 89% or above. These statistics are complied from 11 studies involving students with LD (effect sizes for quality, elements, story grammar, or length were not available for the other two LD studies) and included 19 individual effect sizes. Although this is a relatively small *n* when compared to an area such as phonological awareness (*n* > 700; Bus & van IJzendoorn, 1999), the general consistency of the findings strengthens the conclusion that SRSD provides an effective treatment for addressing the writing difficulties of students with LD. None of the individual PNDs fell below the effective range (70% or higher), and two-thirds of the individual effect sizes for the group design studies were above 1.0, with the other one-third ranging from 0.32 to 0.55 (small to medium effects).

OTHER GROUPS OF STUDENTS

Although the findings for other groups of students must be viewed as more tentative, due to the smaller *n* for effect sizes, the data support the contention that SRSD is an effective writing treatment for students in general. For students who are poor writers (*n* = 11), for example, the average effect size on quality and length at posttest (1.67 and 2.02, respectively) exceeded the average effect size obtained by students with LD (see Table 20.5). Their average effect size for elements was also quite large (ES = 1.42) as was their average PNDs for quality, elements, and length (all PNDs at posttest = 100%).

The available statistics for average writers and good writers suggests that they benefit from SRSD instruction in writing too. For average writers (*n* = 7), PNDs for the four writing variables at posttest ranged from 84% to 100%, and the single effect size for quality from the group design studies was 1.71; the single effect size for length was 0.82 (see Table 20.5). For good writers (*n* = 3), the results from the limited database were not quite as strong but still quite promising. The PND for quality was 100% (i.e., very effective treatment) and 83% for elements (i.e., effective treatment). The impact of SRSD on the length of good writers' compositions was questionable, however, as the PND was just 50% for this variable at posttest.

If a single-participant study by De La Paz (2001) is representative, then SRSD also appears to be an effective writing treatment for mainstreamed students with attention-deficit/hyperactivity disorder (ADHD) and speech/language difficulties. The PND for elements in this study was 100%.

Does SRSD Improve Students' Revising?

The average effect sizes reviewed in the previous section were all based on studies involving the teaching of planning strategies.

The only exception was a single effect size (1.19 for quality) generated by MacArthur, Schwartz, and Graham (1991) in a study in which students with LD were taught a revising strategy. Table 20.4 presents effect sizes for SRSD revising studies. With the exception of one PND (100% for revising time in a study with gifted students), all available effect sizes are from three studies involving students with LD. We did not develop average effect sizes for this data, as the measures used across the LD studies were not equivalent.

The primary objective of these SRSD revising studies was to increase the number of substantive revisions made by students with LD. As noted earlier in the chapter, children with LD focus most of their revising efforts on minor surface-level features of text, such as correcting mechanical errors and substituting one word for another (MacArthur & Graham, 1987: MacArthur, Graham, & Schwartz, 1991). As can be seen in Table 20.4, SRSD had moderate to strong effects on increasing substantive revisions at posttest. In the group design study by MacArthur, Schwartz, and Graham (1991), the effect size for substantive or nonsurface revisions was 0.64, whereas the PNDs for nonsurface as well as meaning-changing nonsurface revisions in the Stoddard and MacArthur (1993) investigation were both 100%. Likewise, the PND for meaning-changing revisions in Graham and MacArthur (1988) was 100%.

Although these studies were primarily designed to increase substantive revisions, each investigation included procedures for bolstering surface-level revisions as well. The effects of SRSD on these types of revisions at posttest were more variable (see Table 20.4). In the group design study by MacArthur, Schwartz, and Graham (1991), the effect size for surface-level revisions was quite large (1.29), but a more moderate PND (75%) was obtained for this variable by Stoddard and MacArthur (1993). In contrast, SRSD was ineffective in increasing meaning-preserving revisions (PND = 30%) in the study by Graham and MacArthur (1988). Finally, small to moderate effects were found for improved punctuation (ES = 0.33) and spelling (ES = 0.54) in revised papers following SRSD instruction in the

MacArthur, Schwartz, and Graham (1991) study, but not for capitalization (ES = 0.14).

Are SRSD Effects Maintained and Generalized?

A major issue in strategy instructional research, especially for students with LD, is whether effects are maintained over time and are generalized to new tasks and situations (Graham & Harris, 1997). Table 20.5 presents average effect sizes for maintenance and generalization. Although average effect sizes were typically not as large at maintenance as they were at posttest for students in general, as well as for poor writers and students with LD in particular, they remained moderate to large for these three groups in terms of overall quality, structure (elements or story grammar), and length. The average effect size for group design studies ranged from 0.74 to 1.60 overall, 0.69 to 1.82 for students with LD, and 0.49 to 1.67 for poor writers. Similarly, average PNDs ranged from 89% to 100% overall, 84% to 100% for students with LD, and 93% to 100% for poor writers. For the revision studies presented in Table 20.4, strong maintenance effects were observed for the number of substantive revisions made by students with LD (all PNDs = 100) but not for the less important surface-level revisions (PNDs ranged from 50% to 83%).

It is interesting to note that maintenance was not much of an issue for average and good writers in the SRSD studies conducted to date. All available PNDs at maintenance ($n = 9$; see Tables 20.1—20.3) for these students were 100%. Furthermore, effect sizes for length for average writers in the De La Paz and Graham (in press) study was higher at maintenance than at posttest (see Table 20.3). Although the effect size for overall quality was smaller at maintenance in this study, it was still quite substantial (ES = 0.74).

Data on generalization from one genre to the next was only available for poor writers and students with LD. In studies in which this generalization was assessed, students were taught how to use a writing strategy in one genre (e.g., opinion essay) and transfer effects to another genre (e.g., stories). For students with LD, SRSD was effective in promoting cross-genre transfer as the average PNDs ($n = 3$) was 84% (see Table 20.5). This was also the case for poor writers, as average effect sizes ($n = 6$) ranged from moderate to large (0.86 to 1.23; PND = 83%).

Transferring SRSD effects from one setting or person to another did not appear to pose much difficulty for students when such data were collected (i.e., for average writers and students with LD), as all average PNDs equaled 100% (see Table 20.5). Students with LD were also generally effective in transferring SRSD revising effects from the word processor to paper and pencil as there was little difference in their PNDs when these two modes of composing were employed (compare posttest vs. generalization in Table 20.4).

Is SRSD Effective with Younger and Older Students?

To answer this question, we computed average effect sizes for students in grades 2 through 6 as well as grades 7 and 8 for writing quality, elements, and length (see Table 20.6). At posttest, all average effect sizes for group design studies exceeded 1.21 (i.e., a large effect) for both groups of students, whereas the average PNDs for each group were within the effective to very effective range (i.e., 71% to 96%). Although average effect sizes for group design studies were smaller at maintenance, they remained above 0.80 (a large effect) for both groups in all but two instances. The average effect size for writing quality for students in grades 7 and 8 was 0.71 at maintenance, while the average effect size (based on an *n* of 1) for length was 0.49 for students in grades 2 through 6. The average PNDs of both groups remained in the effective to very effective range (i.e., 85% to 100%) at this point.

Although SRSD provides an effective writing treatment for both groups of students, comparison between the two age groups were mixed. Average writing quality effects were larger for younger students than for older ones, whereas effects for composition length were stronger for older children. There was no clear-cut difference

for elements (see Table 20.6).

Is SRSD Effective with Different Types of Genres?

Story and personal narratives served as the primary genre of interest in approximately half of all SRSD studies, whereas opinion or explanation essays were the main focus in the other investigations. Table 20.6 presents average effect sizes for narrative writing studies (i.e., stories and personal narratives) and expository writing studies (i.e., opinion and explanatory essays). At posttest, all average effect sizes for group design studies were large (1.44 or greater) for both types of genres, and average PNDs for each genre were within the effective to very effective range (i.e., 71% to 100%). Average effect sizes for both genres were generally lower at maintenance but remained above 0.80 (a large effect) for both genres in all but two instances (0.71 for quality of expository writing and 0.49 for length of narrative compositions). The average PND for elements at maintenance (the only available data for single-participant studies) remained high (89% and 95%).

Although there was no clear-cut difference between genres at posttest and maintenance, generalization to another genre was clearly stronger when the primary focus of SRSD writing instruction was on exposition (see Table 20.6). For narrative writing, average effect sizes ranged from small to moderate (ES = 0.27 and 0.56; PND = 79%), whereas effect sizes for expository writing were much larger (ES = 1.15 and 1.58; PND = 88%). For the available data (i.e., elements), there was no difference between genres in terms of transfer to a different person or place (both PNDs = 100%).

Can Teachers Apply SRSD Effectively?

Of the 18 SRSD writing studies presented in Tables 20.1 through 20.4, slightly more than one-fourth were implemented by teachers. All the rest were carried out by graduate assistants or the researchers themselves. Table 20.6 provides the average effect sizes for teacher as well as graduate assistant (GA)/researcher–implemented SRSD writing instruction. First, SRSD writing in-

TABLE 20.6. Average Effect Sizes for Self-Regulated Strategy Development Studies at Different Grades, Genres, and Instructors

Measures	Grades 2–6	Grades 7–8	Narrative	Expository	GA or researcher	Classroom teacher
Quality						
Group-Post.	1.68 (4)	1.21 (3)	1.52 (3)	1.44 (4)	1.48 (5)	1.45 (2)
Group-Maint.	0.82 (1)	0.71 (3)	0.82 (1)	0.71 (3)	0.73 (3)	0.74 (1)
Group-Gen. genre	—	—	0.56 (1)	1.15 (1)	—	—
Elements						
Group-Post.	1.38 (2)	2.15 (2)	1.76 (1)	1.99 (3)	—	—
Group-Maint.	1.16 (1)	1.82 (2)	1.16 (1)	1.82 (2)	—	—
SP-Post.	96% (7)	85% (4)	100% (3)	89% (8)	94% (5)	90% (5)
SP-Maint.	85% (7)	100% (4)	95% (3)	89% (8)	77% (5)	100% (6)
SP-Gen. genre	—	—	79% (2)	88% (2)	—	—
SP-Gen. P & P	—	—	100% (2)	100% (2)	100% (2)	100% (2)
Story grammar						
SP-Post.	—	—	—	—	100% (2)	100% (2)
SP-Maint.	—	—	—	—	67% (1)	100% (2)
Length						
Group-Post.	2.02 (2)	2.10 (3)	2.21 (1)	2.04 (4)	2.39 (4)	0.82 (1)
Group-Maint.	0.49 (1)	1.01 (3)	0.49 (1)	1.01 (3)	0.82 (3)	1.07 (1)
Group-Gen. genre	—	—	0.27 (1)	1.58 (1)	—	—
SP-Post.	71% (1)	85% (3)	71% (1)	85% (4)	71% (1)	85% (4)

Note. Narratives include stories or personal narratives. Expository included opinion essays and explanation essays. Group, group design; SP, single-participant design; Post., posttest; Maint., maintenance; Gen. Genre, generalization to genre; Gen. P & P, generalization to a different person or place.

struction had moderate to large effects for both implementation groups at posttest and maintenance. All the average effect sizes for group design studies exceeded 0.74 (the majority were above 1.0), and all but one PND was greater than 71%. The exception was the PND (67%) for story grammar at maintenance for the GA/researcher implementation group. This effect size is in the questionable effectiveness range (50–70%).

When the two implementation groups were compared at posttest, the GA/researcher group generally evidenced larger average effect sizes (1.48 to 2.39 vs. 0.82 to 1.45; 94% to 100% vs. 90% to 100%). In contrast, the advantage was held by teachers for maintenance (0.74 to 1.07 vs. 0.73 to 0.82; 100% vs. 67% to 77%) and generalization to a different writing genre (85% to 71%). This is not necessarily surprising, as students are learning to apply the strate-

gies in the context in which they are most likely to use them during teacher-implemented SRSD instruction.

Do Independent Evaluations Support the Effectiveness of SRSD Writing Instruction?

Of the 18 studies reviewed in this chapter, we were authors on all but four of the investigations. Three of these four studies were conducted by former students or colleagues (i.e., De La Paz, 1999, 2001; Stoddard & MacArthur, 1993). With one exception, PNDs for all four of these studies were in the effective to very effective range at posttest, maintenance, and generalization (75% to 100%). The exception involved generalization of surface-level revisions from word processor to paper and pencil in the Stoddard and MacArthur (1993) investigation (PND = 67%). As noted before, promoting surface-level revisions was a secondary goal in this study.

Clearly, more independent evaluations of SRSD are needed. However, the effects for SRSD are consistent with or exceed the findings of other strategy investigators. To illustrate, Gersten and Baker (2001) computed effect sizes for 13 group-designed writing intervention studies involving students with LD. Ten of these studies focused on teaching writing strategies for planning and/or revising. When we removed effect sizes for any SRSD studies (four studies), the average effect size was 1.01. Our average SRSD effect size computed across all posttest indices for group design studies in Tables 20.1 through 20.4 was 1.37 for students with LD.

What Components of SRSD Instruction Are Most Important?

We have conducted several studies to determine the relative effectiveness of SRSD components designed to promote self-regulation. Two studies (Graham & Harris, 1989a; Sawyer et al., 1992) assessed the added value of explicit instruction in three self-regulation components (goal setting, self-monitoring, and self-recording). In both of these studies, students with LD were taught a strategy for planning and writing a story. For the story grammar scale described earlier, the inclusion of these self-regulation procedures had little impact at posttest or maintenance (average ESs = 0.07 and 0.05, respectively) but generated a strong incremental effect on generalization to a new setting (average ES = 1.03). Although effect sizes for writing quality could only be computed for the more recent study (Sawyer et al., 1992), the addition of the three self-regulation procedures produced moderate effects at posttest (ES = 0.42), maintenance (average ES = 0.40), and generalization (ES = 0.75).

Sawyer and colleagues (1992) further decomposed the SRSD model by removing not only explicit instruction in goal setting, self-monitoring, and self-recording but other instructional components thought to induce self-regulation as well (use of personalized self-statements, teacher modeling, etc.). In comparison to this reduced version of the model, full SRSD was much more powerful, as effects for the story grammar measure were quite large at posttest (ES = 1.96), maintenance (average ES =1.51), and generalization (ES = 2.78). Although the effects on writing quality were small at posttest (ES = 0.30), they were strong at maintenance (average ES = 1.15) and generalization (ES = 1.22). Thus, components designed to promote self-regulation in the SRSD model make a significant contribution to improved writing performance for students with LD.

Implications

We started this chapter with the claim that an important goal in writing instruction for students with LD is to help them develop a more sophisticated approach to composing—one that draws on the same types of composing processes and strategies employed by more skilled writers. We further asserted that this problem needs to be tackled "head on" by explicitly teaching students with LD such strategies, and that this instruction should be multifaceted, addressing students' strategic behavior, self-regulation skills, knowledge, and motivational dispositions. To test this proposition, we developed a strategy instructional model, SRSD, designed to meet these specifications. Since the early 1980s, the model has been tested repeatedly by ourselves, colleagues, students, and others to determine if it provides an effective and viable model for improving the writing performance of students with LD as well as other students. In this chapter, we examined the outcomes of this test by computing effect sizes for 18 SRSD intervention studies in writing.

One of the primary findings of our review was that SRSD is an effective approach for improving the writing of students with LD. Following instruction, average effect sizes for four different writing indices each exceeded 1.13, and the average PNDs for these measures were 89% or higher. Impressive effects were also found for maintenance and generalization, as effect sizes ranged from moderate to strong for these variables. These findings, along with the impressive effects obtained by other researchers such as Englert and her colleagues (1991) and Wong and her collaborators (Wong, Butler, Ficzere, & Kuperis, 1996, 1997), makes it clear that an important part of an effective writing program for students with LD is explicit writing strategy instruction.

Although we can provide no definitive answer on the most effective components of such instruction for students with LD, our research demonstrated that the inclusion of procedures that foster self-regulation contributes to these children's writing development. This appears to be especially true for generalization and maintenance. Because maintenance and generalization are such critical issues for students with LD, additional research is needed to determine how each can be fostered and supported. The findings from this review suggest that context and student ability may play an important role in such an analysis. Students evidenced greater maintenance and generalization when teachers rather than researchers or GAs taught writing strategies. Furthermore, average and high-ability students were more likely than weaker writers to maintain strategy effects.

In contrast to strategy instructional research in reading (see Gersten, Fuchs, Williams, & Baker, 2001), our review of SRSD studies found that writing strategies taught to students with LD also had a beneficial impact on the writing of poor, average, and good writers. A similar finding was reported by Englert and colleagues (1991). One reason such effects may be so universal is that almost all students experience difficulty mastering basic writing processes such as content generation, planning, revising, and so forth (Scardamalia & Bereiter, 1986). With the advent of inclusion, it has become increasingly important to identify instructional procedures that are effective with a wide range of students. This review and the research by Englert and colleagues suggest that strategy instruction meets this requirement.

In summary, SRSD appears to be a versatile tool. It was effective with younger and older students as well as different types of students, instructors, and writing genres. Perhaps most important, classroom teachers were able to apply the model effectively, improving the writing performance of a wide range of students, including those with learning disabilities.

Acknowledgments

Preparation of this chapter was supported by the Center to Accelerate Student Learning, funded by the U.S. Department of Education's Office of Special Education Programs (Grant # H324V980001).

References

Abbington, A. (1952). *Bigger and better boners.* New York: Viking Press.

Alexander, P., Graham, S., & Harris, K. R. (1998). A perspective on strategy research: Prospect and progress. *Educational Psychology Review, 10,* 129–154.

Albertson, L. R., & Billingsley, F. F. (1997, March). *Improving young writers' planning and reviewing skills while story-writing.* Paper presented at the annual meeting of the American Educational Research Association, Chicago.

Bednarczyk, A. (1991). *The effectiveness of story grammar instruction with a self-instructional strategy development framework for students with learning disabilities.* Unpublished doctoral dissertation, University of Maryland, College Park.

Berninger, V., Vaughn, K., Abbott, R., Abbott, S., Rogan, L., Brooks, A., Reed, E., & Graham, S. (1997). Treatment of handwriting problems in beginning writers: Transfer from handwriting to composition. *Journal of Educational Psychology, 89, 652–666.*

Berninger, V., Vaughn, K., Abbott, R., Brooks, A., Abbott, S., Rogan, L., Reed, E., & Graham, S. (1998). Early intervention for spelling problems: Teaching functional spelling units of varying size with a multiple-connections framework. *Journal of Educational Psychology, 90, 587–605.*

Bus, A., & van IJzendoorn, M. (1999). Phonological awareness and early reading: A meta-analysis of experimental training studies. *Journal of Educational Psychology, 91, 403–414.*

Case, L. P., Harris, K. R., & Graham, S. (1992). Improving the mathematical problem solving skills of students with learning disabilities: Self-regulated strategy development. *Journal of Special Education, 26,* 1–19.

Collins, R. A. (1993). *Narrative writing of option II students: The effects of combining whole-language techniques, writing process approach, and strategy training.* Unpublished master's thesis, State University of New York at Buffalo.

Danoff, B., Harris, K. R., & Graham, S. (1993). Incorporating strategy instruction within the writing process in the regular classroom: Effects on the writing of students with and without learning disabilities. *Journal of Reading Behavior, 25,* 295–319.

De La Paz, S. (1999). Self-regulated strategy instruction in regular education settings: Improving outcomes for students with and without learning disabilities. *Learning Disabilities Research and Practice, 14,* 92–106.

De La Paz, S. (2001). Teaching writing to students with attention deficit disorders and specific language impairments. *Journal of Educational Research, 95,* 37–47.

De La Paz, S., & Graham, S. (1995). Dictation: Application to writing for students with learning disabilities. In T. Scruggs & M. Matropieri (Eds.), *Advances in learning and behavioral disorders* (Vol. 9, pp. 227–247). Greenwich, CT: JAI Press.

De La Paz, S., & Graham, S. (1997a). Effects of dictation and advanced planning instruction on the composing of students with writing and learning problems. *Journal of Educational Psychology, 89,* 203–222.

De La Paz, S., & Graham, S. (1997b). Strategy instruction in planning: Effects on the writing performance and behavior of students with learning disabilities. *Exceptional Children, 63,* 167–181.

De La Paz, S., & Graham, S. (in press). Explicitly teaching strategies, skills, and knowledge: Writing instruction in middle school classrooms. *Journal of Educational Psychology.*

De La Paz, S., Swanson, P., & Graham, S. (1998). The contribution of executive control to the revising of students with writing and learning difficulties. *Journal of Educational Psychology, 90,* 448–460.

Englert, C., Raphael, T., Anderson, L., Anthony, H., Steven, D., & Fear, K. (1991). Making writing and self-talk visible: Cognitive strategy instruction writing in regular and special education classrooms. *American Educational Research Journal, 28,* 337–373.

Englert, C., Raphael, T., Anderson, L., Gregg, S., & Anthony, H. (1989). Exposition: Reading, writing, and metacognitive knowledge of learning disabled students. *Learning Disabilities Research, 5,* 5–24.

Gersten, R., & Baker, S. (2001). Teaching expressive writing to students with learning disabilities: A meta-analysis. *Elementary School Journal, 101,* 251–272.

Gersten, R., Fuchs, D., Williams, J., & Baker, S. (2001). Teaching reading comprehension strategies to students with learning disabilities. *Review of Educational Research, 71,* 279–320.

Graham, S. (1990). The role of production factors in learning disabled students' compositions. *Journal of Educational Psychology, 82,* 781–791.

Graham, S. (1997). Executive control in the revising of students with learning and writing difficulties. *Journal of Educational Psychology, 89,* 223–234.

Graham, S., & Harris, K. R. (1989a). A component analysis of cognitive strategy instruction: Effects on learning disabled students' compositions and self-efficacy. *Journal of Educational Psychology, 81,* 353–361.

Graham, S., & Harris, K. R. (1989b). Improving learning disabled students' skills at composing essays: Self-instructional strategy training. *Exceptional Children, 56,* 201–214.

Graham, S., & Harris, K. R. (1994). The role and development of self-regulation in the writing process. In D. Schunk & B. Zimmerman (Eds.), *Self-regulation of learning and performance: Issues and educational applications* (pp. 203–228). Hillsdale, NJ: Erlbaum.

Graham, S., & Harris, K. R. (1997). Self-regulation and writing: Where do we go from here? *Contemporary Educational Psychology, 22,* 102–114.

Graham, S., & Harris, K. R. (2000). The role of self-regulation and transcription skills in writing and writing development. *Educational Psychologist, 35,* 3–12.

Graham, S., & Harris, K. R. (in press). Literacy: Writing. In R. Anand (Ed.), *Encyclopedia of cognitive sciences.* London: Macmillan.

Graham, S., Harris, K. R., & Fink, B. (2000). Is handwriting causally related to learning to write? Treatment of handwriting problems in beginning writers. *Journal of Educational Psychology, 93,* 4–88–497.

Graham, S., Harris, K. R., & Fink, B. (in press). Contribution of spelling instruction to the spelling, writing, and reading of poor spellers. *Journal of Educational Psychology.*

Graham, S., Harris, K. R., MacArthur, C., & Schwartz, S. (1991). Writing and writing instruction with students with learning disabilities: A review of a program of research. *Learning Disability Quarterly, 14,* 89–114.

Graham, S., & MacArthur, C. (1988). Improving learning disabled students' skills at revising essays produced on a word processor: Self-instructional training. *Journal of Special Education, 22,* 133–152.

Graham, S., MacArthur, C., Schwartz, S., & Page-Voth, V. (1992). Improving the compositions of students with learning disabilities using a strategy involving product and process goal setting. *Exceptional Children, 58,* 322–334.

Graham, S., Schwartz, S., & MacArthur, C. (1993). Knowledge of writing and the composing process, attitude toward writing, and self-efficacy for students with and without learning disabilities. *Journal of Learning Disabilities, 26,* 237–249.

Harris, K. R., & Graham, S. (1985). Improving learning disabled students' composition skills: Self-control strategy training. *Learning Disability Quarterly, 8,* 27–36.

Harris, K. R., & Graham, S. (1996). *Making the writing process work: Strategies for composition and self-regulation.* Cambridge, MA: Brookline Books.

Harris, K. R., Graham, S. (1999). Programmatic intervention research: Illustrations from the evolution of self-regulated strategy development. *Learning Disability Quarterly, 22,* 251–262.

Harris, K. R., Graham, S., & Deshler, D. (1998). *Teaching every child every day: Learning in diverse schools and classrooms.* Cambridge, MA: Brookline Books.

Harris, K. R., Graham, S., & Mason, L. (2002). [Teaching strategies for writing stories and persuasive essays: The effects of SRSD instruction with young struggling writers]. Unpublished raw data.

Hayes, J. (1996). A new framework for understanding cognition and affect in writing. In M. Levy & S. Ransdell (Eds.), *The science of writing: Theories, methods, individual differences, and applications* (pp. 1–27). Mahwah, NJ: Erbaum.

Hayes, J., & Flower, L. (1980). Identifying the organization of writing processes. In L. Gregg & E. Steinberg (Eds.), *Cognitive processes in writing* (pp. 3–30). Hillsdale, NJ: Erlbaum.

Johnson, L., Graham, S., & Harris, K. R. (1997). The effects of goal setting and self-instruction on learning a reading comprehension strategy among students with learning disabilities. *Journal of Learning Disabilities, 30,* 80–91.

Loranger, D. (2000, December). *Reader's Digest,* p. 126.

MacArthur, C., & Graham, S. (1987). Learning disabled students' composing with three methods: Handwriting, dictation, and word processing. *Journal of Special Education, 21,* 22–42.

MacArthur, C., Graham, S., & Schwartz, S. (1991). Knowledge of revision and revising behavior among students with learning disabilities. *Learning Disability Quarterly, 14,* 61–74.

MacArthur, C., Graham, S., Schwartz, S., & Schafer, W. (1995). Evaluation of a writing instruction model that integrated a process approach, strategy instruction, and word processing. *Learning Disability Quarterly, 18,* 276–291.

MacArthur, C., Schwartz, S., & Graham, S. (1991). Effects of a reciprocal peer revision strategy in special education classrooms. *Learning Disability Research and Practice, 6,* 201–210.

MacArthur, C., Schwartz, S., Graham, S., Molloy, D., & Harris, K. R. (1996). Integration of strategy instruction into a whole language classroom: A case study. *Learning Disabilities Research and Practice, 11,* 168–176.

McCutchen, D. (1988). "Functional automaticity" in children's writing: A problem of metacognitive control. *Written Communication, 5,* 306–324.

Pressley, M., Harris, K. R., & Marks, M. (1992). But good strategy instructors are constructivists! *Educational Psychology Review, 4,* 3–31.

Reeve, R., & Brown, A. (1985). Metacognition reconsidered: Implications for intervention research. *Journal of Abnormal Child Psychology, 13,* 343–356.

Saddler, B., Moran, S., Graham, S., & Harris, K. R. (2002). [Preventing writing difficulties: Strategy instruction for young struggling writers]. Unpublished raw data.

Sawyer, R., Graham, S., & Harris, K. R. (1992). Direct teaching, strategy instruction, and strategy instruction with explicit self-regulation: Effects on the composition skills and self-efficacy of students with learning disabilities. *Journal of Educational Psychology, 84,* 340–352.

Scardamalia, M., & Bereiter, C. (1986). Written composition. In M. Wittrock (Ed.), *Handbook of research on teaching* (3rd ed., pp. 778–803). New York: MacMillan.

Scruggs, T., & Mastropieri, M. (2001). How to summarize single-participant research: Ideas and applications. *Exceptionality, 9,* 227–244.

Sexton, R. J., Harris, K. R., & Graham, S. (1998). The effects of self-regulated strategy development on essay writing and attributions of students with learning disabilities in a process writing setting. *Exceptional Children, 64,* 295–311.

Stoddard, B., & MacArthur, C. (1993). A peer editor strategy: Guiding learning disabled students in response and revision. *Research in the Teaching of English, 27,* 76–103.

Tanhouser, S. (1994). *Function over form: The relative efficacy of self-instructional strategy training alone and with procedural facilitation for adolescents with learning disabilities.* Unpublished doctoral dissertation, Johns Hopkins University.

Thomas, C., Englert, C., & Gregg, S. (1987). An analysis of errors and strategies in the expository writing of learning disabled students. *Remedial and Special Education, 8,* 21–30.

Troia, G., & Graham, S. (in press). The effectiveness of highly explicit and teacher-directed strategy instructional routine: Changing the writing performance of students with learning disabilities. *Journal of Learning Disabilities.*

Troia, G. A., Graham, S., & Harris, K. R. (1999). Teaching students with learning disabilities to mindfully plan when writing. *Exceptional Children, 65,* 215–252.

Wong, B. Y. L., Butler, D. L., Ficzere, S. A., & Kuperis, S. (1996). Teaching low achievers and student with learning disabilities to plan, write, and revise opinion essays. *Journal of Learning Disabilities, 29.*

Wong, B. Y. L., Butler, D. L., Ficzere, S. A., & Kuperis, S. (1997). Teaching adolescents with learning disabilities and low achievers to plan, write, and revise compare-contrast essays. *Learning Disabilities Research and Practice, 12,* 2–15.

Wong, B., Wong, R., & Blenkinsop, J. (1989). Cognitive and metacognitive aspects of learning disabled adolescents' composing problems. *Learning Disability Quarterly, 12,* 310–323.

Zimmerman, B., & Risemberg, R. (1997). Becoming a self-regulated writer: A social cognitive perspective. *Contemporary Educational Psychology, 22,* 73–101.

21

Preventing Written Expression Disabilities through Early and Continuing Assessment and Intervention for Handwriting and/or Spelling Problems: Research into Practice

Virginia W. Berninger
Dagmar Amtmann

Referral of students with written expression problems sharply increases around grade 4, when amount and complexity of written assignments also increases (Levine, Oberklaid, & Meltzer, 1981). Not only do many upper-elementary-grade students have problems in written expression but also a sizable number of middle school students do (Hooper et al., 1993). Writing is the most common problem of 9- to 14- year-old students with learning disabilities (Cobb-Morocco, Dalton, & Tivnan, 1992). Over a decade ago, the first author initiated a systematic research program to identify the developmental origins of these written expression problems early in schooling when the probability of remediation, and therefore prevention, may be greatest. The first wave of this research focused on multivariate process assessment in cross-sectional, unreferred samples (grades 1 to 9) (Berninger, 1994), whereas the second wave focused on early instructional intervention (grades 1 to 3). We launched this research at a time that process writing and integrated reading-writing instruction focused primarily on high-level meaning (e.g., Britton, 1978; Clay, 1982; Graves, 1975). Although both waves of our research extended process to include processes involved in transcription, we also included high-level processes for constructing meaning in both our assessment batteries and instructional protocols.

Early intervention in writing was initially justified on the basis of a longitudinal study documenting the persistence of early spelling problems across the elementary grades (Juel, 1988). We subsequently found that early intervention for at-risk spelling was more likely to result in improved spelling (e.g., Abbott, Reed, Abbott, & Berninger, 1997; Berninger, Vaughan et al., 1998) than later intervention with upper elementary grades for students with spelling problems (e.g., Brooks, Vaughan, & Berninger, 1999). By the end of second grade, children may be impaired in handwriting only, spelling only, or both; those with dual disabilities in handwriting and spelling were the most impaired and responded more slowly to early intervention (Berninger, Abbott, Rogan, et al., 1998).

Transcription skills and related processes are what best differentiates good and poor writers among intellectually talented students in the elementary grades (Yates, Berninger, & Abbott, 1994). Intellectually talented students with impaired transcription or related processes may not be identified for early intervention because their strengths in high-level thinking skills mask the difficulties they initially have with low-level skills. By the time their marked deficiencies in low-level skills are discovered, they may be beyond the critical period in writing development when transcription skills are most easily remediated. Later in schooling, they may be mislabeled as lazy or unmotivated when, in reality, they have underidentified and untreated transcription problems that compromised their ability to learn to express their ideas in writing and complete writing assignments (see Yates et al., 1994).

Early Precursors of Written Expression Problems

The initial hypothesis (Berninger, Mizokawa, & Bragg, 1991) that the developmental origin of written expression problems lay in impaired low-level transcription skills in handwriting and spelling, which in turn were related to developmental variations in related neuropsychological processes, was confirmed. To begin with, confirmatory factor analyses indicated that handwriting, spelling, and composing are separable processes, even though they may be functionally integrated during the writing process (Abbott & Berninger, 1993). Subsequent structural equation modeling documented a direct, significant path from handwriting to compositional length and quality throughout elementary school, and from spelling to composition length and quality primarily in the early elementary grades (Graham, Berninger, Abbott, Abbott, & Whitaker, 1997). Other multivariate analyses identified the associated neurodevelopmental indicators of handwriting and spelling. Both fine motor skills and orthographic coding of written words in short-

term memory accounted for unique variance in handwriting skills in primary-grade children (Berninger & Rutberg, 1992; Berninger, Yates, et al., 1992). Yet the direct path from short-term orthographic coding to handwriting was significant, but the direct path from fine motor skills to handwriting was not significant (Abbott & Berninger, 1993). This finding does not mean that motor skills are not involved in handwriting (see reviews by Berninger, in press, and Graham & Weintraub, 1996, with evidence that they are). Rather, this finding calls attention to the fact that handwriting is more than just a motor act. Handwriting is "language by hand" (Berninger & Graham, 1998), and language by hand is a separate functional system that is on a different developmental trajectory than "language by eye" (reading) (Berninger, 2000).

Orthographic and memory processes may contribute even more than motor skills to handwriting through the following mechanisms: representation of letter forms in short-term and long-term memory, access to and retrieval of these representations in memory, and planning for letter production. Orthographic–motor integration may be more important than motor processes per se in beginning writing (Berninger, 1994; Jones & Christensen, 1999). Failure to replicate the relationship between orthographic coding and handwriting in older students with persisting handwriting problems (Weintraub & Graham, 2000) may be due to one or both of the following factors: (1) Their predictor orthographic processing measure used manuscript letters and the criterion handwriting measure used cursive writing, and (2) primary motor problems may be overrepresented in samples of older students with persisting handwriting problems, as Weintraub and Graham studied, compared to the normal variation in motor skills in samples of beginning at-risk writers, as we studied. If so, generalizations about the neurodevelopmental correlates of handwriting should be qualified by age of students and by whether or not they have comorbid motor disabilities. Longitudinal studies of aural/oral language development and of reading development have shown that different subtypes of reading disabilities surface at different developmental stages (see Berninger, 2001b, for review) and the same may hold for writing disabilities. However, we have replicated our own finding that orthographic coding is directly and significantly related to handwriting, spelling, and composing in a sample carefully recruited for dyslexia (specific reading disability) and/or dysgraphia (specific writing disability) without comorbid primary motor disabilities (Berninger, Abbott, Thomson, & Raskind, 2001). Put another way, students with severe motor problems are likely to have handwriting problems, but children with motor development within the normal range may also have handwriting problems, which are more directly related to orthographic than motor processing skills.

An automaticity factor also contributed to individual differences in beginning writing (Berninger, Yates, et al., 1992; Jones & Christensen, 1999). The more automatic low-level handwriting and spelling are, the more the spatial and temporal resources of working memory are available for high-level composing (Berninger, 1999; McCutchen, 1996). Robust gender differences, in favor of girls, in automaticity of letter production from memory occurred in the primary-grade sample (Berninger & Fuller, 1992) and the intermediate and junior high samples. Removing effects due to individual differences in this automaticity of letter production eliminated the gender difference, in favor of girls, in compositional quality in the junior high grades (Berninger, Whitaker, Feng, Swanson, & Abbott, 1996). Thus, early intervention in increasing automaticity of letter production may have long-range effects on written expression in the junior high years, but further research is needed on this issue.

In contrast to handwriting that draws on orthographic coding, spelling draws on both orthographic and phonological coding (Abbott & Berninger, 1993; Berninger & Abbott, 1994a; Berninger, Cartwright, Yates, Swanson, & Abbott, 1994) and vocabulary knowledge (Berninger, Hart, Abbott, & Karovsky, 1992, Berninger, Yates, et al., 1992; Berninger et al., 1994). Moreover, phonological short-term memory, which is genetically constrained, appears to play a role in learning to spell (Hsu, Berninger, Thomson, Wijsman, & Raskind, 2002).

Effective Early Intervention for Spelling and Handwriting

Handwriting Training followed by Composing in Same Lesson

First-graders at the bottom of their classes on measures of legibility and automaticity of handwriting at the beginning of the year were randomly assigned to a contact control of phonological awareness training or one of five treatments: (1) conventional repeated copying of letters, (2) conventional modeling and imitating of motor components in letter formation, (3) studying visual cues (numbered arrow cues) for a sequential plan for letter formation, (4) writing letters from memory after increasing delays in how long the letter form had to be retained in memory, and (5) combination of (3) and (4). All groups composed and read their compositions to the tutor and other children in the triad. Following 24 lessons distributed over a 4-month period, the combination of studying numbered arrow cues and writing letters from memory was found to be more effective than the control or other conditions in improving handwriting legibility and automaticity and compositional fluency (amount written under timed conditions) (Berninger et al., 1997). Effect sizes ranged from 1.7 for copying letters in text to 1.8 for writing letters from dictation. Graham, Harris, and Fink (2000) and Jones and Christensen (1999) replicated the finding that handwriting training leads to improved compositional fluency.

Spelling Training followed by Composing in Same Lesson

Second-graders at the bottom of their classes on standardized measures for spelling at the beginning of the year were randomly assigned to a contact control treatment of phonological awareness training or one of seven treatments (whole word, alphabetic principle, or onset-rime training, singly or in combinations of two or three strategies for making connections between spoken and written words). All groups composed at the end of the session and shared what they wrote with the tutor and other child in the dyad. Following 24 lessons distributed over

4 months, alphabetic principle training (in isolation) followed by combined whole word and onset rime training in word context resulted in the best learning of taught words (effect size 1.7) *and* transfer to untaught words (effect size 0.35). However, only the combination of training alphabetic principle both in isolation and in word context led to significant improvement in composition length and spelling accuracy in composing. These results replicate the finding that explicit code instruction facilitates beginning spelling in the general education classroom (Foorman, Francis, Novy, & Liberman, 1991). Another study has replicated the transfer of spelling training to compositional fluency (Graham, Harris, & Fink, in press).

By the end of the second-grade intervention, half the sample was at or above grade level (the faster responders) and half had improved but were still below grade level (the slower responders). The faster responders were monitored at the beginning and end of third grade; the slower responders were monitored at the same time points and received continuing intervention in fall of third grade. Both groups maintained their relative gains from end of second to beginning of third grade (Berninger et al., 2000), which is important because normal spellers tend to regress in spelling over the summer months (Allinder, Fuchs, Fuchs, & Hamlett, 1992) and long-term retention is what differentiates good and poor spellers over time (Dreyer, Luke, & Mellican, 1994). Repeated practice in writing specific words in dictated sentences was found to be effective for word-specific learning (Gough, Juel, & Griffith, 1992) for those third-graders who received continuing tutoring (Berninger et al., 2000). An additional study with at-risk third-grade spellers indicated that reflective phonological awareness training aimed at eight syllable types in English, first at the spoken level and then in written words, also had some beneficial effects in improving their spelling (Berninger et al., 2000).

Comparison of Transcription and Composition Training, Singly and Combined

Third-graders at the bottom of their classes on a standardized measure of compositional fluency at the beginning of the year were randomly assigned to one of four time-equated treatments: spelling only training, genre-specific essay composing training, combined spelling and essay composing training, or a contact control of keyboard training without explicit writing instruction. The two treatments that contained spelling instruction were superior in improving spelling of taught words, although only the treatment that focused only on spelling transferred to better spelling in compositions. That spelling treatment had instructional components aimed at both automatization of alphabetic principle and reflection about alphabetic principle. The two treatments that contained composition training were superior in improving persuasive essay writing. Overall, only the combined treatment improved both spelling and composing skills (Berninger et al., 2002). By third grade, it appears to be important to provide at-risk writers with explicit writing instruction for both low-level transcription (e.g., spelling) and high-level composition (e.g., genre-specific strategies for essay writing).

Integrated Handwriting, Spelling, and Composition

Teachers referred children who were having difficulty with written expression during third grade for a summer intervention at the critical transition in writing development between third and fourth grade. In individual 1-hour tutorials, children worked on handwriting automaticity, multiple strategies for spelling, and composing (teacher modeling and scaffolding the planning, translating, reviewing, and revising processes). Both at immediate posttesting and 6-month follow-up, the treated children improved significantly on at least one measure of handwriting, spelling, and composition compared to the untreated control group (Berninger, Abbott, Whitaker, Sylvester, & Nolen, 1995).

Instructional Design Principles

First, there is more than one effective way to implement scientifically supported instructional practices (Berninger, 1998b). However, instructional design principles that cut across commercially available instructional materials are emerging from our instructional studies on writing and reading. The first is that children may benefit from instruction aimed at both low-level and high-level skills within the same lesson. Possible reasons for this benefit include the following:

1. Transfer of low-level skills to support the development of high-level skills, for example, automatizing low-level skills through practice frees up working memory for high-level skills.
2. High-level reflection is motivating and makes children willing to work hard on low-level skills that are necessary but difficult for them.
3. Integrating skills in lessons helps children coordinate components of writing close in time in working memory and thus facilitates development of functional writing systems (Berninger, 1999).

See Berninger and Richards (2002) for further discussion of these possibilities based on both brain research and instructional research.

Second, the goal of composing in the first two grades for at-risk writers should be to encourage them to put their thoughts in writing despite the transcription difficulties they have. Invented spellings (Chomsky, 1979) should be encouraged and the mechanics of writing should not be overemphasized. However, explicit instruction for handwriting and spelling is necessary and conventional spellings should be introduced. The important instructional challenge is to create learning environments in which children with transcription problems begin to think of themselves as writers and are willing to write daily and do not avoid writing, creating a self-perpetuating cycle in which poor writing breeds poor writing through lack of practice. Once these children develop adequate transcription skills and have had some experience in expressing their ideas in writing, the goal of instruction should be to learn the processes of writing—planning, translating, and reviewing/revising (Berninger et al., 1995, 2002; Hayes & Flower, 1980), genre-specific discourse structures (e.g., McCutchen, 1995; Wong, Butler, Ficzere, & Kuperis, 1996) and executive function strategies for regu-

lating the writing process (e.g., Harris & Graham, 1996; Hooper, Swartz, Wakely, deKruif, & Montgomery, 2002).

Third, writing is inherently a social activity (see Englert & Mariage, Chapter 27, in this volume; see also Cobb-Morocco et al., 1992; Wong et al., 1994; Zimmerman & Reisenberg, 1997), and writing instruction may be delivered most effectively to groups. With a few exceptions, our early interventions have been delivered to small groups of two or three at-risk writers, and recently we have scaled up to groups as large as 10 to 12 (unpublished data).

Simple View of Writing

Although transcription plays a fundamental role in beginning writers' ability to translate their ideas into written language, other components of the functional writing system come into play as writing develops (see Berninger & Swanson, 1994, for developmental models of emerging writing components, based on cross-sectional studies in grades 1 to 9, which require further research). These components include working memory (McCutchen, 1996; Swanson & Berninger, 1996), discourse knowledge (e.g., McCutchen, 1995; Wong, 1997), the cognitive processes of planning and reviewing and revising (Hayes & Flower, 1980), and strategies for the executive functions for self-regulating these cognitive processes during writing (e.g., Graham, 1997; Graham & Harris, 1996; Harris & Graham, 1996; Hooper et al., 2002).

To incorporate these various components and the diverse research traditions in the field of writing (educational, cognitive, linguistic, developmental, neuropsychological), Berninger and colleagues (2002) proposed the Simple View of Writing (see Figure 21.1) to capture the most relevant of these components for assessing and teaching students at-risk for developing normal writing skills. According to the Simple View, writing can be represented as a triangle encompassing a short-term, working, and long-term memory environment. At the base supporting the writing process are transcription (left angle) and executive functions (right angle). At the vertex of the triangle is text generation. Early in writing de-

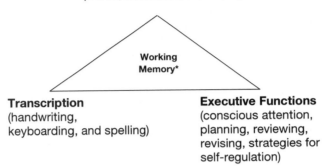

FIGURE 21.1. Simple view of writing. *Activates long-term memory during composing and short-term memory during reviewing.

velopment, the transcription processes provide the foundation from which writing springs; they allow the writer to translate generated ideas and language in his or her mind into visual symbols that represent the language. Across development, the executive functions will play an increasing role in text generation and management of the writing process. Early in writing development, the executive functions that manage the planning, translating, reviewing (monitoring), and revising processes are dependent on other-regulation in the form of guided assistance from parents, teachers, and peers. As writers mature, they transition from other-regulation to self-regulation of these cognitive processes (e.g., Zimmerman & Reisenberg, 1997). This transition from other- to self- regulation is dependent on both brain maturation and instruction, reflecting the nature–nurture interactions in literacy learning (Berninger & Richards, 2002).

We return to components of this Simple View of Writing in the next section as we discuss how computer technology might be used in the instructional program for students with transcription disabilities. This model provides a conceptual framework for (1) thinking about how computer technology may bypass certain transcription problems but pose challenges for the text generation, executive function, and/or working memory components of writing and (2) evaluating the extent to which the computer technology can be used independently by the student or will require considerable oth-

er-regulation from the teacher for writing skills to develop.

Research-Supported Use of Computer Technology

Computer technology has advanced more rapidly than has research on the most effective ways to use computer technology during writing instruction with students with handwriting and/or spelling disabilities. Although computer technology may create the illusion that it is more educationally sound than instructional approaches not using technology, in reality there has been relatively little research on educational applications of hardware and software during composing or teaching composing. This lack of research is especially concerning now that the Individuals with Disabilities Education Act mandates that adaptive technology solutions be considered when developing individualized education plans. Multidisciplinary teams (MDTs) and others who participate in technology selection and purchasing decisions tend to rely on software developers or vendors of computer technology rather than research (Raskind & Higgins, 1995). More research with well-defined populations and educational objectives is needed on the educational applications of computer technology to assist MDTs in making decisions about adaptive technology for students with writing (and reading) problems.

First we review the computer tools available to students with handwriting problems and then those with spelling problems. These tools are conceptualized as an addition (a complement) to and not as a replacement (an alternative) for research-supported instructional interventions, such as those described earlier. Although we are cautiously optimistic about the potential of technology to assist students with specific writing disabilities with writing tasks, we offer caveats to make the point that computer technology may not be the quick fix that many assume it is. When considering technology, educators and parents must (1) take into account a student's profile of developmental and academic skills and stage of writing development, (2) think about how the technology will make specific components of writing easier for the student while possibly making other components more challenging, and (3) consider practical issues of implementation. Regarding the latter, all implementation of computer technology should deal with issues of compatibility of different software tools needed to create an individually tailored system, plan for potential hardware crashes, and take into account the level of technical support available when the system fails. Other implementation factors to consider are the amount of time available for instruction for and practice with the computer tool, the environments in which the tool will be used, the familiarity of adults in those environments with the technology, and the nature of the writing task(s) for which it will be used.

Computer-Based Compensatory Tools for Handwriting

Currently keyboarding, dictation using a voice recognition system, and word prediction programs are the three computer-based strategies for bypassing handwriting problems. Unless keyboarding is automatized, handwriting is the fastest mode of text entry. However, each of these computer tools has been shown to improve the writing accuracy of students with learning disabilities (Lewis, Graves, Ashton, & Kieley, 1998). In each case it is important to remember that these technological tools bypass handwriting difficulties but create new tasks with processing requirements that may or may not be a challenge for an individual student.

KEYBOARDING

Keyboarding changes the task from forming letters by hand to the task of finding and selecting the key. Motor processes are still involved but are less complex than for pencil manipulations. Although selection of the correct key produces a correctly formed letter, the process of automaticity is still relevant. Typing may indeed slow rate of text production compared to handwriting (Lewis et al., 1998; MacArthur & Graham, 1987). Unless a student automatizes the letter finding and key press process, typing may not be sufficiently fluent to support keyboarding as a viable alternative to handwriting. Students who have difficulty with automatizing letter production with a pencil may also have difficulty with automatizing letter finding and selection on the keyboard. Short-term keyboard instruction (e.g., for 6 weeks) does not appear to be effective in increasing typing speed, and close teacher monitoring is needed or students will revert to hunt and peck (Lewis, 1998). Instruction aimed at keyboarding fluency needs to be built into the instructional program and carefully monitored and evaluated (Bryant & Bryant, 1998) because ultimately those students with good keyboarding skills are the ones who are best able to use computer-based strategies for composing (Anderson-Inman, Knox-Quinn, & Horney, 1996). Overall, keyboarding is probably the least restrictive bypass tool for students with handwriting problems, but research is needed on the best predictors of which students, based on well-defined characteristics, will benefit from use of a keyboard as a bypass tool. It is important to remember that keyboarding draws on some of the same processes as handwriting, and students who have trouble learning handwriting may also have trouble learning keyboarding. If used as a bypass strategy, keyboarding requires systematic, sustained instruction until keyboarding skills are automatized.

DICTATION USING VOICE RECOGNITION

Typically developing fifth- or sixth-graders tend to dictate longer but not better-quality compositions than they write with pencil and paper (Scardamalia, Bereiter, & Goelman, 1982). In contrast, for students with learning disabilities, both the length and quality of dictated compositions may be superior to handwritten compositions (Graham, 1990). Speech recognition software is available that directly translates dictated speech into typed text through a program that depends on voice recognition for the individual student. These voice recognition programs are relatively new and rapidly evolving; the literature reviews on the first generation of these programs no longer apply to the newer ones now on the market. However, Reece and Cumming (1996) reported that quality of dictated compositions was enhanced by use of a voice recognition system that generated a written record to review while composing. Although Borgh and Dickson (1992) found no effect of dictation with voice recognition on composition length, they did find that it resulted in improved revising of typically developing second- and fifth-graders.

A number of issues should be considered in deciding whether to use dictation with a voice recognition system as a bypass for handwriting problems. First, keyboards are more transportable across work environments than are voice recognition systems. Second, voice recognition systems may be disruptive to other students in the classroom who are not using such systems, and the accuracy of voice recognition decreases in noisy environments. Third, voice recognition software requires a computer with sufficient processing and storage capacity and a good-quality microphone. Fourth, the system has to be adequately trained on recognizing the student's voice. Although the issue of transporting voice files will be eventually resolved, it is currently difficult to move voice files; thus students have to create a voice file on every computer that will be used. Fifth, the student user must take time to learn to use a number of commands for monitoring and repairing errors. Sixth, although dictating may reduce the time needed to enter text, the time and skills necessary for finding and correcting recognition errors may be considerable. Seventh, the simultaneous processes of dictation, self-monitoring for errors, and effective use of program commands for fixing errors place considerable demands on working memory, which has limited resources for all developing writers, especially in elementary school. In addition, dictation using a voice recognition system may be taxing for the developing executive management system for writing (see Hooper et al., 2002). Nevertheless, for students with transcription problems who sustain use of dictation once the novelty wears off, voice recognition may make it possible to generate longer and better text than they would otherwise be able to write.

WORD PREDICTION

This software provides support by predicting, based on the syntax and spelling of text written so far, frequency of words in the language, and any letters typed so far for the word at hand, what the current word might be; it then generates on the monitor a list of possibilities from which the student can select. Word prediction software was originally developed to reduce the number of keystrokes needed to make keyboarding easier, faster, and less tiring for individuals with severe motor disabilities. More recently, it has been used with individuals with written language but not severe motor disabilities. Word prediction programs that incorporate into their algorithms alternative phonetic spellings for the same word are especially helpful for students with written language disabilities. If the student has a reading problem in addition to a handwriting and/or spelling problem, some word prediction programs provide synthesized speech that reads each of the options on the list to assist in the selection of one of the predicted options. This adaptation can increase the time costs for using word prediction substantially.

Word prediction programs may present challenges for students who have working memory (MacArthur, 1999) or attention or executive function problems along with transcription problems because they must carefully monitor the list of options, which changes with each typed letter. Another limitation of word prediction programs is that they are a slow mode of text entry compared to handwriting for students with learning disabilities (e.g., Lewis et al., 1998). In the Lewis and colleagues (1998) study, students using word prediction only reached 82% of their handwriting speed; moreover, those who also used synthesized speech with the word prediction program only reached 41% of their handwriting speed. At the same time, the decrease in speed was accompanied by an increase in spelling accuracy for these students. The group using word prediction with speech feedback halved the number of spelling errors they made. Thus, in making decisions for individual students, an MDT may need to weigh the trade-off between reduced speed but increased spelling accuracy. Word prediction may serve as an excellent starting point for students with transcription problems, as long as the necessary instruction in handwriting and spelling is in place, but eventually other computer tools that result in faster text entry may have to be introduced as the student is more able to handle them. Younger writers tend to enjoy the multiple supports provided by word prediction that allow them to begin to compose, whereas older writers who face longer writing assignments may find word prediction to be frustratingly slow.

Computer-Based Compensatory Tools for Spelling

SPELL CHECKERS

Many proficient writers use spell checkers as a way to detect errors due to typing and repair the error based on their ability to choose the correctly spelled word. Even for skilled writers, spell checkers are not without their limitations, for example, in detecting incorrectly spelled words for a particular sentence context, as captured in the first verse of the anonymously authored "Ode to a Spell Chequer," which is circulating on the Web:

> Eye halve a spelling chequer,
> It may come with my pea sea,
> It plainly marques for my revue,
> Miss steaks eye kin knot see.

For the students with spelling disabilities, mainstream spell checkers may be of limited use. The major limitations are that their spelling errors are not sufficiently recognized by the spell checkers to even suggest possible correct spellings for severely misspelled words, and the students may not be able to recognize the correctly spelled word in the list of possibilities (MacArthur, Gra-

ham, Haynes, & De La Paz, 1996). Nevertheless, spell checkers (and to a lesser degree grammatical checkers) showed benefits for students in grades 4 to 12 with learning disabilities (Lewis, Ashton, Haapa, Kieley, & Fielden, 2000). In another study, students with learning disabilities increased their spelling error correction rate of 9% without a spell checker to 37% with a spell checker (MacArthur et al., 1996). Some commercially available software packages were developed specifically for people with learning disabilities and generate spell-check options based on phonetic spellings. These programs may be more helpful than mainstream spell checkers to students with spelling problems, who tend to spell words the way they sound, but more research is needed on this topic.

WORD PREDICTION

As already discussed, word prediction programs with text entry may enhance spelling accuracy despite slowing text entry speed. The size and sophistication of a student's vocabulary may influence how effectively a student may be able to use this tool in composing (MacArthur, 1999). Flexible programs that allow users to customize by creating a personal dictionary are most likely to transfer to improved composing. Research is not available on whether training in word prediction transfers to improved, unaided spelling while composing.

SPEECH FEEDBACK SOFTWARE

Users receive auditory feedback about whether they spelled (typed) a word correctly. These programs have a voice synthesizer that pronounces for the user any word that appears on the screen. When the program detects a misspelled word, it attempts to pronounce the word phonetically. Pronounced word sounds that seem odd to the user are a cue that a spelling error has probably been made. At the same time, orthographic feedback highlights the word being pronounced by the speech synthesizer. In some cases the orthographic feedback display consists of color-coded units smaller than the word. The combination of auditory and written feedback may enhance detection of spelling errors (Higgins & Zvi,

1995), but more research is needed on this topic at different stages of writing development and for different well-defined populations.

Integrating Computer Tools in the Instructional Program in Writing

The research on the effect of computers on writing has shifted from a focus on the computer alone to the interaction of the technology and instruction (Cobb-Morocco et al., 1992). Using word processors in the instructional program in writing results in modest gains for typically developing writers (Bangert-Drowns, 1993). Bangert-Drowns differentiated among computer applications for (1) supplanting lower-order processes, (2) modifying higher-order processes, and (3) providing metacognitive prompts. Word processors have been shown to be especially helpful for the higher-order revision process (e.g., Cobb-Morocco et al., 1992). Simply providing the student with adaptive technology does not guarantee that the student will use it effectively unless teacher guidance is provided. See Wise and Olson (1992) for empirical evidence that students are less likely to request feedback when not monitored by an adult. One reason for integrating the computer technology with teacher-guided instruction is that young writers in general and students with learning disabilities in particular have considerable difficulty in self-regulation, including attention-managing and self-monitoring, and benefit from other-regulation provided by teachers, as already discussed. Technology-supported writing instruction may be more likely than technology-supported writing without instruction to transfer to improved, unaided writing, but further research is needed on this issue.

KEYBOARDING INSTRUCTION

Keyboarding instruction should probably start early, as early as first grade, for all beginning writers—not just for the at-risk ones—so that they do not later have to unlearn hunt-and-peck strategies that may become automatized. Compressed keyboards with smaller keys positioned closer together may accommodate smaller hands and fingers of beginning writers. Keyboarding

should not replace handwriting instruction for beginning writers. In the 21st century, children need to become bilingual in language by hand, able to transcribe with a pencil as well as a keyboard. Early keyboard training should also be integrated in the writing instruction program so that children can learn to use the keyboard to compose for authentic communication purposes.

SPELLING INSTRUCTION

One issue to consider in choosing spelling software to integrate into the instructional program is whether it is linguistically correct in providing orthographic and/or phonological feedback for phoneme–spelling correspondences. Many times such programs do not provide accurate feedback for those instances in which phonemes correspond to two letters (e.g., the last sound in h*er*) rather than one letter (e.g., the first sound in *r*ose) and erroneously treat the /er/ and /r/ phoneme as equivalent when they are not (Berninger, 1998c). Such erroneous feedback can be confusing to students who are still learning to make connections between units they perceive in spoken words and corresponding units in written words. Another factor to consider is that software may present letter–sound correspondences for reading words, as if they are the same for spelling words as well. However, in English such correspondences (the alphabetic principle) are applied differently when going from spoken words to written words in spelling than in going from written to spoken words as in reading (Berninger, 1998c). For instance, an *a* in a written word has a corresponding long and short sound or a reduced vowel (schwa), but the long /a/ phoneme may be spelled in many more ways than the single letter *a* (e.g., m*a*de, pl*a*y, p*ai*d, w*eigh*, and th*ey*) and may depend on its placement in an open (e.g., *a*pron) rather than closed syllable. Explicit reflection on these alternations generalized to improved spelling while composing (Berninger et al., 2002). Another factor to consider is that at-risk spellers have problems in word-specific spelling, which requires integrating knowledge of a specific phoneme–spelling correspondence with a specific word context (e.g., which spelling to use in the phrase pl__ with toys). Purportedly Mark Twain told an editor who complained that he had spelled the same word 10 different ways in the same manuscript that he felt sorry for anyone who could not think of 10 different ways to spell the same word. Such knowledge of the alternations of alphabetic principle suggests outstanding linguistic awareness but poor word-specific spelling knowledge. Clearly, as demonstrated by Twain's superb storytelling ability, this kind of word-specific spelling knowledge and ability to generate text are separate writing skills.

The value of computer-assisted orthographic and speech feedback in spelling instruction has been understudied. In an exploratory study, Wise and Olson (1992, 1994) reported null effects. However, computer-assisted immediate feedback as to the accuracy of the spelling appears to be more effective than the delayed feedback on accuracy of handwritten spelling (MacArthur, Haynes, Malouf, Harris, & Owings, 1990). Spelling error correction rate improved when high school students with spelling problems received instruction in strategies for using spell checkers (McNaughton, Hughes, & Ofiesh, 1997). A reasonable goal for spelling instruction is to bring students with spelling problems to the level at which they can use commercial spell checkers effectively and independently.

COMPOSING INSTRUCTION

Computer-based strategies appear to have benefits over handwriting only for extended writing assignments requiring, for example, 4 to 6 weeks to complete (Cobb-Morocco et al., 1992). Integrating instruction in advance planning with dictation has benefits beyond dictation alone (De La Paz & Graham, 1997). Integrating instruction in strategies for planning, drafting, and revising with use of word processing resulted in greater improvement in narrative and essay writing for upper-elementary-grade students with learning disabilities compared to a control group with learning disabilities that did not receive such instruction (MacArthur, Graham, Schwartz, & Schafer, 1995). Computers can assist in writing in more ways than bypassing transcription problems, for example, as supports for planning through prompting, outlining, and

semantic mapping or as networks to support collaboration and problem solving (MacArthur, 1996). Additional research is needed on the most effective ways to incorporate such high-level computer applications most effectively in the instructional program in writing for students with transcription problems.

Application of Research to Practice

Three-Tier Approach to Definition of Learning Disability

The first tier screens students who are at risk for handwriting and spelling problems and provides them with early intervention (Berninger, 2002; Berninger & Abbott, 1994b; Berninger, Stage, Smith, & Hildebrand, 2002). The second tier provides progress monitoring and curriculum modification when needed in the general education writing program (e.g., Fuchs, Fuchs, Hamlett, & Allinder, 1991a, 1991b). The third tier assesses students who fail to respond reasonably well to the first two tiers—both to decide whether the students qualify for special education services and to clarify, through differential diagnosis, the nature of their learning differences, which is important to parents and is relevant to understanding etiology, planning intervention, and gauging prognosis (e.g., Berninger, 1998b, 2002; Berninger et al., 2001). Berninger (1998b) and Berninger, Stage, and colleagues (2001) provide practical recommendations for implementing this conceptual approach. The process measures that were shown to have the best validity in cross-sectional and instructional intervention studies have now been nationally normed (Berninger, 2001a). In general, there is enormous normal variation within and across developmental and academic domains in children with learning differences (see Berninger, Abbott, Billingsley, & Nagy, 2001, for the reading and writing system; Sandler et al., 1992, and Hooper et al., 1994, for the writing system). Thus, we advocate for a flexible approach that serves all children (Berninger, 1998b; Berninger, Hart, Abbott, & Karovsky, 1992) and believe that accomplishing this goal requires a lifespan approach (Wong, 1998) and better cooperation and coordination among general and special education. We use a multidomain profile approach for assessing older students with persisting writing (Berninger, in press) or reading (Berninger, 2001b) disabilities and an approach to instructional intervention based on all the necessary components of functional writing and reading systems (Berninger, 1998b; Berninger & Richards, 2002). Learning outcomes for writing and reading of students without neurological disease or damage depend on nature-nurture interactions (both brain and genetic constraints and quality of instruction) (Berninger & Richards, 2002). We end this section with an illustrative example of how practitioners might apply knowledge of spelling, based on research, to analyzing spelling errors and generating individually tailored spelling accommodations within comprehensive instruction aimed at all components of the functional writing system.

Assessing Spelling Errors for Instructional Clues

Standard scores indicate how well students spell compared to age or grade peers but do not specify how to improve spelling. Analysis of spelling errors can provide instructional clues for improving spelling. Reliability of errors is important, however, and recommended instructional interventions should be based on patterns of errors that occur repeatedly. Table 21.1 contains questions teachers and testers can ask about spelling errors for clues to intervention. The example words are not the test items but illustrate the kinds of spelling errors observed in the standardization sample of the Wechsler Individual Achievement Test—Second Edition (WIAT-2; Psychological Corporation, 2002). Correct spelling is in parentheses. Some errors are double-coded because they reflect more than one kind of error. This scheme can be applied to standardized or informal measures of spelling words from dictation or standardized or informal measures of written composition to evaluate whether the same kinds of errors occur when spelling single words from dictation as when spelling while composing text.

The recommended coding scheme for analyzing spelling errors is based on research showing that multiple language sources influence spelling: phonological, orthograph-

ic, and morphological (Bryant, Nunez, & Bindman, 1997; Carlisle, 1988; Ehri, 1992; Gough et al., 1992; Leong, 2000; Moats, 2000; Treiman, 1997; Treiman & Bourassa, 2000; Tyler & Nagy, 1989; Varnhagen, 1994; Varnhagen, Varnhagen, & Das, 1992; Venezky, 1970, 1999). English spelling varies in predictability of sound–spelling correspondence but is not capricious. Most phonemes (the smallest sound units in spoken words) can be spelled with a small set of alternative one- and two-letter spelling units (alternations) (Venezky, 1970, 1999). Most written words have mostly spelling units that conform to these alternations, especially if the speller has orthographic awareness that in English the functional spelling unit is often a two-letter rather than one-letter unit Berninger (1998c). Thus it is misleading to categorize spelling words as regular *or* irregular for either teaching or testing purposes. Of the many sources of language knowledge contributing to spelling—phonology, orthography, and morphology and their relationships—a word may be irregular in correspondences for one of these language sources but regular for another source.

Conclusions and Future Research Directions

Given the enormous problems at-risk writers face in learning transcription skills, it is not surprising that they become overfocused on the mechanics of writing such as handwriting and spelling (Graham, Schwartz, & MacArthur, 1993; MacArthur, 1999). Based on 12 years of research on prevention of writing problems, we propose that early intervention aimed at teaching handwriting and/or spelling to at-risk writers early in schooling may eliminate or significantly reduce the number of students needing to use computer-based technologies as bypass strategies for low-level processes in writing and increase the number of students able to use computers adaptively for the high-level processes in writing later in writing development. However, research-based evidence currently available suggests that for the students who continue to experience difficulties with transcription processes, in spite of appropriate interven-

TABLE 21.1. Coding of Spelling Errors and Their Links to Intervention[a,b,c]

I. PHONOLOGICAL PROCESSING PROBLEMS: These errors indicate that the student does not have precise phonological representation of all the phonemes in a spoken word that is being translated into its written form. Mixed phonological errors are the most indicative of serious phonological processing problems.

  A. Diagnostic Questions
    1. Are phonemes deleted? Example: The /r/ phoneme is deleted in pinsiss (princess).
    2. Are additional phonemes inserted? Example: The /p/ phoneme is added in abpsent (absent).
    3. Are phonemes transposed? Example: The /d/ and /n/ phonemes are switched in order in ruts (rust).
    4. Are phonemes confused and similar ones substituted? Examples: peg (pig) in which the short e and short i phonemes are confused; apsent (absent) in which the /p/ phoneme is confused with the /b/ phoneme; bug (dug) in which the /b/ and /d/ phonemes are confused. *Note.* Some dialects do not distinguish between short e and short i. Also, b and d confusions may be related to their phonemic rather than graphemic (letter) similarity.
    5. Are there mixed phonological errors? Example: vamlee (family) in which the /v/ phoneme is substituted for the /f/ phoneme and the second syllable (reduced vowel) is omitted.

  B. Intervention
    1. Phonological awareness training (see, e.g., Berninger, 1998b).
    2. Always analyze words in spelling lesson phonologically before spelling them. For example, count the syllables, count the phonemes in syllables, say the word phoneme by phoneme, especially for polysyllabic words. Provide feedback if phonological representation is not perfect. See Berninger and colleagues (2000).

II. PHONOLOGICAL–ORTHOGRAPHIC PROCESSING PROBLEMS

  A. Diagnostic Question
    1. Is a spelling unit implausible given the conventional phoneme–spelling correspondences (and their alternations) in English? Examples: fich (fish), lorchj (large), ridn (riding), sithed (sight). See Berninger and Abbott (1994a).

  B. Intervention
    1. Teach alphabet principle[c] and its alternations in the direction of phonemes to one- or two-letter spelling unit. See Berninger (1998c).

III. WORD-SPECIFIC ORTHOGRAPHIC PROCESSING PROBLEMS (see Gough et al., 1992)

  A. Diagnostic Questions
    1. Is a spelling unit plausible for a conventional phoneme–spelling correspondence (one of the alternations) in English but not appropriate for a specific word context? Examples: cairful (careful), monkee (monkey), anshunt (ancient), wile (while), briet (bright), resine (resign). See Berninger and Abbott (1994a).
    2. Is the schwa (reduced vowel marked in the dictionary with an upside-down backwards e), which can only be spelled correctly by memorizing it for a specific word context, spelled with the correct arbitrary letter? Examples: seperately (separately), sentance (sentence).
    3. Does the misspelled spelling unit involve one or more silent letters that can only be spelled correctly by memorizing the letter(s) for a specific word context? Example: anser (answer).

  B. Intervention
    1. Combine teaching alphabet principle[c] and its alternations in the direction of phonemes to one- or two-letter spelling unit (see Berninger, 1998c) with word-specific training by spelling target word in dictated sentence (see Berninger et al., 2000).

IV. MORPHOLOGICAL PROCESSING PROBLEMS

  A. Diagnostic Questions (see Tyler & Nagy, 1989)
    1. Are there errors in inflectional suffixes or stem changes for tense? Note that there are three spellings for past-tense marker—d, t, or ed; three spellings for plurality, -s /z/, -s/s/, or -es (es or ez). Examples: bumpd (bumped), washs (washes), grow (grew).

(continued)

TABLE 21.1. *Continued*

    2. Are there errors in prefixes? Examples: *ad*cite (excite) or *in*polite (impolite).
    3. Are there errors in derivational suffixes? Examples: reli*gous* (religious), nash*unal* (national).
    4. Is spelling of stem morpheme maintained? Example: bomming (bombing).

  B. Intervention
    1. Combine morphological awareness training[c] with word-specific training by spelling target word in dictated sentence (see Berninger, 1998b).

V. SPELLING CONVENTIONS (RULES)

  A. Diagnostic Questions
    1. Is there an error in doubling final consonant of closed syllables before adding another morpheme? Examples: acomodate (accommodate), begining (beginning).
    2. Is there an error in changing y to i when adding morpheme? Example: busyer (busier).
    3. Is there an error in forming a contraction? Example: woulden't (wouldn't).
    4. Is there an error in twinning for l, s, or f in final position? Example: kised (kissed).
    5. Is there an error in final e for soft c or soft g? Example: dans (dance).

  B. Intervention
    1. Systematically and explicitly teach spelling rules (see Berninger, 1998b, for instructional resources, and Masterson et al., 2002, for strategies).

VI. PHONOLOGICAL/ORTHOGRAPHIC/MORPHOLOGICAL CONFUSIONS

  A. Diagnostic Questions
    1. Is the spelled word a homonym (sounds the same but meaning and spelling are different)? Examples: too (two), him (hymn).
    2. Is the spelled word a homograph (spelled the same but sounds different)? (Can only be evaluated in context.) Examples: "He red the book" for "He read the book."

  B. Intervention
    1. Spelling targeted words in dictated sentences so that sentence context must be taken into account.

VII. PREALPHABETIC PRINCIPLE STAGE OF SPELLING DEVELOPMENT

  A. Diagnostic Questions (see Ehri, 1992; Treiman, 1997; Treiman & Bourassa, 2000)
    1. Does the spelling appear to be random letters rather than attempted representation of speech in writing? Example: utody (train).
    2. Does the spelling appear to represent speech at a phonetic level (invented spelling stage) and is only partially phonemic (based on alphabetic principle)? Example: bz (bees).

  B. Intervention
    1. Phonological Awareness (Berninger, 1998b) and Alphabetic Principle Training[c] (Berninger, 1998c)

VIII. LETTER PRODUCTION ERRORS

  A. Diagnostic Questions
    1. Is there a letter reversal? Example: ma*q* (map).
    2. Is there a letter inversion? Example: *me* (we).
    3. Are letters transposed? Example: to*w* (two).

  B. Intervention
    1. Combine Handwriting Lessons (Berninger, 1998a) and Alphabetic Principle Training[c] (Berninger, 1998c)

---

[a]Some misspelled words can be given more than one code because more than one kind of error is involved.
[b]These kinds of errors were observed in standardization sample for the Wechsler Individual Achievement Test—Second Edition (WIAT-II; Psychological Corporation, 2002). However, the words used to illustrate the error types are not the same as the test items.
[c]A criterion-referenced approach to spelling assessment and intervention that can be used to complement norm-referenced assessment is *A Prescriptive Assessment of Spelling on CD-ROM* (Masterson, Apel, & Wasowitz, 2002).

tions, computer-based bypass strategies should be considered.

Systematic research is needed to assess which computer-based tools, under which circumstances, and for which groups of students with well-specified characteristics are helpful in addressing specific writing difficulties. Just as we studied the development of writing processes using a pencil, we are now studying development of component writing processes using computer technology. Research on effective use of specific writing technologies in teaching specific writing skills may benefit from understanding the underlying processes for learning specific writing skills with specific technologies. For example, research is needed on how to automatize use of technology tools so that they require minimum attention and effort. Research should also address how to predict and plan for the appropriate level of training and support for both students and educators in using technology.

Research on both writing disabilities and educational applications of computer technology to writing is of recent origin, having gained momentum during the last two decades of the 20th century. Progress in generating scientifically supported instructional practices in writing, with and without the support of computer assistance, is most likely to be made during the 21st century if the federal government increases funding for cross-site collaborations designed to replicate study designs across well-defined populations and instructional settings.

Acknowledgments

Grant No. HD25858-11 supported the first author and Grant No. H224A30006 supported the second author in preparation of this chapter. Grant Nos. HD25858-1 to -10 supported the research on writing assessment and intervention conducted at the University of Washington. The authors thank the Psychological Corporation for providing representative spelling errors from the standardization sample of the Wechsler Individual Achievement Test—Second Edition (WIAT II) to use in developing a coding system.

References

Abbott, R., & Berninger, V. (1993). Structural equation modeling of relationships among developmental skills and writing skills in primary and intermediate grade writers. *Journal of Educational Psychology, 85,* 478–508.

Abbott, S., Reed, L., Abbott, R., & Berninger, V. (1997). Year-long balanced reading/writing tutorial: A design experiment used for dynamic assessment. *Learning Disability Quarterly, 20,* 249–263.

Allinder, R., Fuchs, L., Fuchs, D., & Hamlett, C. (1992). Effects of summer break on math and spelling performance as a function of grade level. *Elementary School Journal, 92,* 451–460.

Anderson-Inman, L., Knox-Quinn, C., & Horney, M. (1996). Computer-based study strategies for students with learning disabilities: Individual differences associated with adoption level. *Journal of Learning Disabilities, 29,* 461–484.

Bangert-Drowns, R. (1993). The word processor as an instructional tool: A meta-analysis of word processing in writing instruction. *Review of Educational Research, 63,* 69–93.

Berninger, V. (1994). *Reading and writing acquisition: A developmental neuropsychological perspective.* Madison, WI: W. C. Brown (Distributed by Perseus Books).

Berninger, V. (1998a). Handwriting Lessons Program in *Process of the Learner (PAL) intervention kit.* San Antonio, TX: Psychological Corporation.

Berninger, V. (1998b). *Process assessment of the learner: Guides for reading and writing intervention.* San Antonio, TX: Psychological Corporation.

Berninger, V. (1998c). Talking Letters Program in *Process of the Learner (PAL) intervention kit.* San Antonio, TX: Psychological Corporation.

Berninger, V. (1999). Coordinating transcription and text generation in working memory during composing: Automatized and constructive processes. *Learning Disability Quarterly, 22,* 99–112.

Berninger, V. (2000). Development of language by hand and its connections to language by ear, mouth, and eye. *Topics in Language Disorders, 20,* 65–84.

Berninger, V. (2002). Best practices in reading, writing, and math assessment-intervention links: A systems approach for schools, classrooms, and individuals. In A. Thomas & J. Grimes (Eds.), *Best practices in school psychology IV* (Vol. 1, pp. 851–865). Bethesda, MD: NASP Press.

Berninger, V. (in press). Understanding the graphia in dysgraphia. In D. Dewey & D. Tupper (Eds.), *Developmental motor disorders: A neuropsychological perspective.* New York: Guilford Press.

Berninger, V. (2001a). *Process Assessment of the Learner (PAL) Test Battery for Reading and Writing. (PAL-RW).* San Antonio, TX: Psychological Corporation.

Berninger, V. (2001b). Understanding the lexia in dyslexia. *Annals of Dyslexia, 51,* 23–48.

Berninger, V., & Abbott, R. (1994b). Redefining learning disabilities: Moving beyond aptitude–achievement discrepancies to failure to respond to validated treatment protocols. In G. R. Lyon

(Ed.), *Frames of reference for the assessment of learning disabilities: New views on measurement issues* (pp. 163–202). Baltimore: Brookes.

Berninger, V., & Abbott, R. (1994a). Multiple orthographic and phonological codes in literacy acquisition: An evolving research program. In V. Berninger (Ed.), *The varieties of orthographic knowledge I: Theoretical and developmental issues* (pp. 277–317). Dordrecht, The Netherlands: Kluwer Academic.

Berninger, V., Abbott, R., Billingsley, F., & Nagy, W. (2001). Processes underlying timing and fluency: Efficiency, automaticity, coordination, and morphological awareness. In M. Wolf (Ed.), *Dyslexia, fluency, and the brain* (pp. 383–414). Timonium, MD: York Press.

Berninger, V., Abbott, R., Rogan, L., Reed, L., Abbott, S., Brooks, A., Vaughan, K., & Graham, S. (1998). Teaching spelling to children with specific learning disabilities: The mind's ear and eye beat the computer or pencil. *Learning Disability Quarterly, 21,* 106–122.

Berninger, V., Abbott, R., Thomson, J., & Raskind, W. (2001). Language phenotype for reading and writing disability: A family approach. *Scientific Studies in Reading, 5,* 59–105.

Berninger, V., Abbott, R., Whitaker, D., Sylvester, L., & Nolen, S. (1995). Integrating low-level skills and high-level skills in treatment protocols for writing disabilities. *Learning Disability Quarterly, 18,* 293–309.

Berninger, V., Cartwright, A., Yates, C., Swanson, H. L., & Abbott, R. (1994). Developmental skills related to writing and reading acquisition in the intermediate grades: Shared and unique variance. *Reading and Writing: An Interdisciplinary Journal, 6,* 161–196.

Berninger, V., & Fuller, F. (1992). Gender differences in orthographic, verbal, and compositional fluency: Implications for diagnosis of writing disabilities in primary grade children. *Journal of School Psychology, 30,* 363–382.

Berninger, V., & Graham, S. (1998). Language by hand: A synthesis of a decade of research on handwriting. *Handwriting Review, 12,* 11–25.

Berninger, V., Hart, T., Abbott, R., & Karovsky, P. (1992). Defining reading and writing disabilities with and without IQ: A flexible, developmental perspective. *Learning Disability Quarterly, 15,* 103–118.

Berninger, V., Mizokawa, D., & Bragg, R. (1991). Theory-based diagnosis and remediation of writing disabilities. *Journal of School Psychology, 29,* 57–79.

Berninger, V., & Richards, T. (2002). *Brain literacy for educators and psychologists.* New York: Academic Press.

Berninger, V., & Rutberg, J. (1992). Relationship of finger function to beginning writing: Application to diagnosis of writing disabilities. *Developmental Medicine and Child Neurology, 34,* 155–172.

Berninger, V., Stage, S., Smith, D., & Hildebrand, D. (2001). Assessment for reading and writing intervention: A three-tier model for prevention and remediation. In J. Andrews, D. Saklofske, & H. Janzen (Eds.), *Handbook of psychoeducational assessment. Ability, achievement, and behavior in children* (pp. 195–223). New York: Academic Press.

Berninger, V., & Swanson, H. L. (1994). Modifying Hayes & Flower's model of skilled writing to explain beginning and developing writing. In E. Butterfield (Ed.), *Children's writing: Toward a process theory of development of skilled writing* (pp. 57–81). Greenwich, CT: JAI Press.

Berninger, V., Vaughan, K., Abbott, R., Abbott, S., Brooks, A., Rogan, L., Reed, E., & Graham, S. (1997). Treatment of handwriting fluency problems in beginning writing: Transfer from handwriting to composition. *Journal of Educational Psychology, 89,* 652–666.

Berninger, V., Vaughan, K., Abbott, R., Begay, K., Byrd, K., Curtin, G., Minnich, J., & Graham, S. (2002). Teaching spelling and composition alone and together: Implications for the simple view of writing. *Journal of Educational Psychology, 94,* 291–304.

Berninger, V., Vaughan, K., Abbott, R., Brooks, A., Abbott, S., Reed, E., Rogan, L., & Graham, S. (1998). Early intervention for spelling problems: Teaching spelling units of varying size within a multiple connections framework. *Journal of Educational Psychology, 90,* 587–605.

Berninger, V., Vaughan, K., Abbott, R., Brooks, A., Begay, K., Curtin, G., Byrd, K., & Graham, S. (2000). Language-based spelling instruction: Teaching children to make multiple connections between spoken and written words. *Learning Disability Quarterly, 23,* 117–136.

Berninger, V., Whitaker, D., Feng, Y., Swanson, H. L., & Abbott, R. (1996). Assessment of planning, translating, and revising in junior high writers. *Journal of School Psychology, 34,* 23–52.

Berninger, V., Yates, C., Cartwright, A., Rutberg, J., Remy, E., & Abbott, R. (1992). Lower-level developmental skills in beginning writing. *Reading and Writing: An Interdisciplinary Journal, 4,* 257–280.

Borgh, K., & Dickson, W. P. (1992). The effects on children's writing of adding speech synthesis to a word processor. *Journal of Research on Computing in Education, 24,* 533–544.

Britton, J. (1978). The composing processes and the functions of writing. In C. R. Cooper & L. Odell (Eds.). *Research on composing: Points of departure* (pp. 13–28). Urbana, IL: National Council of Teachers of English.

Brooks, A., Vaughan, K., & Berninger, V. (1999). Tutorial interventions for writing disabilities: Comparison of transcription and text generation processes. *Learning Disability Quarterly, 22,* 183–191.

Bryant, D., & Bryant, B. (1998). Using assistive technology adaptations to include students with learning disabilities in cooperative learning activities. *Journal of Learning Disabilities, 3,* 41–54.

Bryant, P., Nunes, T., & Bindman, M. (1997). Children's understanding of the connection between grammar and spelling. In B. A. Blachman (Ed.), *Foundations of reading acquisition and dyslexia: Implications for early intervention* (pp. 219–240). Mahwah, NJ: Erlbaum.

Carlisle, J. (1988). Knowledge of derivational morphology and spelling ability in fourth, sixth, and eighth graders. *Applied Psycholinguistics, 9,* 247–266.

Chomsky, C. (1979). Reading, writing, and phonology. *Harvard Educational Review, 40,* 287–309.

Clay, M. (1982). Research update. Learning and teaching writing: A developmental perspective. *Language Arts, 59,* 65–70.

Cobb-Morrocco, C., Dalton, G., & Tivnan, T. (1992). The impact of computer-supported writing instruction on fourth grade students with and without learning disabilities. *Reading and Writing Quarterly: Overcoming Learning Difficulties, 8,* 87–113.

De La Paz, S., & Graham, S. (1997). Effects of dictation and advanced planning instruction on the composing of students with writing and learning problems. *Journal of Educational Psychology, 89,* 203–222.

Dreyer, L., Luke, S., & Melican, E. (1994). Children's acquisition and retention of word spellings. In V. W. Berninger (Ed.), *The varieties of orthographic knowledge II: Relationships to phonology, reading, and writing* (pp. 291–320). Dordrecht, The Netherlands: Kluwer Academic.

Ehri, L. (1992). Review and commentary: Stages of spelling development. In S. Templeton & D. Bear (Eds.), *Development of orthographic knowledge and foundations of literacy* (pp. 307–332). Hillsdale, NJ: Erlbaum.

Foorman, B., Francis, D., Novy, D., & Liberman, D. (1991). How letter-sound instruction mediates progress in first-grade reading and spelling. *Journal of Educational Psychology, 83,* 456–469.

Fuchs, L., Fuchs, D., Hamlett, C., & Allinder, R. (1991a). The contribution of skills analysis to curriculum-based measurement in spelling. *Exceptional Children, 57,* 443–452.

Fuchs, L., Fuchs, D., Hamlett, C., & Allinder, R. (1991b). Effects of expert system advice within curriculum-based measurement on teacher planning and student achieving in spelling. *School Psychology Review, 20,* 49–66.

Gough, P., Juel, C., & Griffith, P. (1992). Reading, spelling, and the orthographic cipher. In P. Gough, L. Ehri, & R. Treiman, R. (Eds.), *Reading acquisition* (pp. 35–48). Hillsdale, NJ: Erlbaum.

Graham, S. (1990). The role of production factors in learning disabled students' compositions. *Journal of Educational Psychology, 82,* 781–791.

Graham, S. (1997). Executive control in the revising of students with learning and writing difficulties. *Journal of Educational Psychology, 89,* 223–234.

Graham, S., Berninger, V., Abbott, R., Abbott, S., & Whitaker, D. (1997). The role of mechanics in composing of elementary school students: A new methodological approach. *Journal of Educational Psychology, 89,* 170–182.

Graham, S., & Harris, K. (1996). Addressing problems in attention, memory, and executive functioning: An example from self-regulated strategy development. In G. R. Lyon & N. Krasnegor (1996). *Attention, memory, and executive function* (pp. 349–365). Baltimore: Brookes.

Graham, S., Harris, K., & Fink, B. (2000). Is handwriting causally related to learning to write? Treatment of handwriting problems in beginning writers. *Journal of Educational Psychology, 92,* 620–633.

Graham, S., Harris, K., & Fink, B. (in press). Is spelling causally related to learning to write and read? *Journal of Educational Psychology.*

Graham, S., Schwartz, S., & MacArthur, C. (1993). Knowledge of writing and the composing process, attitude toward writing, and self-efficacy for students with and without learning disabilities. *Journal of Learning Disabilities, 26,* 237–249.

Graham, S., & Weintraub, N. (1996). A review of handwriting research: Progress and prospects from 1980 to 1994. *Educational Psychology Review, 8,* 7–87.

Graves, D. (1975). An examination of the writing processes of seven year-old children. *Research in the Teaching of English, 9,* 227–241.

Harris, K., & Graham, S. (1996). *Making the writing process work: Strategies for composition and self-regulation* (2nd ed.). Cambridge, MA: Brookline Books.

Hayes, J., & Flower, L., (1980). Identifying the organization of the writing process. In L. W. Gregg & E. R. Sternberg (Eds.), *Cognitive processes in writing* (pp. 3–30). Hillsdale, NJ: Erlbaum.

Higgins, E., & Zvi, J. (1995). Assistive technology for postsecondary students with learning disabilities: From research to practice. *Annals of Dyslexia, 45,* 123–142.

Hooper, S., Montgomery, J., Swartz, C., Reed, M., Sandler, A., Levine, M., Watson, T., & Wasileski, T. (1994). Measurement of written expression. In G. R. Lyon (Ed.), *Frames of reference for the assessment of learning disabilities. New views on measurement issues* (pp. 375–417). Baltimore: Brookes.

Hooper, S., Swartz, C., Montgomery, J., Reed, M., Brown, T., Wasileski, T., & Levine, M. (1993). Prevalence of writing problems across three middle school samples. *School Psychology Review, 22,* 608–620.

Hooper, S., Swartz, C., Wakely, M., deKruif, R., & Montgomery, J. (2002). Executive functions in elementary school children with and without problems in written expression. *Journal of Learning Disabilities, 35,* 57–68.

Hsu, L., Berninger, V., Thomson, J., Wijsman, E., & Raskind, W. (2002). Familial aggregation of dyslexia phenotype II: Paired correlated measures. *American Journal of Medical (Neuropsychiatric Genetics Section), 114,* 471–478.

Jones, D., & Christensen, C. (1999). The relationship between automaticity in handwriting and students' ability to generate written text. *Journal of Educational Psychology, 91,* 44–49.

Juel, C. (1988). Learning to read and write. A longitudinal study of 54 children from first through fourth grades. *Journal of Educational Psychology, 80,* 437–447.

Leong, C. K. (2000). Rapid processing of base and derived forms of words and grades 4, 5, and 6 children's spelling. *Reading and Writing: An Interdisciplinary Journal, 12,* 277–302.

Levine, M., Oberklaid, F., & Meltzer, L. (1981). Developmental output failure: A study of low productivity in school-age children. *Pediatrics, 67,* 18–25.

Lewis, R. (1998). *Enhancing the writing skills of students with learning disabilities through technology: An investigation of the effects of text entry tools, editing tools, and speech synthesis* (Final report for H1800G40073, Special Education Programs (ED/OSERS)). Washington, DC.

Lewis, R., Ashton, T., Haapa, B., Kieley, C., & Fielden, C. (2000). Improving the writing skills of students with learning disabilities: Are word processors with spelling and grammar checkers useful? *Learning Disabilities, 9,* 87–98.

Lewis, R., Graves, A., Ashton, T., & Kieley, C. (1998). Word processing tools for students with learning disabilities: A comparison of strategies to increase text entry speed. *Learning Disabilities Research and Practice, 13,* 95–108.

MacArthur, C. (1996). Using technology to enhance the writing processes of students with learning disabilities. *Journal of Learning Disabilities, 29,* 344–354.

MacArthur, C. (1999). Overcoming barriers to writing: Computer support for basic writing skills. *Reading and Writing Quarterly, 15,* 169–192.

MacArthur, C., & Graham, S. (1987). Learning disabled students composing under three methods of text production: Handwriting, word processing, and dictation. *Journal of Special Education, 21,* 22–42.

MacArthur, C., Graham, S., Haynes, J., & De La Paz, S. (1996). Spelling checkes and students with learning disabilities: Performance comparisons and impact on spelling. *Journal of Special Education, 30,* 35–57.

MacArthur, C., Graham, S., Schwartz, S., & Schafer, W. (1995). Evaluation of a writing instruction model that integrated a process approach, strategy instruction, and word processing. *Learning Disability Quarterly, 18,* 278–291,

MacArthur, C., Haynes, J., Malouf, D., Harris, K., & Owings, M. (1990). Computer-assisted instruction with learning disabled students: Achievement, engagement, and other factors that influence achievement. *Journal of Educational Computing Research, 6,* 311–328.

Masterson, J., Apel, K., & Wasowicz, J. (2002). *A prescriptive assessment of spelling on CD-ROM.* Evanston, IL: Learning by Design.

McCutchen, D. (1995). Cognitive processes in children's writing: Developmental and individual differences. In J. S. Carlson (Ed.), *Issues in education: Contributions from educational psychologists* (pp. 123–160). Greenwich, CT: JAI Press.

McCutchen, D. (1996). A capacity theory of writing: Working memory in composition. *Educational Psychology Review, 8,* 299–325,

McNaughton, D., Hughes, C., & Ofiesh, N. (1997). Proofreading for students with learning disabilities: Integrating computer and strategy use. *Learning Disabilities Research and Practice, 12,* 16–28.

Moats, L. (2000). *Speech to print. Language essentials for teachers.* Baltimore: Brookes.

The Psychological Corporation. (2002). *Wechsler Individual Achievement Test—2nd Edition. (WIAT-II).* San Antonio, TX: Psychological Corporation.

Raskind, M., & Higgins, E. (1995). Reflections on ethics, technology, and learning disabilities: Avoiding the consequences of ill-considered actions. *Journal of Learning Disabilities, 28,* 425–438.

Reece, J., & Cumming, G. (1996). Evaluating speech-based composition methods: Planning, dictation, and the listening word processor. In C. M. Levy & S. Ransdell (Eds.), *The science of writing.* Mahwah, NJ: Erlbaum.

Sandler, A., Watson, T., Footo, M., Levine, M., Coleman, W., & Hooper, S. (1992). Neurodevelopmental study of writing disorders of middle childhood. *Journal of Developmental and Behavioral Pediatrics, 13,* 17–23.

Scardamalia, M., Bereiter, C., & Goleman, H. (1982). The role of production factors in writing ability. In M. Nystrand (Ed.), *What writers know: The language, process, and structure of written disc*ourse (pp. 173–210). New York: Academic Press.

Swanson, H. L., & Berninger, V. (1996). Individual differences in children's working memory and writing skills. *Journal of Experimental Child Psychology, 63,* 358–385.

Treiman, R. (1997). Spelling in normal children and dyslexics. In B. Blachman (Ed.), *Foundations of reading acquisition and dyslexia: Implications for early intervention.* Mahwah, NJ: Erlbaum.

Treiman, R., & Bourassa, D. (2000). The development of spelling skill. *Topics in Language Disorders, 20,* 1–18.

Tyler, A., & Nagy, W. (1989). The acquisition of English derivational morphology. *Journal of Memory and Language, 28,* 649–667.

Varnhagen, C. (1994). Children's spelling strategies. In V. W. Berninger (Ed.), *The varieties of orthographic knowledge II: Relationships to phonology, reading, and writing* (pp. 251–290). Dordrecht, The Netherlands: Kluwer Academic.

Varnhagen, C., Varnhagen, S., & Das, J. P. (1992). Analysis of cognitive processing and spelling errors of average ability and reading disabled children. *Reading Psychology: An International Journal, 13,* 217–239.

Venezky, R. (1970). *The structure of English orthography.* The Hague: Mouton.

Venezky, R. (1999). *The American way of spelling.* New York: Guilford Press.

Weintraub, N., & Graham, S. (2000). The contribution of gender, orthographic, finger function, and visual-motor processes to the prediction of handwritten status. *Occupational Therapy Journal of Research, 20,* 121–140.

Wise, B., & Olson, R. (1992). How poor readers and spellers use interactive speech in a computerized spelling program. *Reading and Writing: An Interdisciplinary Journal, 4,* 145–163.

Wise, B., & Olson, R. (1994). Computer speech and the remeditaion of reading and spelling problems. *Journal of Special Education Technology, 12,* 207–220.

Wong, B. (1997). Research on genre-specific strategies for enhancing writing in adolescents with learning disabilities. *Learning Disability Quarterly, 20,* 140–159.

Wong, B. (Ed.). (1998). *Learning about learning disabilities* (2nd ed.). New York: Academic Press.

Wong, B., Butler, D., Ficzere, S., & Kuperis, S. (1996). Teaching low achievers and students with learning disabilities to plan, write, and revise opinion essays. *Journal of Learning Disabilities, 29,* 1978–212.

Wong, B., Butler, D., Ficzere, S., Kuperis, S., Corden, M., & Zelmer, J. (1994). Teaching problem learners revision skills and sensitivity to audience through two instructional modes: Student-teacher versus student-student interactive dialogues. *Learning Disabilities Research and Practice, 9,* 78–90.

Yates, C., Berninger, V., & Abbott, R. (1994). Writing problems in intellectually gifted children. *Journal for the Education of the Gifted, 18,* 131–155.

Zimmerman, B., & Reisenberg, R. (1997). Becoming a self-regulated writer: A social cognitive perspective. *Contemporary Educational Psychology, 22,* 73–101.

22

Science and Social Studies

Thomas E. Scruggs
Margo A. Mastropieri

Science and social studies are significant content areas, incorporating much of what is taught in U.S. public schools. Both areas have been the focus of reform efforts in recent years, reflected most strongly in President George H. Bush's mandate, as part of his *America 2000* goals, that U.S. students should be "first in the world" (p. 63) in science achievement by the year 2000 (U.S. Department of Education, 1991). In most cases, it has been recommended that models of rote learning of facts and principles be abandoned in favor of models that emphasize higher-order thinking skills. The American Association for the Advancement of Science (AAAS), for example, suggested a model of science education that emphasized reorganizing content, promoting the study of common themes, interrelating science, mathematics, and technology with human and social aspects, and developing understanding of the "big picture," rather than supporting details and specialized vocabulary (Rutherford & Ahlgren, 1990). Similarly, it has been recommended that instruction in social studies focus on broad themes and ideas, and less on recitation of names and dates (Brophy, 1990). These views have been challenged in recent years to some ex-

tent by the advent of high-stakes testing, which in many cases has emphasized the acquisition of basic content knowledge (Frase-Blunt, 2000).

In fact, students with learning disabilities have not been heavily involved in educational decision making relevant to science or social studies. For example, the AAAS book, *Science for All Americans* (Rutherford & Ahlgren, 1990) avoided mention of Americans with disabilities, although it did provide discussion of race, gender, language, and economic circumstance as it related to science education. Further, implementation of high-stakes testing has often not carefully considered the needs of students with disabilities (Frase-Blunt, 2000).

Nevertheless, a substantial amount of research has been undertaken in science and social studies education for students with learning disabilities. In this chapter, we provide an overview of research in this area, followed by a discussion of theoretical models relevant to science and social studies for students with learning disabilities. We next provide a review of research in the area conducted by ourselves and colleagues and discuss the cumulative findings and implications of this research.

Research in Science and Social Studies with Students with Learning Disabilities

In spite of a relative lack of attention from mainstream science and social studies educators, some attention has been focused on content-area learning of students with learning disabilities, and to some extent this research has followed the dominant paradigms found in the general education literature. Mastropieri and Scruggs (1992) reviewed research on science instruction with students with disabilities from 1954 to 1992 and identified 25 studies that involved learning disabilities, and (Scruggs, Mastropieri, & Boon, 1998) reviewed science education literature from 1992 to 1998, identifying a number of additional studies involving students with learning disabilities. Much of this research focused on text adaptations, including study guides and graphic organizers (e.g., Benedetti, 1984; Bergerud, Lovitt, & Horton, 1988; Horton, Lovitt, & Bergerud, 1990; Horton, Lovitt, Givens, & Nelson, 1989; Lovitt, Rudsit, Jenkins, Pious, & Benedetti, 1985, 1986). Other research investigated the effectiveness of mnemonic strategy instruction to facilitate recall of science and social studies content (e.g., Mastropieri & Scruggs, 1989a). In addition, research has investigated outcomes associated with hands-on, or activities-oriented models of content-area instruction (e.g., Mastropieri, Scruggs, & Magnusen, 1999; Palincsar, Magnusson, Collins, & Cutter, 2001). Most recently, researchers have developed technological "virtual reality" approaches to science learning (Sprague & Behrmann, 2001). All these areas have reported positive outcomes for students with learning disabilities, as they have influenced both text–vocabulary recall and acquisition of relevant concepts.

Theoretical Models

Theoretical perspectives relevant to this area of inquiry involve analysis of the characteristics of learning disabilities, analysis of the characteristics of curriculum and instruction in science and social studies, and analysis of the interaction of characteristics of the curriculum and characteristics of the learner. Relevant characteristics of students with learning disabilities include problems in language and literacy (Kavale & Forness, 1995), attention (Hallahan & Cottone, 1997), semantic or verbal memory (Swanson, 1987), working memory (Swanson, 1994), metacognition, or awareness of cognitive processes (Montague, 1998), and, in some cases, social skills and peer relations (Sullivan & Mastropieri, 1994). All or any of these characteristics can limit potential for academic success in science and social studies for students with learning disabilities. For individuals with such characteristics, it has often been found that a combination of strategy training and direct instruction has been effective (Swanson & Hoskyn, 2000), and, in fact, many special education programs operate on these principles (Mastropieri & Scruggs, 2002).

It has also been suggested that many if not most problems underlying learning disabilities result from a relative deficit in phonemic awareness, the ability to isolate and discriminate among the smallest meaningful units of speech. Because of such deficits, it is argued, students often do not develop fluent reading skills, which later has a negative impact on comprehending content-area textbooks (Lyon et al., 2001; Sternberg, 1999). Though such problems likely play a role, it seems unlikely that phonemic awareness is in itself responsible for all problems in science and social studies achievement. Such an argument must either ignore or subordinate observed deficits in other areas, including working memory, semantic memory, prior knowledge, and organizational and study skills, all of which have been seen to play a role in academic problems of students with learning disabilities (Scruggs & Mastropieri, 2001). Such an argument also makes the incorrect assumption that study from text is the only medium for content-area learning.

Science and social studies education have been characterized by two major models of instruction (e.g., Mastropieri & Scruggs, 1996). Most professional organizations and university science education programs have advocated constructivist, child-centered models of instruction (e.g., Rutherford & Ahlgren, 1990). In science, these models focus on concrete experiences with relevant hands-on activities and an inductive, inquiry model for constructing content knowledge. Often these activities are undertaken in cooperative learning groups. Social studies professionals often endorse a "Socratic" approach to instruction (Brophy, 1990), which promotes learner inquiry and avoids a direct teaching model of instruction. Such models typically emphasize the process of knowledge construction and promote depth of learning over breadth and comprehension of relevant concepts over recall of factual material.

In contrast to constructivist approaches are content-driven or textbook-based approaches to science and social studies. These approaches, commonly found in public schools, involve substantial vocabulary learning (e.g., *phagocytosis, radial symmetry,* and *hegemony*), learning and recall of large amounts of factual content, lecture and worksheet activities, and independent study from text. Content-driven models typically emphasize breadth over depth of learning and the acquisition of factual material. Content-driven models have gained much momentum during the current era of standards-based learning and high-stakes testing (Frase-Blunt, 2000).

Scruggs and Mastropieri (1993) reviewed science curriculum and characteristics of students with special needs and concluded that there are several potential advantages to constructivist approaches. These advantages include emphasis on concrete, meaningful experiences, emphasis on redundancy and depth of learning, deemphasis of rote verbal learning, and use of performance assessment, in which learners demonstrate their knowledge on relevant materials rather than exclusive reliance on paper-and-pencil tests. Potential challenges may include appropriate interaction with peers and overreliance on learner "discovery" and insight in concept acquisition. Although content-driven models may include fewer of these latter challenges, they have in common the demands on semantic memory and independent learning of often abstract content from texts, areas that are known to be problematic for students with learning disabilities. Mastropieri and Scruggs (1994b) evaluated science curriculum from several school districts and concluded that vocabulary demands were particularly challenging in content-driven approaches. They concluded that strategies for effective science

instruction for students with disabilities may include learning and memory strategies for academic content, strategies for studying from text, adapted hands-on activities, and teacher support for inquiry learning. In the following section, we discuss our own research program in science and social studies.

Our Program of Research

Samples

Throughout our research program, we have employed school-identified samples of students with learning disabilities, although in some cases we have subdivided these samples into subgroups. To this extent, students with learning disabilities have putatively met the state criteria for learning disabilities, which has typically meant a significant discrepancy between ability and achievement (1 standard deviation or more), coupled with exclusionary criteria such as adequate sensory, intellectual, and emotional functioning; lack of cultural disadvantage; and adequate opportunity to learn. However, it is also clear that in many cases, students identified by schools as having learning disabilities have not met state standards (e.g., MacMillan, Gresham, & Bocian, 1998); thus to the extent this is true, it is possible that samples we have employed have not all met state definitional standards and may have performed differently than students identified using different procedures. Typically, we conducted our intervention research on students as they appeared in special education or inclusive classes and reported assessment data as they appeared in school files (which may not always have been the same data on which placement decisions were made), as indicators of current functioning. In addition to IQ and achievement data, we have also included, when available, data on such variables as age, ethnicity, gender, years in special education, and time per day in special education settings. We chose not to exclude any students from participating in classroom interventions, even when, in some cases, smaller numbers of students identified as having mild mental retardation were included in the classes. In most cases, effects were so pronounced (e.g., using mnemonic instruction) that it seemed unlikely that subgroups were not responding. And, in fact, mnemonic instruction has been seen to be effective with many other types of students, including normally achieving and "gifted" (Scruggs & Mastropieri, 1988). When we felt there was reason to anticipate differential responding to treatment (e.g., in our investigations of scientific reasoning), we examined the role of IQ in predicting outcomes.

Designs

Most of our research was conducted as true "laboratory" experiments, classroom applications, or teacher applications. For our initial investigations into the efficacy of particular strategies (e.g., text processing, mnemonic strategies, or coached elaborations), we employed true experimental designs, in which students were assigned at random to individual treatments with researchers. Such designs seemed particularly appropriate at early stages of research. In later studies, when we taught students in small groups, we assigned the groups at random to treatment conditions, and used group performance means as the unit of analysis. For our broader classroom application studies, we used crossover designs, in which classrooms of students received both treatments in counterbalanced order which controlled for the effects of treatment order and relative unit difficulty. In those investigations, each student served as his or her own control, so the effects of differential attrition over the longer course of the treatment were minimized (Mastropieri & Scruggs, 1994a). For teacher applications, a variety of designs were employed, including within-subjects, pre–post, and group-comparative designs. Although these designs typically lacked experimental rigor, they nevertheless provided an important link to actual teacher classroom practice.

Teaching and Learning Strategies

Science and social studies are complex content areas, involving a variety of facts, rules, concepts, procedures, and understandings to be acquired. These may interact with particular characteristics in these same types of learning (Scruggs, 1988). As a consequence, it is not realistic to suggest that one particular model of instruction or instructional strategy will accomplish all instructional objectives in these areas. Instead, instructional strategies must interact appropriately with both the characteristics of learning disabilities and the characteristics of the curriculum or content to be learned. Therefore, our own approach to science and social studies instruction has involved a variety of instructional strategies and materials, depending on the particular instructional objectives being considered. Overall, our approach to facilitating to content learning has involved text-processing strategies, mnemonic strategies, elaborative interrogation, inquiry/oriented and activities-oriented instruction, and peer tutoring.

Text-Processing Strategies

Much of content-area instruction, as employed in schools, requires independent study from texts, an area of great difficulty for students with learning disabilities (Mastropieri & Scruggs, 1997). Although relatively simple summarization strategies have been demonstrated to be effective in promoting text recall (e.g., Malone & Mastropieri, 1992), it seemed that more complex strategies could be useful for processing content area texts. This hypothesis was tested on a sample of 54 eighth-grade students with learning disabilities, who were taught to study science text over 3 days of individually administered sessions. Bakken, Mastropieri, and Scruggs (1997) developed a set of text processing strategies based on the type of text structure being considered (see Cook, 1983). These strategies included those appropriate for studying text with *main idea, list,* or *order* structures. An example of a *main idea* paragraph is a description of acid rain, with supporting statements. An example of a *list* paragraph is a main topic such as runoff, and a list of attributes, such as amount of rain, slope of the land, and amount of vegetation. An example of an *order* paragraph is a main topic, such as sedimentary rocks, followed by specific steps in sequence, such as breaking up rock, moving pieces by water, erosion building layers of material, and pressure from upper layers of rock. Students in the text structure processing condition were taught to identify these different types of text structure and to employ study strategies appropriate to each. All conditions received 3 days of training. For example, if students identified a paragraph as *main idea,* they were taught to locate and underline the main idea, then to write down the main idea and supporting information in the student's own words. If students identified a paragraph as *list,* they were taught to locate and underline the general topic of the passage, then to write down the general topic and subtopics in the student's own words. If students identified a paragraph as *order,* they were taught to locate and underline the general topic of the passage, then to write down the details with respect to the order identified in the passage. Students in the paragraph restatement condition received training in reading the paragraph and writing short restatements of the paragraph in their own words. Over 3 days, they studied the strategy using the same materials studied in the paragraph restatement condition. In the traditional instruction condition, students practiced on the same passages by reading the passages and answering questions. Students were asked to recall the information and were given corrective feedback as necessary.

After 3 days of instruction, all students on the fourth day received a test involving studying new passages. On the fifth day, students were given a transfer test on social studies passages. Students taught to use text structure processing strategies significantly and substantially outperformed students on other conditions on recall of central information and recall of incidental information and on all transfer measures. Student scores were particularly low in the traditional instruction, suggesting that typical methods of promoting content-area study skills are not at all effective with students with learning disabilities. Student survey reports suggest that students also felt that the text structure processing strategy was effective, and that traditional methods were not. Although the passages were developed specifically for this investigation, and therefore may not have been entirely representative of content-area passages typically found in textbooks, the substantial effect sizes obtained suggest that it is important to teach students how to identify the structure of science and social

studies texts when studying for later retrieval.

Mnemonic Instruction

Many school programs in science and social studies instruction actively promote factual content and vocabulary knowledge as critical components of such instruction. Students with learning disabilities, many of whom experience difficulty in verbal learning and memory, may find such programs extremely challenging. Given the strong emphasis on fact and vocabulary learning of such programs (Mastropieri & Scruggs, 1993), we have developed an extended program of applied research on the use of mnemonic strategies to promote such learning. Mnemonic instruction was thought to interact positively with the characteristics of learning disabilities, because it enhances meaningfulness and concreteness in learning, and because it emphasizes relative strengths of students with learning disabilities (memory for pictures, use of acoustic encoding and retrieval) and deemphasizes relative weaknesses (automatic semantic processing, memory for abstract vocabulary) (Scruggs, Mastropieri, & Levin, 1987).

One of the most commonly used mnemonic strategies in this research is the *keyword method* (Atkinson, 1975). Using the keyword method, a concrete, acoustically similar keyword is created for a new vocabulary word. For example, to promote recall that the scientific term ranidae refers to the family of common frogs, a keyword is created. In this case, "rain" would be a good keyword for ranidae, because it sounds like the first part of ranidae and is easily pictured. Next, an interactive illustration is created in which the keyword and the definition are shown interacting. In the present instance, a frog could be shown sitting in the rain. Learners are told to study the picture and when asked the meaning of *ranidae,* first think of the keyword ("rain"), think of the picture with the rain in it (frog in the rain), and retrieve the answer, *frogs* (Mastropieri & Scruggs, 2000, Chapter 10). Mastropieri, Scruggs, Levin, Gaffney, and McLoone (1985) employed the keyword method to teach vocabulary words to students with learning disabilities and found that students instructed mnemonically significantly and substantially outperformed students taught using a direct instruction, rehearsal-based teaching strategy. Mastropieri, Scruggs, Bakken, and Brigham (1992) reported that keywords could be combined to facilitate learning of U.S. states and capitals. Fulk, Mastropieri, and Scruggs (1992) demonstrated that students with learning disabilities could be trained to generate their own mnemonic strategies in science and social studies to outperform students who studied using a rehearsal-based study strategy (see also King-Sears, Mercer, & Sindelar, 1992).

Mastropieri, Scruggs, and Levin (1985) added a pegword strategy to the keyword method to teach hardness levels of North American minerals, according to the Mohs scale, to secondary students with learning disabilities. Pegwords are rhyming proxies for numbers (e.g., one is bun, two is shoe, three is *tree*) and are used in teaching numbered or ordered information. For example, to teach that *wolframite* is hardness level *four,* a keyword was constructed for *wolframite* (wolf), and a pegword was used for *four* (floor). The interactive mnemonic illustration was a wolf on a floor. Students were taught, when asked the hardness level of *wolframite,* to think of the keyword (wolf), think of the picture with the wolf in it, remember there was a *floor* in the picture, and retrieve the answer, *four.* Students taught hardness levels of 14 minerals using this mnemonic technique substantially outscored students taught via direct instruction–rehearsal or a free study control. Students taught mnemonically retained their advantage over comparisons on a 24-hour recall task, remembering even more hardness levels the second day than they had on the day of instruction. The population of students with learning disabilities was subdivided into students who scored relatively higher or lower on tests of reading comprehension. No interactions were observed between treatment and comprehension level. Further research demonstrated the facilitative effect of mnemonic instruction when instruction was delivered in small groups rather than individually (Mastropieri, Scruggs, & Levin, 1986). In that investigation, it was seen in a second experiment that students with mild mental retardation could also benefit from the keyword–pegword strategy. However, in

that experiment overall learning gains were lower in both mnemonic and comparison conditions, and a substantial amount of time was needed to pretrain students in the use of the mnemonic pegwords. In a related investigation, Mastropieri, Scruggs, and Whedon (1997) reported that students with learning disabilities remembered significantly more U.S. Presidents (e.g., Jackson = seventh president) when using a mnemonic keyword–pegword strategy.

To determine how much information could be included on one mnemonic picture, Scruggs, Mastropieri, Levin, and Gaffney (1985) taught multiple attributes of minerals, including hardness level, color, and use, to adolescent students with learning disabilities. For example, to teach that *wolframite* was hardness level *four,* was *black* in color, and used in the manufacture of (tungsten filaments for) *lightbulbs,* students were shown a picture of a *black wolf* standing on a tile *floor,* turning on a *lightbulb.* Students were taught, when asked to recall attributes of *wolframite,* to think of the keyword (wolf), remember with the picture with the wolf in it, and remember the color (*black* wolf), hardness level (*floor* = four), and use (*lightbulbs*). Students mnemonically taught attributes of eight minerals greatly outperformed students taught by direct instruction or free study. In a fourth condition, students were taught attributes of only four minerals via direct instruction and remembered a smaller proportion than students taught attributes of eight minerals mnemonically. Later studies demonstrated that information about minerals could be effectively coded into dichotomies (hard vs. soft, light vs. dark, home vs. industrial use) (Mastropieri, Scruggs, McLoone, & Levin, 1985), and whether such mnemonic illustrations could be incorporated into text to facilitate prose recall (Scruggs, Mastropieri, McLoone, Levin, & Morrison, 1987). Veit, Scruggs, and Mastropieri (1986) demonstrated that mnemonic strategies could be used effectively over multiple lessons with students with learning disabilities, and that color could be used to encode information (green = herbivore, red = carnivore). Mastropieri, Scruggs, and Levin (1987) found that other academic information employing different learning strategies, could be included in mnemonic instructional lessons. Finally, Scruggs, Mastropieri, Levin,

McLoone, Gaffney, and Prater (1985) demonstrated in two experiments that mnemonic instruction of dichotomous or continuous attributes of minerals was superior to conditions employing visuospatial displays as an organizing strategy.

Scruggs and Mastropieri (1989a, 1989b) attempted to broaden mnemonic instructional procedures to include other types of encoding in a model they referred to as reconstructive elaborations. In this model, content is evaluated for concreteness and familiarity, and appropriate strategies are developed to address this content. That is, for information that is unfamiliar (e.g., Eddie Rickenbacker was a World War I flying ace), mnemonic keywords (e.g., linebacker) or pegwords are employed as acoustic reconstructions. For information that is familiar but abstract (e.g., U.S. foreign policy), pictures representing symbols (e.g., Uncle Sam) are employed as symbolic reconstructions. For information that employs familiar and concrete vocabulary (e.g,. many World War I soldiers died of illness contracted in unhealthy trenches), this information is represented literally in mimetic reconstructions (e.g, sick soldiers in trenches). It was found that the model of reconstructive elaborations can be versatile in addressing different types of content and can facilitate learning and recall far better than direct teaching methods which do not employ mnemonics. Although that investigation employed true experimental methodology (students assigned individually, at random, and treated individually), later studies employed classroom applications of reconstructive elaborations in science and social studies to classes of students with learning disabilities, for periods of instruction up to 8 weeks (Mastropieri & Scruggs, 1988, 1989b; Scruggs & Mastropieri, 1992). In an application of reconstructive elaborations in science learning, Scruggs and Mastropieri (1992) reported that students with learning disabilities could effectively create their own mnemonic strategies, but that the classes progressed through the content at only one-third the rate they did when teachers presented already-constructed mnemonic illustrations. Mastropieri, Sweda, and Scruggs (2000) described a teacher application of mnemonic strategy instruction, used by a fourth-grade teacher of an inclusive social studies class, with five students identified as having learning disabilities. The teacher reported that while mnemonic strategies raised test performance of normally achieving students from 83.3% to 88.9%, they raised the performance of students with learning disabilities from 36.7% to 75%.

Scruggs, Mastropieri, Brigham, and Sullivan (1992) investigated whether mnemonic illustrations could be helpful in facilitating recall of spatial information from maps. Students with learning disabilities studied maps with mnemonic pictures for place names (Ticonderoga = tiger) or nonmnemonic pictures (e.g.,. a military fort). Students who had studied the mnemonic maps were much more able to identify the locations of battles of the American Revolution. In another study, Brigham, Scruggs, and Mastropieri (1995) demonstrated that mnemonic maps could be also effectively include narrative information from particular battles (e.g., a tiger with a cannon to represent that American forces captured cannon at Ft. Ticonderoga).

Overall, mnemonic strategy instruction has been associated with substantial positive effects. Scruggs and Mastropieri (2000) conducted a meta-analysis of all mnemonic instructional research with students with special needs (79% of the research studies were conducted with students with learning disabilities) and obtained an average effect size of 1.59 ($SD = .93$) for mnemonic science instruction (n of effect sizes = 13), and an average effect size of 1.53 ($SD = .86$) for mnemonic social studies instruction (n of effect sizes = 13). These highly similar mean effect sizes suggest that mnemonic instruction is similarly facilitative in the two content areas. In each case, the outcomes associated with mnemonic instruction were positive, leading to a nearly 2-to–1 learning advantage for mnemonic instruction over a variety of comparison conditions. Mean effect sizes were also highly similar for investigations conducted by Mastropieri, Scruggs, and colleagues and investigations conducted by other researchers (e.g., King-Sears et al., 1992).

Coached Elaborations

Within special education some debate exists whether information should be presented directly or whether students should be prompted and coached to create knowledge for themselves (Mastropieri & Scruggs, 2002). Learning of information about life science under inquiry or direct instruction procedures was directly investigated in a series of investigations. Scruggs, Mastropieri, Sullivan, and Hesser (1993), investigating the utility of the pegword method in promoting recall of information about dinosaur extinction, found that students with learning disabilities, including a small number of students with mild mental retardation, comprehended better when prompted to explain the reasons given for dinosaur extinction (e.g., "why does this make sense?"). Scruggs, Mastropieri, and Sullivan (1994) taught fourth- and fifth-grade students with learning disabilities, including a small number of students with mild mental retardation, facts about animals, under three conditions. In the no-explanation condition, students were told the fact and asked to repeat it (e.g., "Anteaters have long claws on their front feet. What do anteaters have? Good, anteaters have long claws on their front feet."). In the provided-elaboration condition, students were provided with both the fact and the explanation (e.g., "Anteaters have long claws on their front feet, so that they can dig for ants. What do anteaters have? Good, long claws on their front feet. Why do they have long claws on their front feet? Good, to dig for ants."). In the coached-elaboration condition, students were not directly provided with the explanation but a series of prompts to lead them to the correct answer, as in the following:

EXPERIMENTER: Anteaters have long claws on their front feet. Why does it make sense that anteaters have claws on their front feet?
STUDENT: I don't know.
EXPERIMENTER: Well, let's think. What do we know about anteaters. For example, what do they eat?
STUDENT: Anteaters eat ants.
EXPERIMENTER: Good! And, where do ants live?
STUDENT: In holes in the ground.
EXPERIMENTER: So, why does it make sense that anteaters have long front claws?
STUDENT: So they can dig for ants.
EXPERIMENTER: Good. To dig for ants. (translated from Mastropieri, 1995, pp. 122–123)

After treatment and a brief delay interval, students were asked to recall the fact (e.g., "What did you learn about anteaters?") and the explanation for that fact (e.g, "Why does that fact make sense?"). Scruggs and colleagues (1994) concluded that students scored higher in the coached-elaboration condition than in the other two conditions on immediate and delayed (1-week) recall. Students learned and recalled more information when they were prompted to actively reason through it themselves than when they were directly provided with the same information. Explanation score was particularly low in the no-explanation condition, suggesting the need for students with learning disabilities to practice active thinking about academic content. However, there was not a statistically significant difference on immediate fact recall between the coached-elaborations and provided-elaborations groups; and only about half the students were available for delayed recall testing, because of the end of the school year. Sullivan, Mastropieri, and Scruggs (1995) replicated and extended this study with a sample of 63 students with learning disabilities, who had an average 15-point discrepancy between IQ and language achievement, and a somewhat smaller discrepancy between IQ and reading achievement. In that investigation, students in the coached elaboration condition outperformed students in other conditions on all measures, with the exception that the mean delayed explanation score was not significantly higher than that of the provided-explanation condition. However, even in that comparison, students in the coached-elaboration condition outperformed provided-explanation students by .60 standard deviation units.

In a test of independent use of coached elaborations, Mastropieri and colleagues (1996) presented prose passages containing facts about vertebrate animals to 29 seventh- and eighth-grade students with learning disabilities. Students in the control condition were told to read each sentence and try hard to remember the information. In the experimental condition, students were trained to ask themselves and answer "why" questions about the information presented in each sentence (e.g., "Why would it make sense that camels have two rows of eyelids?"). Results suggested that students in the condition performed similarly in recall of factual information; however, students trained in thinking skills produced significantly more correct explanations of that information than did students in the control condition. Student performance in both conditions was lower than observed in previous studies in which students were directly coached and prompted to reason through school content. Across all investigations, it was concluded that appropriately structured coaching can result in higher performance than direct teaching and rehearsal techniques, and that the constructivist notion of learning can lead to at least some positive outcomes for students with learning disabilities.

Differential Outcomes to Inquiry-Oriented Instruction

It was thought that students with learning disabilities, with relative weakness in vocabulary learning, text processing, and working memory, would potentially benefit from the concrete, nonverbal experiences provided by activities-oriented approaches. However, it was also thought that the emphasis on abstract, inductive thinking found in constructivist approaches may prove to be a source of difficulty for students with learning disabilities. This question was tested in two experiments evaluating possible differential learning outcomes in inquiry learning science tasks. Mastropieri, Scruggs, and Butcher (1997) presented middle school students with learning disabilities, students with mental retardation, and normally achieving students a task in which, in a series of steps, they were expected to infer the relationship between rate of swing of a pendulum and the length of the pendulum (i.e., increasing pendulum length negatively influences rate of swing). All students were seen individually. Students with learning disabilities scored an average of 15.5 standard score points lower in reading achievement than on standardized tests of intelligence, whereas students with mental retardation had an average IQ score of 60. After presentation of pendulums of different lengths and calculation of their rates of swing, students were presented with a number of prompts to elicit the inductive conclusion regarding pendulum movement. These prompts focused attention on string length and rate of swing, had participants rearrange a series of pendulums in order of length and evaluate change in swing rate, and provided direct prompts regarding swing rate and length. Finally, students were provided directly with the rule and asked if they agreed that it was accurate. Students were then given two transfer tasks in which they were asked to apply the rule. Analysis of results revealed that virtually all normally achieving students constructed the appropriate rule either immediately or with only one prompt. Half the students with learning disabilities constructed the rule immediately, but all others required more extensive prompting. However, almost all the students with mental retardation never constructed the rule independently and required explicit provision of the rule to proceed. Performance on the generalization task was mixed. When asked to estimate the rate of swing on a new pendulum, only 50% of the students with learning disabilities were able to do so (compared with 90% of normally achieving students); however, when asked a question about how to slow the speed of a grandfather clock that was running too fast, nearly the same proportion of students with learning disabilities (94.4%) answered correctly as did normally achieving students (95%). In contrast, few students with mental retardation responded correctly to either task.

Since the students with learning disabilities who had exhibited difficulties on the pendulum task tended to be those with lower psychometric intelligence, we planned another study that would examine inquiry learning in science across the range of IQ rather than across disability categories. Mastropieri, Scruggs, Boon, and Carter (2001) examined relative learning efficacy on an inquiry task of principles of buoyancy, in which students were asked to draw relevant inductions about density and flotation (i.e., that more dense substances float on less dense substances). In this investigation, normally achieving students and students with "high-incidence disabilities" (48 were students with learning disabilities, and 3 were students with autism or mild mental retardation) across a range of grade levels (1–6). In this investigation, we were interested in the role of psychometric IQ and grade level as predictors of inquiry science learning. We found that across all students, grade level was significantly correlated with all learning tasks, including preconceptions of density/flotation, density/flotation score on the learning task, and generalization score ($rs = 0.25-0.43$). These findings are consistent with the general science education literature (e.g., Driver, Asoko, Leach, Mortimer, & Scott, 1994). Further, within the special education sample, we found that IQ was significantly correlated with all aspects of the learning task ($rs = 0.40-0.53$). We subdivided the high-incidence disabilities population into IQ > 80 ($n = 40$) and IQ < 80 ($n = 11$) and observed that students in the higher IQ group scored almost identically to the normally achieving students, and significantly higher than the lower IQ group on all measures. These two investigations, taken together, suggested that IQ, rather than learning disability status, predicted learning on constructivist, inquiry-oriented science tasks, and that most students with learning disabilities, perhaps with some additional prompting, could be expected to function adequately on such tasks. Students with mental retardation or lower IQ, unlike students with learning disabilities, may exhibit difficulty with such task presentations (see also Scruggs & Mastropieri, 1995). However, it should be remembered that treatments in these investigations were administered individually, and that the groups may have performed differently in group learning contexts.

Activities-Oriented Instruction

Scruggs, Mastropieri, Bakken, and Brigham (1993) directly tested the relative benefits of textbook and activities-oriented instruction in science learning with four classes of middle school students with learning disabilities. All students studied units involving rocks and minerals and electricity according to textbook-based or activities-oriented instruction. For example, textbook-condition students studied telegraphs and how they operated from textbooks and completed worksheets, while activities-oriented condition students constructed and operated their own telegraphs. In this crossover design, all students completed one unit using textbook-based procedures and one unit using

activities-oriented procedures. After 2 weeks of instruction, it was found that students learned and recalled substantially more in the activities-oriented condition, regardless of the unit being studied. Furthermore, although students recalled more vocabulary in the activities-oriented condition, vocabulary learning in both conditions was very low, suggesting the need for additional vocabulary-enhancement strategies. Mastropieri, Scruggs, and Magnusen (1999) described several teacher applications of activities-oriented instruction with students with learning disabilities and other special needs in areas including human anatomy, rocks and minerals, and the nervous system. In all cases, students outperformed students in textbook conditions, or made significant pre–posttest gains. In a 2-year qualitative study of activities-oriented science instruction in special education classes of students with learning disabilities and mild mental retardation, Scruggs and Mastropieri (1994a) reported that, with sufficient teacher academic and behavioral support, students responded positively to an activities and inquiry-oriented approach to science instruction, which employed questioning techniques similar to those employed in the coached-elaborations investigations (e.g., Sullivan et al., 1995). Similar results were also reported by Bay, Staver, Bryan, and Hale (1992).

In a long-term qualitative investigation of science instruction in inclusive elementary classes, Scruggs and Mastropieri (1994b) found that students with special needs (including students with learning disabilities) participated successfully. Further, it was found that, across classrooms and science content areas, successful inclusive instruction was found to be meaningfully associated with (1) administrative support; (2) support from special education personnel; (3) accepting, positive classroom environment; (4) appropriate (activities-oriented) curriculum; (5) effective general teaching skills; (6) peer assistance; and (7) disability-specific teaching skills.

The quantitative outcomes of activities-oriented instruction were tested in inclusive fourth-grade classes which included students with learning disabilities (in addition to mental retardation, emotional disturbance, and physical disabilities), studying a months-long unit on ecosystems (Mastropieri et al., 1998). In this investigation, students created their own ecosystems, described their properties, and performed experiments on their ecosystems and observed outcomes. Compared with general education fourth-grade classes that spent the same time studying ecosystems from textbooks, worksheets, and paper-and-pencil projects, students using the activities-oriented materials scored much higher on tests of content recall and on performance-based measures. Interestingly, in this investigation, students with disabilities, as a group scored near the average of the inclusive class on all measures, and far above the mean of the textbook-condition classes. Also, in the inclusive class, variables associated with effective inclusion were found to be the same as those identified in the Scruggs and Mastropieri (1994a) investigation.

Peer Tutoring

Mastropieri, Scruggs, Spencer, and Fontana (in press) evaluated the effectiveness of a peer tutoring procedure with embedded strategy questioning, as compared with a guided notes strategy in the study of high school world history by 16 students with special needs, 15 of whom had learning disabilities. Using a procedure similar to that employed by Mastropieri, Scruggs, Mohler, and colleagues (2001) in English classes, students in the tutoring condition were assigned to pairs of "admirals" and "generals." At the beginning of tutoring, admirals read one paragraph while generals listened, and then students reversed roles. Following oral reading, students used summarization strategies to promote reading comprehension. Students asked each other after reading, "What is the most important what or who in the text?," followed by "What is the most important thing about the what or who in the text?," and "What is the summary sentence?" For each paragraph, students worked with their partners to develop responses to the questions, but each student wrote answers to the questions on his or her own accompanying worksheet. The teacher then employed a whole-class review session, during which a blank summarization sheet was placed on the overhead projector and students were asked to supply their responses to the questions. Differing responses were

discussed and students were encouraged to alter their own responses to reflect information based on the class discussion. In the guided-notes condition, whole-class lecture and discussion were employed, and students were provided with guided notes to promote learning. At the end of the 8-week unit, analysis of test scores indicated that students in the tutoring condition significantly outperformed students in the guided-notes condition on chapter tests and on the cumulative unit tests. In addition, analysis of end-of-year testing revealed that students in the tutoring condition scored significantly higher on the content covered during the experimental unit, while students in the guided-notes condition did not. This investigation compares favorably with other peer-tutoring studies in demonstrating the facilitative effect of pairs of students with learning disabilities working together on academic content (e.g., Cook, Scruggs, Mastropieri, & Casto, 1985–1986; Mastropieri, Spencer, Scruggs, & Talbott, 2000; Mathes & Fuchs, 1994; Scruggs & Mastropieri, 1998), and extends it to use of reading comprehension strategies on a secondary content area text.

Mastropieri and colleagues (2002) reported on an investigation that examined the effects of integrating strategies to facilitate the learning of complex chemistry content within a peer tutoring delivery system in inclusive 10th grade chemistry classes. Classes were cotaught by a general education chemistry teacher and a special education teacher with disability-specific expertise along with curriculum adaptation expertise. Participants included 55 students, of whom 15 had disabilities. Fourteen of the students were classified as having learning disabilities and one student was classified as having emotional disabilities and Asperger's syndrome. The mean age of the sample was 197 months ($SD = 8.1$).

Materials consisted of information identified by the teachers as critical for the statewide competency tests that would be administered at the end of the school year. The content was subdivided into relevant units of instruction and further subdivided such that five to seven major ideas were presented together in a single folder. Each separate concept was included on a single tutoring page and consisted of, for example, (a) a question asking the partner, "Who was Mendeleev?"; (b) a strategy to help facilitate the learning of the question; (c) a question asking, "What else is important to know about Mendeleev?"; and (d) questions asking for additional characteristics associated with the original question and answer. Materials were further coded such that if a student knew the answer to the first question, tutoring partners would skip the strategy and move directly to the questions asking for additional relevant information and characteristics.

Students were assigned to work with partners for approximately 15 minutes during each class to practice reviewing the content area information together. Students with disabilities were assigned to work with their typically achieving peers as partners. Students recorded on sheets in their folders when they had practiced and mastered the various items. When they successfully completed a folder containing the five to seven items, they progressed to the next set of materials. Findings suggested that tutoring significantly enhanced performance, with gains over traditional instruction of 16% for normally achieving students and 43% for students with disabilities.

Summary of Consistent Findings

Our program of research has generally supported those of others in identifying a number of treatments that are associated with positive outcomes in science and social studies education for students with learning disabilities. These variables are consistent with the findings of Swanson and Hoskyn (2000), who summarized a great volume of intervention research in learning disabilities and concluded that combinations of direct instruction and strategy instruction were particularly effective. Following are some variables that have been consistently associated with positive outcomes in our research (see also Mastropieri & Scruggs, 2002).

1. *Clearly specified instructional objectives.* Even though a variety of different treatments have been evaluated, all our research to date has involved instruction directed toward specific instructional objectives. It seems clear that teaching to

specific objectives is a critical factor in effective instruction.

2. *Maximized engagement.* In all our investigations, we have made specific efforts to maximize engaged time on task, and, in fact, one specific advantage commonly imputed to peer tutoring is its utility in maximizing opportunities to respond (e.g., Greenwood, Delquadri, & Hall, 1984).

3. *Concreteness and meaningfulness.* From mnemonic instructional strategies to active manipulation of science materials, we have found that efforts to increase concreteness and meaningfulness have led to generally positive outcomes, on verbal as well as nonverbal levels (e.g., Mastropieri & Scruggs, 1998).

4. *Active thinking.* In most of our intervention studies, we have actively promoted active thinking on the part of students with learning disabilities. This thinking has taken many forms, from actively thinking about text structure to actively retrieving steps of a mnemonic strategy to actively reasoning through scientific problems and experiments. In each case, when active thinking is encouraged and carefully supported, learning outcomes are positive.

5. *Explicit provision of learning strategies.* Students with learning disabilities have typically exhibited difficulty in both creation and application of effective learning strategies. However, when task-relevant learning strategies are explicitly demonstrated, practiced, and prompted, significant learning gains have been realized.

Overall, our findings have lent support to the model of effective instruction widely promoted in special education. This model has included careful task analysis and specification, coupled with a variety of strategies targeted to promote engagement, active thinking, and strategic learning. These instructional components appear to interact favorably with the characteristics of learning disabilities.

Competing Models

At present, there are few clearly articulated competing models of content-area instruction for students with learning disabilities. Much of our research has employed elements of behavioral, cognitive, and constructivist models of learning; therefore, alternative approaches may reflect a matter of balance. For example, exclusively behavioral approaches may be beneficial in maximizing student engagement and reinforcing correct responding but may not sufficiently engage active thinking. Cognitive strategy instruction may in some cases promote accurate verbal responding without sufficiently enhancing comprehension of more complex concepts. Activities-based instruction may be beneficial only when on-task behavior is high and students are made clearly aware of the relationship between concrete phenomena and the concepts underlying their interactions. It has been seen, for example, that without the implementation of appropriate teacher-effectiveness variables, activities-oriented science instruction may not be effective. Brigham, Scruggs, and Mastropieri (1992) manipulated teacher enthusiasm across classes of middle school students with learning disabilities, and found that even when an activities-oriented approach to instruction of atmospheric science was undertaken, teacher enthusiasm was the strongest predictor of student learning and behavior.

It is also true that specific instructional strategies are appropriate for specific instructional objectives. For example, mnemonic strategies are particularly effective for promoting recall of relevant vocabulary and factual information in science and social studies. Text structure processing can be helpful when learning involves independent study from text. Activities involving manipulation of content materials and coached elaborations are helpful in promoting comprehension of relevant concepts. Peer tutoring is effective in promoting core content knowledge in practice activities. It seems clear that truly effective teachers will exhibit skills in all these areas, in addition to general teacher effectiveness skills (Mastropieri & Scruggs, 2002).

Conclusions and Future Directions

Overall, our own program of research has convinced us of the need for a variety of teaching strategies, linked to specific instructional objectives, to promote learning of science and social studies in students with learning disabilities. These strategies are particularly effective when they address the characteristics of students with learning disabilities, deemphasizing learning weaknesses, such as independent learning from lecture and text, and promoting relative strengths, such as visual memory, episodic memory for learning activities, and nonverbal comprehension.

Our most recent research has integrated peer tutoring with text comprehension strategies, and to date outcomes have been positive, as compared with such alternatives as guided notes. Some of the challenges for the immediate future include the development of appropriate tutoring materials and learning strategies for more complex areas of learning, such as high school chemistry. Such content is notable not only for difficult vocabulary (*ionic* and *covalent bonding*) but for the complexity of the concepts underlying this vocabulary and the expectations of prior knowledge and understandings. Nevertheless, some of our initial findings in this area have been positive and lead us to be optimistic for the future of research in science and social studies for students with learning disabilities.

References

Atkinson, R. C. (1975). Mnemotechnics in second-language learning. *American Psychologist, 30,* 821–828.

Bakken, J. P., Mastropieri, M. A., & Scruggs, T. E. (1997). Reading comprehension of expository science material and students with learning disabilities: A comparison of strategies. *Journal of Special Education, 31,* 300–324.

Bay, M., Staver, J. R., Bryan, T., & Hale, J. B. (1992). Science instruction for the mildly handicapped: Direct instruction versus discovery teaching. *Journal of Research in Science Teaching, 29,* 555–570.

Benedetti, D. M. (1984). *The effectiveness of an instructional adaptation on the acquisition of science information by middle school learning disabled students.* Unpublished doctoral dissertation, University of Washington, Seattle.

Bergerud, D., Lovitt, T., & Horton, S. (1988). The effectiveness of textbook adaptations in life science for high school students with learning disabilities. *Journal of Learning Disabilities, 21*(2), 70–76.

Brigham, F. J., Scruggs, T. E., & Mastropieri, M. A.

(1992). The effect of teacher enthusiasm on the learning and behavior of learning disabled students. *Learning Disabilities Research and Practice, 7,* 68–73.

Brigham, F. J., Scruggs, T. E., & Mastropieri, M. A. (1995). Elaborative maps for enhanced learning of historical information: Uniting spatial, verbal, and imaginal information. *Journal of Special Education, 28,* 440–460.

Brophy, J. (1990). Teaching social studies for understanding and higher-order applications. *Elementary School Journal, 90,* 351–417.

Cook, L. K. (1983). *Instructional effects of text structure-based reading strategies on the comprehension of scientific prose.* Unpublished doctoral dissertation, University of California, Santa Barbara.

Cook, S., Scruggs, T. E., Mastropieri, M. A., & Casto, G. C. (1985–1986). Handicapped students as tutors. *Journal of Special Education, 19,* 483–492.

Driver, R., Asoko, H., Leach, J., Mortimer, E., & Scott, P. (1994). Constructing scientific knowledge in the classroom. *Educational Researcher, 23*(7), 5–12.

Frase-Blunt, M. (2000). High stakes testing a mixed blessing for special students. *CEC Today, 7*(2), 1, 5, 7, 15.

Fulk, B. J. M., Mastropieri, M. A., & Scruggs, T. E. (1992). Mnemonic generalization training with learning disabled adolescents. *Learning Disabilities Research and Practice, 7,* 2–10.

Greenwood, C. R., Delquadri, J. C., & Hall, R. V. (1984). Opportunity to respond and student academic performance. In W. Heward, T. Heron, D. Hill, & J. Trap-Porter (Eds.), *Behavior analysis in education* (pp. 58–88). Columbus, OH: Merrill.

Hallahan, D. P., & Cottone, E. A. (1997). Attention Deficit Hyperactiviey Disorder. In T. E. Scruggs & M. A. Mastropieri (Eds.), *Advances in learning and behavioral disabilities* (Vol. 13, pp. 27–68). Oxford, UK: Elsevier Science/JAI.

Horton, S., Lovitt, T., & Bergerud, D. (1990). The effectiveness of graphic organizers for three classifications of secondary students in content area classes. *Journal of Learning Disabilities, 23,* 12–29.

Horton, S. V., Lovitt, T. C., Givens, A., & Nelson, R. (1989). Teaching social studies to high school students with academic handicaps in a mainstreamed setting: Effects of a computerized study guide. *Journal of Learning Disabilities, 22,* 102–107.

Kavale, K. A., & Forness, S. R. (1995). *The nature of learning disabilities.* Mahwah, NJ: Erlbaum.

King-Sears, M. E., Mercer, C. D., & Sindelar, P. T. (1992). Toward independence with keyword mnemonics: A strategy for science vocabulary instruction. *Remedial and Special Education, 13,* 22–33.

Lovitt, T., Rudsit, J., Jenkins, J., Pious, C., & Benedetti, D. (1985). Two methods of adapting science materials for learning disabled and regular seventh graders. *Learning Disability Quarterly, 8,* 275–285.

Lovitt, T., Rudsit, J., Jenkins, J., Pious, C., & Benedetti, D. (1986). Adapting science materials for regular and learning disabled seventh graders. *Remedial and Special Education, 7*(1), 31–39.

Lyon, G. R., Fletcher, J. M., Shaywitz, S. E., Shaywitz, B. A., Torgesen, J. K., Wood, F. B., Schulte, A., & Olson, R. (2001). Rethinking learning disabilities. In C. E. Finn, Jr., A. J. Rotherham, & C. R. Hokanson, Jr. (Eds.), *Rethinking special education for a new century* (pp. 259–287). Washington, DC: Thomas B. Fordham Foundation.

MacMillan, D. L., Gresham, F. M., & Bocian, K. M. (1998). Discrepancy between definitions of learning disabilities and school practices: An empirical investigation. *Journal of Learning Disabilities, 31,* 314–326.

Malone, L. D., & Mastropieri, M. A. (1992). Reading comprehension instruction: Summarization and self-monitoring training for students with learning disabilities. *Exceptional Children, 58,* 270–279.

Mastropieri, M. A. (1995). L'instruzione mnemonica é l'interrogazione elaborative: Strategie per recordarsi e per pensare [Mnemonic instruction and elaborative interrogation: Strategies for remembering and for thinking]. In C. Cornoldi & R. Vianello (Eds.), *Handicap e apprendimento: Ricerche e proposte di intervento* [*Handicap and learning: Research and proposals for intervention*] (pp. 117–124). Bergamo, Italy: Juvenilia.

Mastropieri, M. A., & Scruggs, T. E. (1988). Increasing the content area learning of learning disabled students: Research implementation. *Learning Disabilities Research, 4,* 17–25.

Mastropieri, M. A., & Scruggs, T. E. (1989a). Constructing more meaningful relationships: Mnemonic instruction for special populations. *Educational Psychology Review, 1,* 83–111.

Mastropieri, M. A., & Scruggs, T. E. (1989b). Mnemonic social studies instruction: Classroom applications. *Remedial and Special Education, 10*(3), 40–46.

Mastropieri, M. A., & Scruggs, T. E. (1992). Science for students with disabilities. *Review of Educational Research, 62,* 377–411.

Mastropieri, M. A., & Scruggs, T. E. (1993). *A practical guide for teaching science to students with special needs in inclusive settings.* Austin, TX: Pro-Ed.

Mastropieri, M. A., & Scruggs, T. E. (1994a). Issues in intervention research: Secondary students. In S. Vaughn & C. Bos (Eds.), *Research in learning disabilities: Theory, methodology, assessment, and ethics* (pp. 130–145). New York: Springer Verlag.

Mastropieri, M. A., & Scruggs, T. E. (1994b). Text-based vs. activities-oriented science curriculum: Implications for students with disabilities. *Remedial and Special Education, 15,* 72–85.

Mastropieri, M. A., & Scruggs, T. E. (1996). Current trends in science education: Implications for special education. In C. Warger & M. Pugach (Eds.), *Curriculum trends, special education, and reform: Refocusing the conversation* (pp. 42–52). New York: Teachers College Press.

Mastropieri, M. A., & Scruggs, T. E. (1997). Best practices in promoting reading comprehension in students with learning disabilities. *Remedial and Special Education, 18,* 197–213.

Mastropieri, M. A., & Scruggs, T. E. (1998). Constructing more meaningful relationships in the classroom: Mnemonic research into practice. *Learning Disabilities Research and Practice, 13,* 138–145.

Mastropieri, M. A., & Scruggs, T. E. (2000). *The inclusive classroom: Strategies for effective instruction.* Columbus, OH: Prentice Hall/Merrill.

Mastropieri, M. A., & Scruggs, T. E. (2002). *Effective instruction for special education* (3rd ed.). Austin, TX: Pro-Ed.

Mastropieri, M. A., Scruggs, T. E., Bakken, J. P., & Brigham, F. J. (1992). A complex mnemonic strategy for teaching states and capitals: Comparing forward and backward associations. *Learning Disabilities Research and Practice, 7,* 96–103.

Mastropieri, M. A., Scruggs, T. E., Boon, R., & Carter, K. B. (2001). Correlates of inquiry learning in science: Constructing concepts of density and buoyancy. *Remedial and Special Education, 22,* 130–138.

Mastropieri, M. A., Scruggs, T. E., & Butcher, K. (1997). How effective is inquiry learning for students with mild disabilities? *Journal of Special Education, 31,* 199–211.

Mastropieri, M. A., Scruggs, T. E., Graetz, J., Fontana, J., Cole, V., & Gersen, A. (2002, July). *Teacher–researcher partnerships to promote success in inclusive high school science and social studies classes.* Paper presented at the annual U.S. Department of Education Project Director's Meeting, Washington, DC.

Mastropieri, M. A., Scruggs, T. E., Hamilton, S. L., Wolfe, S., Whedon, C., & Canevaro, A. (1996). Promoting thinking skills of students with learning disabilities: Effects on recall and comprehension of expository prose. *Exceptionality, 6,* 1–11.

Mastropieri, M. A., Scruggs, T. E., & Levin, J. R. (1985). Mnemonic strategy instruction with learning disabled adolescents. *Journal of Learning Disabilities, 18,* 94–100.

Mastropieri, M. A., Scruggs, T. E., & Levin, J. R. (1986). Direct vs. mnemonic instruction: Relative benefits for exceptional learners. *Journal of Special Education, 20,* 299–308.

Mastropieri, M. A., Scruggs, T. E., & Levin, J. R. (1987). Learning disabled students' memory for expository prose: Mnemonic vs. nonmnemonic pictures. *American Educational Research Journal, 24,* 505–519.

Mastropieri, M. A., Scruggs, T. E., Levin, J. R., Gaffney, J., & McLoone, B. (1985) Mnemonic vocabulary instruction for learning disabled students. *Learning Disability Quarterly, 8,* 57–63.

Mastropieri, M. A., Scruggs, T. E., & Magnusen, M. (1999). Activities-oriented science instruction for students with disabilities. *Learning Disability Quarterly, 22,* 240–249.

Mastropieri, M. A., Scruggs, T. E., Mantzicopoulos, P. Y., Sturgeon, A., Goodwin, L., & Chung, S.

(1998). "A place where living things affect and depend on each other": Qualitative and quantitative outcomes associated with inclusive science teaching. *Science Education, 82,* 163–179.

Mastropieri, M. A., Scruggs, T. E., & McLoone, B., Levin, J. R. (1985). Facilitating learning disabled students' acquisition of science classifications. *Learning Disability Quarterly, 8,* 299–309.

Mastropieri, M. A., Scruggs, T. E., Mohler, L. J., Baranek, M. L., Spencer, V., Boon, R. T., & Talbott, E. (2001). Can middle school students with serious reading difficulties help each other and learn anything? *Learning Disabilities Research and Practice, 16,* 18–27.

Mastropieri, M. A., Scruggs, T. E., Spencer, V., & Fontana, J. (in press). Promoting success in high school world history: Peer tutoring versus guided notes. *Learning Disabilities Research and Practice.*

Mastropieri, M. A., Scruggs, T. E., & Whedon, C. (1997). Using mnemonic strategies to teach information about U. S. presidents: A classroom-based investigation. *Learning Disability Quarterly, 20,* 13–21.

Mastropieri, M. A., Spencer, V., Scruggs, T. E., & Talbott, E. (2000). Students with disabilities as tutors: An updated research synthesis. In T. E. Scruggs & M. A. Mastropieri (Eds.), *Educational interventions: Advances in learning and behavioral disabilities* (Vol. 14, pp. 247–279). Oxford, UK: Elsevier Science/JAI.

Mastropieri, M. A., Sweda, J., & Scruggs, T. E. (2000). Teacher use of mnemonic strategy instruction. *Learning Disabilities Research and Practice, 15,* 69–74.

Mathes, P. G., & Fuchs, L. S. (1994). The efficacy of peer tutoring in reading for students with mild disabilities: A best-evidence synthesis. *School Psychology Review, 23,* 59–80.

Montague, M. (1998). Research on metacognition in special education. In T. E. Scruggs & M. A. Mastropieri (Eds.), *Advances in learning and behavioral disabilities* (Vol. 12, pp. 247–279). Oxford, UK: Elsevier Science/JAI.

Palincsar, A. S., Magnusson, S. J., Collins, K. M., & Cutter, J. (2001). Making science accessible to all: Results of a design experiment in inclusive classrooms. *Learning Disability Quarterly, 24,* 15–32).

Rutherford, F. J., & Ahlgren, A. (1990). *Science for all Americans.* New York: Oxford University Press.

Scruggs, T. E. (1988). Nature of learning disabilities. In K. A. Kavale (Ed.), *Learning disabilities: State of the art and practice* (pp. 22–43). Boston: Little, Brown/College Hill.

Scruggs, T. E., & Mastropieri, M. A. (1988). Acquisition and transfer of learning strategies by gifted and nongifted students. *Journal of Special Education, 22,* 153–166.

Scruggs, T. E., & Mastropieri, M. A. (1989a). Mnemonic instruction of learning disabled students: A field-based evaluation. *Learning Disability Quarterly, 12,* 119–125.

Scruggs, T. E., & Mastropieri, M. A. (1989b). Reconstructive elaborations: A model for content area learning. *American Educational Research Journal, 26,* 311–327.

Scruggs, T. E., & Mastropieri, M. A. (1992). Classroom applications of mnemonic instruction: Acquisition, maintenance, and generalization. *Exceptional Children, 58,* 219–229.

Scruggs, T. E., & Mastropieri, M. A. (1993). Current approaches to science education: Implications for mainstream instruction of students with disabilities. *Remedial and Special Education, 14*(1), 15–24.

Scruggs, T. E., & Mastropieri, M. A. (1994a). The construction of scientific knowledge by students with mild disabilities. *Journal of Special Education, 28,* 307–321.

Scruggs, T. E., & Mastropieri, M. A. (1994b). Successful mainstreaming in elementary science classes: A qualitative investigation of three reputational cases. *American Educational Research Journal, 31,* 785–811.

Scruggs, T. E., & Mastropieri, M. A. (1995). Science and mental retardation: An analysis of curriculum features and learner characteristics. *Science Education, 79,* 251–271.

Scruggs, T. E., & Mastropieri, M. A. (1998). Peer tutoring and students with special needs. In K. Topping & S. Ehly (Eds.), *Peer assisted learning* (pp. 165–182). Mahwah, NJ: Erlbaum.

Scruggs, T. E., & Mastropieri, M. A. (2000). The effectiveness of mnemonic instruction for students with learning and behavior problems: An update and research synthesis. *Journal of Behavioral Education, 10,* 163–173.

Scruggs, T. E., & Mastropieri, M. A. (2001). *On babies and bathwater: Addressing the problems of identification and assessment of learning disabilities.* Fairfax, VA: George Mason University, Graduate School of Education.

Scruggs, T. E., Mastropieri, M. A., Bakken, J. P., & Brigham, F. J. (1993). Reading vs. doing: The relative effectiveness of textbook-based and inquiry-oriented approaches to science education. *Journal of Special Education, 27,* 1–15.

Scruggs, T. E., Mastropieri, M. A., & Boon, R. (1998). Science for students with disabilities: A review of recent research. *Studies in Science Education, 32,* 21–44.

Scruggs, T. E., Mastropieri, M. A., Brigham, F. J., & Sullivan, G. S. (1992). Effects of mnemonic reconstructions on the spatial learning of adolescents with learning disabilities. *Learning Disability Quarterly, 15,* 154–162.

Scruggs, T. E., Mastropieri, M. A., & Levin, J. R. (1987). Implications of mnemonic strategy research for theories of learning disabilities. In H. L. Swanson (Ed.), *Memory and learning disabilities: Advances in learning and behavior disabilities* (pp. 225–244). Greenwich, CT: JAI Press.

Scruggs, T. E., Mastropieri, M. A., Levin, J. R., & Gaffney, J. S. (1985). Facilitating the acquisition of science facts in learning disabled students. *American Educational Research Journal, 22,* 575–586.

Scruggs, T. E., Mastropieri, M. A., Levin, J. R., McLoone, B. B., Gaffney, J. S., & Prater, M. (1985). Increasing content-area learning: A comparison of mnemonic and visual-spatial direct instruction. *Learning Disabilities Research, 1,* 18–31.

Scruggs, T. E., Mastropieri, M. A., McLoone, B. B., Levin, J. R., & Morrison, C. (1987). Mnemonic facilitation of learning disabled students' memory for expository prose. *Journal of Educational Psychology, 79,* 27–34.

Scruggs, T. E., Mastropieri, M. A., & Sullivan, G. S. (1994). Promoting relational thinking skills: Elaborative interrogation for mildly handicapped students. *Exceptional Children, 60,* 450–457.

Scruggs, T. E., Mastropieri, M. A., Sullivan, G. S., & Hesser, L. S. (1993). Improving reasoning and recall: The differential effects of elaborative interrogation and mnemonic elaboration. *Learning Disability Quarterly, 16,* 233–240.

Sprague, D., & Behrmann, M. (2001). Zoning in on physics: Creating virtual reality environments to aid students with learning disabilities. In T. E. Scruggs & M. A. Mastropieri (Eds.), *Technological applications: Advances in learning and behavioral disabilities* (Vol. 15, pp. 17–38). Oxford, UK: Elsevier Science/JAI.

Sternberg, R. J. (1999). Epilogue: Toward and emerging consensus about learning disabilities. In R. J. Sternberg & L. Spear-Swerling (Eds.), *Perspectives on learning disabilities: Biological, cognitive, contextual.* (pp. 277–282). Boulder, CO: Westview Press.

Sullivan, G. S., & Mastropieri, M. A. (1994). Social competence of individuals with learning disabilities. In T. E. Scruggs & M. A. Mastropieri (Eds.), *Advances in learning and behavioral disabilities* (Vol. 8, pp. 171–214). Oxford, UK: Elsevier Science/JAI.

Sullivan, G. S., Mastropieri, M. A., & Scruggs, T. E. (1995). Reasoning and remembering: Coaching thinking with students with learning disabilities. *Journal of Special Education, 29,* 310–322.

Swanson, H. L. (Ed.). (1987). *Advances in learning and behavioral disabilities: Memory and learning disabilities.* Oxford, UK: Elsevier Science/JAI.

Swanson, H. L. (1994). The role of working memory and dynamic assessment in the classification of children with learning disabilities. *Learning Disabilities Research and Practice, 4,* 190–202.

Swanson, H. L., & Hoskyn, M. (2000). Intervention research for students with learning disabilities: A comprehensive meta-analysis of group design studies. In T. E. Scruggs & M. A. Mastropieri (Eds.), *Educational interventions: Advances in learning and behavioral disabilities* (Vol. 14, pp. 1–153). Oxford, UK: Elsevier Science/JAI.

U.S. Department of Education. (1991). *America 2000: An education strategy.* Washington, DC: Author.

Veit, D. T., Scruggs, T. E., & Mastropieri, M. A. (1986). Extended mnemonic instruction with learning disabled students. *Journal of Educational Psychology, 78,* 300–308.

IV

FORMATION OF
INSTRUCTIONAL MODELS

23

Cognitive Strategies Instruction Research in Learning Disabilities

Bernice Y. L. Wong
Karen R. Harris
Steve Graham
Deborah L. Butler

Cognitive strategies instruction research in learning disabilities (LD) reflects in general the cognitive influence in education, and in particular the influence of cognitive strategies research in cognitive and educational psychologies. "Cognitive strategies are cognitive processes that the learner intentionally performs to influence learning and cognition. Examples include basic processes such as using a rehearsal strategy to memorize a list and metacognitive strategies such as recognizing whether one comprehends a passage" (Mayer, 2001, p. 86). The goal of cognitive strategies instruction research in LD is the design and validation of strategies that enhance learning and performance in students with LD.

Broadly speaking, this research in LD was shaped by the research of Scott G. Paris and the late Ann L. Brown. Specifically, Paris and his associates highlighted the importance of informing students of the rationale of the strategy to be learned, pointing out the link between strategy use and enhanced learning and performance, and the range and conditions of strategy application (Paris, Cross, & Lipson, 1984; Paris & Jacobs, 1984; Paris & Newman, 1990; Paris & Winograd, 1990). Brown and Palincsar

(1982) focused on self-control components in strategy learning: planning and executing the strategy, monitoring, and evaluating strategy use. Brown and Palincsar considered these components to be essential in students' orchestration of strategy use.

With their respective associates, Paris and Brown primed researchers in LD to attend to these metacognitive components, beyond the specific strategy to be learned. Neglecting them would undermine students' strategy acquisition, maintenance, and transfer. Moreover, students must value strategy use, otherwise they would not apply it when needed despite having mastered it previously (Nolen, 1988). This valuing of strategy use appears likely to arise if students perceive not only the link between effective strategy use and subsequent successful learning outcomes but also their own agency in forging the link. Such perceived agency would also lead to correct attributions of successful learning outcome—that it is students' own strategy execution that resulted in their successful learning and not luck or teacher's favor.

This chapter summarizes cognitive strategies instruction research in LD in the last two decades. We organize the research summary according to the age range of participants in the studies: children, adolescents, and young adults, thus resulting in three sections. Unifying/connecting these sections are discernable commonalities in the instructional procedures in cognitive strategies training.

Strategy Instruction for Students with LD in the Elementary Grades

Research involving strategy instruction at the elementary grade levels for students with LD has slowly but steadily increased over the past two decades. Though a comprehensive review of this research is not possible here, we note that this research has primarily focused in several areas: mnemonics, reading, mathematics, and composition. This section focuses primarily on strategies instruction in composition, as this area has received the broadest attention for students with LD. However, we note critical contributions in the other areas first.

Mnemonics, Mathematics, and Reading

MNEMONICS

Research on teaching mnemonic strategies to students with LD has occurred across the elementary through secondary grades. The work of Mastropieri, Scruggs, and their colleagues has been critical in this area. Mnemonic strategy approaches, including keyword, pegword, and symbolic representation strategies, have proven beneficial in the development of language skills and content vocabulary across content areas, and in comprehension of science and social studies concepts (Mastropieri & Scruggs, 1989; Scruggs & Mastropieri, 1990, 1992). In their meta-analysis of 24 studies involving instruction in keyword and keyword–pegword mnemonics, Mastropieri and Scruggs reported an overall mean effect size of 1.62. Although instruction in the use of mnemonics has not always involved full-blown strategies instruction (and indeed may not always need to do so to be effective), the use of strategy instruction stages and procedures has been recommended by these researchers (Fulk, 1994; Scruggs & Mastropieri, 1992).

MATHEMATICS

Several important reviews of intervention research for students with LD and others who have difficulties with mathematics have been published (cf. Mastropieri, Scruggs, & Chung, 1998; Mastropieri, Scruggs, & Shiah, 1991; Miller & Brewster, 1992). Many different approaches have been investigated, yet surprisingly little programmatic research has been done involving the use of multicomponent strategy instruction models at the elementary-grade levels. Researchers have looked at the effects of some of the common components of strategy instruction models, such as reinforcement and goal setting, self-instructions to deal with anxiety, self-instructional cues, self-monitoring, direct or explicit instruction in a math strategy, or the use of mnemonics (cf. Mastropieri et al., 1991). Those few studies where interventions have involved multicomponent strategy instruction models have focused primarily on problem solving (cf. Case, Harris, & Graham, 1992; Jitendra & Hoff, 1995), although in at least one study using a more complete strategies instruction approach the focus was on improved calculation of basic facts (Miller & Mercer, 1993). Further, Montague and her colleagues have demonstrated that strategy instruction models have been successful with middle school and junior high school students (Montague, 1992; Montague, Applegate, & Marquard, 1993; see also Hutchinson, 1993). Given the generally positive results in studies that have involved components common in strategy instruction models and in studies in which strategy instruction models have been used, this appears a fruitful area for future, programmatic research.

READING

Other chapters in this book deal with reading both at the word level and in terms of comprehension. Thus, we do not elaborate on the research in these areas here. We do note, however, that a great deal of strategies instruction research has been conducted in the area of reading, particularly for improving comprehension. Trabasso and Bouchard, authors of the review of reading comprehension research in grades 2 through 8 for the National Reading Panel (National Institute of Child Health and Human Development, 2000), described comprehension strategies as learned procedures that allow active, competent, self-regulated, and intentional reading (Trabasso & Bouchard, 2002). They noted that before the 1970s, explicit instruction in reading comprehension was not conducted, with students learning to comprehend text primarily through reading in the content areas. Initial research in strategies instruction in reading focused on single strategies and then moved to a focus on combinations of strategies taught with multicomponent approaches, as the integrated use of multiple cognitive strategies is critical to skilled reading. Trabasso and Bouchard (2002) found two classes of multiple strategy instruction in comprehension: reciprocal teaching (Palincsar & Brown, 1984) and transactional strategies instruction (Pressley et al., 1992).

Trabasso and Bouchard (2002) concluded, "The bottom line is that readers who are given cognitive strategy instruction make significant gains on comprehension compared with students who are trained with conventional instruction procedures" (p. 177). Much of this research, however, does not specifically involve students with LD. Exceptions include studies of reciprocal teaching by Palincsar and others (cf. Palincsar & Brown, 1984), and the reading comprehension procedure developed by Englert and her colleagues (cf. Englert & Mariage, 1991), and the studies using Harris and Graham's self-regulated strategy development model applied to reading comprehension (Bednarczyk, 1991; Johnson, Graham, & Harris, 1997). As Mann (1998) noted, however, there is little or no attempt to differentiate between children identified as LD and "garden-variety poor readers" in many studies and reviews of reading research. Research indicating a lack of meaningful differences between these two groups in terms of a phonological core deficit is the main reason for this lack of differentiation.

This same research, however, has established differences between LD and other poor readers in terms of receptive vocabulary (perhaps due to the correlation between IQ and vocabulary, as a discrepancy between IQ and reading ability is a defining characteristic for LD) and has also indicated that children labeled as dyslexic or LD possess superior real-world knowledge and

strategic abilities (Mann, 1998). Differences in self-regulatory abilities, as well as other areas, may also exist (Alexander, Garner, Sperl, & Hare, 1998). Thus, strategies instruction in comprehension may neither produce differing results nor require differing components, procedures, or time—for students with LD as compared to other poor readers. However, it may be premature to disregard the differences between these groups when it comes to strategies instruction in reading. Further research on potential differences in responding to strategy instruction appears warranted.

Composition

Harris and Graham and their colleagues and Englert and her colleagues have developed strategy instruction models for composition. Englert and her colleagues refer to their approach as the cognitive strategy instruction writing (CSIW) program (Englert, Raphael, & Anderson, 1992; Englert et al., 1991). Harris and Graham's approach has come to be called self-regulated strategy development (SRSD; see Harris & Graham, 1999, for a more detailed discussion of the evolution of this model). Both models are reviewed here.

SRSD

Harris and Graham's first strategy instruction study for children with LD in the elementary grades was published in 1985. Arising from Harris's early research on cognitive-behavioral interventions for children (Harris, 1980, 1982) and Graham's (1982) early work on children's writing, and their shared concern for children with LD who struggle with writing, this strategy instruction model was initially referred to as self-control strategy training. Though the roots of, and continuing empirical and theoretical bases for this approach are discussed in greater detail elsewhere (Case, Mamlin, Harris, & Graham, 1995; Harris & Graham, 1992), we note several critical influences and components here.

Four theoretical and empirical sources provided the initial foundation for this model in the early 1980s. First, based on Meichenbaum's (1977) cognitive-behavioral intervention model, and its emphasis on Socratic dialogue as well as stages of intervention, Harris and Graham developed their initial stages of instruction and an emphasis on the role of dialogue/discussion in instruction. Second, the work of Soviet theorists and researchers (including Vygotsky, Luria, and Sokolov) on the social origins of self-control and the development of the mind was influential and contributed to the self-regulation and modeling components of the model. Third, the work of Deshler, Schumaker, and their colleagues on the validation of acquisition steps for strategies among adolescents with LD (Deshler, Alley, Warner, & Schumaker, 1981), steps that were also influenced by the work of Meichenbaum and others, strongly influenced, and continues to influence, the SRSD model. Fourth, the work of Brown, Campione, and their colleagues on development of self-control, metacognition, and strategies instruction was also foundational (Brown, Campione, & Day, 1981).

Though current models of strategies instruction have converged in many ways (Pressley & Harris, 2001), in the early stages of its development the SRSD model differed from other strategies instruction models for students with LD in at least two important ways. First, based in part on the research on expertise in writing and research on children's self-regulation (see Alexander et al., 1998; Harris & Graham, 1992, for further detail), explicit instruction in and supported development of critical aspects of self-regulation were integrated throughout the stages of instruction in the SRSD model. These self-regulation components include goal-setting. self-assessment, self-instruction, self-reinforcement, imagery, and managing the writing environment.

Second, Harris and Graham's early experience with strategies instruction with children with LD and the research base indicated these children, though a heterogeneous group, often face additional challenges related to reciprocal relations among academic failure, self-doubts, learned helplessness, low self-efficacy, maladaptive attributions, unrealistic pretask expectancies, and low motivation and engagement in academic areas. Thus, children's attitudes and beliefs about themselves as writers and the strategies instruction they participate in became critical targets for intervention as well as as-

sessment during and after strategies instruction. Throughout SRSD instruction, students are supported in the development of attributions for effort and the use of powerful writing strategies, knowledge of writing genres, self-efficacy, and high levels of engagement (Harris & Graham, 1992). Furthermore, progression through SRSD instructional stages (develop background knowledge and skills, discuss it, model it, memorize the mnemonics, engage in supported/collaborative practice, and demonstrate independent performance) is criterion based rather than time based, so that students have the time they need to attain important outcomes.

Moreover, students with LD often experience difficulties with attention, impulsivity, memory or other areas of information processing, as well as significant academic difficulties. Harris and Graham articulated an underlying premise of SRSD early on—children who face significant and often debilitating difficulties in academic areas would benefit from an integrated approach to intervention that directly addressed their affective, behavioral, and cognitive characteristics, strengths, and needs (Harris, 1982; Harris & Graham, 1992). An intervention model that allows the integration of knowledge gained from multiple theories and models of teaching and learning—even competing models that may appear theoretically incompatible—allows the development of intervention approaches that maximize the strengths of each while addressing the weaknesses in any given model through strengths inherent in others (Harris & Alexander, 1998). Researchers have found, in fact, that a common characteristic of outstanding teachers is their ability to blend models of instruction in just such ways (Pearson, cited in Willis, 1993, p. 8; Pressley, 1998).

Another premise articulated early on in the development of the SRSD model was that children who face serious struggles with learning often need to be meaningfully engaged in more extensive, structured, and explicit instruction to develop skills, strategies (including self-regulation strategies), and understandings that their peers form more easily (Graham, Harris, & Sawyer, 1987). Explicitness and structure, however, do not equate with isolated skills training, decontextualized learning of subskills, passive learning, or the gradual accruing of basic skills (Harris & Graham, 1994). Children's perceptions of what they are doing and why they are doing it, as well as their teacher's intentions, are critical.

Since 1985, more than 30 studies using the SRSD model of instruction have been reported in the area of writing, involving students from the elementary grades through high school. In many of these studies, instruction has been conducted by the special and/or general education teachers in their own classrooms, often as a part of writers' workshop (cf. Danoff, Harris, & Graham, 1993; De La Paz, 1999, 2001; De La Paz & Graham, 2001; MacArthur, Graham, Schwartz, & Shafer, 1995; MacArthur, Schwartz, & Graham, 1991; MacArthur, Schwartz, Graham, Molloy, & Harris, 1996; Sexton, Harris, & Graham, 1998). Teachers have been able to implement SRSD and have found SRSD acceptable and beneficial in their classrooms. Studies have been undertaken to determine the contributions of various components of the SRSD approach and the stages of instruction (Danoff et al., 1993; Graham & Harris, 1989b; Sawyer, Graham, & Harris, 1992). Studies have also been conducted by researchers independently of Graham, Harris, and their colleagues (Albertson & Billingsley, 1997; Collins, 1992; Tanhouser, 1994).

SRSD research has resulted in the development of writing strategies, typically with the assistance of teachers and their students, for a variety of genres; these genres include personal narratives, story writing, persuasive essays, report writing, expository essays, and state writing tests. SRSD has resulted in significant and meaningful improvements in children's development of planning and revising strategies, including brainstorming, self-monitoring, reading for information and semantic webbing, generating and organizing writing content, advanced planning and dictation, revising with peers, and revising for both substance and mechanics (Harris & Graham, 1996).

SRSD has resulted in improvements in four main aspects of students' performance: quality of writing, knowledge of writing, approach to writing, and self-efficacy (Graham, Harris, MacArthur, & Schwartz, 1991; Harris & Graham, 1999). Across a variety of strategies and genres, the quality, length, and structure of students' compositions have improved. Depending on the strategy taught, improvements have been documented in planning, revising, content, and mechanics. These improvements have been consistently maintained for the majority of students over time, with some students needing booster sessions for long-term maintenance, and students have shown generalization across settings, persons, and writing media. Improvements have been found with normally achieving students as well as with students with LD, making this approach a good fit for inclusive classrooms (cf. Danoff et al., 1993; De La Paz, 1999; De La Paz, Owen, Harris, & Graham, 2000; MacArthur et al., 1996). In some studies, improvements for students with LD have resulted in performance similar to that of their normally achieving peers (Danoff et al., 1993; De La Paz, 1999; Sawyer et al., 1992).

CSIW

Englert and her colleagues have published two influential studies with elementary students with LD using their CSIW program (Englert et al., 1991, 1992). In CSIW, "think sheets" are used to prompt students to carry out specific activities during the following writing processes: planning, organizing information, writing, editing, and revising. For example, the think sheet for organizing information when writing directions for completing a task includes prompts to identify where the activity will take place, what materials are needed, and what steps are involved. A variety of features common to strategies instruction models are used to aid students in internalizing the strategies and the framework represented in the think sheet, including teacher modeling, self-instructions, gradually faded support in using the procedures, and guiding students to understand what they are learning, why it is important, and when it can be used.

Results of these studies indicated that both students with and without LD improved their knowledge of the writing process and their writing abilities. In the Englert and colleagues (1991) study, students with LD performed similarly to their peers with disabilities on all five posttest writing variables. In their 1992 study, Englert and colleagues found that the quality of students' metacognitive knowledge was positively related to measures of performance in both reading and writing.

Caveats and Future Directions

As many cognitive strategy instruction researchers have articulated, academic competency and literacy represent a complexity of skills, strategies, processes, and attributes. Clearly, no single intervention approach can effect all aspects of performance or the complex nature of school success or failure (Duffy, 2002; Harris & Graham, 1992; Pressley & Harris, 2001). Strategy instruction is not a panacea but, rather, a powerful component of teachers' instructional repertoires. Furthermore, strategy instruction continues to be an evolving approach, one that must be informed by ongoing research and development in teaching and learning. A final important caveat is that meeting the goals of strategy instruction requires a carefully thought out combination of components, characteristics, and procedures, enacted by reflective, analytical teachers in a meaningful environment (Duffy, 2002; Harris, 1982).

Many questions remain to be answered regarding strategy instruction in the elementary grades for students with LD and others who struggle with writing, and promising directions exist for future research. For example, though some studies and models have shown positive results, further improvements in maintenance and generalization remain to be addressed. Many academic needs of children with LD in the elementary grades have not yet been addressed yet appear appropriate for strategy instruction, such as learning in the content areas, further aspects of mathematics, and homework and study strategies. Two of the most intriguing questions are the long-term results of strategy instruction and the development of self-regulation across the grades and academic disciplines. Parents could also be partners in such long-term intervention. Researchers have argued that a focus on how teachers become adept at, committed to, and supported in strategy instruction is needed, as is more work aimed at filtering this approach into the schools (Duffy, 2002; Harris & Alexander, 1998; Pressley & Harris, 2001). Much more needs to be understood about the relative contributions of the components in these multicomponent approaches. Harris and Graham (1992) noted that strategy instruction provides teachers and students with richly informative assessment data, and research is needed to establish the role and functions of such assessment information for teachers, parents, students, and administrators.

Strategy Instruction for Students with LD in Secondary School

In the 1980s, researchers at the Institute of Research in LD at the University of Kansas (KU-IRLD) spearheaded cognitive strategies development and research with adolescents and young adults with LD. In their research they were guided by the conceptual notion of learning to learn (Alley & Deshler, 1979), which focused on teaching students how to learn instead of tutoring them to complete immediate assignments or pass impending tests. The KU-IRLD researchers developed and field-tested numerous strategies that eventuated in the learning strategies curriculum. The latter contains three strands that promote, respectively, "acquisition, storage, and expression of written information" (Schumaker & Deshler, 1992, p. 28). These strands correspond to task demands that are faced by adolescents with LD in secondary schools. Moreover, KU-IRLD researchers have streamlined the instructional methodology for use in strategy training (see Schumaker & Deshler, 1992, pp. 30–32). We highlight only four of the seven steps because they appear to be the kernel ones. Using a thinking-aloud procedure, the instructor models the cognitive strategy for the adolescent with LD. The adolescent is instructed to verbally rehearse the strategy steps until he or she can internalize them so that self-instruction becomes covert. The adolescent with LD practices the strategy on controlled (reading-age) materials. As he or she attains mastery of it, he or she applies the strategy to grade-level curricular materials and is also given increasing control in strategy learning.

Cognitive strategies developed at KU-

IRLD cover reading comprehension (Schumaker, Deshler, Alley, Warner, & Denton, 1982), paragraph writing (Schumaker & Lyerla, 1991), sentence writing (Schumaker & Sheldon, 1985), error monitoring in writing (Schumaker, Nolan, & Deshler, 1985), content learning (Lenz, Bulgren, & Hudson, 1990), and opinion essay writing (Ellis & Larkin, 1998). Space restrictions precludes summarizing all of them. Instead, for illustration purposes, selective attention is paid to the DEFENDS strategy (Ellis & Colvert, 1996).

DEFENDS (Ellis & Colvert, 1996) is an expository writing strategy for defending a point-of-view or opinion essay. The strategy steps elicit in students both cognitive and metacognitive processes. DEFENDS involve the following steps:

Decide on goals and theme

Decide who will read this and what you hope will happen when they do.
Decide on what kind of information you need to communicate
Decide on what your theme will be about
Note the theme on your planning form.

Estimate main ideas and details

Think of at least two main ideas that will explain your theme.
Make sure the main ideas are different.
Note the main ideas on your planning form.
Note at least three details that can be used to explain each main idea.

Figure best order of main ideas and details

Decide which main idea to write about first, second, etc., & note on the planning form.
For each main idea, note the best order for presenting the details on the planning form.
Make sure the orders are logical.

Express the theme in the first sentence

The first sentence of your essay should state what the essay is about.
Note each main idea and supporting points
Note your first main idea using a complete sentence; explain this main idea using the details you ordered earlier.
Tell yourself positive statements about your writing and tell yourself to write more.
Repeat for each of the main ideas.

Drive home the message in the last sentence

Restate what your theme was about in the last sentence.
Make sure you used working different from the first sentence.

Search for errors and correct

Look for different kinds of errors in your essay and correct them.
> Set editing goals.
> Examine your essay to see if it makes sense.
> **Ask** yourself whether your message will be clear to others.
> **Reveal** picky errors (capitalization, punctuation, spelling, etc.)
> Copy over neatly.
> Have a last look for errors.

The DEFENDS strategy is quite representative of the characteristics of cognitive strategies developed by the researchers from KU-IRLD. Specifically, the strategy steps in each are encapsulated in a mnemonic that facilitates retention by adolescents with LD. More important, each letter in the mnemonic cues students to activate appropriate cognitive and/or metacognitive processes required in the execution of the strategy step. Moreover, the mnemonic guides sequential enactment of the strategy for the adolescent with LD. Finally, to match learning needs of adolescents with LD, the strategies are structured. Obviously, this degree of structure may not be needed by adolescents without LD.

Apart from KU-IRLD, on a much smaller scale and exclusively focused on writing, is Wong's strategy research. Wong's research arose from Graham and Harris's (1993) call for more genre-specific writing strategies research. In three consecutive studies, Wong and her associates validated three writing strategies, respectively, for reportive, opinion, and compare-and-contrast essays (Wong, Butler, Ficzere, & Kuperis, 1996; Wong, Butler, Ficzere, & Kuperis, 1997; Wong, Wong, Darlington, & Jones, 1991). Reportive essays involve adolescents writing about topics such as "the best birthday present I could have" and "the most embarrassing event in my life."

Several instructional principles and factors underlay the design of Wong's genre-specific writing strategies. First and foremost was the focus on instructing the adolescents with LD in both declarative and procedural knowledge of the writing process, as prior research showed that they often lack such knowledge (Englert et al., 1988; Graham, Schwartz, & MacArthur, 1993; Wong, Wong, & Blenkisop, 1989). Of importance was their need to understand the relevance of planning and revising in writing, and the recursive nature of the cognitive processes in planning, writing, and revising (Flower & Hayes, 1980). Then came the consideration of meshing genre-specific strategies with junior high English curriculum. A good fit here was essential if the strategy instruction was to profit those adolescents with LD. Because short stories, novels, plays, and poems comprise the English curriculum in junior high, three matching genres for instruction appeared to be reportive essays, opinion (persuasive) essays, and compare-and-contrast essays.

Moreover, because writing involves metacognitive as well as cognitive processes (Flower & Hayes, 1980), the question arises on what metacognitive aspects of writing to instruct adolescents with LD. Metacognition about writing includes but is not restricted to the following: awareness of audience need for clarity, felicity in choice of words, a powerful introduction/conclusion, cadence, and so on (Wong, 1999). Although these metacognitive aspects are all interesting, they vary in difficulty regarding cultivation in student writers. Furthermore, except for work by Wray (1994), to date there is no developmental research on them. However, one aspect appears to be more amenable to instruction, namely, awareness of audience need for clarity. Research by Graham and Harris (1993), as well as reports from effective teachers, attest to students' increased efficacy in editing and revising after conferencing with teacher or peers. Through interactive dialogues in conferences, teachers and/or peers pinpoint ambiguities in the essay of the student writer, question the latter on his or her communicative intent, or seek more specific information from him or her. Through explanations and/or elaborations, the student writer clarifies his or her communication intent or furnishes the necessary details. Constant repetition of such interactive dialogues in student–teacher/peer conferencing eventu-

ates in students' increased ability and efficacy in editing and revising their own papers. Such enhancements as editors and revisers of their own writings suggest that students may well have developed some awareness of audience's need for clarity (Wong, Butler, Ficzere, Kuperis, & Corden, 1994; Wong et al., 1996, 1997).

Considerations of cognitive and metacognitive components in writing strategy instruction are necessary but insufficient. Echoing the affective emphasis in the SRSD model, these cognitive and metacognitive components underlying the design of Wong's writing strategies need the accompaniment of affective components. Otherwise, the strategy instruction would not escape Zajonc's (1980) criticism of its reflecting cold cognition. Indeed, Borkowski and colleagues (1992) advocated for including affective components in strategy instruction. Heeding Borkowski and colleagues, Wong included self-efficacy and general attitudes toward writing as the affective components to be fostered in their strategy instruction.

Finally, Wong capitalized on educational technology in strategy instruction. The rationale was that adolescents with LD would lose motivation to learn the writing strategies if they had to write and revise with pen and paper. Using a word processing program (Clarisworks) to write and revise on the microcomputer alleviates physical labor entailed in using pen and paper. This, however, necessitated prior training of adolescents with LD on keyboard skills.

Instruction of the three genres of essays differed in the following ways.

1. Only the opinion and compare-and-contrast essays involved the use of plan sheets.
2. The instructional targets differed across the genres. For reportive essays, clarity and thematic salience were targeted for instruction and enhancement. For opinion essays, clarity and cogency of arguments were the instructional targets. For compare-and-contrast essays, clarity, appropriateness of ideas, and organization were the instructional targets. Appropriateness of ideas referred to ideas that pertained to comparisons or contrasts.
3. Only the instruction of reportive essay involved the use of visualizing. Students

were instructed to use three steps in planning of this genre:

a. Search and select from their memory the event they want to write. For example, if they were going to write about the most embarrassing event in their lives, they would have to recall all the embarrassing events that they had experienced and choose, from them, the most embarrassing episode.
b. Having settled on their choice, they would have to relive it in their mind's eye as though they were playing a videotape (with sound) with themselves as the main actors/actresses.
c. They would have to activate the very emotions associated with the event to be described. For the most embarrassing event in their lives, they should feel a burning sensation on their faces/necks!

Wong and colleagues (1994, 1996, 1997) reported that their genre-specific writing strategies increased both quality and quantity of writing in adolescents with LD. However, compared to non-LD peers, the latter needed to write more essays to reach a satisfactory level of the instructional criteria per genre.

At the close of the 1990s, cognitive strategies research in LD showed an exciting development in mathematics problem solving. Designed originally by Montague and Bos (1986), and subsequently honed in two intervention studies (Montague, 1992; Montague et al., 1993), Montague and her associates validated a strategy for mathematics problem solving for adolescents with LD. This strategy consists of both cognitive and metacognitive components. The cognitive processes and specific problem-solving strategies include READ (comprehension), PARAPHRASE (translation), VISUALIZE (transforming), HYPOTHESIZE (planning), ESTIMATE (prediction), COMPUTE (calculation), and CHECK (evaluation). The metacognitive processes and strategies (awareness and regulation of cognitive strategies) include SELF-INSTRUCT (strategy knowledge and use), SELF-QUESTION (strategy knowledge and use), and SELF-MONITOR (strategy control) (Montague, 1997, p. 168). The goal of this strategy is to enable junior and senior high adolescents with LD to solve one-, two-, and three-step mathematical word problems. Montague (1997) acknowledged that more research is needed to validate the component cognitive and metacognitive processes and strategies. But she cited data from her own research that indicated that successful problem-solvers evidenced knowledge and effective use of those processes and strategies. More important, when adolescents with LD were instructed in the use of the combined cognitive and metacognitive processes and strategies, their problem-solving improved to the level of non-LD peers (Montague et al., 1993).

Cognitive strategies instruction in mathematics is a timely new direction in LD because of emergent data on the characteristics of students with LD with mathematics problems (Bryant, Bryant, & Hammill, 2000). But cognitive strategy research in mathematics problem solving in students with LD would profit from a concomitant focus on their substantial math anxiety, because these students suffer from crippling math anxiety that manifests in negative self-talk and perceptions of ability to do well in mathematics (Kamann, 1989).

Kamann and Wong (1993) validated a coping strategy that effectively addressed math anxiety in students with LD in lower and upper intermediate grades and enabled these students to achieve well in mathematics learning and performance. This coping strategy involves the following steps:

1. Student assesses the situation (label the task and plan attack). Student then generates coping self-statements: What is it that I have to do? Look over the task and think about how I will work through it.
2. Student recognizes and controls negative thoughts (Recognize that negative thoughts hurt my work. Control negative thoughts by replacing them with positive thoughts). Coping self-statements include: *Recognition.* OK I feel worried and scared. . . . I'm saying things that don't help. . . . I can stop and think more helpful thoughts. *Controlling.* Don't worry, remember to use my plan. Take it step by step—look at one question at a time. Don't let my eyes wander to other questions. When I feel fear coming on . . .

I take a deep breath, and think I am doing just fine . . . things are going well. I
can do this (I remember having learned
and mastered this kind of problem with
my LD teacher in the resource room). I'll
just think through the questions and do
my best.

3. Self-reinforcement (patting myself on the
back for doing a good job).Reinforcing
self-statements include the following: I
did really well in not letting my anxiety
get the best of me. Good for me I did a
good job! I did a good job in not allowing myself to worry so much.

Strategic Content Learning Instruction for Adolescents and Adults with LD

Strategic content learning (SCL) was developed in the early 1990s to promote strategic
learning and problem solving by students
with LD (see Butler, 1993, 1994, 1995).
Current research evaluates SCL as a model
for supporting adolescents with LD (Butler,
Jarvis, Beckingham, Novak, & Elaschuk,
2001), but early studies were conducted
with adults. This initial focus was selected
because the problems experienced by students with LD extend into adulthood, and
because little research has been available regarding how to support students with LD in
postsecondary settings (Vogel & Adelman,
1990). This section outlines theoretical
strands that converged in the formation of
SCL, SCL instructional guidelines, research
into SCL efficacy, and directions for future
research involving SCL.

SCL's Theoretical Rationale

At least five theoretical strands converged in
the development of SCL. First, one contribution of educational psychology as a field
has been to describe cognitive processes that
can be associated with enhanced performance on academic tasks (e.g., Dole, Duffy,
Roehler, & Pearson, 1991). An implication,
borne out in research, is that student performance should improve when teachers structure instruction and academic work to cue
effective processing. Examples of instructional practices that guide effective learning
include using advance organizers, concept
maps, or procedural facilitators while teach-

ing content (e.g., Andrews & Lupart, 1993;
Larkin & Ellis, 1998). Simultaneously, however, researchers described how independent
and strategic learning also requires students'
explicit awareness and self-direction of cognitive processing (Brown, 1980, 1987;
Flavell, 1976; Wong et al., 1991). As a result, strategy training approaches were developed to foster students' metacognitive reflection on learning activities (Butler,
1998b; Harris & Graham, 1996), thereby
bridging teacher-guided instruction and stu-
dent-directed learning (e.g., Ellis, 1993).
Consistent with these theoretical principles,
in SCL teachers bridge content and process
instruction in order to enhance students'
learning processes, metacognition and self-
direction.

Second, SCL draws on models of self-
regulated learning to characterize effective
cognitive processing (Brown, 1987; Butler
& Winne, 1995; Zimmerman, 1989, 1994).
Models of self-regulation describe strategic
learning as comprising recursive cycles of
task analysis, strategy implementation, and
self-monitoring (Butler & Winne, 1995).
During task analysis, students locate cues
that define task demands and interpret what
is expected. Then they select, adapt, or invent strategies to meet task demands. After
implementing strategies, self-regulated
learners self-monitor progress. They self-
evaluate by comparing outcomes (and feedback) to performance criteria and make
judgments about how to proceed. Research
has shown that students with LD struggle
not only with strategy implementation but
also with interpreting tasks, monitoring,
and self-evaluation (see Butler, 1998b,
1999; Wong et al., 1991). Thus, in SCL,
strategic learning is fostered by guiding students to engage reflectively, recursively, and
successfully in cycles of self-regulation.

Third, SCL builds from research documenting that students' knowledge and beliefs mediate their approaches to learning
(Paris & Paris, 2001). For example,
metacognitive knowledge about tasks and
strategies clearly influence students' approaches to tasks (Butler, 1998b; Wong et
al., 1991). Similarly, students' perceptions
of agency, reflected in task-specific perceptions of self-efficacy (Bandura, 1993;
Schunk, 1994) or attributional beliefs
(Borkowski, 1992; Weiner, 1974), can ei-

ther support or undermine their strategic approaches. Research suggests that meta-cognitive knowledge and self-perceptions of agency are fostered when students observe links between learning activities and outcomes. Thus, in SCL, students are supported to construct productive knowledge and beliefs by guiding them to self-regulate effectively and then to self-monitor learning.

Fourth, SCL derives from an integration of sociocultural and constructivist perspectives. Research suggests that while students actively construct knowledge as they seek to make sense of experience, social contexts provide the language and tools students employ to construct understandings (Butler, 1998a; Stone, 1998). Furthermore, although students do not come to instruction as self-regulating "blank slates" (Butler & Winne, 1995), they do need to learn how to channel extant self-regulating abilities in the context of academic work. In this respect, teachers play a key role in helping students to decipher the demands of academic tasks and shape effective approaches to learning. Building from this perspective, in SCL teachers scaffold instruction by building from students' extant knowledge, beliefs, and skills. Teachers complete ongoing functional and dynamic assessments as a foundation for guiding learning and shaping self-regulation.

Fifth, researchers have defined numerous influences on students' independent transfer of learned strategies. For example, one key influence, already discussed, is students' self-perceptions of agency. Students with strong self-perceptions of agency are more likely to use strategies independently (Bandura, 1993). Other instructional practices associated with transfer, and incorporated in SCL, include embedding strategy training in meaningful work (Palincsar & Brown, 1984; Pressley et al., 1992) and assisting students to recognize the value of strategies given task demands (Borkowski, 1992). SCL also requires students to articulate knowledge about strategic processing, in their own words. Mindful abstraction of knowledge has been linked to a fuller understanding about strategies and their usefulness and thus to strategy transfer (Salomon & Perkins, 1989; Wong, 1994). Finally, in SCL transfer is promoted by involving students in strategy construction.

Research suggests that students feel more ownership over strategies that they are involved in constructing and that are personalized to meet their unique needs (Butler, 1995).

To summarize, SCL is an approach to strategy training that focuses on much more than teaching strategies. Instead, SCL provides instructional principles for integrating content and process instruction (see Butler, in press). Furthermore, by interweaving principles from diverse theoretical strands, SCL provides a simple framework for achieving multiple complementary objectives. By promoting reflective and effective self-regulation, SCL assists students to (1) construct knowledge and beliefs critical to successful performance (e.g., domain-specific knowledge, knowledge about tasks and strategies, positive perceptions of agency), (2) learn how to self-direct learning (e.g., interpret tasks and self-direct learning to achieve task objectives), and (3) learn *how to* select, adapt, or even invent personalized strategies that they transfer across contexts and time and over which they feel ownership.

SCL Instructional Guidelines

Descriptions of SCL instructional guidelines are available elsewhere (see Butler, 1993, 1995, in press; Butler, Elaschuk, & Poole, 2000) and so are only overviewed here. Note, however, that SCL does not provide a strategies "curriculum," nor is it something that can be taught in a separate "lesson." Instead, SCL defines guidelines for integrating content and process instruction within classroom lessons, small- and large-group discussions, or one-on-one support (see Butler, in press; Butler, Elaschuk, Poole, et al., 2000).

SCL shares key instructional features with other empirically validated strategy training approaches. For example, as in reciprocal teaching (Palincsar & Brown, 1988), transactional strategies instruction (Pressley et al., 1992), and SRSD (Harris & Graham, 1996), teachers and students engage in interactive discussions about strategies while engaged in meaningful work. Furthermore, as in SRSD (Harris & Graham, 1996), attention focuses on supporting students' metacognitive control over strategy application. As in Ellis's interactive strategy instruction, SCL can be integrated with content instruction to foster students' explicit awareness of effective learning processes (e.g., Ellis, 1993). And, as in all current instructional models, SCL supports students' construction of metacognitive knowledge and motivational beliefs supportive of strategic learning (Paris & Paris, 2001). However, SCL differs from most strategy training models in that direct instruction of strategies is deemphasized. Instead, students are guided to construct personalized strategies while completing authentic academic tasks.

It follows that the central SCL instructional guideline is for teachers to approach all academic tasks as opportunities to guide self-regulation, so that students learn *how to* analyze tasks; define performance criteria; select, adapt, or invent effective strategies; self-monitor outcomes; and revise learning approaches. For example, when planning classroom lessons, teachers would first think about the lesson purpose, possible tasks and activities, and evaluation criteria. Then, to promote self-regulation, the teachers could weave into a lesson, activities designed to promote students' active self-regulation. For example, they could structure opportunities for students to interpret task demands (e.g., ask students to analyze writing exemplars or interpret an assignment description) and define performance criteria. Similarly, they could ask students to brainstorm strategies for meeting task demands. An alternative would be to support students' effective completion of assignments, in small or large groups, and then to ask students to articulate strategies that appear to be working. To support self-evaluation, students could compare their work to performance criteria (before or after turning it in) and/or actively interpret instructor feedback (Butler & Winne, 1995). Then students could articulate advice to themselves (i.e., strategy revisions) for the next time they complete a similar task. Note that each of these suggestions has been used by teachers to structure classroom instruction (see Butler, Jarvis, et al., 2001).

A second SCL instructional guideline is that teachers should foster students' construction of knowledge and beliefs during cycles of self-regulated processing. This can be accomplished by shifting responsively between working with students to complete tasks on-line and asking students to articulate emerging knowledge as meaningful opportunities arise. For example, when working with a student one-on-one, an instructor might assist students to think through a math problem in order to solve it correctly (working together on-line) and then ask the student to articulate strategies that also might work for the upcoming problem (opportunistic reflection).

A third instructional guideline is to treat students' completion of academic tasks as opportunities for collaborative problem solving. When collaborating, teachers' roles shift from explaining or providing students with solution strategies to guiding students' thinking. Students assume control over their own work and make decisions about strategies to use, whereas teachers' roles are to support students to make effective decisions (e.g., by asking questions that cue effective processing or direct students' attention to important decision making cues) (Kamann & Butler, 1996). Similarly, teachers shift from evaluating student performance to supporting self-evaluation. Note, however, that in SCL, students are not left to discover strategies for themselves. Rather, armed with an understanding about effective cognitive processes for different kinds of tasks, teachers structure assignments, ask questions, and/or guide discussions to cue effective processing (i.e., procedural facilitation), while simultaneously supporting students to articulate and make decisions regarding approaches they will use.

A final SCL instructional guideline is to base instruction on ongoing dynamic assessments of students' knowledge, beliefs, and self-regulated approaches to tasks. Strategies for continuous assessment include asking questions, fostering discussion, observing students' strategic approaches, and collecting traces of students' work (Winne & Perry, 2000). Note that in a recent study (Butler, Novak, Beckingham, Jarvis, & Elaschuk, 2001), secondary teachers learning to use SCL recognized how often they made assumptions and provided directives without understanding students' difficulties, even in one-on-one tutoring situations that they had thought were learner centered. In contrast, after mastering SCL, teachers reported having a greater understanding of student needs, improved listening skills, and more positive relationships with students.

SCL Research

Initial research on SCL efficacy included postsecondary students with LD. A sequence of studies was planned to evaluate SCL efficacy when adapted for use within common service delivery models at the postsecondary level, including one-on-one tutoring by learning disability specialists or teachers, peer tutoring, and small-group discussions. Note that participants in the postsecondary studies were a diverse set of students, ranging in age from 18 years to late adulthood. Only a subset of students were high school graduates pursuing college or university degrees. Many were enrolled in vocational programs or academic upgrading classes at the intermediate or high school level (see Butler, 1993, 1995, 1998c; Butler, Elaschuk, & Poole, 2000; Butler, Elaschuk, Poole, MacLeod, & Syer, 1997).

Across the postsecondary studies, multiple parallel case studies were embedded within a pre–posttest design. Research reports include summaries of outcomes associated with SCL intervention (see Butler, 1993, 1995, 1998d), detailed analyses of instructional interactions (see Butler, Elaschuk, Poole, et al., 2000; Kamann & Butler, 1996), and in-depth case study reports (see Butler, Elaschuk, & Poole, 2000). In general, similar patterns of findings were observed across service delivery models. Analyses of questionnaire and interview data revealed pre- to posttest improvements in students' self-perceptions of competence and control and metacognitive knowledge. Further, case study analyses suggested that students' task performance improved over time, and that students were actively involved in strategy construction, developed personalized strategies linked to their unique strengths and needs, and transferred strategy use across contexts and tasks. These outcomes were apparent in the studies on peer tutoring but were most consistent and powerful when SCL was used to structure one-on-one tutoring and small-group discussions. Overall, empirical research strongly supports SCL as a model for providing support to students with LD at the postsecondary level.

A more recent study evaluated SCL when used to support secondary students with LD. In a 2-year project completed in June 2001, teachers and researchers worked collaboratively to adapt SCL instructional guidelines in learning assistance/resource settings and inclusive classrooms. In the first year of the project, nine teachers from four schools adapted SCL to support 53 students with a variety of learning difficulties (46% with LD) in learning assistance or resource classrooms. A tenth teacher chose to adapt SCL to teach writing in her inclusive English/Humanities 9 classroom. As in previous SCL research, multiple, parallel case studies were embedded within a pre–posttest design. The only addition was collection of data from comparison groups in both learning assistance/resource and inclusive class settings.

Preliminary analyses of the first-year data suggest that SCL is also a promising intervention for students at the secondary level (see Butler, Jarvis, et al., 2001). In end-of-the-year interviews, teachers reported improvements in students' confidence, knowledge of task demands, strategies, self-awareness, independence and self-direction, and task performance. Teachers also described positive shifts in classroom climate when students worked more independently. Preliminary analyses of questionnaire and case study data provide converging evidence for teachers' reports. Improvements were found in students' perceptions of agency, metacognitive knowledge, and strategic approaches to learning.

Directions for Further Research on SCL

One obvious direction for further research on SCL is to conduct additional studies at the secondary level, within inclusive classrooms, learning assistance/resource settings, and/or alternative schools. A second direction is to explore SCL for use in upper elementary or intermediate contexts. A final direction is to examine how SCL instructional principles can be employed to support teachers' professional development (i.e., as they learn to implement SCL) (see Butler, Novak, et al., 2001). Future research in these areas will provide a fuller picture of SCL's applicability for supporting students across contexts and across ages.

Epilogue

The preceding summaries clearly show active cognitive strategy instruction research in LD, primarily in the area of composing, a major cornerstone of which is the research ensuing from the SRSD model. In future years, we foresee continual cognitive strategies instruction research in composing as well as exciting extensions into mathematics, social studies/history, and science.

In addition, we anticipate research in at least two other areas. First, as mentioned earlier, cognitive strategies instruction research is always evolving. We highlight such evolvement by pointing to the degree of structure in strategies. For example, on the one hand, we have more structured cognitive strategies from KU. On the other hand, we have much less structure in Butler's SCL approach. In SCL, there is no set script in strategy instruction because the teacher's application of this approach involves an interaction between the student's strategic repertoire and the task. The essence of applying SCL lies in the teacher's guiding/scaffolding the student to do a task analysis of the task demands, and to guide/scaffold the student in devising a strategy to meet these demands. Subsequently, the focus of SCL shifts from being cognitive to metacognitive. The teacher guides/scaffolds the student in self-monitoring and self-regulating task completion and self-assessment of the learning/performance outcome. Thus, the SCL approach affords the teacher much flexibility as she uses her content, pedagogic, and strategic knowledge and teaching experience to help the student devise a task-appropriate strategy. The approach also affords the student with LD optimal opportunities in developing into a self-regulated learner. However, the effectiveness of this approach appears to depend importantly on the extant strategic repertoire of the student. Because students with LD tend to be deficient in cognitive and metacognitive strategies in learning, conceivably some of them may need more explicit and structured strategy instruction to build up a sufficient strategy repertoire in order to benefit from an approach such as SCL. This contrast between strategy structure in KU strategies and the SCL approach suggests that we should treat/consider strategy structure as a continuum. From this perspective, researchers simply vary structure in their strategy designs as a function of student needs. A parallel line of research would be on the conditions of when more or less structured strategy instruction would fit the needs of particular students with LD.

Second, a persistent research question in cognitive strategy instruction research has been how we can help students with LD to be become strategic learners. We are keenly aware that teaching students one or several cognitive and metacognitive strategies by no means turn them into strategic learners who consistently approach various tasks planfully and strategically and willingly expend effort at learning. A minimum requirement for making students with LD into strategic learners appears to involve immersing them in strategy instruction continuously across curriculum. This had been attempted by Gaskins, Cunicelli, and Satlow (1992). At a private school for students who might well be LD, Gaskins and colleagues ran a 3-year research project in which the school's director and supervisors of teachers all supported strategy instruction across the curriculum. Teachers were actively encouraged to join the project. In the main, Gaskins and colleagues had much success in getting the teachers to learn to teach strategies and enjoy the collaborative spirit and professional growth. However, teachers who did not share the enthusiasm or took longer to join the project felt stressed. They worried that they had fallen out of favor with the director of the school. There were also some students who did not respond positively to the strategy instruction approach. But Gaskins and colleagues' project underscored an important point, namely, wholesale school-based cognitive strategy instruction depends on open and full support from the administrators/principals.

Undeniably, students who learn in the environment such as the Benchmark school of Gaskins and colleagues (1992) have the best opportunities to become strategic learners because of the intensity and extensity of given strategy instruction. However, there is at least another approach that we can adopt, one that may bring us similar results without the negative concerns of teachers who may not wish to experiment with strategy instruction. This approach is forming a community of practice in which university researchers and classroom teachers join to collaboratively develop ways to teach cognitive and metacognitive strategies. Using the community of practice concept in forming such a community, we deviate from the original concept of Lave and Wenger (1991), who described their observations and analyses of established communities of practice such as tailors. But our deviation appears acceptable because we maintain the essence of such a community, that among members there is distributed knowledge/expertise; that knowledge is socially constructed, mediated, and shared; and that meaning is negotiated.

As university researchers, Palincsar, Magnusson, Collins, and Cutter (2000) recruited elementary teachers who shared an interest in using inquiry learning in science education and formed a community of practice. The goal was to collaboratively develop best teaching practices to effect a principled science instructional approach called guided inquiry learning supporting multiple literacies (GIsML). Similarly, Perry and VandeKamp (2000) formed a community of practice with primary teachers interested in fostering self-regulation in the children.

Relating a community of practice to strategy instruction research, university researchers would recruit teachers interested in cognitive strategy instruction. They would all commit time to meet and plan strategy instruction regularly and to share experiences in strategy instruction. Simultaneously, the university researchers would gather data from the teachers' classrooms to assess the efficacy of strategy instruction on student learning and student perceptions of the benefits of strategy instruction. Moreover, teachers' reactions to their experiences in strategy instruction would be analyzed (e.g., through teachers' reflective journals).

A community of practice that pursues strategy instruction with single-mindedness may be a step in the right direction in our attempt to immerse students in strategy instruction because, as community members, supported by university researchers, the teachers will effect sustained and systematic instruction of cognitive strategies. More important, teachers in their own schools can be the best recruiters of peers to join the community of practice because of extant friendship/rapport and because there would be no top-down pressure from administrators to teach strategies. Moreover, the network of colleagual support between university researchers and teachers can withstand the absence of support from administrators. When teachers from different but consecutive grades within the same school become members of this community of practice and engage in strategy instruction across the curriculum, students with LD may have the most optimal environment in developing into more strategic learners. Surely, research is called for on forming a community of practice as one way to fostering strategic learners.

References

Albertson, L. R., & Billingsley, F. F. (1997, March). *Improving young writers planning and reviewing skills while story writing.* Paper presented to the annual meeting of the American Educational Research Association, Chicago.

Alexander, P. A., Garner, R., Sperl, C. T., & Hare, V. C. (1998). Fostering reading competence in students with learning disabilities. In B. Y. L. Wong (Ed.), *Learning about learning disabilities* (pp. 343–366). New York: Academic Press.

Alley, G., & Deshler, D. (1979). *Teaching the learning-disabled adolescent: Strategies and methods.* Denver, CO: Love.

Andrews, J., & Lupart, J. (1993). *The inclusive classroom: Educating exceptional children.* Scarborough, Ontario, Canada: Nelson Canada.

Bandura, A. (1993). Perceived self-efficacy in cognitive development and functioning. *Educational Psychologist, 28,* 117–148.

Bednarczyk, A. (1991). *The effectiveness of story grammar instruction with a self-instructional strategy development framework for students with learning disabilities.* Unpublished doctoral dissertation, University of Maryland, College Park.

Borkowski, J. G. (1992). Metacognitive theory: A framework for teaching literacy, writing, and math skills. *Journal of Learning Disabilities, 25,* 253–257.

Borkowski, J. G., Day, J. D., Saenz, D., Dretmeyer, D., Estrada, T. M., & Groteluschen, A. (1992). Expanding the boundaries of cognitive interventions. In B. Y. L. Wong (Ed.), *Contemporary intervention research in learning disabilities* (pp. 1–21). New York: Springer-Verlag.

Brown, A. L. (1980). Metacognitive development and reading. In R. J. Spiro, B. C. Bruce, & W. F. Brewer (Eds.), *Theoretical issues in reading comprehension: Perspectives from cognitive psychology, linguistics, artificial intelligence, and education* (pp. 453–481). Hillsdale, NJ: Erlbaum.

Brown, A. L. (1987). Metacognition, executive control, self-regulation, and other more mysterious mechanisms. In F. E. Weinert & R. H. Kluwe (Eds.), *Metacognition, motivation, and understanding* (pp. 65–116). Hillsdale, NJ: Erlbaum.

Brown, A., Campione, J., & Day, (1981). Learning to learn: On training students to learn from text. *Educational Researcher, 10,* 14–21.

Brown, A. L., & Palincsar, A. S. (1982). Inducing strategic learning from texts by means of informed, self-control training. *Topics in Learning and Learning Disabilities, 2*(1), 1–17.

Butler, D. L. (1993). *Promoting strategic learning by adults with learning disabilities: An alternative approach.* Unpublished doctoral dissertation, Simon Fraser University, Burnaby, BC.

Butler, D. L. (1994). From learning strategies to strategic learning: Promoting self-regulated learning by post secondary students with learning disabilities. *Canadian Journal of Special Education, 4,* 69–101.

Butler, D. L. (1995). Promoting strategic learning by post secondary students with learning disabilities. *Journal of Learning Disabilities, 28,* 170–190.

Butler, D. L. (1998a). In search of the architect of learning: A commentary on scaffolding as a metaphor for instructional interactions. *Journal of Learning Disabilities,* 31 (4), 374–385.

Butler, D. L. (1998b). Metacognition and learning disabilities. In B. Y. L. Wong (ed.), *Learning about learning disabilities* (2nd ed.) (pp. 277–307). Toronto: Academic Press.

Butler, D. L. (1998c). A Strategic Content Learning approach to promoting self-regulated learning. In B. J. Zimmerman & D. Schunk (Eds.), *Developing self-regulated learning: From teaching to self-reflective practice* (pp. 160–183). New York: Guildford Press.

Butler, D. L. (1998d). The Strategic Content Learning approach to promoting self-regulated learning: A summary of three studies. *Journal of Educational Psychology, 90,* 682–697.

Butler, D. L. (1999, April). *Identifying and remediating students' inefficient approaches to tasks.* Paper presented at the annual meeting of the American Educational Research Association, Montreal, Quebec, Canada.

Butler, D. L. (in press). Individualizing instruction in self-regulated learning. *Theory into Practice.*

Butler, D. L., Elaschuk, C. L., & Poole, S. (2000). Promoting strategic writing by postsecondary students with learning disabilities: A report of three case studies. *Learning Disability Quarterly, 23,* 196–213.

Butler, D. L., Elaschuk, C. L., Poole, S., MacLeod, W. B., & Syer, K. (1997, June). *Teaching peer tutors to support strategic learning by post-secondary students with learning disabilities.* Papaer presented at the annual meeting of the Canadian Society for Studies in Education, St. John's, NF, Canada.

Butler, D. L., Elaschuk, C. L., Poole, S. L., Novak, H. J., Jarvis, S., & Beckingham, B. (2000, April). *Investigating an application of strategic content learning: Promoting strategy development in group contexts.* Paper presented at the annual meeting of the American Educational Research Association. New Orleans, LA.

Butler, D. L., Jarvis, S., Beckingham, B., Novak, H., & Elaschuk, C. L. (2001). *Teachers as facilitators of students' strategic performance: promoting academic success by secondary students with learning difficulties.* Paper presented at the annual meeting of the American Educational Research Association, Seattle.

Butler, D. L., Novak, H., Beckingham, B., Jarvis, S., & Elaschuk, C. L. (2000). *Professional development and meaningful change: towards sustaining an instructional innovation.* Paper presented at the annual meeting of the American Educational Research Association, Seattle.

Butler, D. L., & Winne, P. H. (1995). Feedback and self-regulated learning: A theoretical synthesis. *Review of Educational Research, 65,* 245–281.

Case, L., Harris, K. R., & Graham, S. (1992). Improving the mathematical problem solving skills of students with learning disabilities and self-regulated strategy development. *Journal of Special Education, 26,* 1–19.

Case, L., Mamlin, N., Harris, K., & Graham, S. (1995). Self-regulated strategy development: A theoretical and practical perspective. In T. Scruggs & M. Mastropieri (Eds.), *Research in learning and behavioral disabilities* (pp. 21–46). Greenwich, CT: JAI Press.

Collins, R. (1992). *Narrative writing of option II students: The effects of combining the whole-language techniques, writing process approach and strategy training.* Unpublished thesis, State University of New York, Buffalo.

Danoff, B., Harris, K. R., & Graham, S. (1993). Incorporating strategy instruction within the writing process in the regular classroom. *Journal of Reading Behavior, 25,* 295–322.

De La Paz, S. (1999). Self-regulated strategy instruction in regular education settings: Improving outcomes for students with and without learning disabilities. *Learning Disabilities Research and Practice, 14,* 92–106.

De La Paz, S. (2001). Teaching writing to students with attention deficit disorders and specific language impairment. *Journal of Educational Research, 95,* 37–47.

De La Paz, S., & Graham, S. (2001). *Strategy instruction in planning: Enhancing the planning behavior and writing performance of middle school students.* Manuscript submitted for publication.

De La Paz, S., Owen, B., Harris, K. R., & Graham, S. (2000). Riding Elvis' motorcycle: Using self-regulated strategy development to PLAN and WRITE for a state exam. *Learning Disabilities Research and Practice, 15*(2), 101–109.

Deshler, D., Alley, G., Warner, M., & Schumaker, J. (1981). Instructional practices for promoting skill acquisition in severely learning disabled adolescents. *Learning Disability Quarterly, 4,* 415–421.

Dole, J. A., Duffy, G. G., Roehler, L. R., & Pearson, P. D. (1991). Moving from the old to the new: Research on reading comprehension instruction. *Review of Educational Research, 61,* 239–264.

Duffy, G. G. (2002). The case for direct explanation of strategies. In C. C. Block & M. Pressley (Eds.), *Comprehension instruction: Research-based best practices* (pp. 28–41). New York: Guilford Press.

Ellis, E. S. (1993). Integrative strategy instruction: A potential model for teaching content area subjects to adolescents with learning disabilities. *Journal of Learning Disabilities, 26,* 358–383, 398.

Ellis, E. S., & Colvert, G. (1996). Writing strategy instruction. In D. D. Deshler, E. S. Ellis, & B. K. Lenz (Eds.), *Teaching adolescents with learning disabilities: Strategies and methods* (2nd ed., pp. 127–170). Denver, CO: Love.

Ellis, E. S., & Larkin, M. J. (1998). Adolescents with learning disabilities. In B. Y. L. Wong (Ed.), *Learning about learning disabilities* (2nd ed., pp. 557–584). San Diego, CA: Academic Press.

Englert, C. S., & Mariage, T. V. (1991). Making students partners in the comprehension process: Organizing the reading "POSSE." *Learning Disability Quarterly, 14,* 123–138.

Englert, C. S., Raphael, T. E., & Anderson, L. M. (1992). Socially mediated instruction: Improving students' knowledge and talk about writing. *Elementary School Journal, 92,* 411–449.

Englert, C. S., Raphael, T. E., Anderson, L. M., Anthony, H. M., Fear, K. L., & Gregg, S. L. (1988). A case for writing intervention: Strategies for writing informational text. *Learning Disabilities Focus, 3*(2), 98–113.

Englert, C. S., Raphael, T. E., Anderson, L., Anthony, H., Stevens, D., & Fear, K. (1991). Making writing strategies and self-talk visible: Cognitive strategy instruction in writing in regular and special education classrooms. *American Educational Research Journal, 28,* 337–373.

Flavell, J. H. (1976). Metacognitive aspects of problem solving. In L. B. Resnick (Ed.), *The nature of intelligence* (pp. 231–235). Hillsdale, NJ: Erlbaum.

Flower, L. S., & Hayes, J. R. (1980). The dynamics of composing: Making plans and juggling constraints. In L. W. Gregg & E. R. Steinberg (Eds.), *Cognitive processes in writing* (pp. 31–50). Hillsdale, NJ: Erlbaum.

Fulk, B. M. (1994). Mnemonic keyword strategy training for students with learning disabilities. *Learning Disabilities Research and Practice, 9,* 179–195.

Gaskins, L., Cunicelli, E. A., & Satlow, E. (1992). Implementing an across-the-curriculum strategies program: Teachers' reactions to change. In M. Pressley, K. R. Harris, & J. T. Guthrie (Eds.), *Promoting academic competence and literacy in school* (pp. 407–426). San Diego, CA: Academic Press.

Graham, S. (1982). Written composition research and practice: A unified approach. *Focus on Exceptional Children, 14,* 1–16.

Graham, S., & Harris, K. R. (1989a). A components analysis of cognitive strategy instruction: Effects on learning disabled students' compositions and self-efficacy. *Journal of Educational Psychology, 81,* 353–361.

Graham, S., & Harris, K. R. (1989b). Improving learning disabled students' skills at composing essays: Self-instructional strategy training. *Exceptional Children, 56,* 201–216.

Graham, S., & Harris, K. R. (1993). Teaching writing strategies to students with learning disabilities: Issues and recommendations. In L. J. Meltzer (Ed.), *Strategy assessment and instruction for students with learning disabilities: From theory to practice* (pp. 271–292). Austin, TX: Pro-Ed.

Graham, S., Harris, K. R., MacArthur, C. A., & Schwartz, S. (1991). Writing and writing instruction for students with learning disabilities: Review of a research program. *Learning Disability Quarterly, 14,* 89–114.

Graham, S., Harris, K. R., & Sawyer, R. (1987). Composition instruction with learning disabled students: Self-instructional strategy training. *Focus on Exceptional Children, 20*(4), 1–11.

Graham, S., Schwartz, S. S., & MacArthur, C. A. (1993). Knowledge of writing and the composing process, attitude toward writing, and self-efficacy for students with and without learning disabilities. *Journal of Learning Disabilities, 26*(4), 237–249.

Harris, K. R. (1980). The sustained effects of cognitive modification and informed teachers on children's communication apprehension. *Communication Quarterly, 24,* 47–57.

Harris, K. R. (1982). Cognitive-behavior modification: Application with exceptional students. *Focus on Exceptional Children, 15* (2), 1–16.

Harris, K. R., & Alexander, P. A. (1998). Integrated, constructivist education: Challenge and reality. *Educational Psychology Review, 10*(2), 115–127.

Harris, K. R., & Graham, S., (1992). Self-regulated strategy development: A part of the writing process. In M. Pressley, K. E. Harris, & J. T. Guthrie (Eds.), *Promoting academic competence and literacy in school* (pp. 277–309). New York: Academic Press.

Harris, K. R., & Graham, S. (1994). Constructivism: Principles, paradigms, and integration. *Journal of Special Education, 28,* 233–247.

Harris, K. R., & Graham, S. (1996). *Making the writing process work: Strategies for composition and self-regulation.* Cambridge, MA: Brookline.

Harris, K. R., & Graham, S. (1999). Programmatic intervention research: Illustrations from the evolution of self-regulated strategy development. *Learning Disability Quarterly, 22,* 251–262.

Hutchinson, N. L. (1993). Effects of cognitive strategy instruction on algebra problem solving of adolescents with learning disabilities. *Learning Disability Quarterly, 16,* 34–43.

Jitendra, A. K., & Hoff, K. E. (1995). *Schema-based instruction on word problem solving per-*

formance of students with learning disabilities. East Lansing, MI: National Center for Research on Teacher Training. (ERIC Document Reproduction Service No. ED 381 990)

Johnson, L., Graham, S., & Harris, K. R. (1997). The effects of goal setting and self-instruction on learning a reading comprehension strategy among students with learning disabilities. *Journal of Learning Disabilities, 30*(l), 80–91.

Kamann, M. P., & Butler, D. L. (1996, April). *Strategic content learning: An analysis of instructional features.* Paper presented at the annual meeting of the American Educational Research Association, New York.

Kamann, M. P., & Wong, B. Y. L. (1993). Inducing adaptive coping self-statements in children with learning disabilities through self-instruction training. *Journal of Learning Disabilities, 26*(9), 630–638.

Larkin, M. J. & Ellis, E. S. (1998). Adolescents with learning disabilities. In B. Y. L. Wong (Ed.), *Learning about learning disabilities* (2nd ed., pp. 557–584). Toronto: Academic Press.

Lave, J., & Wenger, E. (1991). *Situated learning: Legitimate peripheral participation.* Cambridge, UK: Press Syndicate of the University of Cambridge.

Lenz, K. B., Bulgren, J., & Hudson, P. (1990). Content enhancement: A model for promoting the acquisition of content by individuals with learning disabilities. In T. E. Scruggs & B. Y. L. Wong (Eds.), *Intervention research in learning disabilities* (pp. 122–165). New York: Springer-Verlag.

MacArthur, C. A., Graham, S., Schwartz, S., & Shafer, W. (1995). Evaluation of a writing instruction model that integrated a process approach, strategy instruction, and word processing. *Learning Disability Quarterly, 18,* 278–291.

MacArthur, C. A., Schwartz, S., & Graham, S. (1991). Effects of a reciprocal peer revision strategy in special education classrooms. *Learning Disabilities Research and Practice, 6,* 201–210.

MacArthur, C., Schwartz, S., Graham, S., Molloy, D., & Harris, K. R. (1996). Integration of strategy instruction into a whole language classroom: A case study. *Learning Disabilities Research and Practice, 11*(3), l68–l76.

Mann, V. (1998). Language problems: A key to early reading problems. In B. Y. L. Wong (Ed.), *Learning about learning disabilities* (pp. 163–201). New York: Academic Press.

Mastropieri, M. A., Scruggs, T. E. (1989). Constructing more meaningful relationships: Mnemonic instruction for special populations. *Educational Psychology Review, 1*(2), 83–111.

Mastropieri, M. A., Scruggs, T. E., & Chung, S. (1998). Instructional interventions for students with mathematics learning disabilities. In B. Y. L. Wong (Ed.), *Learning about learning disabilities* (pp. 425–451). New York: Academic Press.

Mastropieri, M. A., Scruggs, T. E., & Shiah, S. (1991). Mathematics instruction with learning disabled students: A review of research. *Learning Disabilities Research and Practice, 6,* 89–98.

Mayer, R. E. (2001). What good is educational psychology? The case of cognition and instruction. *Educational Psychologist, 36*(2), 83–88.

Meichenbaum, D. H. (1977). *Cognitive behavior modification.* New York: Plenum Press.

Miller, G. E., & Brewster, M. E. (1992). Developing self-sufficient learners in reading and mathematics through self-instructional training. In M. Pressley, K. E. Harris, & J. T. Guthrie (Eds.), *Promoting academic competence and literacy in school* (pp. 169–222). New York: Academic Press.

Miller, S. P., & Mercer, C. D. (1993). Using a graduated word problem sequence to promote problem-solving skills. *Learning Disabilities Research and Practice, 8,* 169–174.

Montague, M. (1992). The effects of cognitive and metacognitive strategy instruction on mathematical problem solving of middle school students with learning disabilities. *Journal of Learning Disabilities, 25,* 230–248.

Montague, M. (1997). Cognitive strategy instruction in mathematics for students with learning disabilities. *Journal of Learning Disabilities, 30*(2), 164–177.

Montague, M., & Bos, C. (1986). The effect of cognitive strategy training on verbal math problem solving performance of learning disabled adolescents. *Journal of Learning Disabilities, 19,* 26–33.

Montague, M., Applegate, B., & Marquard, K. (1993). Cognitive strategy instruction and mathematical problem-solving performance of students with learning disabilities. *Learning Disabilities Research and Practice, 8,* 223–232.

National Institute of Child Health and Human Development. (2000). *Teaching children to read: An evidence-based assessment of the scientific research literature on reading and its implications for reading instruction* [Report of the National Reading Panel] (NIH Publication No. 00–4769). Washington, DC: U.S. Government Printing Office.

Nolen, S. B. (1988). Reasons for studying: Motivational orientations and study strategies. *Cognition and Instruction, 5*(4), 269–287.

Palincsar, A. S., & Brown, A. L. (1984). Reciprocal teaching of comprehension-fostering and comprehension monitoring activities. *Cognition and Instruction, 1,* 117–175.

Palincsar, A. S., & Brown, A. L. (1988). Teaching and practicing thinking skills to promote comprehension in the context of group problem solving. *Remedial and Special Education, 9*(1), 53–59.

Palincsar, A. S., Magnusson, S. J., Collins, K. M., & Cutter, J. (2000). Making science accessible to all: Results of a design experiment in inclusive classrooms. *Learning Disability Quarterly, 24,* 15–32.

Paris, S. G., Cross, D. R., & Lipson, M. Y. (1984). Informed strategies for learning: A program to improve children's reading awareness and comprehension. *Journal of Educational Psychology, 76,* 1239–1252.

Paris, S. G., & Jacobs, J. E. (1984). The benefit of informed instruction for children's reading awareness and comprehension skills. *Child Development, 55,* 2083–2093.

Paris, S. G., & Newman, R. S. (1990). Developmental aspects of self-regulated learning. *Educational Psychologist, 25*(1), 87–102.

Paris, S. G., & Paris, A. H. (2001). Classroom applications of research on Self-Regulated Learning. *Educational Psychologist, 36(2),* 89–101.

Paris, S. G., & Winograd, P. (1990). How metacognition can promote academic learning and instruction. In B. F. Jones & L. Idol (Eds.), *Dimensions of thinking and cognitive instruction* (pp. 15–51). Hillsdale, NJ: Erlbaum.

Perry, N. E., & VandeKamp, K. J. O. (2000). Creating classroom contexts that support young children's development of self-regulated learning. *International Journal of Educational Research, 33,* 821–843.

Pressley, M. (1998). *Reading instruction that works: The case for balanced teaching.* New York: Guilford Press.

Pressley, M., El-Dinary, P. B., Gaskins, I. W., Schuder, T., Bergman, J. L., Almasi, J., & Brown, R. (1992). Beyond direct explanation: Transactional instruction of reading comprehension strategies. *Elementary School Journal, 92,* 513–555.

Pressley, M., & Harris, K. R. (2001). Cognitive strategies instruction. In A. L. Costa (Ed.), *Developing minds: A resource book for teaching thinking* (3rd ed., pp. 466–471). Alexandria, VA: Association for Supervision and Curriculum Development.

Salomon, G., & Perkins, D. N. (1989). Rocky roads to transfer: Rethinking mechanisms of a neglected phenomenon. *Educational Psychologist, 24,* 113–142.

Sawyer, R. J., Graham, S., & Harris, K. R. (1992). Direct teaching, strategy instruction, and strategy instruction with explicit self-regulation: Effects on learning disabled students' composition skills and self-efficacy. *Journal of Educational Psychology, 84,* 340–352.

Schumaker, J. B., & Deshler, D. D. (1992). Validation of learning strategy interventions for students with LD: Results of a programmatic research effort. In B. Y. L. Wong (Ed.), *Contemporary intervention research in learning disabilities: an international perspective* (pp. 22–46). New York: Springer-Verlag.

Schumaker, J. B., Deshler, D. D., Alley, G. R., Warner, M. M., & Denton, P. H. (1982). Multipass: A learning strategy for improving reading comprehension. *Learning Disability Quarterly, 5,* 295–304.

Schumaker, J. B., & Lyerla, K. (1991). *The paragraph writing strategy: Instructor's manual.* Lawrence: University of Kansas Institute for Research in Learning Disabilities.

Schumaker, J. B., Nolan, S. M., & Deshler, D. D. (1985). *The error monitoring strategy.* Learning strategies curriculum, University of Kansas, Lawrence.

Schumaker, J. B., & Sheldon, J. (1985). *The sentence writing strategy: Instructor's manual.* Lawrence, KS: Edge Enterprise.

Schunk, D. H. (1994). Self-regulation of self-efficacy and attributions in academic settings. In D. H. Schunk & B. J. Zimmerman (Eds.), *Self-regulation of learning and performance: Issues and educational applications* (pp. 75–99). Hillsdale, NJ: Erlbaum.

Scruggs, T. E., & Mastropieri, M. A. (1990). The case for mnemonic instruction: From laboratory research to classroom applications. *Journal of Special Education, 24*(1), 7–32.

Scruggs, T. E., & Mastropieri, M. A. (1992). Classroom applications of mnemonics instruction: Acquisition, maintenance, and generalization. *Exceptional Children, 58,* 219–229.

Sexton, M., Harris, K. R., & Graham, S. (1998). Self-regulated strategy development and the writing process: Effects on essay writing and attributions. *Exceptional Children, 64*(3), 295–311.

Stone, C. A. (1998). The metaphor of scaffolding: Its utility for the field of learning disabilities. *Journal of Learning Disabilities, 31*(4), 344–364.

Tanhouser, S. (1994). *Function over form: The relative efficacy of self-instructional strategy training alone and with procedural facilitation for adolescents with learning disabilities.* Unpublished doctoral dissertation, Johns Hopkins University.

Trabasso, T., & Bouchard, E. (2002). Teaching readers how to comprehend text strategically. In C. C. Block & M. Pressley (Eds.), *Comprehension instruction: Research-based best practices* (pp. 176–200). New York: Guilford Press.

Vogel, S. A., & Adelman, P. B. (1990). Intervention effectiveness at the postsecondary level for the learning disabled. In T. Scruggs & B. Y. L. Wong (Eds.), *Intervention research in learning disabilities* (pp. 329–344). New York: Springer-Verlag.

Weiner, B. (1974). An attributional interpretation of expectancy-value theory. In B. Weiner (Ed.), *Cognitive views of human motivation* (pp. 51–69). New York: Academic Press.

Willis, S. (1993). Whole language in the '90s. *ASCD Update, 35*(9), 1–8.

Winne, P. H., & Perry, N. E. (2000). Measuring self-regulated learning. In P. Pintrich, M. Boekarts, & M. Zeidner (Eds.), *Handbook of self-regulation* (pp. 531–566). Orlando, FL: Academic Press.

Wong, B. Y. L. (1994). Instructional parameters promoting transfer of learned strategies in students with learning disabilities. *Learning Disability Quarterly, 17*(2), 110–120.

Wong, B. Y. L. (1999). Metacognition in writing. In R. Gallimore, C. Bernheimer, D. MacMillan, D. Speece, & S. Vaughn (Eds.), *Developmental perspectives on children with high incidence disabilities: papers in honor of Barbara K. Keogh* (pp. 183–198). Hillsdale, NJ: Erlbaum.

Wong, B. Y. L., Butler, D. L., Ficzere, S. A., & Kuperis, S. (1996). Teaching adolescents with learning disabilities and low achievers to plan, write, and revise opinion essays. *Journal of Learning Disabilities, 29*(2), 197–212.

Wong, B. Y. L., Butler, D. L., Ficzere, S. A., & Kuperis, S. (1997). Teaching adolescents with learning disabilities and low achievers to plan, write, and revise compare-and-contrast essays. *Learning Disabilities Research and Practice, 12*(1), 2–15.

Wong, B. Y. L., Butler, D. L., Ficzere, S. A., Kuperis, S., & Corden, M. (1994). Teaching problem learners revision skills and sensitivity to audience through two instructional modes: Student-teacher versus student—student interactive dialogues. *Learning Disabilities Research and Practice, 9*(2), 78–90.

Wong, B. Y. L., Wong, R., & Blenkinsop, J. (1989). Cognitive and metacognitive aspects of learning disabled adolescents' composing problems. *Learning Disability Quarterly, 12*(4), 300–322.

Wong, B. Y. L., Wong, R., Darlington, D., & Jones, W. (1991). Interactive teaching: An effective way to teach revision skills to adolescents with learning disabilities. *Learning Disabilities Research and Practice, 6*(2), 117–127.

Wray, D. (1994). *Literacy and awareness.* London: Hodder & Stoughton.

Zajonc, R. B. (1980). Feeling and thinking: Preferences need no inferences. *American Psychologist, 35,* 151–175.

Zimmerman, B. J. (1989). A social-cognitive view of self-regulated learning. *Journal of Educational Psychology, 81,* 329–339.

Zimmerman, B. J. (1994). Dimensions of academic self-regulation: A conceptual framework for education. In D. H. Schunk & B. J. Zimmerman (Eds.), *Self-regulation of learning and performance: Issues and educational applications* (pp. 3–21). Hillsdale, NJ: Erlbaum.

24

Direct Instruction

Gary Adams
Douglas Carnine

The field of education has a long history of wrangling about educational issues with each side often having little or no research evidence to substantiate their claims. A major change has occurred in the last decade. It seems that there has been a heightened interest in looking at the actual research behind various claims. Some of these efforts have been by researchers (e.g., Chall, 2000) and national organizations both individually (e.g., the American Federation of Teachers, www.aft.org/edissues/whatworks/index) and collectively through funding of reports by research groups such as the American Institutes for Research (*An Educators' Guide to Schoolwide Reform,* www.assa.org/reforms) or the private or publicly funded meta-analyses such as the one conducted by Swanson, Lee, and Hoskyn (1999). Most recently, the Direct Instruction model was selected.

One of the consistent finding of these reviews has been the superiority of Direct Instruction programs for achieving academic success in comparison to other published programs. These results match the meta-analysis about Direct Instruction conducted by Adams (Adams & Engelmann, 1996). With effect sizes in the large range (over 0.75) as described in this chapter, Direct Instruction programs must be considered extremely effective. Though most of these reviews have focused on students who are loosely described as at risk for school failure, this chapter provides a meta-analysis of Direct Instruction with studies that limited to those involving students with learning disabilities.

Any discussion about the research on Direct Instruction has to start with a clarification of its definition. Although the term has been around for decades, it is still misused by many education professors and others. Direct Instruction is *not* teacher-directed instruction with an emphasis on lecturing. Teacher-directed instruction is often contrasted to what is described as "child-centered instruction." Direct Instruction is very teacher-directed, but the terms are not synonymous. Also, Direct Instruction is *not* direct instruction. The term "direct instruction" is often associated with research showing that certain educational techniques and methods (pacing, choral responses, cuing, etc.) have resulted in accelerated academic success. However, as Slavin (1989) notes, the research on Madeline Hunter's program showed that just training teachers to use many direct instruction techniques does not necessarily lead to improved student academic achievement.

When someone says that they have created a Direct Instruction program, it means that the person has mixed up "direct instruction" with "Direct Instruction." They usually describe how they have developed several lessons based on direct instruction principles. In contrast, Direct Instruction refers to published curricula developed by Engelmann and associates. Each curriculum usually contains one-half to 1 school year of lessons. A distinctive feature of these curricula is that have been field-tested with students using a three-stage curriculum-testing process (Adams & Engelmann, 1996). Many teachers assume that most available curricula have been field-tested on students before publication; unfortunately, that is not true. Unfortunately, most curricula are written by curriculum developers and then just published. No effort is made to see if the programs actually work with students. This lack of effort leads to an interesting observation that many important products in our lives must pass certain minimum standards (e.g., automobiles, car seats, and toys), and yet in regard to one of the important activities in our children's lives (their education), the curricula they use are not tested on children before publication.

Over the last three decades, many Direct Instruction programs have been created. Several have had multiple revisions. Appendix 24.1 provides a list of Direct Instruction programs that are frequently used with students with learning disabilities.

For those who are unfamiliar with Direct Instruction programs, the following are many characteristics of Englemann and associates' Direct Instruction (DI) programs.

Before Implementation

Teachers are expected to be trained on how to use each program before implementing the program. Training is important because many features must be implemented in a specific way that may not seem intuitive. For example, when students make errors, teachers tend to slow down the lesson pacing. However, the pacing of DI lessons must be brisk (as supported by research studies).

Competent training requires training teachers to mastery and providing the rationales for the DI features. Many teachers are unable to receive training; training is not required for purchasing. For those teachers, each DI program has a teacher's guide describing how the program should be taught with the program's scope-and-sequence chart describing what will be taught.

The next step is to assess the students using the program's placement test. Students will be at different starting points because of diverse skill levels. Students are grouped homogeneously per program into groups of usually no more than 14 students. The intent of this grouping is to ensure that students are with other students at their current skill level for that subject so that they are not overwhelmed because the content is beyond them or bored because the content is below them.

The Lesson

Lessons last for 35–45 minutes and contain 12–20 tasks. The first part of lesson uses a group format and then students complete their individual workbooks to practice the skill being taught in the lesson. The teacher follows the lesson script, which is in the program's Teacher Presentation Book. What the teacher says is printed in colored ink, what the teacher does is in parentheses, and the expected student response is in italics. Also, the specific correction procedure is given. Corrections are treated as opportunities for reteaching without the often typical negative connotation; instead, the teacher gives the correct answer and the students then take turns to provide the correct response. Some of the reasons scripting is used are that it standardizes the wording from task to task across lessons and the length of each lesson is controlled based on prior program field-testing experience. Through using a script, the teacher can quickly provide many succinct examples that are not too wordy.

Probably one of the notable characteristics of DI lessons is brisk pacing. A lot of information is covered and the rapid pacing has been shown to reduce the number of behavior management problems because students are on task. Also, when complex tasks are presented slowly, students have a more difficult time understanding what is being presented. To ensure that the pacing is brisk, the teacher uses signals to ensure that the entire group responds at the same time. From this pacing, the teacher can tell if the students understand what is being presented and can tell which students need more practice. The specific signals are described in the Series Guide. To ensure that all students understand the information, the teacher asks individual students to respond to designated exercises.

After the group exercises are presented, students complete exercises in individual workbooks. The exercises match the content taught in the group lesson and demonstrates each student's mastery of the content.

Each program has a point system. This system is not only for behavior management but also the basis of student grading. Students track their daily grades and, thus, know how well they are doing. Likewise, teachers can tell when students lack certain content, which needs to be retaught.

An Example: Using Corrective Reading

The Corrective Reading program was developed for upper elementary and secondary students with reading deficits. There are three levels (A, B, and C) of Decoding and Comprehension; the B level is split into two parts (B1 and B2). Table 24.1 provides a summary of content taught at each level as adapted from the Corrective Reading Series Guide (Engelmann, Hanner, & Johnson, 1999).

The following scenario would be appropriate for a special education teacher at above the fourth-grade level. The Corrective Reading Series Guide contains the Corrective Reading Decoding and Comprehension Placement Tests, which can be reproduced. The test is administered individually and it takes approximately 10–15 minutes to administer both tests. In general, most students test one level higher in decoding than in comprehension. Because most students have decoding and comprehension deficits, the teacher must figure out a teaching strategy. If the teacher decides to provide instruction in both decoding and comprehension instruction, each lesson takes approximately 45 minutes. For secondary students with severe reading deficits, this strategy is efficient because students can master the necessary reading skills needed for reading and comprehending English, history, science, and other textbooks. However, this strategy may not fit many school situations. The Series Guide provides several other possible strategies for implementations.

Following in this example, all the students who placed at a B1 Decoding level would be in a group. In most special education programs, this means a group of less than 10 students. The students are grouped in a semicircle around a teacher at the chalkboard with the lowest readers in the middle of the group so that they are easier to monitor. With the B1 Decoding Presentation Guide, the teacher reads the script at a brisk pace. Some of lesson's exercises include practice with segmenting and blending sounds. Other exercises practice word identification on the chalkboard. Every few lessons, the teacher provides individual turns to ensure that all students have mastered the content, and not just parroted other students' responses. What many teachers often do not realize is that the words in the exercise are being systematically introduced. Specific sounds and sound combinations are mastered based on a underlying scope-and-sequence chart and taught in a cumulative manner.

The lesson is kept at a brisk pace because the teacher is using signals to ensure that all students are responding at the same time. If that does not happen, the teacher models the correct response and restarts the task. One of the major noticeable differences between DI programs and other programs is the emphasis on the positive. The assumption of DI programs is that when you are learning something new you make mistakes. Thus the correction involves teacher modeling and then a reintroduction of the task. This is unlike other instruction, which often involves long, wordy corrections, which often interfere with the process of concept teaching. For an observer who does not know the research underpinnings behind Direct Instruction, the use of a script and the rapid pacing during the group instruction time may seem artificial and "drill and kill."

After approximately 30 minutes of group work, each student does independent work. The focus of the independent work involves

TABLE 24.1. Overview of the DI Corrective Reading Program

Level A	Decoding: 65 lessons	Comprehension: 60 lessons
Target students	Nonreaders or those in grades 3–12 who read so haltingly they can't understand what they read	Poor readers in grades 4–12 who can't understand concepts underlying much of the material being taught
What is taught	Word-attack skills: Phonemic awareness, sound–symbol identification, sounding out, regular and irregular words, sentence reading	Thinking skills: Deduction and induction, analogies, vocabulary, true/false, recitation, information (such as calendar skills)
Outcomes	60 wpm, 98% accuracy, reading at about a 2.5 grade level	Some higher-order thinking skills and many word definitions
Level B	Decoding: B1: 65 lessons; B2: 65 lessons	Comprehension: B1: 60 lessons; B2: 65 lessons
Target students	Poor readers in grades 3–12 who do not read at an adequate rate and who confuse words	Poor readers in grades 4–12 who have difficulty with conclusions, contradiction, written directions
What is taught	Decoding skills: Letter and word discrimination, sound and letter combinations, word endings, story reading, literal and inferential comprehension	Comprehension skills: More advanced reasoning, handling information, vocabulary, analyzing sentences, writing skills
Outcomes	B1: 90 wpm, 98% accuracy, reading at about a 3.9 grade level; B2: 120 wpm, 98% accuracy, reading at about a 4.9 grade level	A variety of comprehension skills that can be applied in all school subjects; the ability to read information and learn new facts and vocabulary
Level C	Decoding: 125 lessons	Comprehension: 140 lessons
Target students	Fair readers in grades 4–12 who have trouble with multisyllabic words and typical textbook material	Students in grade 6 and up who do not comprehend sophisticated text, do not learn well from material they read, or have trouble thinking critically
What is taught	Skill application: Additional sound combinations, affixes, vocabulary development, reading expository text, recall of events, sequencing, and building reading rate	Concept applications: Organizing and operating on information, using sources of information, communicating information
Outcomes	Over 150 wpm, reading at about a 7.0 grade level	Ability to apply analytical skill to real-life situations and answer literal and inferential questions based on passages read

the same concepts taught in the just completed lesson and other recently taught concepts using different exercises in their workbooks. From this independent practice, the teacher has an even clearer picture of each student's progress.

Points are earned for both group and individual work and these points are the basis for the student's grade. Also, students are able to chart their reading rate. This process is highly motivating for most students as they make the shift from weak to competent readers.

The example gives highlighted decoding instruction. Reading, of course, is more than decoding. The Corrective Reading Comprehension program uses the same instructional process. The content of this program focuses on information that students will need in school. For example, there is a set of lessons in the B1 and B2 programs that teaches fairly sophisticated anatomy and physiology concepts. After completing B1 and B2, students who take biology should have an excellent chance of success because they should have already mastered much of the course content.

Supplementary Direct Instruction Information

Appendix 24.2 provides the research studies behind the various aspects of the Direct Instruction model. For those who would like more information are referred elsewhere for underlying instructional design concepts (Engelmann & Carnine, 1991), Direct Instruction reading (Carnine, Silbert, & Kameenui, 1997) and Direct Instruction math (Stein, Silbert, & Carnine, 1997).

The Advantage of Meta-Analysis over Subjective Reviews

The publication of reviews using an objective meta-analysis procedure as an alternative to subjective reviews has exploded in the last decade. Rosenthal (1981) provided an early example showing the difference between subjective and objective ways of reviewing research studies. He gave a set of seven research articles to two groups of university professors and graduate students. The research studies were on the topic of gender differences on task perseverance. It is politically correct to assert that there are no differences between males and females in task persistence and, in fact, the majority of the reviewers who were asked to subjectively review the articles said that there were no significant differences. In contrast, another group of reviewers calculated effect sizes for each study. Their accurate conclusion was that there was a gender difference with females being more persistent.

The Process of Conducting a Meta-Analysis

Collecting Studies

The starting point for this review was *Research on Direct Instruction: 25 years beyond DISTAR* (Adams & Engelmann, 1996). For that book, the ERIC and Psych-Lit educational and psychological databases

were reviewed based on appropriate descriptors (e.g., Direct Instruction, DISTAR, directed instruction, Corrective Reading, Reading Mastery, direct teaching, and direct verbal instruction). For this chapter, this search was updated with articles published after 1995. Because the focus of this chapter is students with learning disabilities, only studies involving students with learning disabilities were included in this meta-analysis. This means that studies in which students were described as being in general education courses but receiving remedial services were excluded, as were studies involving students with other disabilities (e.g., mental retardation). The categorization information was somewhat straightforward for studies conducted in the United States. The decision-making process for the three studies that were not conducted in the United States was much more difficult, because the Subjects section did not provide a specific special education designation. The students were usually described as needing remedial reading services. (However, as will be shown later, the results for non-U.S. students were similar.) The result of this effort was to collect all studies with acceptable research methodology involving students with learning disabilities.

Some authors of meta-analyses include as many studies as possible on a topic, especially on topics on which there are few research studies. Other authors argue that including poorly designed studies misrepresents the actual results, because poorly designed studies may add highly variable data and possible bias. The meta-analysis described in this article is based on the latter approach. The following was the criteria for exclusion in this meta-analysis:

- The studies lacked a comparison group.
- The studies lacked pretest scores.
- The pretest scores of the DI and the comparison groups of the studies showed significant differences.
- The studies lacked the necessary mathematical information for analysis (means, standard deviations, and sample sizes).
- The studies lasted only one session.
- The Direct Instruction intervention was combined with incompatible interventions.
- The studies involved single-subject research methodology.

- The studies were analyzing Direct Instruction components (e.g., pacing).
- The studies did not involve published or prepublished Direct Instruction curricula by Engelmann and associates.

Of the more than 300 articles, book chapters, and books on Direct Instruction, only 17 were research studies that met the requirement for inclusion in this meta-analysis. In most meta-analyses, these design requirements excluded the majority of the research articles involving Direct Instruction.

Effect Size

The product of the meta-analysis is a statement about the effect of a particular experimental approach or intervention. The effect is referenced to the normal distribution curve. This curve is divided into standard deviations from the mean. Highest and lowest scores that are possible for any measurable characteristic in nature would be at the extreme ends of the curve.

For educational purposes, an intervention that changes the performance of students by one-quarter standard deviation is considered educationally significant. Educational significance is a much more important concept than traditional statistically significant differences. An outcome that creates a difference in mean scores between two groups of one-quarter standard deviation is both real and important, not a mere artifact of measurement or documentation of an insignificant clinical improvement that is stable over a large population. For example, a relatively small difference in reading program scores may result in a statistically significant difference if the researcher uses two large samples of students, but clinically the difference is insignificant.

The most effective description of the magnitude of effect sizes is by Cohen (1988) and others and has become the common standard. Effect sizes below 0.25 are thought to be insignificant. Educationally, this means that the interventions are those that should not be used in the classroom. Effect sizes that should be used in classrooms should be at least 0.25. Effect sizes between 0.25 and 0.49 are described as small effect sizes. Again, they are described

as "small," but they are educationally significant. Effect sizes from 0.50 to 0.74 are described as in the medium effect size range. Large effect sizes are effect sizes above 0.75. This measurement system is valuable when evaluating educational programs. For example, Stahl and Miller (1989) conducted a meta-analysis on whole-language/language-experience studies. They found that the average effect size was 0.09. Using the effect size framework, this approach to reading would not be recommended because it is well below the 0.25 effect size minimum for inclusion as an effective classroom practice.

Calculating Effect Size

The often-cited formula for calculating effect size is

$$\text{Effect size} = \frac{m_e - m_c}{SD_c}$$

The use of the standard deviation for the control (comparison) group has been suggested by Glass, McGaw, and Smith (1981) because that is the standard deviation scores of the existing traditional condition, and it is fairly stable. However, the use of pooled standard deviation (SD_p) was used in the current meta-analysis as recommended by Hunter, Schmidt, and Jackson (1982). Rosenthal (1992) showed that SD_p is a more stable and accurate and less influenced by population variance. The formula is:

$$\text{Effect size} = \frac{m_e - m_c}{SD_p}$$

An effect size of 0.00 means that there is no difference in mean scores between the experimental condition and the control condition. As mentioned earlier, a 0.25 effect size is described as a small effect size, but it means that it is an educational procedure that teachers should use. An effect size of 0.50 is a medium effect size and 0.75 is a large effect size (and is rare in educational research).

In *Research on Direct Instruction*, the effect sizes were calculated two different ways. Because of the similarity of results no matter which unit of analysis was used (per individual effect size or per study) and size limitations, the decision was made to use the per-study score as the unit of analysis for this meta-analysis.

Meta-Analysis Results

The average effect size for the 17 studies that included students with learning disabilities in this meta-analysis was 0.93. This result is similar to the results for students in general education classrooms (0.82) and all special education categories (0.84) in the original meta-analysis conducted by Adams in 1996.

In the following section, the average study effect size is provided with the number of studies involved in parentheses. Although there are 17 studies involved, sometimes the total number of studies is above 17. This is because some studies involved more than one variable (e.g., math and reading DI interventions).

Variable 1. Age/Grade of the Students: Compares Elementary versus Secondary Students

Studies provided age and/or grade information about the students. Kindergarten students were placed in the Elementary group and middle school/junior high school students and adults in the Secondary/Adult group. The average effect size for the 11 studies for the Elementary group was 0.73. The average effect size for the 6 studies in the Secondary/Adult group was 1.37. Based on the effect size power system described earlier, the effect size of the Elementary group also reached a large effect size and the Secondary/Adult group was a large effect size. A possible reason for the discrepancy in scores is because several of the secondary/adult studies involved the use of DI videodisc programs that proved to be powerful interventions with effect sizes over 1.50.

Variable 2. Subject: Compares Effect Sizes across Reading and Math

The analysis of reading and math effect sizes shows large effect sizes for both subjects. The average effect size for the 12 studies involving reading was 0.81 and the average effect size for the 7 studies involving math was 1.08. Both scores are in the large effect size range. Unfortunately, the data were not analyzed in such a way to parse out the effect sizes specifically in regard to decoding and comprehension in reading achievement or calculation and problem solving in math achievement. However, the effect size scores are sufficiently high to suggest that these programs should be the standard from which other reading and math programs should be compared.

Variable 3. Type of Test: Compares Outcomes Measured on Norm-Referenced and Criterion-Referenced Assessment Instruments

There are two main types of tests. Norm-referenced tests include standardized tests such as the Metropolitan Achievement Test. Criterion-referenced tests include teacher-made tests used mastery of the content being taught. The results of the analysis of test type are shown later. The average effect size for the 8 studies involving criterion-referenced measures was 1.14 and the average effect size for the 11 studies involving norm-referenced measures was 0.77. Both effect size score are in the large range and the discrepancy is expected. Norm-referenced tests usually have a wide range of items; some of which may not cover the content being taught by the specific program. In contrast, criterion-referenced tests measure the content that is being covered by the program.

Variable 4. Type of Research Design: Compares Causal-Comparative to Experimental Research Designs

Two types of research designs were included in this analysis: causal-comparative and experimental. Although there are other variables, the main difference between the two types of designs is that experimental design studies uses random assignment of students into DI or control groups. Causal-comparative design (sometimes described as quasi-experimental design) studies used intact groups without random assignment. The average effect size of the 5 causal-comparative studies was 0.90 and the average effect size of the 12 experimental studies was 0.95. Both effect size scores are in the large range. The difference in scores is insignificant.

Variable 5. Duration of Intervention: Compares Durations up to 1 Year and over 1 Year

The duration of the intervention is an important variable because some approaches produce only short-term effects. The average effect size for nine studies that lasted up to a year was 1.08 and the average effect size for the eight studies that lasted over 1 year was .77. The effect size for Direct Instruction was consistently large (over 0.75) even for interventions that lasted over 1 year. On the surface, this result may seem counterintuitive. It might be expected that the longer the intervention lasts, the larger the effect. This, however, did not occur. A possible reason is that often with interventions lasting more than 1 year, there are multiple teachers, which has the possibility of affecting the fidelity of implementation.

Variable 6. Type of Teacher: Compares Results Achieved by Experimental Teachers and Regular Teachers

An issue of concern is the potential of the intervention across a full range of teachers. If a program is effective only when implemented by highly trained, experimental teachers who are "outsiders" who carry out the specific DI intervention, its usefulness is limited because it may not have implications for the normal classroom setting. These programs are often described as laboratory studies that are often conducted in artificial nonclassroom settings. The average effect size of the 6 studies involving regular teachers was 1.24 and the average effect size of the 11 studies involving experimental teachers was 0.77. One of the complaints by critics is that high achievement scores are accomplished through the use of specially trained instructors, but the actual results show that the studies involving the students' regular teachers had higher effect size scores. A possible reason for this result may be that the regular teachers are more familiar with their students' behavior patterns, which improves the fluidity of the instruction presentations.

Variable 7. Fidelity of Implementation: Compares Studies in Which Classroom Performance Is Monitored and Adjusted to Studies without Monitoring

Even though a particular intervention is supposed to be used in the experimental condition, it is not necessarily being implemented. Studies in laboratory settings tended to have implementation checks. Studies conducted in the "real world" were less likely to include implementation checks to ensure that the planned intervention was conducted without changes in quality over time. Implementation checks include following schedules for starting and stopping instruction; following management procedures; and using designated presentation techniques, correction procedures, firming practices, and informal tests of individual students. The average effect size for the 7 studies with fidelity checks was 1.05 and the average effect size for the 10 studies without fidelity checks was 0.85. Both effect sizes are in the large range.

Variable 8. Country: Compares Results in the United States to Results from Other Countries

An interesting issue is the country in which the study was conducted. In general, studies conducted in the United States tended to have the technical components for inclusion in this meta-analysis. The average effect size for the 14 studies that were conducted in the United States was 0.89 and the average effect size of the 3 studies that were not conducted in the United States was 1.12. Again, both effect sizes are in the large range. It might be questionable to overgeneralize too much from the three non-U.S. studies. However, the result was similar to other comparisons—an effect size score in the large range. There were many non-U.S. studies, especially conducted in Australia. Unfortunately, these studies were not included because they lacked the research methodological requirements to be included in this meta-analysis.

Table 24.2 provides a summary of the results, including the studies that were included per variable.

TABLE 24.2. Summary of DI Statistical Analyses with Citations

Meta-analysis		Effect size	Sample size	Magnitude of effect size
If calculated per study (excludes follow-up studies)		0.93	17 studies	Large
Age/grade of students				
Studies 1, 3, 4, 6, 9, 10, 11, 12, 13, 14, 15	Elementary	0.73	11 studies	Large
Studies 2, 5, 7, 8, 16	Secondary	1.31	6 studies	Large
Academic subject				
Studies 1, 2, 3, 4, 5, 9, 10, 11, 12, 13, 14, 15	Reading	0.81	12 studies	Large
Studies 3, 6 7, 8, 11, 16	Math	1.08	7 studies	Large
Type of test				
Studies 4, 5, 6, 7, 8, 9, 16	Criterion-referenced	1.14	8 studies	Large
Studies 1, 2, 3, 5, 9, 10, 11, 12, 13, 14, 15	Norm-referenced	0.77	11 studies	Large
Type of research design				
Studies 1, 3, 10, 11, 14	Causal-comparative	0.90	5 studies	Large
Studies 2, 4, 5, 6, 7, 8, 9, 12, 13, 15, 16	Experimental	0.95	12 studies	Large
Length of intervention				
Studies 1, 4, 6, 7, 8, 12, 13, 16	Up to 1 year	1.08	9 studies	Large
Studies 2, 3, 5, 9, 10, 11, 14, 15	Over 1 year	0.77	8 studies	Large
Type of teacher				
Studies 4, 6, 7, 8, 16	Experimental	1.24	6 studies	Large
Studies 1, 2, 3, 5, 9, 10, 11, 12, 13, 14, 15	Causal-comparative	0.77	11 studies	Large
Fidelity checks				
Studies 3, 5, 6, 7, 8, 16	Yes	1.05	7 studies	Large
Studies 1, 2, 4, 9, 10, 11, 12, 13, 14, 15	No	0.85	10 studies	Large
Country				
Studies 2, 3, 4, 6, 7, 8, 10, 11, 12, 13, 14, 15, 16	United States	0.89	14 studies	Large
Studies 1, 5, 9	Non-U.S.	1.12	3 studies	Large

Note. See p. 416 for a listing of the studies cited.

Summary

No matter which of the eight variables were analyzed, the results (16 effect sizes) are consistently high favoring Direct Instruction. Almost all the effect sizes were in the large range (over 0.75) from 0.73 to 1.26. These results should quiet critics who make subjective comments about the effectiveness of Direct Instruction. The research evidence is simply overwhelmingly favorable. A review of the research on other educational interventions shows that Direct Instruction programs should definitely be considered as a standard for evidence-based best practices.

There are many reasons why these findings should not be unexpected. The components of Direct Instruction programs are based on research studies. What is being taught is clearly explained in each program series guide. In fact, many special education teachers use the scope-and-sequence chart in each series guide as a source for creating their students' individualized education plan goals and objectives. Also, many of the programs (e.g., Corrective Reading) have been revised several times with modifications based on the newest educational research.

One of the main reasons that these programs are successful is that they are field-tested on students. Many original lessons are modified many times or abandoned during the field-testing process. Teacher or student confusion or the lack of student mastery results in revision until the confusion is resolved and mastery is demonstrated. Then the curriculum is published. In contrast, other curricula are just published. When teachers and students start using those curricula, they become product testers without a way of having "bug fixes." The bugs result in teacher and student frustration and also a lack of student achievement.

Though the findings in this meta-analysis clearly indicate the potential of the Direct Instruction programs to serve as powerful instructional tools to assist teachers in improving the performance of students identified as learning disabled, using Direct Instruction is not a panacea. The student learning that occurs for children in Direct Instruction programs depends on how well the programs are taught, which in turn often depends on how well a school is organized to support the use of the Direct Instruction programs. For example, when students begin the Corrective Reading program, a placement test is given to determine the level at which students are to begin instruction. Once the students begin instruction, some students may progress at a much faster rate than others. Ideally, these students should be grouped with other children who can progress at the same rate. Schools which are organized to allow for flexible grouping will allow for maximum progress by all students.

To ensure that Direct Instruction is well taught from classroom to classroom, an infrastructure of trainers and coaches skilled with Direct Instruction should be established. Teachers will need varying degrees of support in learning the techniques incorporated into the Direct Instruction programs. For some teachers, a good deal of coaching will be needed to help them spot and immediately correct student errors, pace the lesson quickly, and use positive behavior management techniques. Districts and schools that can provide this support will find more consistent increases in student performance with Direct Instruction.

On a purely scientific basis, it would be expected that Direct Instruction programs would be highly accepted based on probable achievement scores. Instead, they are often highly scorned. A major reason is one of the main features of Direct Instruction programs—the use of scripts. It is apparent that many teachers hate to follow a script. Some teachers have never been told the rationale behind the use of scripts (e.g., consistency of wording within and across lessons). Other teachers believe that following a script makes them less of a teacher because it is not their wording; it is the program's.

This dislike for the scripting or other DI program features has led to some interesting phone calls and e-mails to the first author (G. A.) since the publication of *Research on Direct Instruction* in 1996. A teacher or administrator will call or write and ask whether there are any studies involving a particular Direct Instruction program (e.g., Reading Mastery) with a particular type of student (Hispanic) with a particular characteristic (e.g., middle class) in a particular setting (e.g., suburban schools). If the answer is "no," his or her response is often "Good, because I was to use the _____ program." Of course, as this meta-analysis shows, the results of Direct Instruction programs have consistently high effect sizes and yet the teacher or administrator wants a rationale for using a different program that has no evidence to show that it works.

The consistency of findings leads to the idea that Direct Instruction programs should be a standard for comparison to other programs. That is, when a curriculum director wants to evaluate a proposed curriculum, an action research study should be designed to compare the proposed curriculum to the equivalent Direct Instruction curriculum. The study should involve the collection of student progress data and use the parameters expected of sound research methodology and be done on a small scale. After the results are analyzed, a plan of school- or districtwide implementation can be created. This is not assuming that the Direct Instruction program will be superior; it does assume that the evidence should drive the decision-making process, instead of the common practice of shifting from program to program based on the fad at that time. The suggested process results in a scientific approach to program selection. The current process results in using teachers and students as guinea pigs for educational decision making.

Appendix 24.1. Direct Instruction Curricula

The following curricula are available through SRA (1-888-772-4543 or *http://sra4kids.com/product_info/direct/*).

Reading

- Reading Mastery—Levels I–VI (Elementary): The complete elementary reading program that includes teaching both decoding and comprehension skills. A student's placement is not based grade level; rather, placement is based on a student's placement test results.

- Corrective Reading—Decoding and Comprehension—Levels A–C (Remedial third grade to adult): Each strand (decoding and comprehension) has four levels. Placements into the decoding and comprehension programs are based on student placement testing. In most cases, students will be at two different program levels.

Language

- Language for Learning—Levels A–B (Elementary): This program teaches the language skills needed classroom instruction (using complete sentences, answering questions, and following directions).
- Language for Thinking (Grades 1–3): This program builds on Language for Learning and teaches making inferences, retelling accounts, and determining means of sentences, and other concepts.
- Reasoning and Writing—Levels A–F (Elementary, but has been used at a secondary level): This program combines the teaching of language, thinking, and writing skills.

Math

- Connecting Math Concepts—Levels A–F (Elementary, but has been used at a secondary level): This program teaches all math skills up to pre-algebra. Student placement should be based on placement test results.
- Corrective Mathematics—7 Levels from Addition to Ratios and Equations (Remedial third grade to adult): These seven self-contained programs teach Addition; Subtraction; Multiplication; Division; Basic Fractions; Fractions, Decimals, Percents; and Ratios and Equations.

Writing

- Expressive Writing—Levels I–II (fourth grade and above): This program teaches writing skills from sentence writing through sophisticated paragraph writing with copyediting.

Spelling

- Spelling Mastery—Levels A–F (Elementary): This spelling program teaches high-utility words, sound–symbol principles, and general spelling strategies. This program is by grade level (grades 1–6).

- Corrective Spelling through Morphographs (fourth grade and above): This program teaches 500 predictable highly generalizable rules.

Cursive Writing

- Cursive Writing Program (Grades 3 and 4): This program teaches clear cursive writing skills.

Appendix 24.2. Direct Instruction Component Analysis

DI versus Non-DI Component Comparison

Carnine, D. (1981). High and low implementation of Direct Instruction teaching techniques. *Education and Treatment of Children, 4,* 43–51.

Correction Procedure

Carnine, D. (1980). Phonic versus whole word correction procedures following phonic instruction. *Education and Treatment of Children, 3,* 323–330.

Meyer, L. A. (1982). Relative effects of word-analysis and word-supply correction procedures with poor readers during word-attack training. *Reading Research Quarterly, 17,* 544–555.

Group Size

Fink, W. T., & Sandall, S. R. (1978). One-to-one vs. group academic instruction with handicapped and nonhandicapped preschool children. *Mental Retardation, 16,* 230–240.

Massed versus Spaced Practice

Kryzanowski, J., & Carnine, D. (1980). Effects of massed versus spaced formats in teaching sound–symbol correspondences to your children. *Journal of Reading Education, 12,* 225–229.

Pacing

Carnine, D. W. (1976). Effects of two teacher presentation rates on off-task behavior, answering correctly, and participation. *Journal of Applied Behavior Analysis, 9,* 199–206.

Carnine, D., & Fink, W. T. (1978). Increasing the rate of presentation and use of signals in elementary classroom teachers. *Journal of Applied Behavior Analysis, 11,* 35–46.

Darch, C., & Gersten, R. (1985). Effects of teacher presentation rate and praise on LD students' oral reading performance. *British Journal of Educational Psychology, 55,* 295–303.

Positive and Negative Examples

Carnine, D. (1980). Correcting word identification errors of beginning readers. *Education and Treatment of Children, 3,* 323–330.

Carnine, D. (1980). Three procedures for presenting minimally different positive and negative instances. *Journal of Educational Psychology, 72,* 452–456.

Carnine, D., Gersten, R., Darch, C., & Eaves, R. (1985). Attention and cognitive deficits in learning-disabled students. *Journal of Special Education, 19,* 319–331.

Gersten, R. M., White, W. A. T., Falco, R., & Carnine, D. (1982). Teaching basic discriminations to handicapped and non-handicapped individuals through a dynamic presentation of instructional stimuli. *Analysis and Intervention in Developmental Disabilities, 2,* 305–317.

Granzin, A. C., & Carnine, D. (1977). Child performance on discrimination tasks: Effects of amount of stimulus variation. *Journal of Experimental Child Psychology, 24,* 332–342.

Horner, R. H., Albin, R. W., & Ralph, G. (1986). Generalization with precision: The role of negative teaching examples in the instruction of generalized grocery item selection. *Journal of the Association of Persons with Severe Handicaps, 11,* 300–308.

Horner, R. H., Eberhard, J. M., & Sheehan, M. R. (1986). Teaching generalized table bussing: The importance of negative teaching examples. *Behavior Modification, 10,* 457–471.

Horner, R. H., & McDonald, R. S. (1982). Comparison of single instance and general case instruction in teaching a generalized vocational skill. *TASH Journal, 8,* 7–20.

Ross, D., & Carnine, D. (1982). Analytic assistance: Effects of example selection, students' age and syntactic complexity. *Journal of Educational Research, 75,* 294–298.

Sprague, J. R., & Horner, R. H. (1984). Effects of single instance, multiple instance, and general case training on generalized vending machine use by moderately and severely handicapped students. *Journal of Applied Behavior Analysis, 17,* 273–278.

Preteaching

Carnine, D. (1980). Preteaching versus concurrent teaching of the component skills of a multiplication algorithm. *Journal for Research in Mathematics Education, 11,* 375–379.

Carnine, D. W. (1981). Reducing training problems associated with visually and auditorily similar correspondences. *Journal of Learning Disabilities, 14,* 276–279.

Kameenui, E. J., & Carnine, D. W. (1986). Preteaching versus concurrent teaching of component skills of a subtraction algorithm to skill-deficient second graders: A components analysis of direct analysis. *Exceptional Child, 33,* 103–115.

Sequences

Carnine, D. (1980). Two letter discrimination sequences: High-confusion-alternatives first versus low-confusion-alternatives first. *Journal of Reading Behavior, 12,* 41–47.

Williams, P., Granzin, A., Engelmann, S., & Becker, W. C. (1979). Teaching language to truly naive learner: An analog study using a tactual vocoder. *Journal of Special Education Technology, 2,* 5–15.

Sound Separation

Carnine, D. (1976). Similar sound separation and cumulative introduction in learning letter sound correspondences. *Journal of Educational Research, 69,* 368–372.

Use of Overt Steps

Adams, A., Carnine, D., & Gersten, R. (1982). Instructional strategies for studying content area texts in the intermediate grades. *Reading Research Quarterly, 18,* 27–55.

Carnine, D., Kameenui, E., & Maggs, A. (1982). Components of analytic assistance: Statement saying, concept training, and strategy training. *Journal of Educational Research, 75,* 374–377.

Carnine, D., Kameenui, E., & Woolfson, N. (1982). Training of textual dimension related to text-based inference. *Journal of Reading Behavior, 14,* 335–340.

Darch, C., Carnine, D., & Gersten, R. (1984). Explicit instruction in mathematics problem solving. *Journal of Educational Research, 77,* 350–359.

Dommes, P., Gersten, R., & Carnine, D. (1984). Instructional procedures for increasing skill-deficient fourth graders' comprehension of syntactic structures. *Educational Psychologist, 42*(2), 155–165.

Hollingsworth, M., & Woodward, J. (1993). Integrated learning: Explicit strategies and their role in problem-solving instruction for students with learning disabilities. *Exceptional Children, 59,* 444–455.

Paine, S., Carnine, D., & White, W. A. T. (1982). Effects of fading teacher presentation structure (covertization) on acquisition and maintenance of arithmetic problem-solving skills. *Education and Treatment of Children, 5,* 93–107.

Patching, W., Kameenui, E., Carnine, D., Gersten, R., & Colvin, G. (1983). Direct instruction in critical reading skills. *Reading Research Quarterly, 18,* 406–418.

Visual Displays

Darch, C., & Eaves, R. C. (1986). Visual displays to increase comprehension of high school learning-disabled students. *Journal of Special Education, 20,* 309–318.

Sprick, R. S. (1979). *A comparison of recall scores for visual–spatial, visual–serial, and auditory presentation of intermediate grade content.* Unpublished doctoral dissertation, University of Oregon, Eugene.

Wording

Carnine, D. (1980). Relationships between stimulus variation and the formation of misconceptions. *Journal of Educational Research, 74,* 106–110.

Williams, P. B., & Carnine, D. (1981). Relationship between range of examples and of instructions and attention in concept attainment. *Journal of Educational Research, 74,* 144–148.

References

Adams, G. L., & Engelmann, S. (1996). *Research on Direct Instruction: 25 years beyond DISTAR.* Portland, OR: Educational Achievement Systems.

Carnine, D. W., Silbert, J., & Kameenui, E. J. (1997). *Direct instruction reading* (3rd ed.). Upper Saddle River, NJ: Merrill.

Chall, J. S. (2000). *The academic achievement challenge: What really works in the classroom?* New York: Guilford Press.

Cohen, J. (1988). *Statistical power analysis for the behavior change* (2nd ed.). Hillsdale, NJ: Erlbaum.

Engelmann, S., & Carnine, D. (1991). *Theory of instruction.* Eugene, OR: Association of Direct Instruction.

Engelmann, S., Hanner, S., & Johnson, G. (1999). *Corrective reading: Series guide.* Columbus, OH: SRA McGraw-Hill.

Glass, G. V., McGaw, B., & Smith, M. L. (1981). *Meta-analysis in social research.* Beverly Hills, CA: Sage.

Hunter, J. E., Schmidt, F. L., & Jackson, G. B. (1982). *Meta-analysis: Cumulating research findings across studies.* Beverly Hills, CA: Sage.

Rosenthal, R. (1992). *Meta-analysis procedures for social research* (2nd ed.). Beverly Hills, CA: Sage.

Slavin, R. (1989). PET and the pendulum: Fads in education and how to stop it. *Phi Delta Kappan, 70,* 752–758.

Stahl, S. A., & Miller, P. D. (1989). Whole language and language experience spproaches for beginning reading: A qualitative research synthesis. *Research of Educational Research, 59,* 87–116.

Stein, M., Silbert, J., & Carnine, D. (1997). *Designing effective mathematics instruction: A Direct Instruction approach (3rd ed.).* Upper Saddle River, NJ: Merrill.

Swanson, H. L., Hoskyn, M., & Lee, C. (1999). *Interventions for students with learning disabilities: A meta-analysis of treatment outcomes.* New York: Guilford Press.

Studies Cited in Table 24.2

1. Branwhite, A. B. (1983). Boosting reading skills by Direct Instruction. *British Journal of Educational Psychology, 53,* 291–298.

2. Campbell, M. (1981). *A study of Corrective Reading as an effective and appropriate program for reading disabled, learning handicapped secondary students.* Report presented to Faculty of School of Education, San Diego State University.

3. Darch, C., Gersten, R., & Taylor, R. (1987). Evaluation of Williamsburg County Direct Instruction Program: Factors leading to success in rural elementary programs. *Research in Rural Education, 4,* 111–118.

4. Darch, C., & Kameenui, E. J. (1987). Teaching LD students critical reading skills: A systematic replication. *Learning Disability Quarterly, 10,* 82–91.

5. Gregory, R. P., Hackney, C., & Gregory, N. M. (1982). Corrective Reading programme: An evaluation. *British Journal of Educational Psychology, 52,* 33–50.

6. Hasselbring, T., Sherwood, R., Bransford, J., Fleenor, K., Griffith, D., & Goin, L. (1987–1988). Evaluation of a level-one instructional videodisc program. *Journal of Educational Technology Systems, 16,* 151–169.

7. Kelly, B., Carnine, D., Gersten, R., & Grossen, B. (1986). Effectiveness of videodisc instruction in teaching fractions to learning-disabled and remedial high school students. *Journal of Special Education Technology, 8,* 5–9.

8. Kelly, B., Gersten, R., & Carnine, D. (1990). Student error patterns as a function of curriculum design: Teaching fractions to remedial high school students and high school students with learning disabilities. *Journal of Learning Disabilities, 23,* 23–29.

9. Lewis, A. (1982). Experimental evaluation of a Direct Instruction programme (Corrective Reading) with remedial readers in a comprehensive school. *Educational Psychology, 2,* 121–135.

10. Lloyd, J., Cullinan, D., Heins, E. D., & Epstein, M. (1980). Direct Instruction: Effects on oral and written language comprehension. *Learning Disability Quarterly, 3,* 70–76.

11. Lloyd, J., Epstein, M. H., & Cullinan, D. (1981). Direct Instruction for learning disabilities. In J. Gottlieb & S. S. Strickart (Eds.), *Developmental theory and research in learning disabilities* (pp. 41–45). Baltimore: University Park Press.

12. Richardson, E., Dibenedetto, B., Christ, A., Press, M., & Winsberg, B. (1978). An assessment of two methods for remediating reading deficiencies. *Reading Improvement, 15,* 82–94.

13. Sexton, C. W. (1989). Effectiveness of the Distar Reading I program in developing first graders' language skills. *Journal of Educational Research, 82,* 289–293.

14. Stein, C. L., & Goldman, J. (1980). Beginning reading instruction for children with minimal brain dysfunction. *Journal of Learning Disabilities, 13,* 52–55.

15. Summerell, S., & Brannigan, G. G. (1977). Comparison of reading programs for children with low levels of reading readiness. *Perceptual and Motor Skills, 44,* 743–746.

16. Woodward, J., Carnine, D., & Gersten, R. (1988). Teaching problem solving through a computer simulation. *American Educational Research Journal, 25,* 72–86.

17. Woodward, J., Carnine, D., Gersten, R., Gleason, M., Johnson, G., & Collins, M. (1986). Applying instructional design principles to CAI for mildly handicapped students: Four recently conducted studies. *Journal of Special Education Technology, 8,* 13–26.

25

Cooperative Learning for Students with Learning Disabilities: Evidence from Experiments, Observations, and Interviews

Joseph R. Jenkins
Rollanda E. O'Connor

Cooperative learning (CL) refers to "the instructional use of small groups so that students work together to maximize their own and each other's learning" (Johnson, Johnson, & Holubec, 1993, p. 6). CL originated in theories of group dynamics (Deutsch, 1962; Lewin, 1935) and social interdependence (Johnson, 1970). It is based on the idea that establishing positive interdependence among members of a learning group encourages individuals to help each other learn (Johnson, 1970). Different theoretical perspectives offer different interpretations of how CL facilitates learning. Behaviorists emphasize the reward-produced motivational aspects of CL in which reinforcement for any group member is contingent upon all members meeting a learning criterion, thereby increasing the likelihood that members will engage in behaviors that lead to mutual learning. In contrast, social constructivists emphasize how scaffolded, dialogical interactions among more and less skilled peers lead to the construction of new knowledge and ways of thinking (Vygotsky, 1978).

Among approaches to classroom instruction, CL stands out by virtue of its extraordinarily large research base, which rivals if not surpasses that of any other approach to teaching. A decade ago, Johnson and Johnson (1992) tallied over 550 experimental and 100 correlational studies on this instructional approach, and those numbers have surely grown since. CL has captured the interest of researchers and practitioners because of its potential for both promoting academic learning and teaching a host of interpersonal skills and dispositions that foster social competence, friendships, and tolerance.

In addition, CL offers teachers a unique strategy for managing instruction in heterogeneous classrooms, where learners' abilities, knowledge, and backgrounds vary broadly, and the range of achievement levels in typical classrooms exceeds five grade levels (Jenkins, Jewell, Leicester, Jenkins, & Troutner, 1990). Faced with such heterogeneity, teachers confront a difficult challenge in attempting to engage *all* students in high-quality learning activities, even the lowest achievers (e.g., those with learning disabilities) who *on their own* are unable to perform some of the more difficult classroom assignments. Not many approaches to instruction are built for classroom conditions this demanding. Indeed, most instructional approaches view individual differences as a nuisance to be controlled through individualized instruction (Wang & Birch, 1984) or ability groups (Carnine, Silbert, & Kameenui, 1990). By contrast, in CL individual differences are viewed as resources that can be exploited in the pursuit of learning (Johnson & Johnson, 1986; Slavin, 1990; Stevens & Slavin, 1995a, 1995b).

The peer support inherent in CL serves as a compensatory mechanism, enabling struggling learners to overcome obstacles they might not overcome working alone. Peer support can materialize in a variety of forms, as when more capable or better-informed peers clarify the nature of an assignment, interpret complex instructions, model performance, explain ideas, give feedback and corrections, take responsibility for difficult parts of the assignment, scaffold problem-solving efforts, and provide encouragement.

More than other disability groups, students with learning disabilities (LD) have been caught in the cross-currents of three reform movements: more rigorous academic standards, access to the general education curriculum, and inclusion of students with disabilities in general education classrooms. In these circumstances, finding effective ways to help students with LD has not been easy. Researchers have sought answers in various forms of peer-mediated instruction (Englert et al., 1995; Fuchs et al., 1997; Palincsar & Brown, 1984), of which CL is one alternative. Many educators perceive CL as special education–friendly, providing the kind of supportive learning environment students with LD need to succeed in the educational mainstream (Alberg, 1991; Johnson & Johnson, 1980; Mainzer, Mainzer, Slavin, & Lowry, 1993; Slavin, 1990; Slavin & Stevens, 1991; Slavin, Stevens, & Madden, 1988; Thousand & Villa, 1991; Will, 1986, Wood, Algozzine, & Avett, 1993)— thus, the continuing interest in CL for students with LD.

In this chapter we review research on the use and effectiveness of CL for students with LD, considering three sources of information. These include (1) experimental studies conducted in general and special education settings that compare academic learning with and without CL, (2) observational studies of teachers' and students'

classroom behavior during CL, and (3) interviews with teachers who use CL or cooperative group work. In these studies, students with LD are school identified using state guidelines.

Experimental Studies of Cooperative Learning for Students with LD

Students with disabilities were rarely included in studies of CL in the 1960s and 1970s, perhaps because the movement toward mainstreaming and inclusion was barely under way. Through the late 1980s, researchers and practitioners tested CL approaches with more diverse kinds of students, including students with disabilities. They found that the outcomes for students with disabilities were not uniformly superior under this arrangement. Tateyama-Sniezek (1990) reviewed studies in which separate analyses were performed on the outcomes of children with disabilities. Only seven of these studies compared the learning of students with high incidence disabilities across cooperative and noncooperative instructional formats, and of these seven, only three reported significant differences favoring CL over independent conditions for students with LD. Of the three reporting significant differences, only two held students with LD individually accountable for their learning.

Tateyama-Sniezek (1990) wrote, "The only firm conclusion is that the opportunity for students to study together does not guarantee gains in academic achievement" (p. 436). Despite her warning to proceed with caution, Wood and colleagues (1993) claimed that there was ample support for using CL in the classroom as an inclusion strategy for students with disabilities. But of the benefits they cited from reviews by Lehr (1984), Slavin (1983a, 1983b), and Johnson and Johnson (1987), none addressed academic improvement for students with learning disabilities. Since Tateyama-Sniezek's review was published, more experimental studies have been conducted to examine the effects of CL for students with LD.

Mathematics

In a pair of studies, Xin (1996) compared the math outcomes of 211 third- and fourth-graders, including 41 with LD, following 20 weeks of instruction on the computer in which students worked either individually or in cooperative teams. First, students in each condition received 30 minutes of teacher-led instruction, which was jointly planned by the general and special education teacher and included a worksheet that students completed independently. Next, children worked either individually (the control) or in cooperative dyads (CL) for 20 minutes in the computer lab, using software that was coordinated with their class textbook. In the CL treatment, the computer lab time was followed with groups of four students (two partner teams) that checked answers to worksheets and provided support for making corrections. In the control condition, teachers conducted the checking. The teaching teams shifted between cooperative and individual practice conditions weekly to decrease the potential for teacher effects. In the third-grade study, outcomes favored children in CL groups; in the fourth-grade study, no differences were found. The results for children with LD were not analyzed separately at either grade level; however, means and standard deviations for the children with LD were reported. For third-graders with LD, a moderate effect (ES = 0.35) appeared to favor children who worked in CL teams; for fourth-graders with LD, that trend was strongly reversed (ES = –1.3). Thus, it is difficult to generalize about CL's effectiveness from these studies.

Homework affects grades and achievement (Foyle & Bailey, 1988), and many students with LD have difficulty completing homework assignments correctly, if at all. To help middle school students with LD complete homework, O'Melia and Rosenberg (1994) used Cooperative Homework Teams (CHT), a form of Team Assisted Individualization (TAI; Slavin, Madden, & Leavey, 1984) that incorporates individual accountability and team rewards. CHT built on TAI by providing collaborative opportunities for students to grade and make corrections to mathematics homework. In an 8-week study, students with high-incidence disabilities (primarily LD) received math instruction from special education teachers and completed their homework independently. On the following day, students met in CHTs to check homework, report

grades, and assist each other with corrections as needed. Although accuracy (ES = 0.55) and completion of assignments (ES = 0.64) improved for CHT students relative to controls who completed the same homework by themselves, the groups did not differ in mathematics achievement on the California Achievement Test (ES = –0.44, favoring the control). Eight weeks of intervention, however, are rarely sufficient to yield significant effects on standardized achievement tests, regardless of the treatment.

Writing

Students with disabilities tend to have difficulties in writing mechanics, such as capitalization and punctuation, as well as with production of essays, stories, and reports. Targeting writing mechanics, Malouf, Weizer, Pilato, and Grogan (1990) tested CL in the context of computer-assisted writing practice. Working in pairs, 36 middle school students with LD received teacher-led grammar instruction, introductory worksheets, and computer games in which they applied the taught skills. Experimental and control groups differed in the structure of the pair work. In the control group, pairs were told to work independently and were taught independent work skills, such as paying attention, working carefully, and taking turns on the computer. Quizzes were scored individually and rewards given for individual scores. In the experimental group, pairs were taught CL skills (e.g., asking questions, catching partners' errors, and explaining). During teacher-led guided practice, students were encouraged to work together on their worksheets. During the computer games, they generated a single score for their shared session, and rewards on the quizzes were given for the averaged score across the two papers. Although both groups improved on writing mechanics, they did not differ significantly (ES = 0.23).

In a second study, Malouf and colleagues (1990) replicated the experiment with 66 fourth-, fifth-, and sixth-grade students with LD in self-contained special education classrooms. Again, CL did not significantly add to students' learning of writing mechanics (ES = 0.09). In both studies, CL pairs engaged in significantly more interactions and keyboard sharing than did pairs who worked independently. Thus, it appears that CL had indeed occurred but did not improve the performance of the students over independent learning conditions.

Wong and colleagues conducted several studies of CL as an arrangement to encourage students to write better structured and more elaborate essays. In a study of middle school students with LD who had poor writing skills, Wong, Butler, Ficzere, and Kuperis (1996) restructured special education English classes from independent work to work in cooperative dyads. The instructional vehicle was an essay-writing strategy that included models of generating opinions and evidence, plan sheets for structuring arguments, prompt cards, and peer editing. After instruction from their teachers, students used the procedures in pairs to write six essays spaced across the school year. Their performance was compared with that of students with LD in special education English classes that used the same curriculum, without the essay-writing strategy and the cooperative grouping. On posttests that students took independently, differences clearly favored the students who worked cooperatively on their essays (ES = 2.5), and these results maintained on a follow-up test 1 week later. Unfortunately, the design of this study did not allow the researchers to tease apart the influence of the cooperative dyads from the strategy instruction.

In another study of strategic writing, Wong, Butler, Ficzere, and Kuperis (1997) applied a modification of their genre-specific essay structure to teach high school students with LD to collaboratively plan compare-and-contrast essays. Following the phases of modeling and collaborative planning, students wrote essays independently and revised them after meetings with their teacher. The analysis of results was based on writing improvement, rather than comparison with a control group or a non-CL condition. Although writing quality improved (ES = 1.33), again the design could not distinguish between the contributions of strategy training and CL. The authors acknowledged this confound and suggested that the observed changes resulted from the dialogue and negotiation that occurred during the planning and revising processes—whether with peers or with teachers.

Utay and Utay (1997) combined CL with cross-age peer tutoring to improve the writing skills of students with LD in grades 2 to 6. The 72 children all received instruction in word processing and writing skills in a computer lab. The researchers formed matched pairs of students based on pretests of writing ability and randomly assigned one student from each pair to one of two forms of writing practice: either independent work on the computer (the control) or cross-age writing teams that were supposed to assist each other with their storywriting assignments. The specific elements of the CL were not specified. Although the children working in cross-age pairs appeared to enjoy this experience, their writing ability at the close of the experiment did not differ significantly from that of students who worked more independently.

Reading

Most studies of CL in reading have been conducted in the context of Cooperative Integrated Reading and Composition (CIRC) and Success for All (SFA). Although we introduce these studies here, they confound CL with other instructional variables, resulting in a mix of treatments.

Slavin (1996) recommended an intensive preventive approach he termed "never-streaming," in which students would be identified early in their school careers and receive immediate and continued intervention as needed to prevent large achievement lags from developing in the early years. SFA (Slavin, Madden, Dolan, & Wasik, 1992) was modeled on that philosophy. The reading package included schoolwide regrouping across grades for 90 minutes daily so that children read materials at appropriate reading levels, comprehension lessons taught at the level of children's receptive language, shared reading with teachers, and cooperative learning. Tutorial support for 20 minutes daily was also offered immediately to children who made less than average progress in the first years of school. Slavin and colleagues (1992) reported decreased incidence of referrals to special education; however, children who were identified for special education services needed additional support beyond that offered by SFA.

In a 2-year study using the same approach in reading along with CL in math, Stevens and Slavin (1995a) reported that, following 1 year of treatment, elementary students with disabilities did not differ significantly in achievement from controls. At the end of the second year, however, they significantly outperformed controls in reading vocabulary (ES = 0.24) and comprehension (ES = 0.26) and in mathematics computation (ES = 0.59), but not math applications. In a similar quasi-experiment that employed CL in the context of CIRC, Stevens and Slavin (1995b) found significant reading effects for both general and special education students in the CIRC treatment, relative to control students who received traditional reading instruction. For students with disabilities (primarily in LD), effects on reading vocabulary and comprehension were 0.33 and 0.20, respectively, after 2 years in the program. CIRC includes 90 minutes of daily reading instruction using materials at appropriate reading levels, instruction in word lists, word meanings, spelling, comprehension, reading-related writing, the writing process, reading at home, and CL. In this study, the special and general educators co-taught for 30 minutes, in addition to CIRC. The authors attributed gains for mainstreamed students to the coaching, feedback, and instructional models provided by peers without disabilities. However in this study, students in CIRC classrooms received small-group reading instruction from the general educator, 30 minutes of in-class support from the special educator, *and* CL groups across the school year, whereas control students received 30 minutes of pullout instruction from the special educator.

In one of the few studies that compared CL to another form of peer mediation, Klingner and Vaughn (1996) compared CL and cross-age peer tutoring, using reciprocal teaching to develop reading comprehension. Participants were 26 seventh- and eighth-grade students with LD who spoke English as a second language. For 2 days, researchers modeled the comprehension strategy, guided students in discussions of key features of the strategy, and used a cue sheet to prompt the strategy. For the next eight sessions, researchers provided guidance and feedback to students as students took turns "teaching" with the strategy. For the last five instructional sessions, researchers gave limited guidance as students took turns with the teaching role. After students achieved competence with the procedures, they were randomly assigned either to cross-age tutoring (in which trained students tutored a sixth grader) or to CL groups of three to five students who practiced the comprehension strategy for an additional 12 days. The two peer-assisted approaches did not differ significantly in outcomes (ES = −0.06 and −0.38 on the Gates–McGinitie and comprehension passages, respectively), although both groups gained in reading comprehension Scores from weekly comprehension tests were graphed across all phases of the experiment, and students made small, steady gains across both treatments. The steepest increases, however, occurred across the 15 days of training, in which instruction was delivered by the researcher.

Mixed Models

Jenkins, Jewell, Leicester, Jenkins, and Troutner (1991) tested CIRC (Stevens, Madden, Slavin, & Farnish, 1987) for students with LD in grade 6. The school restructured instructional arrangements in the general education classes, but despite fundamental changes observed in the delivery of services (in-class services from a special educator combined with daily CL groups), students with disabilities in CL classes did not differ from counterparts in a control school (that used traditional pullout instruction) on social behavior or on most academic measures. The only significant effects favored children in traditional pullout classes on a MAZE task (a measure of reading rate and comprehension, ES = −1.2)).

In a subsequent study, Jenkins, Jewell, Leicester, O'Connor, Jenkins, and Troutner (1994) implemented CIRC, peer tutoring in reading, and in-class support from special education staff in grades 2–6 classrooms, along with small-group direct instruction for the lowest readers in grades 1 and 2. At the end of 1 year, special education students in the experimental school did not differ from controls on two of three reading measures but did register significantly larger gains than controls on Metropolitan Achievement Test reading vocabulary (ES = 0.72) and comprehension (ES = 0.71). The behavior of students in special education, as measured on the Walker McConnell scale, did not differ as a result of long-term use of CL.

In a study of collaborative strategic reading, Klingner, Vaughn, and Schumm (1998) assigned fourth-grade classes that included students with LD to a condition which combined strategy instruction and CL, or to a control condition in which students received instruction based on the teacher's manual. Both conditions used the same history textbook unit for 11 instructional sessions. The researchers spent three sessions teaching students collaborative strategic reading, which consists of a preview of the material for the day, "click and clunk" to monitor comprehension of words and concepts, "get the gist" to restate the main idea of each paragraph, and "wrapup" to summarize the day's reading. Although experimental and control groups did not differ significantly on an end-of-unit test, the CL group significantly outperformed controls on the Gates–McGinitie reading test. In a separate analysis of outcomes for students with LD, differences were not significant.

Klinger and colleagues (1998) analyzed audiotapes of students' conversations to determine groups' use of the various strategy components. Students spent considerably more time discussing content during CL, although peers provided little feedback or modeling for lower achievers during the previewing step of the strategy. Groups made good use of the "click and clunk" and "get the gist" portions of the strategy. The authors noted the importance of a knowledgeable teacher or adult for clarifying meanings of unfamiliar vocabulary and concepts and suggested that monitoring the multiple CL groups was sometimes difficult.

In these mixed models, cooperative learning was one feature of a complex treatment that usually included other features with solid research evidence to support them, such as peer tutoring (Delquardi, Greenwood, Whorton, Carta, & Hall, 1996; Fuchs et al., 1997), cross-age tutoring (Jenkins & Jenkins, 1981), or strategy instruction (Graham & Harris, 1997; Palincsar & Brown, 1986). In none of these models was cooperative learning tested as the independent variable. Moreover, in the cases in which CL was tested against other forms of

peer-assisted support, no significant differences were found.

Based on findings of experimental studies, it is difficult to gauge the extent to which CL advances the achievement of students with LD. To begin with, there are too few studies of CL implemented over an extended period in which its contributions can be isolated from other instructional variables. A larger research base is also needed to assess the influence of participants' age and grade level, types of learning activities, and the CL model used.

In addition, LD researchers have overlooked CL's effects on retention, and transfer to new learning tasks has been generally ignored. If Vygotsky's (1978) notion of socially constructed knowledge and thinking extends to school learning, we might expect CL (with its encouragement of peer discourse) to assist students with LD in connecting new ideas to an array of diverse knowledge structures, and in acquiring generalized thinking strategies that they can apply to a broad range of problems. However, there is little evidence in the LD research base for better retention and transfer of knowledge and skills learned through CL, mainly because so few studies have attended to these dimensions of learning. These issues deserve examination. Considering the extant research base on LD, we find ourselves in agreement with McMaster and Fuchs (2002), who concluded, "The evidence of CL's impact on students with LD remains inconsistent" (p. 19).

Observational Studies of Cooperative Learning for Students with LD

Working in peer-mediated teams is expected to contribute to the development of social competence, interpersonal attraction, and friendships (Cohen, Lotan, & Catanzarite, 1990). Wood and colleagues (1993), in their review of the uses of CL in literacy instruction for students with LD, concluded that "perhaps the greatest benefit of cooperative learning is that when it is used effectively, no student is ignored or forgotten" (p. 375). Some researchers have designed studies to investigate specifically what happens among students who work in CL groups.

Concerned about the variable results reported for children with disabilities in CL arrangements, O'Connor and Jenkins (1996) examined factors related to how students with LD engaged in CIRC-based CL reading lessons. Across 2 years, they observed children with LD who were paired with average-performing children (grades 3–6) in the same general education classrooms. To assess the quality of CL participation for students with LD, O'Connor and Jenkins noted types of learning activities, amount and kind of help students received (and from whom), and amount and kind of contributions they made to group efforts. Students with disabilities offered fewer contributions than did students without disabilities and received more help.

Nevertheless, the assistance provided by peers during CL may not be sufficient to enable the participation of students with LD in the group's activities. Against expectations, O'Connor and Jenkins observed several instances of adults (most often a teaching assistant or special educator) joining a CL group in which a student with LD appeared to have difficulty with the reading requirements of the group's work. When this occurred, it invariably altered the character of the group's participation. Sometimes the adult directed the student's work, cutting the child off from his or her teammates. Sometimes the adult assumed the role of group leader, controlling the structure and character of the other group members' participation.

Overall, O'Connor and Jenkins (1996) classified only 40% of these students (first year) and 44% (second year) as participating successfully in cooperative groups. Analyses disclosed that differences in classroom practices (e.g., selection of partners, the establishment of a cooperative ethic, and teacher monitoring) and individual differences among special education students (reading performance and social competence) were related to successful CL experiences for students with disabilities. For teachers, finding suitable partners for children with LD was among their stiffest challenges, and in this endeavor they were not always successful. Moreover, although most of the teachers taught cooperative behaviors early in the school year, teachers of the more successful students with LD reinforced these behaviors frequently. Related to establishing

cooperative behaviors, teachers' skill in monitoring CL groups distinguished more and less successful student experiences. Some teachers provided ways for groups to monitor their own instances of participation and helping. As they monitored child and group functioning, some teachers also made public statements validating the contributions of the children with LD, which served to raise the status of students who may be less valued by their classmates (Cohen, 1994). Unless teachers succeeded in establishing cooperative norms, groups tended to exclude lower-skilled children from participation.

O'Connor and Jenkins also observed a potentially significant side effect of using CL as an inclusion strategy for students with LD. To prepare students for participation in their group, teachers sometimes exchanged reading practice for listening to a story read by an adult or with a tape recorder. To finish partner reading in time to complete written assignments, the more skilled partner sometimes performed most of the reading aloud while the student with LD looked on. The cognitive abilities and academic skills of students with LD place them at risk for immediate difficulties in the classroom and influence their ability to contribute to team assignments. In these cases, the very procedures that enabled students with LD to participate in CL robbed them of opportunities to build reading skill.

In another observational study, Beaumont (1999) examined the interactions of students with disabilities in a second-grade bilingual, full-inclusion classroom, in which students were heterogeneously grouped for academic work and encouraged through room rules and mottos to help each other and to ask for help from peers when it was needed. About one-third of the students in this class had a disability, and Beaumont rotated observations across these children during 150 hours spread across the school year. After the first 3 months of documenting conversations among students, requests for help, and help received and denied, she concentrated her observations on three students with disabilities, including one boy with a diagnosis of LD. This boy, despite his strong verbal ability and outgoing nature, was identified as a social isolate in the classroom, as were the other two children Beaumont observed closely. Of the 70 helping episodes she coded (defined as an episode beginning with a request for help or offer of help by one student, followed by acceptance or rejection of help from another student), 21 involved pairs of students with disabilities, 9 occurred in groups with only general education students, and 40 occurred in heterogeneous groups of general and special education students. Every instance of denial of help was directed at a special education student. These rejections occurred despite a positive classroom climate and culture that encouraged and rewarded students assisting one another.

Beaumont (1999) also noted that the quality of the interchanges among general education students, which tended to be harmonious, with most help given without criticism or impatience, contrasted sharply with those between general and special education students, which were frequently characterized as impatient, corrective, or critical. Moreover, help, when it was offered, was often unsolicited. Considering all the helping episodes, Beaumont characterized only 40% as successful, which she defined as enabling the student who requested help to proceed with a task.

If children with LD received more training in how to cooperate with one another, would the quality of helping interactions improve? Gillies and Ashman (2000) randomly assigned third-grade teachers of inclusive social studies classes to conditions in which their class was either taught specifically how to interact (structured CL) or encouraged to cooperate but without specific instruction about how to do so (unstructured CL). These classes included 152 students, 22 of whom had LD. The teachers used CL during social studies three times weekly across the school year, and each group was videotaped twice to observe the interactions among students. Interactions were coded by behavior state (cooperative or noncooperative behavior, individual task-oriented or non-task-oriented behavior) and verbal interactions (directives, solicited or unsolicited explanations, solicited or unsolicited terminal responses, interruptions, and nonspecific interactions). The only significant treatment difference for behavior state was a decrease in individual non-task-oriented behavior in structured CL

groups. For verbal interactions, children in structured CL gave more directives over time (e.g., points finger and says, "Look, this is how it's done." [Gillies & Ashman, 2000, p. 22]), and fewer solicited explanations over time. Learning outcomes were also assessed, with a small but reliable difference on a comprehension questionnaire (which did not measure reading comprehension, per se), favoring students in the structured condition. No differences were found on word reading scores. The authors report that the students with LD exhibited more group involvement in the structured CL, which may have contributed to their gain on the comprehension questionnaire.

Interviews of General Education Teachers Who Use CL with Students with LD

Classroom Teachers' Use of CL

As with any approach that originates with researchers, CL's potential for benefiting students with LD depends on teachers' receptivity and willingness to adopt it. Although we know of no data on CL's prevalence in special education settings, many elementary general education teachers appear to organize their classrooms around CL principles. In fact, a study of educational opportunity covering 3 million third-grade students (Puma, Jones, Rock, & Fernandez, 1993) found that a majority of teachers reported using CL in math (79%) and reading and language arts (74%). Another survey of 85 elementary school teachers in two school districts found that 93% indicated they used cooperative learning (Antil, Jenkins, Wayne, & Vadasy, 1998). An in-depth interview of 21 of the teachers who said they used CL disclosed that 81% stated they conducted CL lessons every day in a typical week, with 100% reporting use of the strategy for reading, and 81% for math. In other subjects, 62% teachers reported using CL for social studies, 52% for science, 43% for writing, 33% for language arts, and 24% for spelling. On average, teachers said they regularly used cooperative learning in four subjects, with reported use ranging from one to seven subjects (Antil et al., 1998).

These figures appear to be good news for students with LD, assuming CL works as advertised. However, Antil and colleagues (1998) detected a potentially important discrepancy in the conception of CL held by their respondents and that held by CL researcher–developers. Specifically, when does group work qualify as CL and when is it just group work? From the perspective of CL researcher–developers, CL requires that teachers organize instruction in ways that promote (1) positive interdependence (i.e., create the perception that students must work together to accomplish their goal) and (2) individual accountability (i.e., testing the performance of group members against a standard and feeding this information to the group so that members can help each other raise their performance) (Johnson & Johnson, 1987; Kagan, 1989–1990; Sharan, 1980; Slavin, 1990). For their brand of CL, Johnson and Johnson (1987) specify three *additional* requirements. Teachers must also (3) arrange seating to promote student interactions, (4) teach students interpersonal skills needed to work together, and (5) require groups to reflect on their collaborative efforts and decide on ways to work together more effectively.

When Antil and colleagues (1998) tested their teachers' descriptions of CL against Johnson and Johnson's (1991) five-element standard, nearly all the teachers earned credit for promoting student interaction, establishing positive interdependence, and explicitly teaching students interpersonal and small-group skills. However, considerably fewer had groups reflect on and evaluate their processes (33%), or required individual accountability (24%). Most of the teachers indicated using several elements (mode = 4 elements), but only one of 21 teachers incorporated all five criteria. In contrast, 24% satisfied Slavin's (1990) two-element standard for CL (i.e., positive interdependence and individual accountability). Nearly all those who missed the two-element standard omitted individual accountability in the sense this term is used by CL researcher–developers (i.e., informing individuals and their partners about the status of their knowledge, their possible need for peer assistance, and their contribution to meeting the group's goal). Teachers held students individually accountable in another sense, however. To monitor individuals' learning, they required students to produce individual products ei-

ther in place of or in addition to a group product. Thus, students were individually accountable to the teacher rather than to the group. As one teacher said,

> I want the group product to be spectacular, but the whole point of it is for the individual student to learn and grow and produce something. It's important for me to know how each student is doing. I need some kind of project or activity that demonstrates their knowledge. A lot of times, I'll insert that after they've done a cooperative project to get the knowledge and skills. Then I can evaluate individual students. (Antil et al., 1998, p. 440)

These teachers omission of individual accountability (in the CL sense) to their groups may be important because Slavin's (1990) meta-analysis of CL indicated that the effects of CL were negligible when individual accountability was omitted from the treatment. McMaster and Fuchs's (2002) review produced a similar finding. However, it is important to note that the effect size for individual accountability given by Slavin and McMaster and Fuchs is not based on experiments that systematically vary individual accountability. Such experiments are notably lacking.

Special and Remedial Education Students in CL

Teachers have more opportunities than perhaps anyone to gauge how students with learning problems respond to CL. Their perspective adds an important dimension to the knowledge base on how CL works for students with learning disabilities. As part of the interview conducted by Antil and colleagues (1998), Jenkins, Antil, Wayne, and Vadasy (2003) questioned the same teachers about the benefits remedial and special education students derive from CL, the percentage of these students who consistently participated in CL, the effectiveness of CL for struggling students, and modifications they made in CL for these students. Most of the special education students had a learning disability.

Perceived Benefits

All CL teachers indicated multiple ways that special education students were helped by CL. For example, one fourth-grade teacher said, "They gain a lot more, they finish more, they learn more and gain self-esteem" (Jenkins et al., in press). However, some benefits were more prominent than others.

The three most frequently cited benefits, each mentioned by more than half the respondents (52%) were (1) self-esteem, (2) the security that comes from being part of a group, and (3) higher success rates and/or better products. Illustrating the safe learning environment claim, one teacher said, "They (special education students) like the feeling of success that come out a lot in CL ... there's less frustration and anxiety" (Jenkins et al., 2003).

Along with contributing to students' self-esteem and providing a safe learning environment, teachers also said CL helped struggling students to succeed more often and to create better products. Teachers usually linked increased productivity with feelings of success, as illustrated by the teacher who said, "I think they get a lot more work done. Their self esteem is built up," and the teacher who responded, "Those kids that struggle really feel good about themselves when they've produced a final product. . . . The fact they are able to achieve success through the help of their peers, and perhaps accomplish things they could not accomplish by themselves" (Jenkins et al., 2003).

Thirty-eight percent said that CL gave special education students greater voice and improved their participation levels. One first-grade teacher remarked, "They can be part of a learning group and they can contribute. It might not be a lot, but they have their voice" (Jenkins et al., 2003). Thirty-three percent of the respondents said that CL resulted in better learning for remedial and special education students, usually stating that cooperative groups provide low-achieving students another way to learn. In the words of one third-grade teacher, "They are free to find a better way to learn if they don't get it the way I teach it ... what they need to learn is met easier in a group" (Jenkins et al., 2003).

Participation in CL

Teachers estimated that the percentage of special and remedial education students who participated consistently in CL activities ranged from 50% to 100% with a median estimate of 78%. Remarkably, 43% said that *all* their special and remedial education students consistently participated in CL groups.

Perceived Effectiveness

Fifty-two percent of the teachers said CL worked well for their special and remedial education students, with several remarking that CL especially benefited this group, for example: "I don't think I could do my job if I couldn't do cooperative groups with those kinds of kids. I mean, as far as mainstreaming is concerned there's no better teacher than the kids who are sitting right there beside them" (Jenkins et al., 2003).

The rest of the teachers, while generally positive about CL's effectiveness with special and remedial students, noted that CL was sometimes effective and sometimes not, or effective with some students but not others. When teachers spoke of special education students who failed to thrive in CL, they often mentioned personal characteristics that students brought to the learning task. Among the student characteristics that undermined CL, behavior and attention problems were most cited, but teachers also mentioned other attributes (e.g., the tendency to become discouraged easily). One fifth-grade teacher tied the success of CL to students' motivation to learn: "For some, it [CL] is an excuse to not participate, to hide out, but there are some with special needs who have that desire to learn. They pair themselves up with someone they know will do better" (Jenkins et al., 2003).

Modifying CL for Special and Remedial Education Students

All but 2 of the 21 teachers described steps they took to facilitate special education students' performance in CL. One-third of the teachers said they deliberately selected helpful partners and groupmates for struggling learners. Two of these said they considered the reading and writing skills of their struggling learners, along with the reading and writing requirements inherent in the task: "I most definitely assigned a reader with a non-reader or a writer with a non-writer so that the non-reader or non-writer would not feel hindered by their lack of ability in that area," and "We would take into account group placement.... If it's an activity where we need a writer, we make sure we draw a writer" (Jenkins et al., 2003).

Only three teachers mentioned modifying the task for struggling students. One said, "I'd give them an easy job.... If I was doing reading, I would give them an easy part." Another spoke of changing the mode of response, "Sometimes I'll have a child do dictation for another if it's a written assignment" (Jenkins et al., 2003).

Two teachers reported assisting struggling students outside the CL group so that they would be more successful in the CL group. One said:

> Sometimes when we are doing writing, I do help him a lot, have him read a story to me and we meet together just the two of us first and then I help him elaborate on his story. So I pull a little bit out of him, and we write together before he goes back to his group so he goes back with a good product, so he always has success within his group. (Jenkins et al., 2003)

Two teachers who claimed not to make adjustments for students with disabilities said that the CL group was responsible for making adjustments for struggling students. One responded, "I think in a CL situation the whole point is to help each other be the best you can be, and if a child needs help, group members will step in and assist him" (Jenkins et al., 2003).

In summary, these general education teachers saw CL as one of the strongest means available for teaching special education students. When asked to compare CL with eight other approaches (e.g., tutoring, individualized instruction, and teacher-led small group instruction), 16 of 20 teachers ranked CL first or second in effectiveness in meeting special education students' needs. Although teachers gave generally favorable reviews to the effectiveness of CL for students with learning problems, nearly half acknowledged that CL did not always work well and they had to make adjustments (usually in composing groups) to facilitate these students' performance. The teachers also considered more aspects of efficacy than academic learning, emphasizing benefits such as self-esteem, a safe learning environment, higher success rates, and better classroom products and participation levels, as well as academic achievement.

One finding that cuts across the observation studies and teacher interviews is that students with LD differ in their response to CL. Why do some students fare better than others? O'Connor and Jenkins's (1996) research suggests that the way teachers implement CL *and* the characteristics of the students themselves play a role in success. Other studies suggest that characteristics of students with LD and the way these students are perceived by their classmates must be considered when using CL in general education settings (Beaumont, 1999). Putnam, Markovchick, Johnson, and Johnson (1996) found that long-term involvement in CL groups (twice weekly over 8 months) improved perceptions of students with disabilities in grades 5 through 8; however, students *without* disabilities were still perceived as more desirable work partners. Moreover, many students with LD prefer not to work in groups (Elbaum, Moody, & Schumm, 1999) where their reading difficulties are more apparent to their peers, the noise and distractions make completing work more difficult, and the number of groups in the classroom can increase the time it takes to get appropriate help from a teacher.

Donohue (1994) suggests that some of the difficulties in peer relationships and acceptance found across studies may relate to oral language problems and difficulty in discerning discourse patterns that students with LD experience. For example, many students with LD have difficulty with tactfulness (Pearl, Donahue, & Bryan, 1985) and the negotiations needed to resolve social conflicts (Holder & Kirkpatrick, 1991; Pearl, 1992). Unfortunately, these social skills may be prerequisites to accomplishing tasks in CL groupings.

CL is a blunt instrument that depending on its form and implementation may or may not help students with LD. CL comes in many forms (e.g., Heads together, Jigsaw, Group investigation, TAI, CIRC, Student Teams–Achievement Divisions, Teams–Games–Tournaments, formal and informal versions of Learning Together; not to mention individual teachers' infinite variations on these methods). CL may run from large-scale group projects to collaborative homework, from rehearsal of math and science facts to discussion-oriented literature circles, from completing grammar exercises to writing and presenting reports. Teachers may engage students in learning activities that boost achievement or in activities that are merely engaging. Teachers may incorporate some or all of researcher–developers' criteria for CL. They may induce individual accountability, by using Slavin's (1990) suggestions (e.g., administering tests, computing individual students' improvement scores, and summing improvement points to represent group performance), by using less exacting procedures (e.g., randomly selecting individual students to represent their groups), or by inculcating an ethic of team work (e.g., using modeling, object lessons, admonitions, and rewards), any of which may be implemented more or less efficiently, more or less successfully. Teachers may instruct students in interpersonal and team skills for as long as it takes, or teach and hope. Teachers may effectively monitor groups to ensure that everyone participates and benefits, or fail to notice and intervene with underperforming groups. They may pair struggling learners with under- or oversupportive peers who provide too little or too much help. In any number of ways, subtle and not so subtle differences in the form and implementation of CL may be as important for students' learning and development as is the difference between implementing CL or another instructional approach.

References

Alberg, J. (1991). Models for integration. In J. W. Lloyd, N. N. Singh, & A. C. Repp (Eds.), *The Regular Education Initiative: Alternative perspectives on concepts, issues, and models* (pp. 211–221). Sycamore, IL: Sycamore.

Antil, L. R., Jenkins, J. R., Wayne, S. K., & Vadasy, P. F. (1998). Cooperative learning: Prevalence, conceptualizations, and the relation between research and practice. *American Educational Research Journal, 35,* 419–454.

Aronson, E., Blaney, N., Stephan, C., Sikes, J., & Snapp, M. (1978). *The jigsaw classroom.* Beverly Hills, CA: Sage.

Beaumont, C. J. (1999). Dilemmas of peer assistance in a bilingual full inclusion classroom. *Elementary School Journal, 99,* 233–254.

Carnine, D., Silbert, J., & Kameenui, E. J. (1990). *Direct instruction reading* (2nd ed.). New York: Merrill.

Cohen, E., Lotan, R., & Catanzarite, L. (1990). Treating status probelsm in cooperative classrooms. In S. Sharan (Ed.), *Cooperative learning: Theory and research* (pp. 203–230). New York: Longman.

Delquardi, J., Greenwood, C. R., Whorton, D., Carta, J., & Hall, R. V. (1996). Classwide peer tutoring. *Exceptional Children, 52,* 535–542.

Deutsch, M. (1962). Cooperation and trust: Some theoretical notes. In M. R. Jones (Ed.), *Proceedings of the Nebraska Symposium on Motivation* (pp. 275–319). Lincoln: University of Nebraska Press.

Donohue, M. (1994). Differences in classroom discourse styles of students with learning disabilities. In D. N. Ripich & N. A. Creaghead (Eds.), *School discourse problems* (pp. 229–260). San Diego, CA: Singular.

Elbaum, B., Moody, S. W., & Schumm, J. S. (1999). Mixed ability grouping for breading: What students think. *Learning Disabilities Research and Practice, 14,* 61–66.

Englert, C. S., Garmon, A., Mariage, T., Rozendal, M., Tarrant, K., & Urba, J. (1995). The Early Literacy Project: Connecting across the literacy curriculum. *Learning Disability Quarterly, 18,* 253–275.

Foyle, H. C., & Bailey, G. D. (1988). Research homework experiments in social studies: Implications for teaching. *Social Education, 52,* 292–298.

Fuchs, L. S., Fuchs, D., Hamlett, C. L., Phillips, N. B., Karns, K., & Dutka, S. (1997). Enhancing students' helping behavior during peer mediated instruction with conceptual mathematical explanations. *Elementary School Journal, 97,* 223–249.

Gillies, R. M., & Ashman, A. F. (2000). The effects of cooperative learning on students with learning difficulties in the lower elementary school. *Journal of Special Education, 34,* 19–27.

Graham, S. & Harris, K. R. (1997). It can be taught, but it does not develop naturally: Myths and realities in writing instruction. *School-Psychology-Review, 26,* 414–424.

Holder, H., & Kirkpatrick, S. (1991). Interpretation of emotion from facial expressions in children with and without learning disabilities. *Journal of Learning Disabilities, 24,* 170–177.

Jenkins, J. R., Antil, L. R., Wayne, S. K., & Vadasy, P. F. (2003). How cooperative learning works for special education and remedial students. *Exceptional Children, 69,* 3.

Jenkins, J. R., & Jenkins, L. M. (1981). *Cross-age and peer tutoring: Help for children with learning problems.* Reston, VA: Council for Exceptional Children.

Jenkins, J. R., Jewell, M., Leicester, N., Jenkins, L., & Troutner, N. (1990, April). *Develop-*

ment of a school building model for educating handicapped and at risk students in general education classrooms. Paper presented at the meeting of the American Educational Research Association, Boston.

Jenkins, J. R., Jewell, M., Leicester, N., Jenkins, L., & Troutner, N. (1991). Development of a school building model for education students with handicaps and at-risk students in general education classrooms. *Journal of Learning Disabilities, 24,* 311–320.

Jenkins, J. R., Jewell, M., Leicester, N., O'Connor, R. E., Jenkins, L. & Troutner, N. (1994). Accommodations for individual differences without classroom ability groups: An experiment in school restructuring. *Exceptional Children, 60,* 344–358.

Johnson, D. W. (1970). *The psychology of education.* New York: Holt, Rinehart, and Winston.

Johnson, D. W., & Johnson, R. T. (1980). Integrating handicapped children into the mainstream. *Exceptional Children, 47,* 90–98.

Johnson, D. W., & Johnson, R. T. (1986). Mainstreaming and cooperative learning strategies. *Exceptional Children, 52,* 553–561.

Johnson, D. W., & Johnson, R. T. (1987). *Learning together and alone: Cooperative, competitive, and individualistic learning* (2nd ed.). Boston: Allyn & Bacon.

Johnson, D. W., & Johnson, R. T. (1991). *Learning together and alone: Cooperative, competitive, and individualistic learning* (3rd ed.). Boston: Allyn & Bacon.

Johnson, D. W., & Johnson, R. T. (1992). Implementing cooperative learning. *Contemporary Education, 63*(3), 173–180.

Johnson, D. W., Johnson, R. T., & Holubec, E. J. (1993). *Circles of learning: Cooperation in the classroom* (4th ed.). Edina, MN: Interaction.

Kagan, S. (1989–90). The structural approach to cooperative learning. *Educational Leadership, 47*(4), 12–15.

Klingner, J. K., & Vaughn, S. (1996). Reciprocal teaching of reading comprehension strategies for students with learning disabilities who use English as a second language. *Elementary School Journal, 96,* 275–293.

Klingner, J. K., Vaughn, S., & Schumm, J. S. (1998). Collaborative strategic reading during social studies in heterogeneous four-grade classrooms. *Elementary School Journal, 99,* 3–22.

Lehr, F. (1984). Cooperative learning. *Journal of Reading, 27,* 458–460.

Lewin, K. (1935). *A dynamic theory of personality.* New York: McGraw-Hill.

Mainzer, R. W., Mainzer, K. L., Slavin, R. E., & Lowry, E. (1993). What special education teachers should know about cooperative learning. *Teacher Education and Special Education, 16*(1), 42–50.

Malouf, D. B., Wizer, D. R., Pilato, V. H., & Grogan, M. M. (1990). Computer-assisted instruction with small groups of mildly handicapped students. *Journal of Special Education, 24,* 51–68.

McMaster, K. N., & Fuchs, D. (2002). Effects of cooperative learning on the academic achievement of students with learning disabilities: An update of Tateyama-Sniezek's review. *Learning Disabilities Research and Practice, 17,* 107–117.

Moskowitz, J. M., Malvin, J. H., Schaeffer, G. A., & Schaps, E. (1983). Evaluation of a cooperative learning strategy. *American Educational Research Journal, 20,* 687–696.

O'Connor, R. E., & Jenkins, J. R. (1996). Cooperative learning as an inclusion strategy: A closer look. *Exceptionality, 6,* 29–51.

O'Melia, M. C., & Rosenberg, M. S. (1994). Effects of cooperative homework teams on the acquisition of mathematics skills by secondary students with mild disabilities. *Exceptional Children, 60,* 538–548.

Palincsar, A., & Brown, A. L. (1984). Reciprocal teaching of comprehension-fostering and monitoring activities. *Cognition and Instruction, 1,* 117–175.

Palincsar, A. S, & Brown, A. L (1986). Interactive teaching to promote independent learning from text. *Reading–Teacher, 39,* 771–777.

Pearl, R. (1992). Psychosocial characteristics of learning disabled students. In N. Singh & I. Beale (Eds.), *Current perspectives in learning disabilities: Nature, theory, and treatment* (pp. 96–117). New York: Springer-Verlag.

Pearl, R., Donahue, M., & Bryan, T. (1985). The development of tact: Children's strategies for delivering bad news. *Journal of Applied Developmental Psychology, 6,* 141–149.

Puma, M. J., Jones, C. C., Rock, D., & Fernandez, R. (1993). *Prospects: The congressionally mandated study of educational growth and opportunity* (Interim Report). Bethesda, MD: Abt.

Putnam, J., Markovchick, K., Johnson, D. W., & Johnson, R. T. (1996). Cooperative learning and peer acceptance of students with learning disabilities. *Journal of School Psychology, 136,* 741–752.

Sharan, S. (1980). Cooperative learning in small groups: Recent methods and effects on achievement, attitudes, and ethnic relations. *Review of Educational Research, 50,* 241–271.

Slavin, R. E. (1983a). *Cooperative learning: Theory, research, and practice.* Englewood Cliffs, NJ: Prentice-Hall.

Slavin, R. E. (1983b). When does cooperative learning increase student achievement? *Psychological Bulletin, 94,* 429–445.

Slavin, R. E. (1990). *Cooperative learning: Theory, research, and practice.* Boston: Allyn & Bacon.

Slaven, R. E. (1996). Neverstreaming: Preventing learning disabilities. *Educational Leadership, 53,* 4–7.

Slavin, R. E., Madden, N., Dolan, L. J., &

Wasik, B. A. (1992). *Success for all: A relentless approach to prevention and early intervention in elementary schools.* Arlington, VA: Educational Research Service.

Slavin, R. E., Madden, N. A., & Leavey, M. (1984). Effects of team assisted individualization on the mathematics achievement of academically handicapped students and nonhandicapped students. *Journal of Educational Psychology, 76,* 813–819.

Slavin, R. E., & Stevens, R. J. (1991). Cooperative learning and mainstreaming. In J. W. Lloyd, N. N. Singh, & A. C. Repp (Eds.), *The Regular Education Initiative: Alternative perspectives on concepts, issues, and models* (pp. 177–191). Sycamore, IL: Sycamore.

Slavin, R. E., Stevens, R. J., & Madden, N. A. (1988). Accommodating student diversity in reading and writing instruction: A cooperative learning approach. *Remedial and Special Education, 9,* 60–66.

Stevens, R. J., Madden, N. A., Slavin, R. E., & Farnish, A. M. (1987). Cooperative integrated reading and composition: Two field experiments. *Reading Research Quarterly, 22,* 433–454.

Stevens, R. J., & Slavin, R. E. (1995a). The cooperative elementary school: effects on students' achievement, attitudes, and social relations. *American Educational Research Journal, 32,* 321–351.

Stevens, R. J., & Slavin, R. E. (1995b). Effects of a cooperative learning approach in reading and writing on academically handicapped and nonhandicapped students. *Elementary School Journal, 95,* 241–262.

Tateyama-Sniezek, K. M. (1990). Cooperative learning: Does it improve the academic achievement of students with handicaps? *Exceptional Children, 56,* 426–437.

Thousand, J. S., & Villa, R. A. (1991). A futuristic view of the REI: Response to Jenkins, Pious, and Jewell. *Exceptional Children, 57*(6), 556–562.

Utay, C., & Utay, J. (1997). Peer-assisted learning: The effects of cooperative learning and cross-age tutoring with word processing on writing skills of students with learning disabilities. *Journal of Computing in Childhood Education, 8,* 165–185.

Vygotsky, L. S. (1978). *Mind in society: The development of higher psychological processes.* Cambridge, MA: Harvard University Press.

Wang, M. C., & Birch, J. W. (1984). Comparison of a full-time mainstreaming program and a resource room approach. *Exceptional Children, 51,* 33–40.

Will, M. (1986). *Educating students with learning problems: A shared responsibility.* Washington, DC: Office of Special Education and Rehabilitation Services, U. S. Department of Education.

Wong, B. Y. L., Butler, D. L., Ficzere, S. A., & Kuperis, S. (1996). Teaching low achievers and students with learning disabilities to plan, write, and revise opinion essays. *Journal of Learning Disabilities, 29,* 197–212.

Wong, B. Y. L., Butler, D. L., Ficzere, S. A., & Kuperis, S. (1997). Teaching adolescents with learning disabilities and low achievers to plan, write, and revise compare and contrast essays. *Learning Disabilities Research and Practice, 12,* 2–15.

Wood, K. D., Algozzine, B., & Avett, S. (1993). Promoting cooperative learning experiences for students with reading, writing, and learning disabilities. *Reading and Writing Quarterly, 9,* 369–376.

Xin, F. (1996). *The effects of computer-assisted cooperative learning in mathematics in integrated classrooms for students with and without disabilities.* Glassboro: Rowan College of New Jersey. (ERIC Document Reproduction Service No. ED 412696)

26

Identifying Children at Risk for Reading Failure: Curriculum-Based Measurement and the Dual-Discrepancy Approach

Douglas Fuchs
Lynn S. Fuchs
Kristen N. McMaster
Stephanie Al Otaiba

This chapter begins with two uncontested facts: (1) Reading is a foundational skill for virtually all learning (Lyon et al., 2001; Snow, Burns, & Griffin, 1998), and (2) it must be mastered sooner rather than later. Juel's (1988) research has underscored this latter point; she determined that as many as 88% of unsuccessful readers in her first-grade sample remained poor readers in fourth grade. In addition, the gap between poor readers and their more accomplished peers widens over the elementary grades (e.g., Greenwood, Hart, Walker, & Risley, 1993; Stanovich, 1986), partly because remediation becomes increasingly challenging after third grade (e.g., Fletcher & Foorman, 1994).

Moreover, struggling readers do not merely lag behind their peers in reading and other academic areas; they are also more likely to be referred to special education (e.g., Mastropieri, Leinart, & Scruggs, 1999; Riley, 1996) and to suffer low self-esteem, break school rules, and drop out of school (e.g., Juel, 1996). Because many poor readers will someday become illiterate adults, it is noteworthy that this adult group accounts

for 75% of the unemployed, 33% of mothers receiving aid to families of dependent children, and 60% of prison inmates (Orton Dyslexia Society, cited in Adams, 1990).

Treatment Nonresponders

Because reading failure is closely related to so much human misery, and can require so many costly resources from society to deal with its repercussions in adulthood, policymakers are currently supporting various reading initiatives, such as "Reading First," that rely on research-validated early reading programs. One acknowledged research-validated approach is phonological awareness training (e.g., Bradley & Bryant, 1985; Lundberg, Frost, & Peterson, 1988), especially when it is linked to decoding instruction (e.g., Ball & Blachman, 1991; Byrne & Fielding-Barnsley, 1993; Fuchs, Fuchs, Thompson, Al Otaiba, et al., 2001; Hatcher, Hulme, & Ellis, 1994). Bus and van IJzendoorn's (1999) meta-analysis of this literature reported strong short-term effects for phonological awareness training on phonological measures (ES = 0.73) and reading measures (ES = 0.70).

Whereas phonological awareness training helps many to learn to read, it does not help all. Indeed, researchers have reported that as many as 30% of children at risk for reading difficulties (e.g., Blachman, 1994, 1997; Brown & Felton, 1990; Fuchs, Fuchs, Mathes, & Simmons, 1997; Juel, 1994; Mathes, Howard, Allen, & Fuchs, 1998; Shannahan & Bahr, 1995; Torgesen, Morgan, & Davis, 1992), and 50% or more of children with special needs (e.g., Fuchs, Fuchs, Thompson, et al., 2002; O'Connor, 2000; O'Connor, Jenkins, Leicester, & Slocum, 1993; O'Connor, Jenkins, & Slocum, 1995), do not benefit from research-backed phonological awareness programs. Such students have been dubbed treatment "resisters" and "nonresponders."

There are several reasons why children unresponsive to generally effective treatments are the focus of much current research (e.g., Foorman, Francis, Fletcher, Schatschneider, & Mehta, 1998; Torgesen, Wagner, & Rashotte, 1997; Torgesen et al., 1999; Vellutino et al., 1996). First, they are seen as truly having reading disabilities (or learning disabilities [LD]), as opposed to students who read poorly because of poor school instruction (see Vellutino et al., 1996). Whereas both kinds of poor readers should be of concern to educators, studying nonresponders, it is believed, may reveal specific cognitive and linguistic mechanisms responsible for reading disabilities. This, in turn, may help researchers discover precursors of the condition, which would help practitioners in earlier identification and in the formulation of earlier interventions that may even obviate reading failure in the first place. Second, increasing numbers of researchers and policymakers (e.g., Lyon et al., 2001) prefer the unresponsiveness-to-treatment paradigm to traditional methods of identifying poor readers, namely, the IQ–achievement discrepancy approach, which has been used for a quarter century to identify children with LD. This approach has been criticized for many reasons, including that IQ tests allegedly do a poor job of estimating intelligence; that poor readers with an IQ–achievement discrepancy are presumably no different than poor readers without an IQ–achievement discrepancy on

most reading-related measures; and, maybe most persuasive, students must read poorly for several years before they demonstrate an IQ–achievement discrepancy that legitimizes them as proper recipients of special education services. (See Fuchs, Fuchs, Mathes, Lipsey, & Roberts, 2001, for a more complete discussion of the concerns about conventional definitions and operationalizations of the LD construct.)

There is a third reason for interest in nonresponders. A small but growing number of special education academics are arguing that such children should be the responsibility of special educators. If so, goes the argument, special education teachers and trainers of teachers will need to reorient toward instructional concerns and away from "co-teaching," "collaborative consultation," and other endeavors that, however well meaning, have caused many to lose sight of the fact that their field's traditional raison d'être and strength was to provide expert instruction to students with unique learning needs.

Defining Nonresponsiveness

Because researchers have only recently begun using treatment unresponsiveness as a means of identifying poor readers, problems still exist with the approach. Chief among them is an absence of a definition of nonresponsiveness on which many can agree. This absence may seem strange because, on its face, the definition would appear self-evident: "Nonresponsiveness refers to a failure to respond to generally effective instruction." But what precisely does it mean to be "nonresponsive" to instruction? Al Otaiba and Fuchs (2002) conducted an extensive review of this literature and Table 26.1 is a simplification of their tables. Table 26.1 lists 23 studies meeting Al Otaiba and Fuchs's criteria for inclusion in their review. For each study, our table briefly describes respective participants and the definitions of unresponsiveness used by the authors.

Authors have defined unresponsiveness in one of two basic ways: level of performance or rate of growth. More obvious in the table is the considerable variation associated with each of these definitions. With respect to "level of performance," for example, Torge-

TABLE 26.1. Studies Conducted to Explore Characteristics of Unresponsive Children

Article	Demographics	Treatment	Definition and percentage of unresponsive students
		Studies conducted primarily to explore characteristics	
Berninger et al. (1999)	*M* age = 7 years 2% black, 8% Hispanic, 2% Asian, 4% Native American, *M* Verbal IQ = 91.60 Lowest 15% in reading and phonological awareness	Whole word vs. subword (phonemic) vs. whole word + subword training. 8–30 minute tutorials Total = 4 hours	No growth on words trained: 52% No growth on WRMT-R WA: 63% No growth on WRMT-R WI: 75%
Hatcher & Hulme (1999) (see primary study: Hatcher, Hulme, & Ellis, 1994)	*M* age = 7 years *M* IQ = 68–122 Lowest 25% of reading	Phonology (P) vs. Reading (R) vs. Phonology & Reading (P + R) vs. control Individual 30–40 minute tutorial Sessions, 20 weeks Total = 20 hours	Not defined. No percentage reported. Reported predictors of growth in reading accuracy and comprehension.
Schneider, Ennemoser, Roth, & Kuspert (1999) (see primary study: Schneider, Kuspert, Roth, Vise, & Marx, 1997)	*M* age = 5 years, 7 months German	Phonological awareness training using Lundberg's curriculum Classroom instruction Daily 10–15 minute sessions for 6 months Total = 20 hours	No gains. No percentage reported.
Torgesen & Davis (1996)	Age: 5–6 years 73% black, low SES *M* Verbal IQ = est. 91 Lowest 20% on phonological awareness	Phonological awareness training Small group format 4, 20-minute sessions per week 3-month duration Total = 16 hours	No gains. Segmenting: 30% Blending: 10%
Torgesen et al. (1999)	Age: 5–6 years 26% black, 2.1% Other, Verbal IQ > 75 Lowest 12% phonological processing	Phonological awareness + synthetic phonics (PASP), Embedded phonics (EP), regular classroom support (RCS) Individual tutorial 2, 20-minute sessions with tutor, 2, 20-minute sessions with instructional aide Total = 88 hours	WRMT-R standard score < 85 WA, WID, or PC, respectively Controls: 53%, 53%, 56% PASP: 24%, 21%, 36% EP: 47%, 28%, 47% RCS: 44%, 31%, 56%

(continued)

433

TABLE 26.1. *Continued*

Article	Demographics	Treatment	Definition and percentage of unresponsive students
	Studies conducted primarily to explore characteristics (cont.)		
Uhry & Shepherd (1997)	Age: 5–8 years 17% black, middle SES IQ > 90 Significant discrepancy between IQ and decoding and low phonological processing performance	Phonological awareness, reading, and writing Individual tutorial 2, 1-hour sessions per week 5-month duration Total = 40 hours	No gain in WRMT-R WID; 8%
Vellutino et al. (1996)	Age: 5–8 years Mostly white, middle SES IQ > 90 Poor readers in 15th percentile	Phonological awareness, reading, and writing Individual tutoring 5, 30-minute sessions per week for 1–2 semesters Total = 35–40 hours	Very limited growth: students with lowest growth slopes on WRMT-R WID & WAT from kindergarten—Fall of second grade: 26% Did not improve beyond 30th percentile on WRMT-R WID & WAT: 33%
	Studies exploring treatment effectiveness: Beginning readers without disabilities		
Ehri & Robbins (1992)	Age: 5–7 years Middle SES	Analogy training Individual tutorial 4, 15-minute sessions 1-month duration Total = 1 hour	Unable to read transfer words: 80% of students who could not segment & blend nonsense words; 0% of students who could segment.
Fox & Routh (1976)	M age = 4 years Middle SES M IQ =112	Decoding training Individual tutorial 2, half-hour sessions 1-week duration Total = 1 hour	Did not improve performance on decoding; 50% overall; 100% of students who could not segment
Peterson & Haines (1992)	Age: 5–6 years, PPVT > 85	Analogy training Individual tutorial 7, 15-minute sessions 1-month duration Total = 2 hours	Did not significantly improve word-reading: 33% overall; 100% of low-segmenters.

Study	Sample	Intervention	Findings
Vandervelden & Siegel (1997)	Age: 5–7 years Low SES	Phonological awareness and analogy training Individual or small-group training 1, 30–45-minute session/week 3-month duration Total = 6–9 hours	No gains in phonological awareness (PA): 13% overall; 18% of students with low PA. Could not read more than 1 word: 27% overall; 36% of students with low PA.

Studies exploring treatment effectiveness: Preliterate children with disabilities

Study	Sample	Intervention	Findings
Fazio (1997)	Age: 4–6 years M Nonverbal IQ = 85–115	Phonological encoding Individual tutoring 4, 15-minute sessions 1-month duration Total = 1 hour	Difficulty learning and recalling a rhyming poem: Percentage not reported.
Kasten (1998)	M age = 5 years White, low SES Mild mental retardation	Phonics training in resource room setting; whole language classroom instruction 3-year duration No total reported	Did not make significant growth on reading achievement on Woodcock Johnson Reading subtests. No percentage reported.
O'Connor et al. (1993)	Age: 4–6 years	Rhyming, blending, or segmenting Small-group training 4, 10-minute sessions per week 7-week duration Total = 4.5 hours	Did not learn to identify rhyming oddities: 8% Did not learn to blend onset-rime: 36% Did not learn to segment first sound: 46%
O'Connor, Notari-Syverson, & Vadasy (1996, 1998)	Age: 5–7 years 56% black, 2% other, M Verbal IQ = 67, Mild mental retardation; 90, learning disabled; 91, behavior disordered	Phonological awareness training in classroom 100–281 sessions 6-month duration No total reported	Made less than half the M gain in phonological awareness: General education students: 18% Students with disabilities: 33% Mild mental retardation: 66% Learning disabled: 38% Behavior disordered: 50%

(continued)

TABLE 26.1. *Continued*

Article	Demographics	Treatment	Definition and percentage of unresponsive students
		Studies exploring treatment effectiveness: Older children	
Foorman et al. (1997)	Age: 7–9 years 32% black, 24% low SES, Verbal IQ > 79 Lowest 25th percentile on reading	Synthetic phonics, analytic phonics, or sightword Whole class instruction 1 hour daily Resource room instruction 6-month duration Total = 120 hours	Not defined. No percentage reported.
Foorman, Francis, Fletcher, Schatschneider, & Mehta (1998)	Grades 1–2 60% black, 20% hispanic, low SES Lowest 18% in reading	Classroom instruction: Direct (DC), Embedded (EC), or Implicit Code delivered by School (IC-S) or by Research staff (IC-R) for 90 mins. daily; plus 30 mins. daily small group or tutorial instruction for 6 mos. No total reported	Learned fewer than 2.5 words on a 50-word list 46% IC-R 38% IC-S 44% EC 16% DC
Hurford (1990)	Age: 7–9 years IQ > 90 Lowest 35th percentile for reading	Phonemic discrimination	Posttreatment segmentations skills remain inferior to students without disabilities. No percentage reported.
Snider (1997)	Age: 7–9 years 10% low SES All students with LD	Code-emphasis reading instruction in resource room 30–45-minute daily 9-month duration Total = 90 hours	Did not significantly improve reading rate and accuracy on oral reading fluency: 10%
O'Shaughnessy & Swanson (2000)	M age = 7 years, 8 mos. 4.4% black, 2.2% Asian, 28.9% Hispanic, low SES M IQ = 89.9 Lowest 10% on reading and phonological awareness	Phonological Awareness Training (PAT) vs. Word Analogy Training (WAT), vs. a math training (MAT) condition Small-group format 3, 30-minute sessions across 6 weeks	Did not significantly improve the rate and accuracy on oral reading fluency: PAT: 20% WAT: 27%
Vadasy, Jenkins, Antil, Wayne, & O'Connor (1997)	Age: 5–8 years 50% Low SES	Phonological awareness and reading Individual tutorial 100 sessions 6-month duration Total = 54 hours	Gained less than 8 points on the Wide Range Achievement Test—Revised Reading and Spelling: 35%

Note. WRMT-R, Woodcock Reading Mastery Tests—Revised; WA, Word Attack; WI, Word Identification; SES, socioeconomic status.

sen and Davis's (1996) unresponsive students segmented only one word correctly and blended only two words or less than two words correctly. In contrast, Torgesen and colleagues' (1999) definition of unresponsiveness was a performance level that was one standard deviation below the mean of the standardization population on Word Attack (WA) and Word Identification (WI) tests from the Woodcock Reading Mastery Tests (WRMTs). For Hurford (1990), posttreatment segmentation scores less than those of students with disabilities distinguished nonresponders. In terms of "rate of growth," Hatcher and Hulme (1999) defined treatment nonresponsiveness as no growth whatsoever on reading accuracy, whereas Foorman and colleagues (1998) set growth at less than 2.5 words read correctly per minute over an academic year as their nonresponsiveness criterion (see Table 26.1).

We believe that there are serious limitations to both the performance-level and growth-rate definitions. Understanding unresponsiveness only in terms of performance level would appear problematic for low-performing students because performance level is insensitive to growth. In other words, performance may be at a relatively low level, but the student may have demonstrated admirable growth nonetheless. Likewise, conceptualizing nonresponsiveness by growth alone would seem to ignore the possibility that high-performing students may show comparatively little of it but may be performing at acceptable levels. Low-performing students, including many with disabilities, may make relatively impressive growth and still have unacceptably low levels of performance.

What is needed is a criterion-referenced framework that provides growth cut-points, below which meaningful long-term functional reading competence is jeopardized. At this time, the cut-points are unknown. Nevertheless, we believe that there is a desirable alternative to performance-level-only and growth-rate-only approaches. We call this alternative the dual-discrepancy approach (Fuchs & Fuchs, 1998a, 1998b). As its name implies, it combines both performance level and growth rate in identifying nonresponders. Before explaining and illustrating the dual-discrepancy approach, we turn our attention to curriculum-based mea-surement (CBM), which is at the heart of our method of identifying students unresponsive to generally effective instruction.

Curriculum-Based Measurement

CBM is a set of methods for indexing academic competence and progress. In developing CBM, Deno and colleagues (see Deno, 1985) sought to establish a measurement system that (1) teachers could use efficiently; (2) would produce accurate, meaningful information with which to index standing and growth; (3) could answer questions about the effectiveness of programs in producing academic growth; and (4) would provide information that helped teachers plan better instructional programs. To accomplish this goal, a systematic program of research, conceptualized as a 3 × 3 matrix (see Deno & Fuchs, 1987), was undertaken. The rows in this matrix specified three questions for developing a measurement system (what to measure, how to measure, and how to use the resulting database); the columns provided three criteria against which answers to those questions could be formulated (technical adequacy, treatment validity, and feasibility). A 20-year research program, undertaken by independent investigators at multiple sites, has addressed the cells in this matrix with multiple studies for four academic domains: reading, spelling, mathematics, and written expression.

In each domain, CBM deliberately integrates key concepts from traditional measurement theory and from the conventions of classroom-based observational methodology to forge an innovative approach to assessment. As with traditional measurement, every assessment samples a relatively broad range of skills by sampling each dimension of the annual curriculum on each weekly test. Consequently, each repeated measurement is an alternate form, of equivalent difficulty, assessing the same constructs. This sampling strategy differs markedly from typical classroom-based assessment methods, where teachers assess mastery on a single skill and, after mastery is demonstrated, then move on to a different, presumably more difficult skill (see Fuchs & Deno, 1991; Fuchs & Fuchs, 1999). CBM also reflects a traditional psychometry by incorporating conventional notions of reliability and validity: Standardized test administration and scoring methods have been designed to yield accurate and meaningful information.

By sampling broadly with standardized administration and scoring procedures, the CBM score can be viewed as a "performance indicator": It produces a broad dispersion of scores across individuals of the same age, with rank orderings that correspond to important external criteria, and it represents an individual's global level of competence in the domain. Practitioners can use this performance indicator to identify discrepancies in performance levels between individuals and peer groups, which helps inform decisions about the need for special services or the point at which decertification and reintegration of students with disabilities might occur.

At the same time, however, CBM departs from conventional psychometric applications by integrating concepts of standardized measurement and traditional reliability and validity with key features from classroom-based observational methodology: repeated performance sampling, fixed time recording, graphic displays of time-series data, and qualitative descriptions of student performance. Reliance on these classroom-based observational methods permits slope estimates for different time periods and alternative interventions for the same individual. This creates the necessary database for describing growth and testing the effects of different treatments for a given student. Research also suggests that when combined with prescriptive decision rules, these time-series analytic methods result in better instruction and learning: Teachers raise goals more often and develop higher expectations (Fuchs, Fuchs, & Hamlett, 1989a), they introduce more adaptations to their instruction (Fuchs, Fuchs, & Hamlett, 1989b), and they produce better student learning (Fuchs, Fuchs, Hamlett, & Stecker, 1991).

In addition, because each assessment simultaneously samples the multiple skills embedded in the annual curriculum, CBM can yield qualitative descriptions of student performance to supplement graphed quantitative analyses of CBM total scores. These diagnostic profiles demonstrate reliability and validity (see Fuchs, Fuchs, Hamlett, & Allinder, 1991; Fuchs, Fuchs, Hamlett,

Thompson, et al., 1994), offer the advantage of being based on the local curriculum, provide a framework for determining strategies for improving student programs, and result in teachers planning more varied, specific, and responsive instruction to meet individual student needs (Fuchs, Fuchs, Hamlett, & Allinder, 1991).

Consequently, CBM bridges traditional psychometric and classroom-based observational assessment paradigms and represents an innovative approach to measurement. Through this bridging of frameworks, CBM simultaneously yields information about standing as well as change; about global competence as well as skill-by-skill mastery. CBM, therefore, can be used to answer questions about interindividual differences (e.g., How different is Henry's academic level and growth from that of other students in the class, school, or district?); questions about intraindividual improvement (e.g., How successful is an adapted regular classroom in producing better academic growth for Henry?); and questions about how to strengthen individual students' programs (e.g., On which skills in the annual curriculum does Henry require instruction?).

Next, we discuss research demonstrating the psychometric features of CBM; then we examine CBM's capacity to evaluate treatment effects; and finally, we describe how CBM may be used to identify children who do not profit from generally effective instruction.

CBM's Psychometric Features

We illustrate the psychometric strengths of CBM by briefly summarizing information in the area of reading. In mathematics, spelling, and written expression, similar data exist; however, the vast majority of independent replications occur in reading. We discuss the technical adequacy of CBM in terms of the features necessary for describing performance at one point in time versus the features required to model growth over time.

Describing Student Competence at One Point in Time

To provide the basis for sound decision making about a student's performance level, an assessment score (or an average across several scores) must provide an accurate and meaningful estimate of competence. Therefore, traditional psychometric methods for investigating technical adequacy apply. To achieve these traditional psychometric criteria, assessment methods typically sample behavior broadly, rely on standardized administration and scoring procedures, and are thereby viewed as "performance indicators." This is true for CBM, which illustrates how a classroom-based assessment can achieve traditional psychometric standards.

There are two CBM assessments in reading: number of words read aloud and correctly from text (1 minute) and number of correct replacements restored to text in which every seventh word has been deleted (2.5 minutes). For each assessment, studies demonstrate strong criterion validity with respect to widely used commercial reading tests (Fuchs & Fuchs, 1992; Marston, 1989), informal reading measures involving question answering, cloze completion, and recall of passages (Fuchs & Fuchs, 1992; Fuchs, Fuchs, & Maxwell, 1988), and teachers' judgments of reading competence (Fuchs & Fuchs, 1992; Fuchs, Fuchs, & Deno, 1982). In addition, there is evidence of (1) construct validity; (2) discriminative validity with respect to special education status (Deno, Mirkin, & Chiang, 1982; Shinn, Tindal, Spira, & Marston, 1987) and grade level (Deno, 1985; Fuchs & Deno, 1992; Fuchs, Fuchs, Hamlett, Walz, & Germann, 1993); (3) stability (Fuchs, Deno, & Marston, 1983; Fuchs & Fuchs, 1992); and (4) interscorer agreement (Fuchs, Fuchs, Hamlett, & Ferguson, 1992; Marston & Deno, 1981).

In a recent study of CBM's psychometric features, Hosp and Fuchs (2001) had 74 first-graders, 81 second-graders, 79 third-graders, and 75 fourth-graders read two CBM grade-appropriate passages; had the students complete the Woodcock Reading Mastery Tests Word Identification (WI), Word Attack (WA), and Passage Comprehension subtests; and readministered the CBM passages 2 to 3 weeks later to a subsample of the participants (i.e., 29, 30, 30, and 30 at grades 1–4, respectively). At these respective grades, criterion validity between CBM and WI was .89, .88, .89, and .79; between CBM and WA, .70, .82, .82, and .74; between CBM and Passage Comprehension, .76, .83, .83, and .83. Test–retest reliability was .96, .97, .93, and .93.

Modeling Academic Growth

There are two reasons why performance indicators commonly associated with commercial tests are also important to classroom-based assessment methods, such as CBM, for modeling growth. First, performance indicators provide a broad range of scores required for demonstrating change over time. Second, the traditional standards of psychometric adequacy on which performance indicators are based provide necessary evidence for presuming that differences between an individual's data points represent meaningful change.

Although these traditional psychometric criteria are necessary to identify a behavior to use within CBM, they are insufficient evidence that a measure can adequately depict growth. As discussed by Francis, Shaywitz, Steubing, Shaywitz, and Fletcher (1994), instruments for modeling longitudinal individual change must demonstrate certain technical features, which are illustrated in CBM. First, the instrument must provide equal scaling of individuals throughout the range of behavior measured over time (i.e., produce data with interval scale properties, free from ceiling or floor effects). With CBM, a common test framework is administered to children within a fixed age range; thus, it is possible to judge performance over an academic year on the same raw score metric. And when performance is measured on the appropriate instructional level of the curriculum, floor and ceiling effects do not occur.

Second, the construct and the difficulty level measured over time must remain constant. CBM taps constructs that are qualitatively constant over an academic year, for which the difficulty level remains the same. The third technical requirement for modeling growth is that a sufficient number of alternate forms must be available to obtain accurate estimates of change parameters. With CBM, one can sample the curriculum repeatedly to create as many alternate forms as necessary, and research (Fuchs, 1993) suggests that 7–10 data points are adequate for fitting data to a model.

Current techniques for measuring change help researchers and practitioners to reconceptualize growth as a continuous rather than an incremental process. The goal is to describe trajectories, or continuous time-dependent curves, which reflect the change process. An initial step in such a process is to develop a change model at the individual level. Examination of individual and group time-series CBM data provides the basis for an empirical approximation of the shape of CBM growth curves (Francis et al., 1994). Fuchs and colleagues (1993), for example, examined students' academic growth rates when CBM was conducted for 1 school year in students' grade-appropriate curriculum level. Unweighted "weekly" slopes were calculated using a least-squares regression between scores and calendar days; a quadratic component was included in the analysis, as slope was calculated for each individual, to determine whether it contributed to the modeling of student progress. For many students on each CBM measure, a linear relationship adequately modeled student progress within one academic year. When significant quadratic terms occurred, for 0–21% of students, growth was almost consistently described by a negatively accelerating pattern in which student performance continues to improve over the course of a year but the amount of that progress gradually decreases. As suggested in cross-sectional data, this negatively accelerating pattern may also characterize growth across academic years. These findings, in combination with corroborating evidence (Good, Deno, & Fuchs, 1995; Good & Shinn, 1990), support a conceptualization of annual CBM growth characterized by a linear relationship, where slope is a primary parameter describing change. Consequently, CBM appears to be a tenable measurement tool for modeling academic growth.

Evaluating Treatment Effectiveness with CBM

To function as a tool for evaluating treatment effectiveness, CBM must provide data to answer questions such as, "Is regular classroom instruction promoting adequate student growth?" Do adaptations to instruction in the regular classroom result in a stronger growth rate? And, Does the provision of specialized services enhance learning? To answer these and other treatment-effectiveness questions, assessment must be sensitive to student growth and to relative treatment effects, and it must facilitate comparisons of the effectiveness of alternative service delivery options. Researchers and practitioners have shown that CBM can do all of this.

Sensitivity to Academic Change

In an early study addressing sensitivity to academic change, Marston, Fuchs, and Deno (1986) tested students both on traditional commercial achievement tests and on curriculum-based reading and written language measures. Students were tested early in October and again 10 weeks later in December. CBM registered more student growth than did the traditional commercial tests, suggesting that CBM was more sensitive to student growth.

Additional research has directly compared the sensitivity of CBM pre–post performance levels to that of CBM slopes. For example, while investigating the effects of a 3-week winter break on students' math performance, Allinder and Fuchs (1994) contrasted (1) CBM performance levels before and after the break with (2) pre- and postbreak slopes of progress. Results differed by type of analysis. Effects of winter break were not demonstrated when performance level was assessed, but an examination of slopes showed that students with positive prebreak trends were affected adversely by the break, whereas students with negative prebreak trends were not.

Studies have also demonstrated that slopes based on ongoing CBM data are more sensitive indices of treatment effects than traditional measures administered on a pre–post basis. Fuchs and colleagues (1989b) showed that on the Stanford Achievement Test—Reading Comprehension subtest, administered to detect incremental change between two points in time, change scores of the treatment groups were not significantly different, and the effect size was a relatively low 0.36. By contrast, on CBM slope data, differences between groups achieved statistical significance and were associated with a larger effect size of

0.86 standard deviations. This pattern of substantially larger effect sizes for CBM slope data has been corroborated in other treatment effectiveness research (e.g., Fuchs, Fuchs, Hamlett, Phillips, & Bentz, 1994; Fuchs, Fuchs, Hamlett, & Stecker, 1991). Evidence, therefore, suggests that CBM slopes may be sensitive to student growth and to the relative effects of alternative treatments.

Comparing Student Progress under Alternative Service Delivery Options

CBM, therefore, is a sensitive measurement system. Nevertheless, the question remains whether it is useful when comparing student progress under alternatived service delivery options. Two CBM studies illustrate this type of decision making. Marston (1987–1988) compared the relative effectiveness of regular and special education by analyzing slope on weekly CBM reading scores. An initial pool of 272 fourth-, fifth-, and sixth-graders were selected for the yearlong study on the basis of performance at or below the 15th percentile on the Minneapolis Benchmark Test. The CBM reading performance of these 272 children was measured weekly. Eleven students who spent at least 10 weeks in regular education, were referred to and placed in special education, and spent at least 10 weeks in special education were the focus of the analysis.

To determine relative treatment effects of the two service delivery arrangements (i.e., general education and special education), a repeated-measures analysis of variance was applied to the CBM slope data. Slopes were statistically significantly greater in special than in regular education, with the average slopes increasing from .60 to 1.15 words across the two service delivery settings. For 10 of 11 students, slopes were larger in special education; in 7 of the 10 cases, the difference was rather dramatic (see Fuchs & Fuchs, 1995; Marston, 1987–1988).

In a similar way, Fuchs, Fuchs, and Fernstrom (1993) used slope to examine the relative effectiveness of special and regular education for individual students as they moved in the opposite direction; that is, as they reintegrated into general education classrooms. Twenty-one special education students had been randomly assigned to a condition designed to facilitate their successful return to regular classrooms for math instruction through a deliberate and systematic process involving transenvironmental programming and CBM. Special educators used CBM to strengthen their math instruction. At the same time, they monitored each special education student's CBM growth and that of three low-performing (without disabilities) members of the mainstream classroom targeted for the special education student's return. When the special education student's performance level approximated that of the three low-performing peers, reintegration occurred and the responsibility for math instruction was transferred to the regular classroom teacher. After reintegration, CBM data continued to be collected for both the special education student and the low-performing peers.

Within special education, the averaged slope for the 21 experimental students was significantly greater than that of the low-performing peers in the mainstream. However, after reintegration, the slope of the special education students plunged and was significantly lower than that of the comparison students. On average, 63% of the reintegrated students' CBM data points in regular education fell below trend lines that had been projected on the basis of their progress in special education. This compared to only 44% for the comparison peers, a statistically significant difference. As with the Marston (1987–1988) study, this database indicates the relative effectiveness of special education over general education for many students with disabilities. Both studies demonstrate CBM's capacity to document the relative effects of service delivery options (see also Fuchs, Roberts, Fuchs, & Bowers, 1996).

Identifying Nonresponders with CBM: The Dual-Discrepancy Approach

The traditional assessment framework for identifying students with LD relies on discrepancies between intelligence and achievement tests to operationalize "unexpected underachievement." As mentioned, this traditional identification procedure has been criticized for measurement and conceptual difficulties. An alternative approach conceptulizes LD as nonresponsiveness to generally effective instruction. It requires that special education be considered only when a child's performance reveals a dual discrepancy— that is, a performance level and growth rate below that of classroom peers (Fuchs & Fuchs, 1998a, 1998b).

To explain dual discrepancy as a concept, we draw on pediatric medicine. The endocrinologist monitoring a child's physical growth is interested not only in height at one point in time but also in growth velocity over time (Rosenfeld, 1982). Given a child whose current height places her below the third percentile, the endocrinologist considers the possibility of underlying pathology and the need to intervene only if, in response to an adequately nurturing environment, the child's growth trajectory is flatter than that of appropriate comparison groups. Based on long-term, large-scale normative information, this criterion is typically operationalized as an annual growth rate of less than 4 cm at age 7. Consequently, the endocrinologist judges a child who manifests a large discrepancy in height status, but who nonetheless is growing at least 4 cm annually in response to a nurturing environment, to be deriving available benefits from that environment and to be an inappropriate candidate for special intervention.

The endocrinologist's decision-making framework reflects three assumptions. First, genetic variations underlie normal development, producing a range of heights across the population. Second, in response to a nurturing environment, a short but growing child does not present a pathological profile indicative of a need for special treatment to produce growth. Instead, such a profile suggests an individual who may legitimately represent the lower end of the normal distribution of height—an individual whose development is commensurate with his or her capacity to grow. Third, under these circumstances, special intervention is unlikely to increase adult height sufficiently to warrant the risks associated with intervention. Of course, when questions about the quality of the environment arise, the first-level response is to remove those uncertainties by enhancing nurturance (Wolraich, 1996), so that growth can be tested under adequate environmental conditions.

Applied to education, this decision-making framework translates into three related propositions. First, because student capacity varies, educational outcomes will differ across a population of learners. A low-performing child who is learning, albeit slowly, may ultimately perform less well than peers. After all, we do not expect all children to achieve the same degree of reading competence: Some will become acclaimed critics of literature; others will achieve a level of competence necessary to assume the roles of responsible parent, employee (or employer), and citizen.

Second, if a low-performing child is learning at a rate similar to the growth rates of other children in his or her classroom, that child is demonstrating the capacity to profit from that environment. Additional intervention may be unwarranted, even though a discrepancy in performance level may exist. In other words, given that the child is benefiting from classroom instruction, the child may be achieving commensurate with his or her capacity to learn and might not require a unique form of (special education) instruction. Moreover, the risks and costs associated with entering the special education system may be deemed inappropriate and unnecessary in this case because it is unlikely, in light of the growth already occurring, that a different long-term educational outcome could be achieved as a function of special education. Of course, the converse is also assumed. When low-performing children are not demonstrating growth and their classmates are, consideration of special intervention is warranted. Alternative instructional methods must be tested to address the apparent mismatch between the students' learning requirements and those represented by classroom instruction.

A third assumption: When most students in a classroom are achieving inadequate growth rates (in comparison to local or national norms on valued achievement tests), one must question the adequacy of instruction in that environment before making decisions about individual student responsiveness. In such a case, classwide intervention should be implemented, which is aimed at enhancing the overall quality of the instructional program. Growth under more nurturing conditions must be indexed before any child's need for special intervention can be assessed.

Dual discrepancy as an index of "failure to thrive" has an intuitive and empirical appeal. This index deals directly with the problem at hand (e.g., poor reading and poor math skills), reflects a dynamic rather than a static approach to learning and assessment, and is data based. However, it also requires a major shift in beliefs, attitudes, and practices. Implementing a treatment validity approach with dual discrepancy requires (1) assessment of every child in every classroom weekly (or biweekly), (2) evaluation of progress on a regular basis, (3) formulating interventions within general education classrooms for children identified as dually discrepant, (4) implementing those interventions with fidelity, and (5) evaluating effects. CBM is a promising tool for indexing treatment responsiveness due to its capacity to model student growth, to evaluate treatment effects, and to simultaneously inform instructional programming.

Nonresponders as Students with Dual Discrepancies: An Illustration

McMaster, Fuchs, Fuchs, and Compton (2002)

McMaster, Fuchs, Fuchs, and Compton's (2002) nonresponder study took place in 22 classrooms in 8 public elementary schools in Nashville, Tennessee, which were participating in a large-scale investigation of the First-Grade PALS Reading Program (Fuchs, Fuchs, Thompson, Svenson, et al., 2001; Fuchs, Fuchs, Thompson, Al Otaiba, et al., 2000, 2002; Fuchs, Fuchs, Yen, et al., 2001). Eleven of the classrooms were using a standard version of First-Grade PALS, and 11 were implementing a new PALS + Fluency version in which reading fluency was deliberately taught and practiced by students working with each other. An additional 11 classrooms served as no-treatment controls; however, none of the students from the control classes were involved in this nonresponder study. On average, there were 19 children in each of the 22 treatment classrooms, totaling 418 children. From previous PALS Reading research, we knew that there would be nonresponders, as many as 20% of students in the general population (e.g., Fuchs et al., 1997; Mathes et al., 1998). We wished to identify this subgroup relatively quickly to create for ourselves an opportunity to modify PALS, thereby (we hoped) making it more appropriate for a greater number of students.

Treatment nonresponders were selected by a three-step process: (1) selecting a risk pool among the students in the 22 classrooms, (2) monitoring their progress during PALS implementation, and (3) identifying nonresponders. Nonresponders were then assigned randomly to one of three groups: a group that continued to participate in their standard PALS or PALS + Fluency program; a group that participated in a modified PALS or modified PALS + Fluency program, which provided for more individualization within the context of ongoing standard PALS or PALS + Fluency; and a group that received one-to-one tutoring instead of PALS.

IDENTIFICATION OF THE RISK POOL

In October 2000, all students in the 22 PALS classrooms were given a Rapid Letter Naming (RLN) test as part of the pretest battery. Because RLN is a useful predictor of future reading achievement (Torgesen et al., 1997), it was used to identify the lowest-performing readers in each class. Within each class, students' RLN scores were rank-ordered. The teachers were then consulted to determine whether these rankings were consistent with their judgment of students' reading performance. Adjustments in the rankings were made based on teacher response. The eight lowest-performing students in each class were identified as at risk for not responding to the PALS program. Across the 22 classes, this totaled 176 low-performing students. By choosing eight low-performers from each class, we deliberately overselected the number of children we expected to be unresponsive. This overselection reduced the possibility of false negatives (i.e., excluding students from the study who should have been included) and also reflected our expectation that an unknown number of students and their families would move. In addition to the low-performing students, four average-performing students were identified in each class (using the RLN rankings and teacher judgment) to serve as a comparison for the low-performing students, totaling 88 average-performing students (22 classrooms × 4 students).

MONITORING PROGRESS OF THE RISK POOL

For the first 7 weeks of PALS implementation, the 176 low-performing and 88 average-performing students were administered weekly measures to monitor their reading progress. These included weekly "chapter tests," and two CBM assessments: Dolch word probes and Nonword Fluency probes (NWF; Good, Simmons, & Kame'enui, 2001). The *chapter tests* were designed as direct measures of students' progress in the PALS curriculum. They were cumulative and untimed and the chapter-test score was the percentage of sounds and words read correctly. The *Dolch word probes* are equivalent forms of 100 sight words selected randomly from a pool of 126 words from the preprimer, primer, and first-grade levels. Dolch words are common sight words designated for mastery at each grade level. The probes were considered a "near transfer" measure because most of the words appear in First-Grade PALS lessons, and all are taught in the first-grade curriculum of the Metro-Nashville Public Schools. The score is the number of words read correctly in 1 minute. The *NWF probes* (Good et al., 2001) consist of consonant–vowel–consonant and vowel–consonant nonwords. Students read them by saying the individual sounds of the letters (e.g., "s-i-m") or the whole word (e.g., "sim"). The score is the total number of phonemes said correctly in 1 minute. The Dolch and NWF scores were graphed and level and slope were calculated across the 7 weeks for each of the 176 low-performing and 88 average-performing students.

IDENTIFICATION OF THE NONRESPONDERS

Following the seventh week of treatment, nonresponders were identified. First, we calculated means and standard deviations on the average students' slopes and levels from the Dolch and NWF probes. Second, we identified all students from each class who had scored 90% or less on the last chapter test. If none of the students in a class scored less than 90%, we identified the lowest-scoring students from that class. Third, z-scores were calculated on the Dolch and NWF slopes and levels of this subgroup of low-performing students, based on the performance of all the average students.

Generally, students were identified as nonresponders if they scored 1 standard deviation below their average-achieving peers in terms of performance level and slope (growth) on the Dolch and/or NWF measures. However, the decision to identify a student as a nonresponder was made on an individual basis. If a student's performance level on one or both measures was below that of the average-achieving students but his or her growth was similar to or greater than those of the average students, the student would not be identified as nonresponders. Alternatively, if a student performed at a "borderline" level (i.e., within one standard deviation of the average students) but had made no growth or even negative growth on the Dolch or NWF measures, the student would likely be identified as a nonresponder. Sixty-six students were identified as nonresponders. This represented 15.8% of all students in the 22 treatment classrooms.

As indicated, nonresponders were chosen randomly (1) to remain in the PALS (or PALS + Fluency) treatment, (2) to participate in a modified PALS (or modified PALS + Fluency) treatment that permitted more individualization, and (3) for one-to-one tutoring in lieu of PALS. Following a 12-week treatment, nonresponders in the tutoring program outperfomed nonresponders in the other two groups by .2 to .5 standard deviations, depending on the reading measure. Nonresponders in the modified PALS program did least well, suggesting that our attempts to modify PALS resulted in a less effective treatment than did the standard PALS or PALS + Fluency versions.

Is There Value to the Dual-Discrepancy (or Nonresponder) Approach to LD Identification?

Clearly, the dual-discrepancy model as defined by McMaster and colleagues (2002) and others requires much effort and vigilance, especially compared to diagnostic procedures that rely on the identification of IQ–achievement discrepancies or simple low achievement. An obvious and important question becomes, "Is it worth it?"

One way of addressing the question is by directly comparing this approach to other LD identification procedures. Speece and her colleagues (Speece & Case, in press;

Speece, Molloy, & Case, 2000) did precisely this. They compared the dual-discrepancy method to IQ–reading–achievement discrepancy and to simple low-reading-achievement methods of identifying LD in an epidemiological sample of first- and second-grade children. Dual-discrepancy status was based on CBM read-aloud measures collected across approximately 6 months of a school year.

Compared to the IQ-discrepant group, the dual-discrepant (DD) children were more impaired on every measure (including IQ, phonological awareness, and teacher ratings of academic competence, problem behavior, and social skills) except for word reading efficiency. There were fewer and more modest differences between the DD group and the group of simple low achievers. Additional analyses conducted by Speece and her colleagues indicated that the DD children were younger than members of the other two groups and that they become more impaired over time. This suggests that the dual-discrepancy method may facilitate early identification and intervention. In addition, according to Speece and her associates, the DD and simple-low-achieving groups each had racial distributions reflecting the proportions of majority and minority children in the schools, whereas the IQ-discrepant group had a disproportionately high number of majority children.

In short, recent research seems to support the notion that dual-discrepant children have a greater number of more severe problems with skills that underlie beginning reading (e.g., Speece & Case, in press; Speece et al., 2000), and that a specific set of procedures exist for identifying such children (e.g., McMaster et al., 2002). Whether these procedures may be "scaled up" so that all teachers in a district and all districts in a state can use them is a question requiring considerably more research.

Acknowledgments

Our research on nonresponders was funded by Grant # H324D000033 and Grant #H324B0049 from the Office of Special Education Programs in the U.S. Department of Education to Vanderbilt University. This chapter does not necessarily reflect the position or policy of the funding agency and no official endorsement by it should be inferred. Portions of this chapter were presented at the annual meetings of the Society for the Scientific Study of Reading in Boulder, CO, and Council for Exceptional Children in Kansas City, MO, both in 2001.

References

Adams, M. J. (1990). *Beginning to read: Thinking and learning about print.* Cambridge, MA: MIT Press.

Allinder, R. M., & Fuchs, L. S. (1994). Alternative ways of analyzing effects of a short school break on students with and without disabilities. *School Psychology Quarterly, 9,* 145–160.

Al Otaiba, S., & Fuchs, D. (2002). Characteristics of children who are unresponsive to early literacy intervention: A review of the literature. *Remedial and Special Education, 23(5),* 300–316.

Ball, E. W., & Blachman, B. A. (1991). Does phoneme awareness training in kindergarten make a difference in early word recognition and developmental spelling? *Reading Research Quarterly, 26,* 49–66.

Berninger, V. W., Abbott, R. D., Zook, D., Ogier, S., Lemos-Britton, Z., & Brooksher, R. (1999). Early intervention for reading disabilities: Teaching the alphabet principle in a connectionist framework. *Journal of Learning Disabilities, 32,* 491–503.

Blachman, B. A. (1994). What we have learned from longitudinal studies of phonological processing and reading, and some unanswered questions: A response to Torgesen, Wagner, and Rashotte. *Journal of Learning Disabilities, 27,* 287–291.

Blachman, B. A. (1997). Early intervention and phonological awareness: A cautionary tale. In B. Blachman (Ed.), *Foundations of reading acquisition and dyslexia* (pp. 408–430). Mahwah, NJ: Erlbaum.

Bradley, L., & Bryant, P. E. (1985). *Rhyme and reason in reading and spelling.* (International Academy for Research in Learning Disabilities Monograph Series No. 1). Ann Arbor: University of Michigan Press.

Brown, I. S., & Felton, R. H. (1990). Effects of instruction on beginning reading skills in children at risk for reading disability. *Reading and Writing: An Interdisciplinary Journal, 2,* 223–241.

Bus, A. G., & van IJzendoorn, M. H. (1999). Phonological awareness and early reading: A meta-analysis of experimental training studies. *Journal of Educational Psychology, 91,* 403–414.

Byrne B., & Fielding-Barnsley, R. F. (1993). Evaluation of a program to teach phonemic awareness to young children: A 1-year follow-up. *Journal of Educational Psychology, 85,* 104–111.

Deno, S. L. (1985). Curriculum-based measurement: The emerging alternative. *Exceptional Children, 52,* 219–232.

Deno, S. L., & Fuchs, L. S. (1987). Developing curriculum-based measurement systems for data-based special education problem solving. *Focus on Exceptional Children, 19*(8), 1–16.

Deno, S. L., Mirkin, P., & Chiang, B. (1982). Identifying valid measures of reading. *Exceptional Children, 49,* 36–45.

Ehri, L. C., & Robbins, C. (1992). Beginners need some decoding skill to read words by analogy. *Reading Research Quarterly, 27,* 13–26.

Fazio, B. B. (1997). Learning a new poem: Memory for connected speech and phonological awareness in low-income children with and without specific language impairment. *Journal of Speech, Language, and Hearing Research, 40,* 1285–1297.

Fletcher, J. M., & Foorman, B. R. (1994). Issues in definition and measurement of learning disabilities: The need for early intervention. In G. R. Lyon (Ed.), *Frames of reference for the assessment of learning disabilities: New views on measurement issues* (pp. 185–200). Baltimore: Brookes.

Foorman, B. R., Francis, D. J., Fletcher, J. M., Schatschneider, C., & Mehta, P. (1998). The role of instruction in learning to read: Preventing reading failure in at-risk children. *Journal of Educational Psychology, 90,* 37–55.

Foorman, B. R., Francis, D. J., Winikates, D., Mehta, P., Schatschneider, C., & Fletcher, J. M. (1997). Early interventions for children with disabilities. *Scientific Studies of Reading, 1,* 255–276.

Fox, B., & Routh, D. K. (1976). Phonemic analysis and synthesis as word-attack skills. *Journal of Educational Psychology, 68,* 70–74.

Francis, D. J., Shaywitz, S. E., Stuebing, K. K., Shaywitz, B. A., & Fletcher, J. M. (1994). The measurement of change: Assessing behavior over time and within a developmental context. In G. R. Lyon (Ed.), *Frames of reference for the assessment of learning disabilities: New views on measurement issues* (pp. 29–58). Baltimore: Brookes.

Fuchs, D., & Fuchs, L. S. (1995). What's "special" about special education? *Phi Delta Kappan, 76,* 522–530.

Fuchs, D., Fuchs, L. S., & Fernstrom, P. J. (1993). A conservative approach to special education reform: Mainstreaming through transenvironmental programming and curriculum-based measurement. *American Educational Research Journal, 30,* 149–178.

Fuchs, D., Fuchs, L. S., Mathes, P. G., Lipsey, M. W., & Roberts, P. H. (2001, August). *Is "learning disabilities" just a fancy term for low achievement? A meta-analysis of reading differences between low achievers with and without the label.* Paper presented at the Office of Special Education Programs' LD Initiative Conference, Washington, DC.

Fuchs, D., Fuchs, L. S., Mathes, P., & Simmons, D. (1997). Peer-Assisted Learning Strategies: Making classrooms more responsive to diversity. *American Educational Research Journal, 34,* 174–206.

Fuchs, D., Fuchs, L., Thompson, A., Al Otaiba, S., Nyman, K., Yang, N. & Svenson, E. (2000). *Strengthening kindergartners' reading readiness in Title I and non-Title I schools.* Paper presented a the Pacific Coast Research Conference, La Jolla, CA.

Fuchs, D., Fuchs, L., Thompson, A., Al Otaiba, S., Yen, L., Yang, N., Braun, M., & O'Connor, R. (2001). Is reading important in reading-readiness programs? A randomized field trial with teachers as program implementers. *Journal of Educational Psychology, 93,* 251–267.

Fuchs, D., Fuchs, L., Thompson, A., Al Otaiba, S., Yen, L., Yang, N., Braun, M., & O'Connor, R. (2002). Exploring the importance of reading programs for kindergartners with disabilities in mainstream classrooms. *Exceptional Children, 68,* 295–311.

Fuchs, D., Fuchs, L. S., Thompson, A., Svenson, E., Yen, L., Al Otaiba, S., Yang, N., McMaster, K. N., Prentice, K., Kazdan, S., & Saenz, L. (2001). Peer-Assisted Learning Strategies in reading: Extensions for kindergarten, first grade, and high school. *Remedial and Special Education, 22,* 15–21.

Fuchs, D., Fuchs, L., Yen, L., McMaster, K., Svenson, E., Yang, N., Young, C., Morgan, P., Gilbert, T., Jaspers, J., Jernigan, M., Yoon, E., & King, S. (2001). Developing first-grade reading fluency through peer mediation. *Teaching Exceptional Children, 34*(2), 90–93.

Fuchs, D., Roberts, P. H., Fuchs, L. S., & Bowers, J. (1996). Reintegrating students with learning disabilities into the mainstream: A two-year study. *Learning Disabilities Research and Practice, 11,* 214–229.

Fuchs, L. S. (1993). Enhancing instructional programming and student achievement with curriculum-based measurement. In J. J. Kramer (Ed.), *Curriculum-based assessment* (pp. 65–104). Lincoln: Buros Institute of Mental Measurements, University of Nebraska.

Fuchs, L. S., & Deno, S. L. (1991). Paradigmatic distinctions between instructionally relevant measurement models. *Exceptional Children, 57,* 488–501.

Fuchs, L. S., & Deno, S. L. (1992). Effects of curriculum within curriculum-based measurement. *Exceptional Children, 58,* 232–243.

Fuchs, L. S., Deno, S. L., & Marston, D. (1983). Improving the reliability of curriculum-based measures of academic skills for psychoeducational decision making. *Diagnostique, 8,* 135–149.

Fuchs, L. S., & Fuchs, D. (1992). Identifying a measure for monitoring student reading progress. *School Psychology Review, 21,* 45–58.

Fuchs, L. S., & Fuchs, D. (1998a). Curriculum-based measurement: A unifying framework for conceptualizing learning disability. *Learning Disability Research and Practice, 13,* 204–219.

Fuchs, L. S., & Fuchs, D. (1998b). Treatment validity: A unifying concept for reconceptualizing the identification of learning disabilities. *Learning Disabilities Research and Practice, 13* (4), 204–219.

Fuchs, L. S., & Fuchs, D. (1999). Monitoring student progress toward the development of reading competence: A review of three forms of classroom-based assessment. *School Psychology Review, 28,* 659–671.

Fuchs, L. S., Fuchs, D., & Deno, S. L. (1982). Reliability and validity of curriculum-based informal reading inventories. *Reading Research Quarterly, 18,* 6–26.

Fuchs, L. S., Fuchs, D., & Hamlett, C. L. (1989a). Effects of alternative goal structures within curriculum-based measurement. *Exceptional Children, 55,* 429–438.

Fuchs, L. S., Fuchs, D., & Hamlett, C. L. (1989b). Effects of instrumental use of curriculum-based measurement to enhance instructional programs. *Remedial and Special Education, 10*(2), 43–52.

Fuchs, L. S., Fuchs, D., Hamlett, C. L., & Allinder, R. M. (1991). Effects of expert system advice within curriculum-based measurement on teacher planning and student achievement in spelling. *School Psychology Review, 20,* 49–66.

Fuchs, L. S., Fuchs, D., Hamlett, C. L., & Ferguson, C. (1992). Effects of expert system consultation within curriculum-based measurement using a reading maze task. *Exceptional Children, 58,* 436–450.

Fuchs, L. S., Fuchs, D., Hamlett, C. L., Phillips, N. B., & Bentz, J. (1994). Classwide curriculum-based measurement: Helping general educators meet the challenge of student diversity. *Exceptional Children, 60,* 518–537.

Fuchs, L. S., Fuchs, D., Hamlett, C. L., & Stecker, P. M. (1991). Effects of curriculum-based measurement and consultation on teacher planning and student achievement in mathematics operations. *American Educational Research Journal, 28,* 617–641.

Fuchs, L. S., Fuchs, D., Hamlett, C. L., Thompson, A., Roberts, P. H., Kubec, P., & Stecker, P. M. (1994). Technical features of a mathematics concepts and applications curriculum-based measurement system. *Diagnostique, 19*(4), 23–49.

Fuchs, L. S., Fuchs, D., Hamlett, C. L., Walz, L., & Germann, G. (1993). Formative evaluation of academic progress: How much growth can we expect? *School Psychology Review, 22,* 27–48.

Fuchs, L. S., Fuchs, D., & Maxwell, L. (1988). The validity of informal reading comprehension measures. *Remedial and Special Education, 9*(2), 20–29.

Good, R. H., Deno, S. L., & Fuchs, L. S. (1995, February). *Modeling academic growth for students with and without disabilities.* Paper presented at the third annual Pacific Coast Research Conference, Laguna Beach, CA.

Good, R., Kaminski, R., & Shinn, M. (1999, January). *Growth and development indicators: From development to refinement and back again.* Paper presented at the Pacific Coast Research Conference, San Diego, CA.

Good, R. H., & Shinn, M. R. (1990). Forecasting accuracy of slope estimates for reading curriculum-based measurement: Empirical evidence. *Behavioral Assessment, 12,* 179–194.

Good, R. H. III, Simmons, D. C., & Kame'enui, E. J. (2001). The importance of decision-making utility of a continuum of fluency-based indicators of foundational reading success for third grade high-stakes outcomes. *Scientific Studies of Reading, 5,* 257–288.

Greenwood, C. R., Hart, B., Walker, D., & Risely, T. (1993, April). *The importance of opportunity to respond in children's academic success.* Paper presented at the Second Conference on Behavior Analysis in Education, Ohio State University, Columbus.

Hatcher, P. J., & Hulme, C. (1999). Phonemes, rhymes, and intelligence as predictors of children's responsiveness to remedial reading instruction: Evidence from a longitudinal study. *Journal of Experimental Child Psychology, 72,* 130–153.

Hatcher, P. J., Hulme, C., & Ellis, A. W. (1994). Ameliorating early reading failure by integrating the teaching of reading and phonological skills: The phonological linkage hypothesis. *Child Development, 65,* 41–57.

Hosp, M., & Fuchs, L. S. (2001). *Revising technical features of curriculum-based measurement's reading aloud task in the early grades.* Manuscript submitted for publication.

Hurford, D. P. (1990). Training phonemic segmentation ability with a phonemic discrimination intervention in second- and third-grade children with reading disabilities. *Journal of Learning Disabilities, 23,* 564–569.

Juel, C. (1988). Learning to read and write: A longitudinal study of fifty-four children from first through fourth grade. *Journal of Educational Psychology, 80,* 437–447.

Juel, C. (1994). At risk university students tutoring at-risk elementary school children: What factors make it effective? In E. H. Herebert & B. M Taylor (Eds.), *Getting reading right from the start: Effective early interventions.* (pp. 39–62). Boston: Allyn & Bacon.

Juel, C. (1996). What makes literacy tutoring effective? *Reading Research Quarterly, 31,* 268–289.

Kasten, W. C. (1998). One learner, two paradigms. *Reading and Writing Quarterly, 14,* 335–353.

Lundberg, I., Frost, J., & Petersen, O. (1988). Effects of an extensive program for stimulating phonological awareness in preschool children. *Reading Research Quarterly, 23,* 263–284.

Lyon, G. R., Fletcher, J. M., Shaywitz, S. E., Shaywitz, B. A., Torgesen, J. K., Wood, F. B., Schulte, A., & Olson, R. (2001). *Rethinking learning disabilities.* Washington, DC: Hudson Institute.

Marston, D. (1987–1988). The effectiveness of special education: A time-series analysis of reading performance in regular and special education settings. *Journal of Special Education, 21*(4), 13–26.

Marston, D. B. (1989). A curriculum-based measurement approach to assessing academic performance: What it is and why do it. In M. R. Shinn (Ed.), *Curriculum-based measurement: Assessing special children* (pp. 18–78). New York: Guilford Press.

Marston, D., & Deno, S. L. (1981). *The reliability of simple, direct measures of written expression* (Research Report No. 50). Minneapolis: University of Minnesota Institute for Research on Learning Disabilities.

Marston, D., Fuchs, L. S., & Deno, S. L. (1986). Measuring pupil progress: A comparison of standardized achievement tests and curriculum-related measures. *Diagnostique, 11,* 71–90.

Mastropieri, M. A., Leinhart, A., & Scruggs, T. E. (1999). Strategies to increase reading fluency. *Intervention in School and Clinic, 34,* 278–283, 292.

Mathes, P. G., Howard, J. K., Allen, S. H., & Fuchs, D. (1998). Peer-assisted learning strategies for first-grade readers: Responding to the needs of diversity. *Reading Research Quarterly, 31,* 268–289.

McMaster, K. N., Fuchs, D., Fuchs, L. S., & Compton, D. L. (2002). *An experimental analysis of the effects of alternative instructional programs for students unresponsive to beginning reading instruction.* Paper presented at the Society for the Scientific Study of Reading, Chicago.

O'Connor, R. (2000). Increasing the intensity of intervention in kindergarten and first grade. *Learning Disabilities Research and Practice, 15,* 43–54.

O'Connor, R. E., Jenkins, J. R., Leicester, N., & Slocum, T. A. (1993). Teaching phonological awareness to young children with learning disabilities. *Exceptional Children, 59,* 532–546.

O'Connor, R. E., Jenkins, J. R., & Slocum, T. A. (1995). Transfer among phonological tasks in kindergarten: Essential instructional content. *Journal of Educational Psychology, 87,* 202–217.

O'Connor, R. E., Notari-Syverson, A., & Vadasy, P. F. (1996). Ladders to literacy: The effects of teacher-led phonological activities for kindergarten children with and without disabilities. *Exceptional Children, 63,* 117–130.

O'Connor, R. E., Notari-Syverson, A., & Vadasy, P. F. (1998). First-grade effects of teacher-led phonological activities in kindergarten for children with mild disabilities: A follow-up study. *Learning Disabilities Research and Practice, 13,* 43–52.

O'Shaughnessy, T. E., & Swanson, H. L. (2000). A comparison of two reading interventions for children with reading disabilities. *Journal of Learning Disabilities, 33,* 257–277.

Peterson, M. E., & Haines, L. P. (1992). Orthographic analogy training with kindergarten children: Effects on analogy use, phonemic segmentation, and letter–sound knowledge. *Journal of Reading Behavior, 24,* 109–127.

Riley, R. (1996). Improving the reading and writing skills of America's students. *Learning Disability Quarterly, 19,* 67–69.

Rosenfeld, R. G. (1990). Short stature. In M. Green & J. Haggerty Eds.), *Ambulatory pediatrics—IV.* Philadelphia: W. B. Saunders.

Schneider, W., Ennemoser, M., Roth, E., & Kuspert, P. (1999). Kindergarten prevention of dyslexia: Does training in phonological awareness work for everybody? *Journal of Learning Disabilities, 32,* 429–436.

Schneider, W., Kuspert, P., Roth, E., Vise, M., & Marx, H. (1997). Short- and long-term effects of training phonological awareness in kindergarten: Evidence from two German studies. *Journal of Experimental Child Psychology, 66,* 311–340.

Shannahan, T., & Barr, R. (1995). Reading Recovery: An independent evaluation of the effects of an early intervention for at-risk learners. *Reading Research Quarterly, 30,* 958–996.

Shinn, M. R., Tindal, G., Spira, D., & Marston, D. (1987). Practice of learning disabilities as social policy. *Learning Disability Quarterly, 10,* 17–28.

Snider, V. E. (1997). Transfer of decoding skills to a literature basal. *Learning Disabilities Research and Practice, 12,* 54–62.

Speece, D. L., & Case, L. P. (in press). Classification in context: An alternative approach to identifying early reading disability. *Journal of Educational Psychology.*

Speece, D. L., Molloy, D. E., & Case, L. P. (2000, February). *Toward validating a model of reading disability identification based on response to treatment.* Paper presented at the annual Pacific Coast Research Conference, La Jolla, CA.

Snow, C. E., Burns, M. S., & Griffin, P. (Eds.). (1998). *Preventing reading difficulties in young children.* Washington, DC: National Academy Press.

Stanovich, K. E. (1986). Matthew effect in reading: Some consequences of individual differences in the acquisition of literacy. *Reading Research Quarterly, 21,* 360–406.

Torgesen, J. K., & Davis, C. (1996). Individual difference variables that predict response to training in phonological awareness. *Journal of Experimental Child Psychology, 63,* 1–21.

Torgesen, J. K., Morgan, S., & Davis, C. (1992). The effects of two types of phonological awareness training on word learning in kindergarten children. *Journal of Educational Psychology, 84,* 364–370.

Torgesen, J. K., Wagner, R. K., & Rashotte, C. A. (1997). Prevention and remediation of severe reading disabilities: Keeping the end in mind. *Scientific Studies of Reading, 1,* 217–234.

Torgesen, J. K., Wagner, R. K., Rashotte, C. A., Lindamood, P., Rose, E., Conway, T., & Garvan, C. (1999). Preventing reading failure in young children with phonological processing disabilities: Group and individual responses to instruction. *Journal of Educational Psychology, 91,* 579–593.

Uhry, J. K., & Shepherd, M. (1997). Teaching phonological recoding to young children with phonological processing deficits: The effect on sight word acquisition. *Learning Disability Quarterly, 20,* 104–125.

Vadasy, P. F., Jenkins, J. R., Antil, L. R., Wayne, S. K., & O'Connor, R. E. (1997). Community-based early reading intervention for at-risk first graders. *Learning Disabilities Research and Practice, 12,* 29–39.

Vandervelden, M. C., & Siegel, L. S. (1997). Teaching phonological processing skills in early literacy: A developmental approach. *Learning Disability Quarterly, 20,* 63–81.

Vellutino, F. R., Scanlon, D. M., Sipay, E. R., Small, S., Chen, R., Pratt, A., & Denckla, M. B. (1996). Cognitive profiles of difficult-to-remediate and readily remediated poor readers: Early intervention as a vehicle for distinguishing between cognitive and experiential deficits as basic causes of specific reading disability. *Journal of Educational Psychology, 88,* 601–638.

Wolraich, M. (Ed.). (1996). *Disorders of development and training: A practical guide to assessment and management* (2nd ed.). St. Louis, MO: Mosby.

27

The Sociocultural Model in Special Education Interventions: Apprenticing Students in Higher-Order Thinking

Carol Sue Englert
Troy Mariage

This chapter focuses on social constructivism as a theoretical model for designing and implementing instructional programs for students with disabilities. Lev Vygotsky, one of the architects of social constructivism, developed the model to explain the nature of learning, especially among students with disabilities (Gindis, 1999; Vygotsky, 1993). Although many educators associate social constructivism with discovery approaches to learning or whole-language approaches, the model shares many features with the other instructional models in this section. Though many models assume competence resides within the individual, the sociocultural perspective shifts attention to the role of social context in accounting for the development of students' competence (Rueda, Gallego, & Moll, 2000; Vygotsky, 1978).

This chapter provides a focused and in-depth portrayal of a few studies in order to articulate the "big ideas" of the sociocultural model, provide examples, and relate their implications. This approach has been likened to a cognitive apprenticeship, which "establishes a teaching and learning relationship in which interactions between 'expert' learners and 'novice' learners support the movement of the novice toward the expert end of the learning continuum" (Hock, Schumaker, & Deshler, 1999, p. 9). In the first part of the chapter, we describe the essential features and characteristics of the model. In the second part, we present an illustrative example from each of three domains: reading, writing, and science. Our goal is to help readers extrapolate and generalize the model across subject matter areas. Finally, we conclude this chapter with a discussion of the implications of this work for teaching and learning in applied settings.

Situated Activity

One of the central features of the sociocultural model is the assumption about the nature and context of learning. Vygotsky's approach describes an activity approach to knowledge acquisition (Engestrom, Miettinen, & Punamaki, 1999). Cognitive activities, like many of life's activities, have both internal and external sides that must be mastered by novices. Competence goes beyond mere book learning as a novice is mentored into a set of practices, languages, and artifacts that characterize effective disciplinary knowledge and problem-solving performance. Scientists, for example, coordinate themselves (mind and body) with psychological tools, "instruments, tools, symbolic and linguistic expressions, people, objects being studied, and places like laboratories so as to chain all these together into a coherent pattern or configuration" (Gee, 1997, p. 238).

In educational applications, students must have similar opportunities to participate in the "ways of knowing" specific to a particular discipline. To return to the science example, teachers may tend to want to "tell students about science," but teachers need to involve them in the "practice of science" for mastery. Countervailing educational trends that focus on the decomposition of complex mental processes into elemental units or facts, proponents of social constructivism argue that when abstractions are removed from their anchoring activity settings, students are denied access to the higher-order thinking and metacognitive processes that underlie skilled problem solving and academic competence. The purpose and meaning of artifacts, the mental and physical actions related to the tools that produce the artifacts, and the integrated sequence of individual actions in a task are brought into sharp relief in the context of one's performance of meaningful and authentic activity (Englert & Dunsmore, 2002; Roth, 1998).

Apprenticeship in Social Contexts

The emphasis on activity also underscores a second aspect of the sociocultural model, namely, the role of the teacher or expert in the apprenticeship of higher mental functions. Human psychological processes are acquired in the course of *joint-mediated activity* and, thus, are social in their origin (Gee, 1997). Teachers apprentice their students into cognitive activity in several ways. Foremost, teachers guide learning by making visible and explicit the ways of doing and knowing that are not necessarily apparent in the routine actions of experts but are nonetheless requisite for full participation (Wells, 2000). Lave (1997) stresses the need for artifacts and activities to be "transparent" to learners—that is open to inspection.

Likewise, effective instruction occurs when teachers think aloud to make visible their inner thoughts in a more conscious way (Englert & Mariage, 1996). Forging such concrete links between thought, speech, and action can bring the relationship between "knowing and doing" into a plane of active consciousness within an individual (Shotter, 1995).

An apprenticeship approach to learning also assumes a developmental shift in the relationships and roles assumed by the expert and novice in their performance of the activity. Initially, tasks are too difficult for novices to accomplish alone, so they work side by side with more knowledgeable members to accomplish the task jointly. At this point, the novices sometimes assume a peripheral role as they participate in some aspects of the activity, but the expert performs the more difficult aspects that are beyond the learners' immediate grasp and control (Wenger, 1998). Between the participants, the performance of the cognitive process and actions are distributed as they jointly perform the task on a social plane that Vygotsky (1978) called the "interpsychological or intermental" plane.

Gradually, learners appropriate and perform the talk and actions previously modeled by others, as they assume increasing responsibility for the disciplinary moves and practices. Talk and conversation that was enacted on the social plane are anticipated by the learner in the form of egocentric speech (thinking out loud) and, finally, inner speech (talking to oneself). Ultimately, the cognitive process is performed on the intramental plane (within an individual's mind), as the processes and practices that were once jointly produced are internalized, and the social dialogue is turned inward to guide the learner's thoughts and actions. Once mastered, there remains the quality of hidden dialogicality, insofar as the traces of the talk and actions performed by others surface to influence the inner talk and behavioral repertoire of the learner (Wertsch, 1995). What is considered as part of one's mental life has its roots in the conversations that took place in one's "social life" (Toulmin, 1999). Discourse and mental processes are acquired and transformed as any other social practice by participating in them with others (Wenger, 1998).

Tools and Mediational Means

Vygotsky suggested that learning entails the use and appropriation of artifacts, strategies, technologies, and tools that mediate human thought and behavior in the context of activity (Nardi, 1996). Mediational tools include symbols, instruments, language, diagrams, maps, writing implements, procedures, rules of thumb, and any tool used in the transformation and construction process of which speech is among the most important (Wertsch, 1995, 1998).

Although we have described the importance of discourse as an aspect of social learning, it is also a tool that both supports mental reasoning and transforms the mind over time. There are several examples of language-related tools and symbol systems that influence performance. For example, the presentation of strategies provides direct access to the language and procedures that mediate performance. Speech genres and text structures are other examples of symbolic tools that mediate both the production and comprehension of oral and written texts (Cope & Kalantzis, 1993). Artifacts and tools, such as diagrams and maps, are carriers of mental reasoning that organize performance by offloading thought onto the tool and by making elements of the activity more visible (Roth, 1998). Once understood, these tools become "objects to think with" and "objects to talk with," supporting the participation by students with disabilities in the language, cognitive, and communication aspects of a particular discipline (Roth, 1998).

Zone of Proximal Development

Vygotsky's (1978) model provides a conceptual lens for understanding both the instructional and acquisition paths for students with disabilities. With Vygotsky's emphasis on the participation of novices in the full range of activity, it is apparent that students will not be able perform the whole of the activity without support and assistance. The mechanisms for supporting students involve the provision of mediational tools within a sensitive region of assisted performance known as the zone of proximal development.

The zone of proximal development is the distance between the level of performance attained by the child in independent problem-solving activity and the level attained by the child in collaboration with others or with mediational tools. It is a zone of joint action that is in advance of what the child can manage alone (Wells, 1999), making it a particularly rich site for learning and cognitive development. By providing scaffolds at this point of intellectual challenge, teachers can accommodate gaps in learning and induct students into new processes and knowledge (Stone, 2002). The challenge for teachers is to develop participation structures that provide access to developmental data about learners so that performance can be scaffolded on a contingent basis (Schaffer, 1996; Stone, 2002).

Teaching moves that scaffold performance encompass techniques that are well-known in the literature, including prompts, questions, feedback, instruction, and modeling (Hogan & Pressley, 1997; Stone, 2002). Ultimately, effective scaffolds are judged by the degree of fit to the learner, such as (1) contingency to the students' knowledge and social needs; (2) addition or withdrawal of supports based on the success or failure of prior attempts; (3) responsiveness to emergent interpretations and solutions; and (4) presentation of challenging material that calls on problem solving, as well as permitting the identification of cognitive or social tools that can continue the evolutionary path of development (Tobin, 1998). Finally, effective scaffolding requires a delicate balance between modeling, coaching, scaffolding, and fading (Collins, Brown, & Holum, 1991). Vygotsky's work is clear that effective teachers must give and take in tune with their students—not only must they give support by responding to the novice's evolving conception of the task with additional cognitive resources, but they must simultaneously fade or take back support for other aspects of the task for which students show evidence of appropriation and mastery.

Collaborative Participation Structures

Finally, Vygotsky's theory has been expanded by recent work on social mediation that emphasizes the participation of students in collaborative groups or communities of practice. Vygotsky believed that social mediation could ameliorate cognitive and social disabilities. Recent research has confirmed the power of collaboration in four specific areas: (1) promoting greater involvement in the academic discourse and social practices by offering a participation structure that promotes the transfer of control from teachers to students; (2) increasing the contribution of students in the joint solution of problems while offering them support and assistance from others on an ongoing basis (Wells, 2000); (3) providing a motivational context to further students' desire to participate and endure in intellectually rigorous activity (Vaughn & Klingner, 1999); and (4) creating "zones of proximal development" by expanding the potential for students to experience and appropriate the varied ideas, knowledge, resources and strategies of group members.

Collaborative problem solving can optimize learning opportunities for students with disabilities. In collaboration with peers, there is the potential for students with disabilities to reverse the typical interactional roles transacted in a teaching–learning situation, insofar as the "learner" can reposition him- or herself as the one who asks questions as well as answers them, gives directions to others as well as follows them, and becomes the teacher for others rather than the learner (Biemiller & Meichenbaum, 1998). Typically, however, the conferral of task responsibility and leadership roles to students with disabilities is remote or attenuated, leading them to experience academic tasks as something that "others do, but that I need help with" (Biemiller & Miechenbaum, 1998, p. 368). Biemiller and Meichenbaum (1998), in fact, suggest that more attention needs to be directed to the creation of settings in which learners are assigned executive or leadership roles in performing the task and the language that will lead them to exercise the self-regulatory metacognitive skills associated with skilled performance.

Social (De)Construction of Disability

Vygotsky's (1978) model provides several perspectives on disability. First, Vygotsky believed that the differences between persons with and without disabilities were qualitative, and the school must play a decisive role in this "approximation" through social compensation. Vygotsky proposed that a "child is full of unrealized potentials, and these offer a wealth of creative resources on which a handicapped child, or any child, may and must build" (cited in Vygotsky, 1993, p. 13). Further, he suggested that development stems not from biological and inner sources alone but from the interaction of the child with the sociocultural world (Vygotsky, 1993).

Second, with an emphasis on the social construction of ability, Vygotsky (1993) called attention to two aspects of compensation and, hence, assumptions about the possible sites of human differences. He recommended that educators needed to provide special or different symbolic tools suitable to the psychological makeup of the learner, and ways of mastering those tools through special pedagogical methods. In this respect, his work highlights the possibility that disability might be considered (1) differences in the learners' abilities to recognize or implement psychological tools, or to monitor their use, and/or 2) the failure of educators to support compensation by the provision of symbolic systems and tools matched to the students' psychological and biological needs. At the same time, Vygotsky recognized that disability affected the individual's relationship with people, resulting in social dislocation, which can further disturb the trajectory of cognitive and psychological development. Thus, he emphasized the corollary relationship between disabilities and symbolic or social mediation as both the source and resolution of the educational challenges experienced by students with disabilities.

Third, Vygotsky's theory of sociocultural perspectives opens the door for an alternative view for conceptualizing disability. As Gutierrez and Stone (1997) suggest, if competence is related to children's access to and participation in varying forms of learning activities, then changing the nature of participation is essential to make space for less experienced learners to replace those who served in prior roles as experts. To develop new identities of academic competence requires an expansion of the range of roles and interactional acts needed for knowledge development and successful participation (Gutierrez & Stone, 1997). Where disability is mitigated, several aspects seem to be at play, including (1) a social organization that minimizes differences; (2) access to the cognitive and social resources of the classroom; (3) customized assistance based on individual needs; (4) interdependent arrangements that are not solely dependent upon adults; (5) competent performance that is more broadly defined to include individuals operating with mediational means; and (6) the strategic handing over of learning to students (Gutierrez & Stone, 1997).

Educational Applications

Research related to applications of the sociocultural model to educational problems has an early and late history. Early, Vygotsky and his students applied the model to the study and treatment of cognitive and sensory disabilities. More recently, we have seen disciplinary-based studies that have tested many of Vygotsky's assumptions in applied settings with children and youth with disabilities. It is this later research that we review in this section. These studies have in common their focus on higher-order rather than lower-order psychological processes. Furthermore, though many special education scholars believe that sociocultural theory has enormous potential for advancing the instructional efficacy of special education programs (Artiles, Trent, Hoffman-Kipp, & Lopez-Torres, 2000; Gindis, 1999; Rueda et al., 2000; Stone, 2002), we also recognize that this theoretical model has steep connections to the rich traditions of strategy and metacognitive interventions for special education students. This more familiar body of work includes a number of contributing scholars in the area of *reading* (Goatley, Brock & Raphael, 1995; Klingner, Vaughn, & Schumm, 1998; Morocco, Hindin, Mata-Aguilar, & Clark-Chiarelli, 2001; Pressley, El-Dinary, & Afflerbach, 1995), *mathematics* (Goldman, Hasselbring, & Cognition and Technology Group at Vanderbilt, 1996; Woodward & Baxter, 1997), *writing* (De La Paz, 1999; Graham & Harris, 1989a, 1989b; Wong, 1997a, 1997b, 2000), and *social studies* (Ferretti,

MacArthur, & Okolo, 2001; Okolo & Ferretti, 1997). For the illustrative purposes of this chapter, however, we focus on three research programs that have specifically identified the sociocultural model as their guiding framework for designing and evaluating their instructional interventions in reading, writing, and science.

Reading: Reciprocal Teaching

One of the primary sociocultural studies was conducted by Palincsar and Brown (1989). They designed an intervention, reciprocal teaching, to assist poor readers who possessed adequate decoding skills but lacked adequate comprehension and problem-solving strategies. They based their reading methods on studies of poor readers that showed their difficulties in organizing, monitoring, and modifying their reading behaviors.

Four strategies were taught to poor readers to support their comprehension of expository text. These strategies included *Summarizing* (identifying the gist of the text), *Questioning* (asking a question about the main idea), *Clarifying* (clarifying vocabulary or ideas that did not make sense), and *Predicting* (using text information to predict what will happen next). These strategies were selected to enhance students' comprehension and comprehension-monitoring abilities (Brown & Palincsar, 1989; Palincsar, 1986). Furthermore, each strategy was introduced in ways designed to enhance its metacognitive potential by informing students why it was important and in what situation it was to be used.

Reciprocal teaching epitomized the features of the sociocultural model in several key respects. First, the entire set of strategies was taught and practiced in situated activity contexts, during the reading of authentic texts, as opposed to being introduced separately, or in isolated skill exercises (Brown & Palincsar, 1989). Following the reading of expository texts, the four strategies were applied by members of a small collaborative group, while they received coaching, guidance, and feedback from their peers and the teacher. Thus, reciprocal teaching offered a set of language tools or heuristics that might enable students to read more efficiently and self-regulate their comprehension (Palincsar & Brown, 1989).

Second, the strategies represented a form of discourse that encapsulated a repertoire of strategic processes that structured the students' interpersonal social interactions. In essence, reciprocal teaching provided students with particular ways of talking about texts through the employment of the strategies, endowing them with a set of cognitive tools, and offering a communication and symbolic system by which the group could organize and mediate their activities, as well as consider the meaning of the text as an object of attention and reflection. The dialogue was first exercised on an interpsychological plane (between individuals), laying traces for the subsequent internalization of the dialogue in directing reading activity on the intrapsychological plane (within the individual) (Palincsar & Brown, 1989).

Third, the pedagogical process underlying reciprocal teaching provided a dramatic form of apprenticeship that emphasized the developmental shifts in instructor–student positions that reflected the deepening expertise of students. At first, the teacher served as a model of expert reading behavior by overtly modeling the use of the four strategies while thinking aloud. However, reciprocal teaching provided a mechanism for the transfer of control to students. Students took turns assuming the role of leader of the group as each member led the group in the use of the reading strategies. Student leaders summarized text sections, asked questions about main ideas, called on the group for clarifications about text confusions, and predicted what was coming next. The other members of the group elaborated on, answered, or gave feedback on the leader's contributions. The teacher interceded when a student missed a point and the other group members did not catch it, or when a strategy was not applied effectively. In this way, the responsibility for comprehending and problem solving did not lie on the shoulders of individual learners or the teacher because the group shared the responsibility for thinking. This zone of joint action often exceeded what an individual could manage alone (Brown & Palincsar, 1989).

Fourth, through students' discursive participation, the teacher could assess students'

knowledge, fading into the background and acting as a sympathetic coach when students could handle and lead their own learning (Palincsar & Brown, 1989). Likewise, the teacher could take up the leadership when students needed feedback that was tailored to their existing levels of performance. The teacher *provided scaffolded assistance* in a number of ways, including (1) linking students' prior knowledge and contributions to the text; (2) requesting elaborations on ideas or confusions; (3) modeling strategic responses; and (4) questioning, paraphrasing, and reformulating contributions to construct comprehension. The teacher assessed students' knowledge during the discussions and then guided and shaped the course of the conversations to provide support on a moment-to-moment or student-to-student basis.

Reciprocal teaching is an elegant example of how social constructivism can inform the design of instructional interventions. It revolutionized how many came to view reading interventions and demonstrated a process for teaching students how to read and comprehend in the situated context of reading activity. The question, of course, is how effective was reciprocal teaching in positively influencing student outcomes?

The results of several studies revealed the powerful effects of the apprenticeship model on students' reading comprehension. Initially, Brown and Palincsar (1989) instituted the reciprocal teaching procedures in the context of reading groups consisting of seventh- and eighth-graders. In this study, several procedures were adhered to: (1) students were selected on the basis of their low reading comprehension scores; (2) the intervention was fairly extensive, consisting of no fewer than 10 days of discussions, and usually continuing for 20 days; (3) progress was measured by changes in the students' participation in the discussions and by daily tests of their retention on transfer passages; and (4) long-term maintenance, transfer, and generalization were all measured.

In addition, independent raters read transcripts of discussions and rated students' use of the four strategies. Analyses showed large and reliable improvements in students' strategy use (Brown & Palincsar, 1989). Over time, there was a shift from teacher-directed instructional formats to student-controlled interactions, reflecting a more active student role in the dialogues as they increasingly took the lead in directing and monitoring their own and others' understandings of the text (Palincsar & Brown, 1989). The changes seen in the dialogues seemed to reflect a process of internalization, as reflected in independent probes of reading behavior: students who began the program by scoring 30–40% correct reached a stable level of 70–80% correct on the daily independent probes of comprehension. A nearly identical result was obtained in another study when peer tutors taught the procedure to small groups of poor readers. Overall, the examination of reciprocal teaching revealed large and stable quantitative improvements on measures of comprehension; the effects of the intervention were durable on measures of maintenance (2 and 6 months later); and improvement transferred to the classroom and criterion-referenced measures of comprehension (Brown & Palincsar, 1989; Palincsar & Brown, 1984).

These results showed the powerful effects of reciprocal teaching. What are especially noteworthy are the converging findings from a later series of studies that yield support for the role of the sociocultural model in the design of efficacious interventions (Palincsar, 1986). Four findings are consistent with the theoretical assumptions of the model. First, the results are clear that the higher-order cognitive activities associated with reading are best acquired and practiced in situated activity. Teacher modeling followed by skill practice in isolated or noninteractive contexts did not yield the same results as those that featured the transfer of control and the applied use of the comprehension strategies in the context of situated reading activity (Brown & Palincsar, 1989). Second, the results speak to the power of teaching students to use strategies in an integrated fashion rather than decontextualizing or teaching strategies as skill components. Third, the findings suggest that students' participation in social dialogues can advance students' abilities to use these tools to direct their own independent reading activity. Finally, studies of the nature of reciprocal teaching dialogues suggest that the teachers who taught students responsively (e.g., linking students' ideas to new knowledge, transforming partially correct

to more correct understandings) produced greater student gains on transfer measures. Taken together, these results show strong support for Vygotsky's central ideas of the importance of the apprenticeship model and the primary role of the teacher in providing modeling, coaching, scaffolding, and fading.

Writing: Cognitive Strategy Instruction in Writing

Writing is another discipline that requires higher-order thinking and abstraction. Many of the transparent features of spoken language that convey meaning (inflection, tempo, expression, gesture, pause) must be codified and objectified in written language using abstract symbols, marks, or conventions. Globally and locally, written text must be staged at the macro (text-level) and micro (paragraph, sentence, word) levels through the provision of organizational cues and devices to assist the reader in identifying, structuring and understanding the meaning and relationships among the ideas (Spivey, 1997). Furthermore, whereas spoken language is embedded in a shared social situation, written language appears solitary and detached from the experiential world. From the outset, the student undertaking to learn to write must confront the machinery of the language; "he has to become aware of its components and of the various operations required to produce or comprehend it" (Scribner, 1997, p. 169). Quite simply, unlike many automatized skills, the act of writing remains a deliberate mental act throughout life, requiring the conscious attention and reflection of the author (Scribner, 1997).

Comparative studies show that good and poor writers are distinguished in several respects, including their use of metacognitive knowledge to plan, draft, monitor, and revise texts (Englert, Raphael, Fear, & Anderson, 1988; MacArthur, Graham, & Schwartz, 1993); their ability to relate ideas into organizational patterns that correspond to text structures (Mastropieri & Scruggs, 1997; Swanson, 1999); and their ability to monitor and regulate performance (Wong & Jones, 1982; Wong & Wilson, 1984). Good writers are differentiated because they seem to have acquired strategic and metacognitive knowledge about the craft of writing (e.g., tools, conventions, processes, and practices), including a knowledge of what to do, when to do it, why it is important, and when it should be done.

One program that was intentionally designed to provide a cognitive apprenticeship in writing based on a sociocultural framework was Cognitive Strategy Instruction in Writing (CSIW). Teachers in the CSIW program sought to make visible the tacit processes that writers undertake in the act of planning, composing, and editing expository text (Englert et al., 1991). CSIW was designed for implementation in resource and general education classrooms to support the writing performance of elementary students with learning disabilities.

As characterized by reciprocal teaching, CSIW incorporated specific features that were illustrative of the theoretical model of Vygotsky. First, CSIW highlighted the teacher's role in making visible the internal and external sides of writing activity in the situated context of composing and interrogating text. Teachers involved students directly in the practice of writing by composing group stories and by following a process approach to writing that engaged students in the application of various writing strategies specific to each facet of writing. Teachers, for example, involved students in planning their texts by modeling and engaging the students in a collaborative dialogue guided by self-questions, such as "Why am I writing this?" (purpose), "Who is my audience?" "What do I know about my topic?" (activating background knowledge). Similar self-questions were modeled through think-alouds to make available the discourse and self-regulating processes associated with an inquiry approach to writing, including how writers gather information, organize ideas, write, edit, and revise their papers (see Englert et al., 1996; Englert, Raphael, Anderson, Gregg & Anthony, 1989).

Second, teachers actually composed group stories in real time to make explicit the relationships between the specific writing actions that writers take and their associated talk, thoughts, questions, and purposes. Through these public demonstrations, teachers made it possible for students to witness and experience the bottlenecks, false starts, dilemmas, actions, thoughts,

and corrections of writers in the process of text monitoring and construction rather than experience the skills in isolated contexts (Englert & Mariage, 1996). The shared reading and writing of texts involved students in the co-construction of meaning, as well as provided an anchoring context for modeling writing tactics, conventions, structures, strategies, and purposes (Wells, 1999).

Third, the teachers provided specific symbol systems and language tools to mediate and scaffold performance. For example, teachers displayed the acronym POWER to remind students of the *p*lanning, *o*rganizing, *w*riting, *e*diting, and *r*evising processes that good writers employ to compose well-organized texts (Mariage, Englert, & Garmon, 2000). The use of acronyms for supporting strategy use has figured prominently in the work of many writing researchers (Troia, Harris & Graham, 1999). In addition, "think sheets" were provided to externalize the self-questions, strategies, and key language that had been modeled. Students used these think sheets to support their thinking as they planned, organized, composed, and edited their own texts (Englert & Raphael, 1989). Similarly, to assist students in organizing their texts, teachers provided graphic organizers to represent the text structure (see Graham & Harris, 1989a, 1989b) and explicitly taught the conventions of each writing genre or structure (e.g., compare–contrast, explanations, superordinate–subordinate). All these aforementioned tools served as procedural facilitators to make visible and accessible the language and procedures of writers (Vaughn, Gersten, & Chard, 2000). The intention was that the individual(s) operating with such mediational means would be able to perform at levels superior to that which they could achieve otherwise, thereby supporting them in their zones of proximal development (Wertsch, 1995).

Fourth, teachers actively apprenticed students in the writing discourse by promoting a developmental shift in the relationships and roles assumed by teachers and students. Initially, teachers did the modeling. However, students were asked to assume increasing responsibility for whatever aspects of the dialogue or process they were able to execute on succeeding paragraphs, texts, or lessons

(Englert, 1992). Each time a section of a group text was composed, teachers paused to allow students time to question, challenge, support, monitor, revise, or extend the form and meaning of the ideas. Thus, texts were treated as thinking devices that might provoke other meanings, interpretations, and responses (Wertsch & Toma, 1995). The interaction between texts, readers, and authors placed students in explicit dialogical relationships with other writers and audience members, helping them to hear and internalize the dialogue and questions of others that might be reenacted to guide their own problem-solving performance in the future. In this manner, it was intended that the cognitive process and dialogue that were performed on a social plane would be gradually anticipated by writers and turned inward to guide and influence their conversations with texts or readers on the intramental or inner mental plane. Only when students lacked the ability to recognize problems or to provide relevant feedback, did teachers intervene to introduce or prompt the language and strategies to compose or fix the text. Thus, teachers directly engaged writers in the craft of writing while offering technical assistance and coaching them while they were actually engaged in writing and monitoring processes (Wells, 1999).

This problem-solving orientation to ideas and meanings accomplished several important objectives: It (1) provided a foundation for the development of critical thought, executive monitoring functions, and metacognition; (2) prompted internalization and rehearsal of the writing discourse and strategies through an enlargement of the role of students in the dialogues; (3) made visible the rules of discourse and forms of the written register; (4) promoted a consciousness of the dialectical relationship between authors and audience; (5) supported the introduction of new writing procedures; and (6) produced artifacts with visible reminders of the array of cultural artifacts and tools which may be used to mediate the creation of texts and text solutions (Wells, 1999). Over time, in fact, participating students became increasingly capable of exchanging points of view, evaluating the viability of ideas and suggestions, working out text problems, and engaging in an academic discourse in the problem-centered text construction activity (Englert & Mariage, 1996; Jakubowski, 1993; Mariage, 2001; Roth, 1993).

Finally, CSIW was expanded over time to incorporate collaborative structures involving partner or small-group writing. Teachers progressed from interacting with students in teacher-directed whole-class discussions to establishing small-group or partner writing activities, and finally, to occasions when students wrote independently. These spaces offered a range or continuum of assistance and scaffolds made available to students. These collaborative arrangements transferred control to students and placed them in the position of the ones who asked questions rather than merely answered them, gave directions rather than simply followed them, thought aloud rather than simply listened, and challenged ideas to bring all participants into deeper discussions about meaning and practices (Englert & Dunsmore, 2002; Mariage, 2001). While students typically engage with written texts when they are alone, the collaboration afforded an occasion for students to move back and forth between text, talk, and action and engaged them in reciprocal roles as authors, readers, and respondents, as part of a deepening apprenticeship into the spoken and written discourse of writers (Wells, 1999).

As described by Confrey (1993), therefore, the CSIW approach to writing instruction could be likened to an apprenticeship in a more traditional crafts or labor industry based on the following features: (1) the preparation of a product (written text) that represented a shared collaborative enterprise, and that both constrained the interactions and supported their goal-directed activities; and (2) the creation of an artifact that, at the termination of the activity, participants could point to, discuss, and locate their sense of shared goals and tools applied in the course of making the product. To this list, we add two additional traits: (3) a deepening and recursive cycle of apprenticeship that offered challenges and increasing complexity for all participants, while offering mechanisms of support until individuals became capable of fuller participation in all parts of the activity; and (4) the involvement of participants with varying degrees of skill and mastery in the use of the cultural tools (Wells, 1999; Wenger, 1998).

The results of several studies over the course of a number of years revealed some key findings that are noteworthy in understanding this approach. First, a study was conducted of the efficacy of CSIW with 128 fourth- and fifth-grade subjects and 55 students with learning disabilities (Englert et al., 1991). The results revealed significant differences between the treatment conditions. CSIW students significantly surpassed control students in their ability to write well-formed expository texts. On measures of transfer to an untaught text structure, students in the CSIW condition again significantly surpassed control students, whereas control students showed an actual decrease in their writing ability over time. Furthermore, when comparisons were made of the performance of CSIW students with learning disabilities relative to a nonparticipating group of general education students, the results revealed that preintervention differences disappeared over the course of students' participation in CSIW. After participation in CSIW, the writing and reading performance of students with learning disabilities (LD) was similar to that of a group of nonintervention grade-level peers. Finally, analyses further showed that teachers who promoted the greatest gains and transfer (1) modeled the writing strategies, (2) involved students in classroom dialogues, (3) promoted strategy flexibility, and (4) relinquished control of strategies to students (Anderson, Raphael, Englert & Stevens, 1991).

A second study was conducted as part of a later project known as the Early Literacy Project, which expanded CSIW instruction to include a total reading–writing literacy curriculum, and that involved teachers and researchers in a collaborative partnership in a community of practice (Englert & Mariage, 1996; Englert, Raphael, & Mariage, 1998). The Early Literacy Project incorporated a number of reading-related activities, although a central core of the project remained the writing intervention described in this section. We focus on the writing results because of the similar nature of this work to CSIW in both the type of the intervention and the findings.

One research finding was the power of the expository writing treatment. Analyses revealed statistically significant differences (greater than 0.001) between experimental and control students on two different types of text structures (explanations, reports) for nearly all dependent variables. Students of the most experienced experimental teachers significantly surpassed control students on nearly all writing facets, with performance differences between the groups ranging from 0.78 to 1.0 standard deviations on all writing variables.

A second finding related to the complexity of the intervention for teachers to master, requiring a number of years for newcomers to fully understand. Analyses revealed that, in the hands of first-year teachers (first year of implementing the intervention), the treatment was less powerful than in the hands of second-year teachers (second year of implementing the intervention) (Englert et al., 1996). This result was found for two consecutive years of the project (Englert, 1995). Interviews and classroom observations revealed that a key difference between the first- and second-year intervention teachers was their understanding of the principles associated with the sociocultural approach. Englert and Dunsmore (2002), in fact, followed the teaching performance and writing dialogues of one of the more skilled project teachers over the course of several years of her project participation—from the start of her participation to its conclusion. They found several changes in the teacher's instructional moves that were reflective of the patterns found in the larger body of research. At the start of the teacher's participation, for example, she undertook the preponderance of the intellectual work associated with the actions and language of writing, as she named the writing tools and practices, and directed students in their use. However, the teacher was less skilled in providing insight into the inner thoughts that mediated the actions. As the teacher gained experience, she not only became more successful in modeling her inner thoughts, but even more strikingly, she became more skilled in stepping back from the leadership position to share her authority with students. Through public questions about what to do, when to do it, and why it should be done, she artfully positioned her students to think aloud to make their writing practices accessible to others, furthering the exchange of expertise among students and fostering a type of "shop talk" or "laboratory talk" that brought her students to a deeper common understanding of their writing craft (see Roth, 1998). She had learned to transform her largely teacher-directed discourse to a more balanced instructional discourse that incorporated teacher mediation and a student-centered discourse that was further bolstered by responsive and contingent instruction. She became more skilled in responding to students' errors or partially correct understandings with a hierarchy of prompts that were adjusted to support the development of knowledge at points just beyond students' current levels. Her ability to provide a cognitive apprenticeship, therefore, had markedly improved. Concurrently, analyses of the concomitant student moves revealed large increases from the early to later years in the extent to which her students were able to appropriate and practice the writing language, practices, and tools, as well as increases in their participation and leadership in initiating and regulating problem-solving processes during text construction and revision.

Finally, Englert and her colleagues (Englert, Berry, & Dunsmore 2002; Englert & Dunsmore, 2002; Mariage, 2000) examined the nature of students' participation in partner writing and small-group collaborative activity. Their analysis of the talk between writing partners showed several dimensions of social collaboration that furthered the development of higher-order mental functions, as evidenced by four findings: (1) peer collaboration pushed the fuller participation and practice by students in the community's writing discourse and practices, that is, individuals working in collaborative groups exceeded the level of performance and participation obtained in either the teacher-directed lesson or independent writing activities (see Englert & Dunsmore, 2002); (2) peer collaboration provided an acquisition space that was different than that afforded students during teacher-directed lessons, motivating students to try out and regulate challenging writing practices in ways and degrees that were not entirely possible in either teacher-led or independent learning arrangements (Englert & Dunsmore, 2002); (3) a range of participation

roles (author, writer, reader, editor) influenced the type of executive, cognitive, writing, and social skills that were exercised and developed by collaborating students (Mariage, 2001); (4) conversations among students offered teachers valuable opportunities to acquire new insights and data about students' developmental levels and emerging abilities that were not possible to ascertain through an analysis of students' written texts alone; and (5) teacher mediation remained an important aspect that furthered students' development, even while students worked in collaboration with each other. The combined results supported the conclusion of Vaughn and colleagues (2000) that peer collaboration helped students persevere in the face of difficult tasks, and that the feedback from peers may have a salutary effect on performance.

Guided Inquiry in Science through Multiple Literacies

Sociocultural theory may be particularly efficacious for teaching science to students. In developing guidelines to inform their Guided Instruction in Science through Multiple Literacies (GIsML) program, Palincsar, Magnusson, Collins, and Cutter (2001) identify four instructional features that draw directly from sociocultural theory, including (1) emphases on students' participation in a learning community in which there is distributed expertise and overlapping zones of proximal development; (2) acceptance of the multiple ways in which students can represent what they know (i.e., documenting one's learning with the use of writing, drawing, and other graphic representations); (3) participation in authentic cycles of investigation during which students experience learning as a recursive process in which one's knowledge and reasoning are refined over time; and (4) opportunity to engage in problem solving through situated scientific activity (e.g., manipulating the phenomena they are investigating).

GIsML emphasizes the importance of creating a community of practice at the level of both professional development and among students in inclusive settings. These communities of practice use a recursive process for constructing meaning with one another, including (1) *engaging* with the big ideas of a scientific content area (e.g., "How does light interact with matter?" and "Why do things sink or float?"); (2) *investigating* scientific phenomena through the use of firsthand investigations (e.g., experimentation, collaboration, and authentic problem-solving), as well as through the use of secondhand accounts of other scientists' investigations (e.g., reading texts, scientist notebooks, and graphs); (3) *explaining* scientific phenomena through multiple linguistic forms, including writing, speaking, demonstrating; and (4) *reporting* findings to others. The heuristic serves an orienting function that can be thought of as a conceptual map that guides decision making regarding curriculum, instruction, student understanding, and assessment (Palincsar, Magnusson, Marano, Ford, & Brown, 1998).

One of the most innovative aspects of the work involves the conscious manipulation and study of scientific texts to mediate learning in combination with firsthand scientific investigations. In schools, canonical knowledge is primarily disseminated in written texts, making the qualities of those texts a critical feature of science teaching. Yet a number of limitations of traditional texts in elementary science teaching were identified by the GIsML teachers, including (1) concentration on facts, rather than on generative understanding; (2) emphasis on the products of science rather than the nature and process of science; (3) presentation of information in familiar, but not scientifically conventional ways; and (4) linear presentation of text that tends to inhibit the importance of cumulative reference, knowledge building, and reflection on knowledge.

In response to these challenges and based on several quasi-experimental studies, the GIsML researchers developed alternative text formats that would help address deficiencies in traditional texts (Palincsar & Magnusson, 2000). They designed an innovative text genre known as the "scientist notebook" format to cultivate and model scientific "habits of thought" as well as to bridge the gap between traditional texts and scientific journals or notebooks. The hybrid text, scientist notebook, allowed for multiple ways of representing data (e.g., tables, figures, and diagrams), modeled the forms of language and inscriptional conventions used by a fictitious scientist (e.g., "Lesley Park") to make scientific practices accessible, prompted the science teacher to think aloud and model scientific reasoning, provided graphic representations of scientific problems (e.g., providing pictures of a ball rolling down various slopes and hitting a can), and provided first-person accounts of a scientist's thoughts and questions (e.g., "I also saw that a speedier ball from a higher ramp moved a can at the bottom of the ramp further. So the ball had more energy to give the moving can").

To assess the impact of the innovative genre, a quasi-experimental study was conducted in which students read a scientific text and performed a related experiment in their classroom. Seven fourth-grade GIsML classrooms in two districts (rural, urban) participated in a within-subject, across-group design where all students read both a traditional expository text and the innovative science notebook text. The two text types were counterbalanced across classrooms and scientific topics (reflection or refraction). The results of this study indicated that both versions of the scientific text supported learning. However, the results indicated statistically significant gains in favor of the scientist notebook in three of four conditions studied. Students in the scientist notebook condition engaged in more instructional conversations during their own inquiry process, reflected on the text in terms of the inquiry reported in the scientist's notebook, and drew on textual information to inform their own firsthand investigations. Finally, when students used the science notebook, they were better able to carry on instructional dialogues relative to their understanding of the scientific topic (e.g., light), whereas in the traditional text condition, students primarily engaged in paraphrasing the text. The researchers concluded that (1) conceptualizing instruction as guided inquiry teaching consisting of first- and secondhand experiences can help students contextualize the language and practices associated with scientific discourse and inquiry; (2) text features and genres (i.e., those that constituted the notebook genre) support both the participation of students in first- and secondhand investigations, and support the acquisition of scientific reasoning; and (3) classroom contexts must intentionally and carefully structure instruction to support effective inquiry-based teaching and meaningful learning by positioning students in a scientific discourse where the inner thoughts, language, and notations of scientists are made transparent and accessible (Palincsar & Magnusson, 2000, pp. 10). Changing the nature of the text altered the cognitive tools, dispositions, and understandings that were constructed in the classroom community of GIsML classrooms.

A second study was conducted to examine what instructional conditions would be necessary to support students with disabilities in GIsML classrooms (Palincsar et al., 2001). To examine the effectiveness of the GIsML approach for students with learning disabilities and emotional disorders, a 2-year study was conducted. In Phase 1 (Year 1), the researchers conducted a careful observational study of the cognitive, linguistic, and social demands of students with learning disabilities and/or emotional disorders as they participated in each phase of the GIsML inquiry process, but teachers implemented the GIsML instruction based on the suggested framework. At the conclusion of Phase 1, the results indicated that normally achieving students showed statistically significant gains in three of the four GIsML classrooms. However, identified students with disabilities showed statistically significant gains in only one of the four classrooms. The participation of students with disabilities in a process of scientific inquiry did not automatically improve their scientific performance.

In Phase 2, a series of "advanced instructional features" were identified and implemented that were designed to support the performance of students with disabilities in GIsML. Three sets of teaching practices were incorporated into GIsML, including (1) teaching processes for monitoring, facilitating, and scaffolding student thinking; (2) development of print literacy and the acceptance of multiple representational forms; and (3) processes for changing the social organization to support participation. To better monitor, facilitate, and scaffold student thinking, for example, a number of strategies were generated, including *rehearsal* and *mini-conferences*. During rehearsal, students practiced reporting what they would

share with classmates either alone or with a paraprofessional. In addition, teachers held mini-conferences with individuals or small groups to monitor their scientific understanding and to prepare them to participate in a scientific dialogue with peers. These conferences enabled teachers to scaffold individual students' performance by bridging the gap between what was known and not known, by supporting oral expression and communication abilities, and by engaging students in reflecting on the scientific goals of the investigation.

A second set of teaching practices focused on enhancing teachers' acceptance and development of students' scientific literacy by emphasizing and supporting students' use of the symbolic and multiple representational forms used in science. One technique entailed the provision of a specialized vocabulary or the lexicon of scientists, including the use of a glossary of terms that was posted in class. This glossary typically contained terms that were germane to the scientific inquiry process (e.g., evidence, claim, and conclusion) as well as terms unique to the topic of study (e.g., reflect, absorb, and transmit). In addition, teachers encouraged students to represent their knowledge through the use of multiple literacies, including written texts, diagrams, graphic representations, and so forth, as well as partnered students with written expression difficulties with others (peers, aids, teacher) to support them in advance of independent writing performance.

A final set of teaching practices focused on the social norms for effective collaboration, ranging from the provision of procedures for equitable turn taking to a more formal set of practices that that allowed teachers to monitor the groups' interactions and provide feedback about the quality of their collaborations.

Results of the Phase 2 design experiment revealed shifts in the teachers' effectiveness with students with disabilities. Students with disabilities showed statistically significant gains in two of the four classrooms during the advanced teaching practices conditions, and a third classroom approached statistical significance. The same teachers who were not effective in advancing the scientific knowledge of students with disabilities during the general GIsML instruction generated significantly improved outcomes when they incorporated advanced practices that allowed them to assess students' knowledge in a dynamic way, furthering students' access to and participation in the scientific tools related to reporting their scientific understanding, and ensuring their participation in collaborative groups.

Though these data suggest the use of advanced teaching procedures with identified students, the implementation of the procedures did not have a negative impact on either low- or normally achieving students, a particularly efficacious finding. Most important, this study indicated the importance of understanding how individual teachers mediate students' learning, particularly those students with identified needs. When teachers began to consciously reflect on and use advanced instructional features, they provide identified students with the instructional conditions that help ensure social participation and have a positive impact on the learning of *all* students.

The GIsML research program represents the application of sociocultural theory to inform teaching and learning in science. First, detailed attention was given to the nature of *situated activity* and the conscious manipulation of content, discourse, textual, and social resources for all members of the community as they have attempted to participate in the real work of scientists in the school setting. Second, an *apprenticeship* approach toward instruction was employed that allowed students to experience complete cycles of scientific inquiry, including engaging with big ideas, experimenting, explaining, and reporting their findings through iterative phases of development. Third, the program provided community members with access to the *tools and mediational means* used to understand the inquiry process, making visible the unique social practices engaged in by scientists and their texts, as well as involved students in firsthand investigations that directly involved them in a community of practice in the use of particular ways of thinking, acting, and knowing. Fourth, the program provided access to students' thinking through the frequent publication of ideas in multiple semiotic systems (e.g., speaking, small-group collaboration, science notebooks, drawings, and graphical displays of data).

In this sense, the community of practice provided multiple opportunities for students to both assimilate and apply their understandings in iterative cycles of activity. Finally, community members participate in a range of *collaborative participation structures* where there are expectations for social participation

Discussion

In the 21st century, core-curriculum standards have been reconceptualized and redefined to change "what counts" as conventional knowledge. Simultaneously, we have litigated that students with learning disabilities be held accountable to these new standards, even though the cognitive, linguistic, and social demands required to meet these standards have increased exponentially—areas that have often been sources of difficulty for countless students identified as having learning disabilities. The challenges are great, but the sociocultural model may be well suited to offer forms of teaching and learning that satisfy these new content standards by focusing on higher-order thinking and problem solving.

Sociocultural theory has advanced our knowledge about teaching for understanding and conceptual change for students with and without learning disabilities. This review has outlined three programs of research that have at their center the participation of students and teachers in communities of social practice that simulate the communities of real authors and scientists. In all three research programs, domain-specific skills, strategies, discourses, and practices were made available to students in iterative cycles of activity that gradually ceded increasing control for meaning making and performance to students through apprenticeships and collaborations with teachers and peers in the community. Furthermore, in all three programs, teacher modeling and thinking aloud provided access to the knowledge, dispositions, and metacognition required for competent performance in the subject matter discipline. Finally, the provision of tools for creating and comprehending texts as well as other disciplinary artifacts were critical mediators of cognitive and social performance. These key components of effective instruction have been noted in other researchers' syntheses of the research literature in special education (Vaughn et al., 2000). There is agreement that these teaching practices have importance for teaching students with disabilities.

We believe this theory also extends the ways that we have traditionally thought about "adapting and modifying" curriculum and instruction. The use of mnemonic devices, text structure frameworks, and cognitive strategies are often employed to compensate for a variety of visual or auditory processing deficits, organizational challenges, short- or long-term memory difficulties, or a variety of written or oral expression problems that students with learning disabilities often bring to the classroom. These instructional methods are vitally important in helping students with learning disabilities participate more effectively in school settings. In addition, the programs reviewed in this chapter add to these teaching toolkits the notion of assisted development from a broad perspective, including the "big ideas" that organize a field of study, apprenticeship into the social practices of a discipline, making visible the language in use of the cognitive tools and artifacts used to construct meaning in particular communities of practice, and the use of heuristics that delimit and make understandable complex and multistage processes in recursive cycles of activity to members of the community. The notion of assisting development in complex fields of study such as reading, writing, and scientific inquiry are likely to be more effective when we expand our definitions of assisting development to include the unique needs of the cognitive, linguistic, and social demands of learning at every phase of instruction.

In considering the limitations of this body of work for general teaching applications, we recognize that the model is most effective in teaching higher-order thinking and cognitive processes. Basic direct instruction and rehearsal techniques may be more effective in promoting skill acquisition and mastery. However, skills must be recontextualized in situated contexts of use for transfer and generalization to occur. We also recognize that this research is emergent in its developmental history in the field of special education. Although the model has existed for some time, there has been little direct application of this paradigm in instructional research in special education settings. Given this limited number of studies, there is little information about the effect sizes, transfer, or generalization of cognitive processes to new settings or academic disciplines. However, the rich potential of the sociocultural model in explaining teaching and learning could provide researchers with new conceptual and methodological lenses to develop and interpret the interactions and effects of members' participation within classrooms.

References

Anderson, L. M., Raphael, T. E., Englert, C. S., & Stevens, D. D. (1991, April). *Teaching writing with a new instructional model: Variations in teachers' practices and student performance.* Paper presented at the annual meeting of the American Educational Research Association, Chicago.

Artiles, A., Trent, S. C., Hoffman-Kipp, P., & Lopez-Torres, L. (2000). From individual acquisition to cultural-historical practices in multicultural teacher education. *Remedial and Special Education, 21*(2), 79–89, 120.

Biemiller, A., & Meichenbaum, D. (1998). The consequences of negative scaffolding for students who learn slowly—A commentary on C. Addison Stone's "The metaphor of scaffolding: Its utility for the field of learning disabilities." *Journal of Learning Disabilities, 31*(4), 365–369.

Brown, A. L., & Palincsar, A. S. (1989). Guided, cooperative learning and individual knowledge acquisition. In L. Resnick (Ed.), *Knowing, learning, and instruction* (pp. 393–451). Hillsdale, NJ: Erlbaum.

Collins, A., Brown, J. S., & Holum, A. (1991). Cognitive apprenticeship: Making thinking visible. *American Educator,* pp. 6–11.

Confrey, J. (1993). Learning to see children's mathematics: Crucial challenges in constructivist reform. In K. Tobin (Ed.), *The practice of constructivism in science education* (pp. 299–324). Hillsdale, NJ: Erlbaum.

Cope, B., & Kalantzis, M. (1993). The power of literacy and the literacy of power. In B. Cope & M. Kalantzis (Eds.), *The powers of literacy: A genre approach to teaching writing* (pp. 63–89). Pittsburgh, PA: University of Pittsburgh Press.

De La Paz, S. (1999). Self-regulated strategy instruction in regular education settings: Improving outcomes for students with and without learning disabilities. *Learning Disabilities Research and Practice, 14*(2), 92–106.

Engestrom, Y., Miettinen, R., & Punamaki, R. (Eds.). (1999). *Perspectives on activity theory.* New York: Cambridge University Press.

Englert, C. S. (1992). Writing instruction from a sociocultural perspective: The holistic, dialogic, and social enterprise of writing. *Journal of Learning Disabilities, 25*(3), 153–172.

Englert, C. S., Berry, R. A., & Dunsmore, K. L. (2001). A case study of the apprenticeship process: Another perspective on the apprentice and the scaffolding metaphor. *Journal of Learning Disabilities, 34*(2), 152–171.

Englert, C. S., & Dunsmore, K. (2002). Social constructivist teaching: Affordances and constraints. In J. Brophy (Ed.), *Advances in research on teaching* (Vol. 9). Amsterdam: JAI Press.

Englert, C. S., Garmon, A., & Mariage, T. V. (1995, April). *A multi-year literacy intervention: Exploring issues that impact special education students.* Paper presented at the annual meeting of the American Educational Research Association, San Francisco.

Englert, C. S., Garmon, A., Mariage, T. V., Rozendal, M. S., Tarrant, K., & Urba, J. (1996). The Early Literacy Project: Connecting across the literacy curriculum. *Remedial and Special Education, 19*(3), 142–159, 180.

Englert, C. S., & Mariage, T. V. (1996). A sociocultural perspective: Teaching ways-of-thinking and ways-of-talking in a literacy community. *Learning Disaiblities Research and Practice, 11*(3), 157–167.

Englert, C. S., & Raphael, T. E. (1989). Developing successful writers through cognitive strategy instruction. In J. Brophy (Ed.), *Advances in research on teaching* (Vol. 1, pp. 105–151). Greenwich, CT: JAI Press.

Englert, C. S., Raphael, T. E., Anderson, L. M., Anthony, H. M., Stevens, D. D., & Fear, K. L. (1991). Making writing strategies and self-talk visible: Cognitive strategy instruction in writing in regular and special education classrooms. *American Educational Research Journal, 28*, 337–372.

Englert, C. S., Raphael, T. E., Anderson, L. M., Gregg, S. L., & Anthony, H. M. (1989). Exposition: Reading, writing and the metacognitive knowledge of learning disabled students. *Learning Disabilities Research, 5*(1), 5–24.

Englert, C. S., Rapheal, T. E., Fear, K. L., & Anderson, L. M. (1988). Students' metacognitive knowledge about how to write informational texts. *Learning Disability Quarterly, 11*, 18–46.

Englert, C. S., Raphael, T. E., & Mariage, T. V. (1998). A multi-year literacy intervention: Transformation and teacher change in the community of the early literacy project. *Teacher Education and Special Education, 21*(4), 255–277.

Ferretti, R. P., MacArthur, C. D., & Okolo, C. M. (2001). Teaching for historical understanding in inclusive classrooms. *Learning Disability Quarterly, 24*, 59–71.

Gee, J. P. (1997). Thinking, learning, and reading: The situated sociocultural mind. In D. Kirschner & J. A. Whitson (Eds.), *Situated cognition: Social, semiotic, and psychological perspectives* (pp. 235–259). Hillsdale, NJ: Erlbaum.

Gindis, B. (1999). Vygotsky's vision reshaping the practice of special education for the 21st century. *Remedial and Special Education, 20*(6), 333–340.

Goatley, V., Brock, C., & Raphael, T. E. (1995). Diverse learners participating in regular education "Book Clubs." *Reading Research Quarterly, 30*(3), 352–380.

Goldman, S. R., Hasselbring, T. S., & Cognition and Technology Group at Vanderbilt. (1996). Achieving meaningful mathematics literacy for students with learning disabilities. *Journal of Learning Disabilities, 30*(2), 198–208.

Graham, S., & Harris, K. R. (1989a). Components analysis of cognitives strategy instruction: Effects on learning disabled students' compositions and self-efficacy. *Journal of Educational Psychology, 81*(353–361).

Graham, S., & Harris, K. R. (1989b). Improving learning disabled students' skills at composing essays: Self-instructional strategy training. *Exceptional Children, 56*(201–214).

Gutierrez, K. D., & Stone, L. D. (1997). A cultural-historical view of learning and learning disabilities: Participating in a community of learners. *Learning Disabilities Research and Practice, 12*(2), 123–131.

Hock, M. F., Schumaker, J. B., & Deshler, D. D. (1999). Closing the gap to success in secondary schools: A model for cognitive apprenticeship. In D. D. Deshler, J. Schumaker, K. R. Harris, & S. Graham (Eds.), *Teaching every adolescent every day: Learning in diverse middle and high school classrooms* (pp. 1–52). Cambridge, MA: Brookline.

Hogan, K., & Pressley, M. (Eds.). (1997). *Scaffolding student learning: Instructional approaches & issues.* Cambridge, MA: Brookline.

Jakubowski, E. (1993). Constructing potential learning opportunities in middle grades mathematics. In K. Tobin (Ed.), *The practice of constructivism in science education* (pp. 135–144). Hillsdale, NJ: Erlbaum.

Klingner, J. K., Vaughn, S., & Schumm, J. S. (1998). Collaborative strategic reading during social studies in heterogeneous fourth-grade classrooms. *Elementary School Journal, 99*(1), 3–22.

Lave, J. (1997). The culture of acquisition and the practice of understanding. In D. Kirschner & J. A. Whitson (Eds.), *Situated cognition: Social, semiotic, and psychological perspectives* (pp. 17–36). Hillsdale, NJ: Erlbaum.

MacArthur, C., Graham, S., & Schwartz, S. (1993). Knowledge of revision and revising behavior among learning disabled students. *Learning Disability Quarterly, 14*, 61–73.

Mariage, T. V. (2001). Features of an interactive writing discourse: Conversational involvement, conventional knowledge, and internalization in "Morning Message." *Journal of Learning Disabilities, 34*(2), 172–196.

Mariage, T. V., Englert, C. S., & Garmon, M. A. (2000). The teacher as "more knowledgeable other" in assisting literacy learning with special needs students. *Reading and Writing Quarterly, 16,* 299–336.

Mastropieri, M., & Scruggs, T. E. (1997). Best practices in promoting reading comprehension in students with learning disabilities: 1976–1996. *Remedial and Special Education, 18,* 197–213.

Morocco, C. C., Hindin, A., Mata-Aguilar, C., & Clark-Chiarelli, N. (2001). Building a deep understanding of literature with middle-grade students with learning disaiblities. *Learning Disability Quarterly, 24*(1), 47–58.

Nardi, B. A. (1996). Activity theory and human–computer interaction. In B. A. Nardi (Ed.), *Context and consciousness: Activity theory and human-computer interaction* (pp. 7–16). Cambridge, MA: MIT Press.

Okolo, C. M., & Ferretti, R. P. (1997). Knowledge acquisition and multimedia design in the social studies for children with learning disabilities. *Journal of Special Education Technology, 13*(2), 91–103.

Palincsar, A. S. (1986). The role of dialogue in providing scaffolded instruction. *Educational Psychologist, 21*(1&2), 73–98.

Palincsar, A. S., & Brown, A. L. (1989). Classroom dialogues to promote self-regulated comprehension. In J. E. Brophy (Ed.), *Advances in research in teaching* (Vol. 1, pp. 35–71). Greenwich, CT: JAI Press.

Palincsar, A. S., & Magnusson, S. J. (2000, March). The interplay of firsthand and text-based investigations in science education (CIERA Report No. 2-007). Ann Arbor, MI: Center for the Improvement of Early Reading Achievement.

Palincsar, A. S., Magnusson, S. J., Collins, K. M., & Cutter, J. (2001). Making science accessible to all: Results of a design experiment in inclusive classrooms. *Learning Disability Quarterly, 24,* 15–32.

Pressley, M. B., R., El-Dinary, P. B., & Afflerback, P. (1995). The comprehension instruction that students need: Instruction fostering constructively responsive reading. *Learning Disabilities Research and Practice, 10,* 215–224.

Roth, W. M. (1993). Construction sites: Science labs and classrooms. In K. Tobin (Ed.), *The practice of constructivism in science education* (pp. 145–170). Hillsdale, NJ: Erlbaum.

Roth, W. M. (1998). *Designing communities.* Boston: Kluwer Academic.

Rueda, R., Gallego, M. A., & Moll, L. C. (2000). The least restrictive environment: A place or a context? *Remedial and Special Education, 21*(2), 70–78.

Schaffer, H. R. (1992). Joint involvement episodes as context for development. In H. McGurk (Ed.), *Childhood social development: Contemporary perspectives* (pp. 99–129). Hillsdale, NJ: Erlbaum.

Scribner, S. (1997). The cognitive consequences of literacy. In E. Tobach, R. J. Falmagne, M. B. Parlee, L. M. W. Martin, & A. S. Kapelman (Eds.), *Mind and social practice: Selected writings of Sylvia Scribner* (pp. 160–189). New York: Cambridge University Press.

Shotter, J. (1995). In dialogue: Social constructionism and radical constructivism. In L. P. Steffe & J. Gale (Eds.), *Constructivism in education* (pp. 41–56). Hillsdale, NJ: Erlbaum.

Spivey, N. (1997). *Constructivist metaphor: Reading, writing, and the making of meaning.* San Diego, CA: Academic Press.

Stone, C. A. (1993). What's missing in the metaphor of scaffolding? In E. A. Forman, N. Minick, & C. A. Stone (Eds.), *Contexts for learning: Sociocultural dynamics in children's development* (pp. 169–183). New York: Oxford University Press.

Stone, C. A. (2002). Promises and pitfalls of scaffolded instruction for students with language learning disabilities. In K. G. Butler & E. R. Sillman (Eds.), *Speaking, reading, and writing in children with language learning disabilities: New paradigms for research and practice* (pp. 175–198). Mahwah, NJ: Erlbaum.

Swanson, H. L. (1999). Reading research for students with LD: A meta-analysis of intervention outcomes. *Journal of Learning Disabilities, 32,* 504–532.

Tobin, K. (1998). Sociocultural perspectives on the teaching and learning of science. In M. Larochelle, N. Bednarz, & J. Garrison (Eds.), *Constructivism and education* (pp. 195–212). New York: Cambridge University Press.

Toulmin, S. (1999). Knowledge as shared procedures. In Y. Engestrom, R. Miettinen, & R. Punamaki (Eds.), *Perspectives on activity theory* (pp. 53–64). New York: Cambridge University Press.

Troia, G.A., Harris, K. R., & Graham, S. (1999). Teaching students with learning disabilities to mindfully plan when writing. *Exceptional Children, 65*(2), 235–252.

Vaughn, S., Gersten, R., & Chard, D. (2000). The underlying message in LD intervention research: Findings from research syntheses. *Exceptional Children, 67,* 99–114.

Vaughn, S., & Klingner, J. K. (1999). Teaching reading comprehension through collaborative strategic reading. *Intervention in School and Clinic, 34*(5), 284–292.

Vygotsky, L. S. (1978). *Mind in society: The development of higher psychological processes.* Cambridge, MA: Harvard University Press.

Vygotsky, L. S. (1993). The collected works of L. S. Vygotsky. Vol. 2: *The fundamentals of defectology* (R. W. Rieber & A. S. Carton, Eds.; J. E. Knox & C. B. Stevens, Trans.). New York: Plenum Press.

Wells, G. (1999). *Dialogic inquiry: Toward a sociocultural practice and theory of education.* New York: Cambridge University Press.

Wells, G. (2000). Dialogic inquiry in education: Building on the legacy of Vygotsky. In C. D. L. P. Smagorinsky (Ed.), *Vygotskian perspectives on literacy research: Constructing meaning through collaborative inquiry* (pp. 51–85). New York: Cambridge University Press.

Wenger, E. (Ed.). (1998). *Communities of practice: Learning, meaning and identity*. New York: Cambridge University Press.

Wertsch, J. V. (1995). The need for action in sociocultural research. In J. V. Wertsch, P. D. Rio, & A. Alvarez (Eds.), *Sociocultural studies of the mind* (pp. 56–74). New York: Cambridge University Press.

Wertsch, J. V. (1998). *Mind as action*. New York: Oxford University Press.

Wertsch, J. V., & Toma, C. (1995). Discourse and learning in the classroom: A sociological approach. In L. P. Steffe & J. Gale (Eds.), *Constructivism in education* (pp. 159–174). Hillsdale, NJ: Erlbaum.

Wong, B. Y. L. (1997a). Research on genre-specific strategies for enhancing writing in adolescents with learning disaiblities. *Learning Disability Quarterly, 20*(2), 140–159.

Wong, B. Y. L. (1997b). Teaching adolescents with learning disaiblities and low achievers to plan, write and revise compare-and-contrast essays. *Learning Disabilities Research and Practice, 12*(1), 2–15.

Wong, B. Y. L. (2000). Writing strategies instruction for expository essays for adolescents with and without learning disaiblities. *Topics in Language Disorders, 20*(4), 29–44.

Wong, B. Y. L., & Jones, W. (1982). Increasing metacomprehension in learning disabled and normally achieving students through self-questioning training. *Learning Disability Quarterly, 5*, 228–240.

Wong, B. Y. L., & Wilson, M. (1984). Investigating awareness of and teaching passage organization in learning disabled children. *Journal of Learning Disabilities, 17*(8), 447–482.

Woodward, J., & Baxter, J. (1997). The effects of an innovative approach to mathematics on academically low-achieving students in mainstreamed settings. *Exceptional Children, 63*, 373–388.

V

METHODOLOGY

28

Exploratory and Confirmatory Methods in Learning Disabilities Research

Robert D. Abbott
Dagmar Amtmann
Jeff Munson

This chapter explores a selection of exploratory and confirmatory methods used in our research on learning disabilities in reading and writing. We emphasize the strengths and limitations of each method within the contexts of competing theoretical explanations for the data and have minimized the number of equations included in the text, instead referring readers to the relevant sources in the statistical literature. Readers interested in single-subject designs, growth curve analysis, or qualitative research methods are directed to other chapters in this handbook as we minimize discussion of these methods.

Data Structure, Data Management Systems, and Missing Data

Researchers need to develop facility with a variety of statistical and data management software applications. Most researchers are familiar with the row (subject) by column (measurement) data structures commonly found in statistical packages such as SPSS. Such "flat file" databases are consistent with many types of research questions. Flat file databases, however, are limiting when data are nested, such as data on multiple children within each of several classrooms or repeated measures on individual children. Maintaining and preparing such data for analysis are more easily handled with "relational" databases such as Access. Such programs easily allow the linking of data across linked hierarchies such as *repeated measurements* on a child (fall, winter, and spring scores on the Process Assessment of the Learner (PAL) [Berninger, 2001] orthographic coding task), *child* measurements (gender, IQ), *classroom* variables (class size, teacher experience), and *school* characteristics (number of students, public/private, rural/suburban/urban). Using relational databases to manage the data in such hierarchies also reminds the researcher of the large increase in Type I error rates when the data are not treated as nested and the standard errors are incorrectly calculated (e.g., if a single-level regression analysis is being done and each child in the same classroom is assigned the same value on teacher experience) (Raudenbush & Bryk, 2002; Snijders & Bosker, 1999). In addition, in complex studies with multiple data collection sessions and multiple data sources, relational database structures can facilitate scheduling, data collection, and data management. For example, following is a description of a system developed by Munson to manage data within the Autism Program Project.

This system uses Microsoft Access and stores the information in a centralized secure location. Individual staff members then have access, on a password-protected basis, to the relevant sections of the database for their particular responsibilities. Integrating information such as appointment scheduling and data collection status provides up-to-date information to staff members across the project and minimizes the tracking of redundant information. For example, as one family may have as many as 10 or more scheduled appointments, this information is entered into Access a single time, then automatically integrated into confirmation letters to the family, daily schedules for the reception staff, an internet-based testing calendar, and comprehensive subject-specific data collection reports. This system also allows complex data entry and management tasks to be carried out on several computers simultaneously. This architecture enables staff who are working directly with families immediate access to clinically relevant data while simultaneously accomplishing accurate data entry. As a result, data are always saved in the correct format in the same central location for direct import into SPSS and other analysis packages. This system shown in Figure 28.1 has been implemented across a local area network of 13 PCs located in different locations. Ongoing appointment schedules are exported to an Internet-based calendar organized by both date and staff member. Data files and their documentation created for use across projects are placed on a password-protected web site. Other electronic documents, such as testing protocols, data collection forms, digital photos, and so on, are similarly centralized to provide ready access to all staff members. A web page serves as a master catalogue of these resources that currently has over 100 links to specific documents related to the project (e.g., Word, Excel, Access, PowerPoint, and SPSS files). Information from this shared database and document system is continually archived using the AutoSave software program. Immediately after any file is modified, a duplicate of this file is saved on another computer. The AutoSave program is configured to save the last three versions of every file. Furthermore, all data are backed up on read–write CDs once a week that are stored offsite.

Such a system is flexible, allows easy updating and transformation of data, ensures correct linking of up-to-date data across sources, and produces data files that are readily accessible for statistical analysis. Though many of these activities can be accomplished through the careful use of syntax files in SPSS, we often encounter researchers using multiple versions of their data with each version containing some nonoverlapping subset of data revisions and

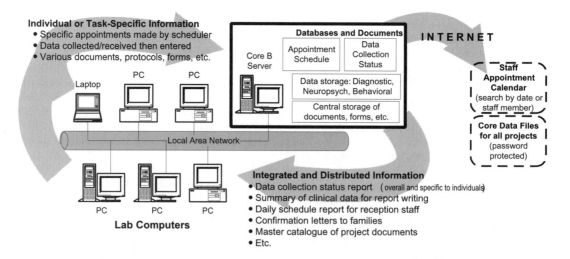

FIGURE 28.1. Example of an integrated relational database system.

transformations, making it difficult to identify a version with all the relevant correctly calculated variables.

Even with the best of management systems, missing data for a person occasionally occurs during data collection, especially in repeated-measure designs or in survey research with large sample sizes. Current statistical approaches view the mechanisms underlying such missing data as either accessible or inaccessible (Graham & Schafer, 1999). Additionally, accessible mechanisms have been viewed as missing completely at random (MCAR) and missing at random (MAR) (Little & Rubin, 1987).

The limitations of traditional approaches to handling missing data are now widely recognized (Schafer, 1997). *Listwise deletion*, where the person, with one or more observations missing, is dropped from all analyses, assumes MCAR (the most stringent mechanism) and often dramatically reduces power. *Pairwise deletion* where the person with missing observations is dropped only from analyses of variables on which the person is missing, often produces correlation/covariance matrices that are non-Gramian and creates problems for analyses that assume such matrices are the result of minor product moment multiplication. In practical terms, the magnitude of the correlations may be inconsistent with each other because they are based on different subsets of the participants. *Mean imputation*, where the missing data point is replaced by the mean on the variable, biases the variances and covariances as estimates of population values.

Contemporary statistical approaches utilize all the available data to estimate the covariance matrix of the measurements (the focus in many analyses) using direct maximum likelihood methods (AMOS 4.0; Arbuckle & Wothke, 1999), multiple imputation (Schafer, 1997, 2001), or empirical Bayes (Raudenbush & Bryk, 2002) approaches. For most data, all of these approaches are superior to listwise, pairwise, and mean imputation methods (Shafer & Graham, 2002). Under certain assumptions, these contemporary approaches lead to the same estimated covariance matrix. For analyses that focus on individual data, such as repeated-measures analyses, growth curve modeling, and survival analyses, estimates of the individual-level missing data values are needed. Schafer (1997) recommends the following steps: (1) *multiple* imputed data sets are estimated (the number of data sets depends on the amount and pattern of missing data), (2) the same statistical models are run on each data set, and (3) the resulting parameter estimates and standard errors are then averaged taking both within- and between-imputation variability into account. Schafer provides free programs for doing these estimations in a windows environment (e.g., Norm) or in SAS (e.g., PAN for panel data; Schafer, 2001). Recent comparisons (Collins, Schafer, & Kam, 2001) of maximum likelihood and multiple imputation approaches suggest including all available auxiliary variables in the imputation procedure because there will be a decreased chance of omitting an important cause of missingness.

These approaches are making maximal use of the available data. They are not creating data. For example, in repeated-measures designs, the methods base their estimates on all the *available* data for all persons and do not delete the available data for a person just because the person is missing data on one variable at one time point. Modeling growth using hierarchical linear models allows growth to be modeled even when the data are not time structured (all children measured at the same time) and some children are missing data (Raudenbush & Bryk, 2002).

Exploratory Methods of Analysis

Once developed, a flexible data management system and missing data approach can be used to readily prepare data for graphical and quantitative exploratory analysis. Exploratory analyses can be used for many purposes. In this chapter we describe some of the exploratory methods we have used to (1) examine the consistency of the data with assumptions made by confirmatory inferential statistical methods, (2) explore measurement structures in the context of new theories of a construct or the relationships among constructs, and (3) develop a better understanding of the heterogeneous nature of growth in our growth modeling efforts.

Exploratory methods are often linked to

the assumptions made when we are going to use a confirmatory method. For example, many of our instructional studies focus on modeling the growth of children during multisession tutorial interventions (Berninger et al., 1998) and comparing the effects of different interventions on parameters of the growth curve such as the slope. As a first step in the confirmatory modeling of the data we examine the variances and covariances of repeated measures using HLM (Bryk & Raudenbush, 1992; Raudenbush, Bryk, Cheong, & Congdon, 2000) to decide whether the compound symmetry assumptions of homogeneous variances and spherical covariances are consistent with the data on the repeated measures or whether these simplifying assumptions should not be made and more complex confirmatory models with heterogeneous variances and autoregressive-structured covariances should be included in the confirmatory model when standard errors are estimated. With respect to repeated-measures designs, examination of assumptions and the choice of subsequent analysis plans have been nicely summarized in recent chapters by Raudenbush (2001a, 2001b). Other examples include the exploration of data relative to such assumptions as normality of distributions of residuals and linearity of relationship.

Selected Graphical Methods of Exploratory Analysis

The uses of graphical exploratory methods have been greatly enhanced by the development of powerful desktop-based graphical interfaces. Starting with programs such as Data Desk and MacSpin, the options for desktop exploratory graphical analysis have been greatly expanded with the development of microprocessors and software such as Splus (MathSoft, 2000; StatSci, 2000), SYSTAT, and recent versions of SPSS. Such approaches as scatterplot brushing and pivot tables have become standard practice in our research for many reasons (e.g., to identify and interpret bivariate extreme scores). These approaches and many others are described in the manuals of the statistical packages as well as various books (e.g., Cook, 1998).

For example, in our work with growth models we have found the graphing capabilities of MLwiN (Goldstein et al., 1998) helpful. Plots of individual growth curve slopes with confidence intervals are available within MLwiN with a few "mouse" clicks. Serpentine graphs of individual growth curve slopes have been helpful as a way to explore the presence of qualitatively different subgroups of children with potentially different growth processes. Examination of the width of confidence intervals helps us identify children with highly variable data and begin to understand the sources of that variability. We have then used this information in *subsequent* studies to design varying instructional treatments and confirmatory data analyses.

Standard references for graphical representations for exploratory analyses include Tufte (1983, 1990, 1997), Cleveland (1993), and Wainer (1997). We have also found the book by Wilkinson (1999) helpful in thinking about potential graphical representations not yet appearing in the standard statistical packages.

Some Quantitative Methods for Exploratory Analysis

A variety of quantitative methods are available for exploratory analysis (Cook, 1998). Some approaches, such as using various symbols to plot the influence or leverage of points in scatter diagrams, combine graphical and quantitative analysis. Others, such as the examination of unplotted studentized residuals in linear regression or the sorting of Mahalanobis statistics in HLM (Raudenbush & Bryk, 2002), are largely based on quantitative analysis.

Since their development in the early 1900s, exploratory factor analysis (EFA) and exploratory principal components analysis (PCA) are among the most widely used methods in psychological research. They have been used in the early stages of scale development (to examine the dimensionality of a set of questions thought to represent a unitary underlying dimension) and in explorations of covariance and correlation matrices among measures to examine the consistency of these relationships with the theoretical predictions derived from the theory of the constructs.

Although widely used, the exploratory

uses of EFA and PCA have been criticized in terms of both theory and practice. Fabrigar, Wegener, MacCallum, and Strahan (1999) summarized and critiqued current practice in using EFA and PCA and offered guidelines for their appropriate use. Key decisions in the appropriate use of these methods include choices about (1) study design (e.g., including enough reliable indicators [3–5 is a common recommendation] of each of the theoretically expected dimensions; defining and sampling the appropriate population); (2) decisions to use EFA (scaling based on common variance estimated via commonalities; factor scores only estimated), or PCA (scaling based on total variance; component scores linear combinations of the measured variables); (3) if using EFA, decisions about the loss function to be maximized (e.g., principal axis factor analysis vs. maximum likelihood factor analysis); (4) decisions about the number of factors or components to retain for subsequent examination; and (5) decisions about how to rotate the initial EFA factors or PCA components to more theoretically interpretable positions (e.g., orthogonal versus oblique rotations). These issues are explored more fully in books on factor analysis and latent variable modeling (Comrey, 1992; Loehlin, 1998)

We agree with Fabrigar, Wegener, MacCallum, and Strahan (1999), and we have found these methods useful at the early stages of our conceptualization and research. For example, in our current work on the use of morphological knowledge by poor and good readers, we have used exploratory PCA (Berninger, Abbott, Billingsley, & Nagy, 2001). In doing so, we first developed multiple measures of each of our theoretical dimensions of morphological knowledge, we administered these multiple measures to a diverse group of readers, and we then explored their measurement structure using PCA with Varimax orthogonal rotation. We used PCA and VARIMAX rotation because scores on each measure had a reasonable degree of reliability and shared common variance with scores on the other measures. We were interested in the independent contribution of each dimension in explaining the covariation of individual differences on the measures so we used orthogonal rotation to retain the independence of the dimensions. Results of this analysis

helped us to conceptualize the dimensions and develop new and more factorially pure measures of each dimension. We also explored changes in interpretation if we used EFA or varied the number of dimensions retained for interpretation. Consistent with the findings of others for data with multiple reliable indicators of each theoretical construct, we found that after rotation, interpretations were highly consistent whether the initial dimensions had been derived using PCA or EFA.

This discussion has emphasized the constant interplay of theory, exploratory methods, and subsequent use of confirmatory methods on new data. In our view, the use of exploratory methods should be guided by theory as much as possible, replicated and extended to a new data set to strengthen their use, and performed so that Type I error rates are tightly controlled so that overgeneralization and Type I errors are minimized. As we use exploratory methods, we constantly keep in mind implications for (1) the construct validity of our measures and manipulations, (2) the influences on the internal validity of the conclusions we draw from our study design, (3) the ways in which our statistical conclusion validity will be influenced by the assumptions we will be making in our confirmatory analyses, and (4) the effects of characteristics of our research context and participants on the external validity of our generalizations about contexts and participants.

Confirmatory Methods of Analysis

A variety of confirmatory methods are available to compare the consistency of data with models derived from competing theories. Methods for normally distributed measured dependent variables range from analyses based on standard univariate linear model analyses using analysis of variance (ANOVA) and regression to multivariate linear model analyses using such methods as multivariate analysis of variance (MANOVA) and discriminant functions (Lunneberg & Abbott, 1983). Methods for binary and categorical dependent variables range from survival methods to exact tests based on permutation and randomization. Methods for latent variable linear models

(Bentler, 1980; Bollen, 2002) range from confirmatory factor (CFA) analysis to structural equation modeling (SEM) of latent variables. In this chapter we can only briefly discuss a few confirmatory methods that we have found useful in our research. Because many of our research questions focus on the covariation of individual differences and growth over time in reading and writing processes we have often used CFA and SEM with multiple indicators to provide a more complete mapping of the theoretical construct and a modeling of measurement error. We therefore focus our discussion on these methods. Again, we have provided readers with citations to overviews and statistical articles that elaborate our discussion.

Typically, the researcher allows the research questions and distributional properties of the data to guide the choice of a CFA method. Often, however, there is not a one-to-one correspondence between a research question and a confirmatory statistical method. For example, in a designed experiment including multiple dependent variables with normally distributed residuals, measured independent variables, and factorially designed randomly assigned treatments, the investigator has a wide choice of approaches ranging from methods used to test competing hypotheses about means (MANCOVA; structural equation modeling of mean structures) to methods used to test competing hypotheses about covariation (canonical correlation; structural equation modeling of covariance structures). While the measured variable linear model-based approaches are standard in research, using multiple indicator SEM methods provides an approach to modeling the reliability of the outcome, allows the modeling of correlated measurement error (perhaps due to method effects), and provides the opportunity to examine competing models of mediating processes.

Modeling of random and correlated measurement error in the SEM methods can provide more accurate estimates of the effects of the experimental treatments (Bollen, 1989). Rigdon (1994) illustrates how failing to model the measurement error in the predictors and criteria of regression models can change the researcher's conclusions about the results. When there are multiple dependent variables in an experiment, the power of the statistical test can be dramatically affected by choice of analysis (Cole, Maxwell, Arvey, & Salas, 1993). If the multiple dependent variables are indicators of a latent variable, then SEM of mean structures provides a more powerful test of the hypothesis of mean differences due to treatment than does MANOVA. If the multiple dependent variables are not indicators of a latent variable, then MANOVA can have greater power. However, the power of the MANOVA test of treatment effects depends on the pattern of correlations among the dependent variables and the direction of the experimental effects (Cole et al., 1993). For example, if the experimental effects are concentrated in a single dimension, then significance tests based on the greatest characteristic root test (e.g., Roy's gcr test) may be more powerful than those based on all roots (e.g., Wilks Lambda).

Another use of a SEM framework for thinking about designed experiments is that the researcher can include potential mediators in the SEM model to directly model threats to internal validity such as resentful demoralization (when control subjects become aware they are not receiving the benefits of the treatment and consequently perform at a lower level than they would have) or poor fidelity of implementation of the treatment that can threaten conclusions drawn from randomized experiments (Cook & Campbell, 1979; Shadish, Cook, & Campbell, 2002). Measuring fidelity of implementation and taking variations in fidelity into account in the statistical analysis is especially important in studies done in schools where contexts and classroom dynamics may vary widely leading to varying implementation of the instructional strategies.

As a context for exploring some of these confirmatory methods, consider a series of our research questions concerning the structural relationships among orthographic knowledge, phonological knowledge, and reading acquisition (Abbott & Berninger, 1995). These questions have included the following: Are covariations among measures of orthographic coding at the letter level, letter cluster level, and word level more consistent with a theoretical model hypothesizing that all these measures reflect a single dimension or a theory that hypothesizes that multiple dimensions are needed to model the covariances among these measures (CFAs of measures for varying developmental levels and genders)? Do orthographic measures account for unique variance in reading and writing acquisition beyond that accounted for by phonological measures and print experience (structural equation modeling of latent variables)? Is orthographic processing important only in word recognition in isolation or also when reading in context? Many of these questions relate to the construct validity of measures of orthographic knowledge. Others relate to the structural relationships of orthographic knowledge, phonological knowledge, and reading and writing (Abbott & Berninger, 1993).

Central to each of these questions is construct validity. In their classic paper, Cronbach and Meehl (1955) suggested that the evaluation of the construct validity of measures should consider both convergent evidence (Are the measures correlated with other measures they theoretically should be correlated with?) and discriminant evidence (Are the measures little correlated with other measures from which they are theoretically distinct?). A well-designed study investigating the construct validity of measures of orthographic knowledge would therefore include measures that are theoretically distinguishable as well as measures that are theoretically related. According to this view, if orthographic knowledge and phonological knowledge are the result of the same process, their correlation should be one, restricted only by our ability to reliably measure the constructs. Exploratory analyses can inform this research as Olsen, Forsberg, and Wise (1994) included measures of orthographic knowledge and phonological knowledge and found a correlation of $r = .43$ between phonological and orthographic factors in their exploratory PCA with oblique rotation. A second aspect of examining whether orthographic knowledge and phonological knowledge are identical is to examine if, when used as predictors of a common criterion, they make unique contributions to the prediction of the criterion.

Though the results derived from such analyses are informative, analysis approaches based on measured variables can be enhanced by incorporating multiple measures of a construct into the research design. By including multiple measures of each construct, CFA allows the researcher to statistically test the degree that the covariances among measures are consistent with relationships predicted by varying theories of the phenomenon. For example, the theory that hypothesizes that orthographic knowledge and phonological knowledge are identical processes would specify that the correlation between standardized factors would have been 1.00 in Olsen and colleagues' (1994) study. CFA of multiple indicators allows us to extend this work by examining this relationship with measurement error modeled and to statistically compare the fit to the data of such a one-factor theory as compared to a theory that hypothesizes the two factors are correlated but not identical.

In contrast to exploratory factor analysis, *confirmatory* factor analysis allows the researcher to statistically test different measurement models underlying the covariations among the indicators. If multiple methods of measuring conceptually similar and distinct constructs are included in a study, CFA can also be used to investigate method effects as well as covariation among the measures due to the underlying construct. In our example, developing measurement models based on multiple indicators will result in factors that are more reliable and provide a more complete operationalization of orthographic and phonological knowledge than can be achieved by a single measurement of each. Subsequent tests of structural relationships among these latent variables or factors will then provide a picture of the nature of relationships among the theoretical constructs less influenced by measurement error and the narrowness of a single measurement of a theoretical construct.

Many resources are available for guiding such latent variable structural modeling efforts (Bentler, 1980; Bentler & Wu, 2001; Bollen, 1989; Byrne, 2001, or earlier versions; Hayduk, 1987). The following discussion outlines some of the steps to consider when using latent variable SEM. First, the researcher clearly specifies the predictions derived from the competing theories of the meaning of the constructs and their structural relationships. To address questions about orthographic knowledge, phonological knowledge, and reading acquisition, for example, the researcher needs to decide on the *measurement* models for orthographic knowledge, phonological knowledge, and reading acquisition (Berninger, 1994). The competing hypotheses about the *structural* relationships among the constructs need to be specified; for example, two such theoretical hypotheses would be one that models the relationship between orthographic coding and reading as completely mediated through phonological coding and a second that includes an additional direct path from orthographic coding to reading hypothesizing that all the relationship between orthographic coding and reading is not accounted for by the relationship of orthographic and phonological coding.

Second, for an appropriately sized sample (Bentler & Yuan, 1999; Curran, West, & Finch, 1996; MacCallum, Browne, & Sugawara, 1996) the researcher needs to measure multiple reliable indicators of each construct, ideally using multiple methods of measurement. In deciding how many indicators to include in a study, the competing elements of practicality and the need to obtain multiple indicators of a factor must be balanced. Obtaining at least three measures of each construct allows the testing of most structural hypotheses, although four measures are necessary for some questions (e.g., to test whether two measures are parallel rather than just the equivalent). This principle will ensure that the paths in many models are identified, but some models (those with many covariances among factors or covariances among the residuals of the measured variables or nonrecursive relationships) and data structures (those with highly correlated redundant indicators) may have some underidentified paths (see Bollen, 1989, and Brito & Pearl, 2002, for a discussion of identification in structural equation models).

Third, the researcher needs to examine whether the measured indicators are reflecting the latent variables consistent with theory. Indicators should have significant loadings on their hypothesized latent variables and the intercorrelations among latent variables should be within the range expected by theory. The fit of competing measure-

ment models (i.e., 5 factors vs. 4 factors) can be hierarchically compared statistically and a decision made about the best-fitting measurement model. Most researchers use a combination of goodness-of-fit statistics (differences in χ^2; Gonzalez & Griffin, 2001), incremental fit indices, model parsimony adjusted statistics, expected parameter change statistics, root mean square error of approximation (RMSEA), confidence intervals, and Lagrangian Multiplier tests to evaluate the fit of hierarchically related competing measurement models. The length of this (incomplete) list attests to current research interest in the development of fit indices of competing models! Byrne (2001) clearly discusses the strengths and weaknesses of this "smorgasbord."

Fourth, the researcher compares the fit of competing theories of the structural relationship among the factors. We argue strongly that attention focuses on the relative fit of relevant, competing theoretical models. In most cases, adding post hoc paths to those specified in the theoretical models will improve the absolute fit in a sample but may not cross-validate well and will not necessarily lead to the population structure that generated the data (MacCallum, 1986; MacCallum, Roznowski, & Necowitz, 1992). In our experience, adding post hoc additional paths such as correlated measurement errors often improves the absolute fit of *both* the competing models and thus their *relative fit* remains the same. The researcher should also consider the possible existence of other theoretically meaningful "equivalent" models that achieve the same degree of overall fit to the matrix of covariances as the model being fitted (MacCallum, Wegener, Uchino, & Fabrigar, 1993). Carefully applying the approaches of MacCallum, and colleagues (1993) or the tracing rules (Loehlin, 1998) will help us recognize some of the likely theoretical alternatives. The approaches described in Pearl (2000) and Spirtes, Glymour, and Scheines (1993) can also be used to identify equivalent models. Some of these alternative models can be removed from consideration if longitudinal data have been collected where the time structure of the data makes some theoretical statements about the relationships among variables untenable. Care must be taken that the tested models evaluate the relevant theoretical hypotheses. For example, cross-sectional panel SEM models evaluate autoregressive patterns of growth. However, without explicit modeling of individual growth in these latent variable models (Duncan, Duncan, Strycker, Li, & Alpert, 1999), some types of treatment effects (e.g., fan-spread growth) will not be detectable. Five, the generalization of the structural and measurement models should be examined for new (or hold-out) samples (MacCallum, Roznowski, Mar, & Reith, 1994) and models should be compared for different groups where theory suggests that the relationships might differ.

When group membership is categorical (e.g., female/male), confirmatory tests that the paths for male and females are equivalent can be carried out using multiple group SEM (Byrne, 2001). When such hypotheses of moderation include continuous variables moderating relationships among constructs, then SEM needs to directly include product terms in a similar fashion to multiple regression. Unfortunately, the process is much more complicated in moderated SEM (in part because the product terms are not multivariate normal) and specialized approaches need to be implemented (Li et al., 2001).

Another form of moderation (or interaction) arises when children have differential growth curves within a treatment. We have found that growth mixture modeling using SEM (Muthen, 2001a, 2001b) can be helpful in differentiating children in our instructional experiments who benefit significantly and quickly from instruction from children who gained little from a particular instructional intervention.

New Directions in Confirmatory Methods

In current research, our confirmatory modeling of data has been enhanced by three statistical developments that might inform others' research. First, our research with MRI (magnetic resonance imagery) brain scanning using PEPSI protocols (Richards et al., 2000) to examine processing differences of children with phonological and orthographic reading problems and typically developing (age- and IQ-matched) children has benefited from the use of permutation-based tests of differences in distributions. In this research, after taking into account the

relevant controls and baseline activation, measuring whether or not a brain regions is activated beyond a chance level is a commonly used outcome. One approach would be to use χ^2 to evaluate the difference in the 2 × 2 table of proportions of dyslexic and typically developing readers showing activation in a brain region. Unless the researcher tested a large number of children, however, he or she might quickly encounter problems because of small sample size, the number of cells relative to sample size, or low expected values in a cell of the table (Cochran, 1954). While various rules for using χ^2 have been proposed (Agresti, 1990), they all rely on using χ^2 and asymptotic theory to estimate a p value. Rather than relying on the asymptotic theory, it is now possible to calculate an exact p value based on permutations of the data (Agresti, 1992). These statistical tests involve permuting the data and determining where the obtained data fall within the population of possible permutations of the data. It is easy to construct examples where the asymptotic χ^2 test gives a $p > .05$ and the exact $p < .05$ or vice versa. Fisher illustrated such cases in his development of the exact test for the 2 × 2 table. Furthermore, even in this simple example, assumptions about the marginals of the table are important. For a 2 × 2 table, using Barnard's test that assumes only one of the marginals is fixed results in greater power for detecting alternative hypotheses than the more widely available but less powerful Fisher's exact test that assumes that both marginals are fixed.

Permutation tests based on enumeration are available today for a great variety of types of data, and research questions including ordered categorical (Agresti, Mehta, & Patel, 1990) and recent statistical and computing developments in Monte Carlo estimation have made accurate approximation of exact tests and estimation of distributional characteristics and confidence intervals for a variety of data types computationally feasible (Senchaudhuri, Mehta, & Patel, 1995). Given that much research about children with learning disabilities only includes a small number of children or measurements with nonnormal error distributions, statistical tests that do not rely on asymptotic, large sample theory may be more appropriate and in many cases may be more powerful when asymptotic assumptions are not consistent with the data. StatXact (2001) and LogXact (1993) are two statistical software packages that provide researchers with modern approaches to calculating these exact *p* values.

A second statistical innovation that we think will prove useful in the future to researchers in learning disabilities is the set of theorems and statistical approaches derived from graph-theoretic representations of relationships among constructs (Edwards, 1995; Pearl, 2000). These approaches provide support for both exploratory identification and examination of equivalent models (Spirtes et al., 1993; Spirtes, Richardson, Meek, & Scheines, 1998) and approaches to confirmatory testing of competing models (Shipley, 2000a, 2000b). Although these methods focus the researcher on equivalent models that have the same overall fit to the covariance matrix, they also suggest ways to describe the distinguishing theoretical predictions of these models (Pearl, 2000; Shipley, 2000a).

A third set of statistical tools that greatly enhances the planning of CFAs includes software packages that compute power for a variety of statistical methods. The ones we use include packages for linear model analyses (Power and Precision 2.0 ; Borenstein, Rothstein, & Cohen, 2001), rates and proportions (StatXact and LogXact), hierarchical models (Optimal Design; Raudenbush & Feng, 2003), and latent variable structural equation models (EQS 6.0, Bentler & Wu, 2001; Mplus, Muthen & Muthen, 2002). Use of these tools greatly assists in the planning of research designs with adequate power.

Summary

In this chapter we have provided an overview of the exploratory and confirmatory methods we have found useful in our research programs and describe some of the strengths and weaknesses of these methods. Other research programs with different, or even the same, research questions may choose to use other methods. If we have touched on methods new to readers, we hope they will consider how these methods might help them clarify research questions and examine the consistency of data with the models derived from competing theoretical perspectives.

We have also pointed readers to a variety of statistical software applications. Each application has complementary strengths and weaknesses. We believe that our readers will benefit by learning about this diversity and using it in their attempts to answer a variety of exploratory and confirmatory research questions.

Acknowledgments

Robert D. Abbott's work on this chapter was supported by (1) Statistics Core for the Learning Disciplinary Center: Links to Schools and Biology, Grant No. P50 HD33812-07; (2) Interventions for Component Writing Disabilities, Grant No. HD25858-11; and (3) the Statistics Core of the Autism Program Project: Neurobiology and Genetics of Autism, Grant No. HD 35465. Dagmar Amtmann's work on this chapter was supported by Grant No. H224A930006 from the U.S. Department of Education, National Institute on Disability and Rehabilitation Research. Jeff Munson's work was supported by Grant No. HD35465.

References

Abbott, R. D., & Berninger, V. W. (1993). Structural equation modeling of relationships among developmental skills and writing skills in primary and intermediate grade writers. *Journal of Educational Psychology, 85*, 478–508.

Abbott, R. D., & Berninger, V. W. (1995). Structural equation modeling and hierarchical linear modeling: Tools for studying the construct validity of orthographic process in reading and writing development. In V. W. Berninger (Ed.), *The varieties of orthographic knowledge: relationships to phonology, reading, and writing (pp. 321–354)*. Dordrecht, The Netherlands: Kluwer Academic.

Agresti, A. (1990). *Categorical data analysis*. New York: Wiley.

Agresti, A. (1992). A Survey of exact inference for contingency tables. *Statistical Science, 7*, 131–177.

Agresti, A., Mehta, C. R., & Patel, N. R. (1990). Exact inference for contingency tables with ordered categories. *Journal of the American Statistical Association, 85*, 453–458.

Arbuckle, J. L., & Wothke, W. (1999). *Amos 4.0 user's guide*. Chicago: Smallwaters.

Bentler, P. M. (1980). Multivariate analysis with latent variables: Causal modeling. *Annual Review of Psychology, 31*, 419–456.

Bentler, P. M., & Wu, E. (2003). *EQS Structural*

equations program manual, version 6.0. Encino, CA: Multivariate Software.

Bentler, P. M., & Yuan, K.-H. (1999). Structural equation modeling with small samples: Test statistics. *Multivariate Behavioral Research, 34,* 181–197.

Berninger, V. W. (1994). *Reading and writing acquisition: A developmental neuropsychological perspective.* Madison, WI: Brown & Benchmark.

Berninger, V. W. (2001). *Process assessment of the learner (PAL) test battery for reading and writing.* San Antonio, TX: Psychological Corporation.

Berninger, V. W., Abbott, R. D., Billingsley, F., & Nagy, W. (2001). Processes underlying timing and fluency: Efficiency, automaticity, coordination, and morphological awareness. In M. Wolf (Ed.), *Dyslexia, fluency, and the brain* (pp. 383–414). Timonium, MD: York Press.

Bollen, K. A. (1989). *Structural equations with latent variables.* New York: Wiley.

Bollen, K. A. (2002). Latent variables in psychology and the social sciences. *Annual Review of Psychology, 53,* 605–634.

Borenstein, M., Rothstein, H., & Cohen, J. (2001). *Power and Precision 2.0.* Teaneck, NJ: Biostat.

Brito, C., & Pearl, J. (2002). A new identification condition for recursive models with correlated errors. *Structural Equation Modeling, 9,* 459–474.

Bryk, A., & Raudenbush, S. W. (1992). *Hierarchical linear models in social and behavioral research: Applications and data analysis methods.* Newbury Park, CA: Sage.

Byrne, B. M. (2001). *Structural equation modeling with AMOS: Basic concepts, applications, and programming.* Mahwah, NJ: Erlbaum.

Cleveland, W. S. (1993). *Visualizing data.* Summit, NJ: Hobart Press.

Cochran, W. G. (1954). Some methods for strengthening the common χ^2 tests. *Biometrics, 10,* 417–454.

Cole, D., Maxwell, S., Arvey, R., & Salas, E. (1993). Multivariate group comparisons of variable systems: MANOVA and structural equation modeling. *Psychological Bulletin, 114,* 174–184.

Collins, L. M., Schafer, J. L., Kam, C.-M. (2001). A comparison of inclusive and restrictive strategies in modern missing data procedures. *Psychological Methods, 6,* 330–351.

Comrey, A. L. (1992). *A first course in factor analysis.* Hillsdale, NJ: Erlbaum.

Cook, R. D. (1998). *Regression graphics: Ideas for studying regressions through graphics.* New York: Wiley.

Cook, T. D., & Campbell, D. T. (1979). *Quasi-experimentation: Design and analysis for field settings.* Chicago: Rand-McNally.

Cronbach, L. J., & Meehl, P. (1955). Construct validity in psychological tests. *Psychological Bulletin, 52,* 281–302.

Curran, P. J., West, S. G., & Finch, J. F. (1996). The robustness of test statistics to nonnormality and specification error in confirmatory factor analysis. *Psychological Methods, 1,* 16–29.

Duncan, T. E., Duncan, S. C., Strycker, L. A., Li, F., & Alpert, A. (1999). *An introduction to latent variable growth curve modeling: Concepts, issues, and applications.* Mahwah, NJ: Erlbaum.

Edwards, D. (1995). *Introduction to graphical modeling.* New York: Springer-Verlag.

Fabrigar, L. R., Wegener, D. T., MacCallum. R. C., & Strahan, E. J. (1999). Evaluating the use of exploratory factor analysis in psychological research. *Psychological Methods, 4,* 272–299.

Goldstein, H., Rasbash, J., Plewis, I., Draper, D., Browne, W., Yang, M., Woodhouse, G., & Healy, M. (1998). *A user's guide to MlwiN.* Bath, UK: Multilevel Models Project.

Gonzalez, R., & Griffin, D. (2001). Testing parameters in structural equation modeling: Every "one" matters. *Psychological Methods, 6,* 258–269.

Graham, J. W., & Schafer, J. L. (1999). On the performance of multiple imputation for multivariate data with small sample size. In R. Hoyle (Ed.), *Statistical strategies for small sample research* (pp. 1–29). Thousand Oaks, CA: Sage.

Hayduk, L. (1987). *Structural equation modeling with LISREL: Essentials and advances.* Baltimore: Johns Hopkins University Press.

Li, F., Duncan, T. E., Duncan, S. C., Wallentin, F. Y., Acock, A. C., & Hops, H. (2001). Interaction models in latent growth curves. In G. A. Marcoulides & R. E. Schumacker (Eds.), *New developments and techniques in structural equation modeling* (pp. 173–202). Mahwah, NJ: Erlbaum.

Little, R. J. A., & Rubin, D. B. (1987). *Statistical analysis with missing data.* New York: Wiley.

Loehlin, J. C. (1998). *Latent variable models: An introduction to factor, path, and structural analysis* (3rd ed.). Mahwah, NJ: Erlbaum.

LogXact. (1993). *Software for exact logistic regression.* Cambridge, MA: Cytel Software.

Lunneborg, C., & Abbott, R. D. (1983). *Elementary multivariate analysis for the behavioral sciences: Application of Basic structure.* New York: Elsevier Science.

MacCallum, R. C. (1986). Specification searches in covariance structure modeling. *Psychological Bulletin, 100,* 107–120.

MacCallum, R. C., Browne, M. W., & Sugawara, H. M. (1996). Power analysis and determination of sample size for covariance structure modeling. *Psychological Methods, 1,* 130–149.

MacCallum, R. C., Roznowski, M., Mar, M., & Reith, J. V. (1994). Alternative strategies for cross-validation of covariance structure models. *Multivariate Behavioral Research, 29,* 1–32.

MacCallum, R. C., Roznowski, M., & Necowitz, L. B. (1992). Model modifications in covariance structure analysis: The problem of capitalization on chance. *Psychological Bulletin, 114,* 490–504.

MacCallum, R. C., Wegener, D. T., Uchino, B. N., & Fabrigar, L. R. (1993). The problem of equivalent models in applications of covariance structure analysis. *Psychological Bulletin, 114,* 185–199.

MathSoft. (2000). *S-PLUS-2000 user's guide.* Seattle, WA: Author.

Muthen, B. (2001a). Latent variable mixture modeling. In G. A. Marcoulides & R. E. Schumacker (Eds.), *New developments and techniques in structural equation modeling* (pp. 1–34). Mahwah, NJ: Erlbaum.

Muthen, B. (2001b). Second-generation structural equation modeling with a combination of categorical and continuous latent variables: New opportunities for latent class-latent growth modeling. In L. M. Collins & A. G. Sayer (Eds.), *New methods for the analysis of change* (pp. 289–322). Washington, DC: American Psychological Association.

Muthén, L. K., & Muthén, B. O. (2001). *Mplus 2.0 User's Guide*. Los Angeles: Muthen & Muthen.

Muthén, L. K., & Muthén, B. O. (2002). How to use a Monte Carlo study to decide on sample size and determine power. *Structural Equation Modeling, 9*, 599–620.

Olsen, R., Forsberg, H., & Wise, B. (1994). Genes, environment, and the development of orthographic skills. In V. W. Berninger (Ed.), *The varieties of orthographic knowledge: Theoretical and developmental issues* (pp. 27–71). Dordrecht, The Netherlands: Kluwer Academic.

Pearl, J. (2000). *Causality*. Cambridge: Cambridge University Press.

Raudenbush, S. W. (2001a). Comparing personal trajectories and drawing causal inferences from longitudinal data. *Annual Review of Psychology, 52*, 501–525.

Raudenbush, S. W. (2001b). Toward a coherent framework for comparing trajectories of individual change. In L. M. Collins & A. G. Sayer (Eds.), *New methods for the analysis of change* (pp. 33–64). Washington, DC: American Psychological Association.

Raudenbush, S. W., & Bryk, A. S. (2002). *Hierarchical linear models: Applications and Data analysis methods* (2nd ed.). Thousand Oaks, CA: Sage.

Raudenbush, S. W., Bryk, A. S., Cheong, Y. F., & Congdon, R. (2000). *HLM-5: Hierarchical linear and nonlinear modeling*. Chicago: Scientific Software, International.

Raudenbush, S. W., & Feng, L. X. (2001). Effects of study duration, frequency of observation, and sample size on power in studies of group differences in polynomial change. *Psychological Methods, 6*, 387–401.

Richards, T., Corinna, D., Serafini, S., Steury, K., Dager, S., Marro, K., Abbott, R. D., Maravilla, K., & Berninger, V. W. (2000). Effects of a phonologically-driven treatment for dyslexia on lactate levels as measured by proton MR Spectroscopic imaging. *American Journal of Neuroradiology, 21*, 916–922.

Rigdon, E. E. (1994). Demonstrating the effects of unmodeled random measurement error. *Structural Equation Modeling, 1*, 375–380.

Schafer, J. L. (1997). *Analysis of incomplete multivariate data*. London: Chapman & Hall.

Schafer, J. L. (2001). Multiple imputation with PAN. In L. M. Collins & A. G. Sayer (Eds.), *New methods for the analysis of change* (pp. 357–377). Washington, DC: American Psychological Association.

Schafer, J. L., & Graham, J. W. (2002). Missing data: Our view of the state of the art. *Psychological Methods, 7*, 147–177.

Senchaudhuri, P., Mehta, C. R., & Patel, N. R. (1995). Estimating exact p-values by the method of control variables, or Monte Carlo rescue. *Journal of the American Statistical Association, 90*, 640–648.

Shadish, W. R., Cook, T. D., & Campbell, D. T. (2002). *Experimental and quasi-experimental designs for generalized causal inference*. New York: Houghton Mifflin.

Shipley, B. (2000a). *Cause and correlation in biology: A user's guide to path analysis, structural equations and causal inference*. Cambridge, UK: Cambridge University Press.

Shipley, B. (2000b). A new inferential test for path models based on direct acyclic graphs. *Structural Equation Modeling, 7*, 206–218.

Snijders, T. A. B., & Bosker, R. J. (1999). *Multilevel analysis: An introduction to basic and advanced multilevel modeling*. Thousand Oaks, CA: Sage.

Spirtes, P., Glymour, C., & Scheines, R. (1993). *Causation, prediction, and search*. New York: Springer-Verlag.

Spirtes, P., Richardson, T., Meek, C., & Scheines, R. (1998). Using path diagrams as a structural modeling tool. *Sociological Methods and Research, 27*, 182–225.

StatSci. (2000). *S–PLUS guide to statistical and mathematical analysis, version 2000*. Seattle, WA: StatSci.

StatXact. (2001). *StatXact–5.0 statistical software*. Cambridge, MA: Cytel Software.

Tufte, E. R. (1983). *The visual display of quantitative information*. Cheshire, CT: Graphics Press.

Tufte, E. R. (1990). *Envisioning information*. Cheshire, CT: Graphics Press.

Tufte, E. R. (1997). *Visual explanations: Images, quantities, evidence and narrative*. Cheshire, CT: Graphics Press.

Wainer, H. (1997). *Visual revelations: Graphical tales of fate and deception from Napoleon Bonaparte to Ross Perot*. New York: Springer-Verlag.

Wilkinson, L. (1999). *The grammar of graphics*. New York: Springer-Verlag.

29

Designs for Applied Educational Research

Jean B. Schumaker
Donald D. Deshler

Following is an excerpt from a recent letter sent to a researcher at the University of Kansas Center for Research on Learning (KU-CRL).

> You will never know what a difference the Content Enhancement Routines have made in my teaching and in the success that my students are having! Let me give you a little background. I have taught high school science for 18 years. As the makeup of our school district has changed in recent years, my classes have become increasingly diverse. For the most part, I did okay as the composition of my classes changed, but five years ago, when our school adopted inclusion for students with disabilities, things began to fall apart on me. If I tried to do things to meet the needs of the students with LD in my classes, I would lose my highly capable students. When I would use things that worked well in the past, more often than not, they didn't work at all—especially with the students with disabilities. After a while, I felt totally frustrated. That following summer, I attended a district workshop on Content Enhancement Routines that were developed at your research center. As I sat through the workshop, a whole new set of possibilities opened up to me. When the school year began, I started using several of the routines I had learned in my classes—they

> changed how I thought about the content that I taught, how I viewed student learning, and what I saw my role being as a teacher. While I don't always succeed with all of my students, I can't begin to tell you how significant the changes have been! Rather than dreading teaching—especially the classes with the most difficult to teach students—I now look forward to the challenge of seeing if I can meet the needs of both the brightest as well as the ones who struggled the most. The things I learned about Content Enhancement have transformed my life as a teacher. More importantly, they have changed how students in my classes learn—and that's why I got into teaching in the first place!

This type of letter is clearly encouraging and the kind of message any educational researcher longs to receive from those who use the products of his or her research and development work. However, for every letter like this that is received, there are probably many other unwritten ones that could be written by teachers who are frustrated because a supposed "research-validated practice" has fallen short of its expectations.

Not surprisingly, researchers at the KU-CRL do everything they can to prevent such disappointment. Indeed, over the past 24 years, researchers at the KU-CRL have been devoted to the goal of creating instructional interventions that are palatable for teachers to use and sufficiently powerful to affect the performance of students with learning disabilities (LD). What is important to understand about their work is that in the process of designing and field-testing a broad array of instructional interventions, they have, more often than not, come up short on an *initial* attempt with regard to producing the results they had in mind. What often has seemed logical to those on the initial design team frequently falls considerably short of the mark when it is taken into the classroom. These "misfires" have led to the KU-CRL motto: "We must be willing to go back to the drawing board!" Indeed, going back to the drawing board on many occasions has been necessary to fine tune an intervention to a point at which it finally starts to make sense to teachers and produces the kinds of results with students that KU-CRL researchers (and the students!) would deem worthwhile.

Not surprisingly, given the enormous complexity of student learning (especially for students who are saddled with a learning disability) and the complex dynamics that exist in most schools (particularly secondary schools), designing interventions that are powerful, practical, and robust is a great challenge. The magnitude of this challenge has been exacerbated in recent years with the expectations set forth in PL 105-17 that programming for students with disabilities be outcome based within the context of successfully mastering (and not merely gaining access to) the general education curriculum (Turnbull, Rainbolt, & Buchele-Ash, 1997). In essence, the requirements of the law demand that students with disabilities not only acquire a significant array of skills that will enable them to compete within rigorous general education classes but that they acquire these skills to such a degree that the skills can be generalized to a host of circumstances and settings *and* be maintained over time.

Since its inception in 1977, the staff of the KU-CRL (initially known as the Institute for Research on Learning Disabilities—it was one of five Office of Special Education Programs-funded LD research institutes), has

had as their overriding goal to design an array of interrelated interventions that would enable adolescents with LD to compete within the context of mainstream environments. To realize that goal, they adopted five standards against which they judge the design and field-testing of new interventions. Each intervention must (1) be practical for teachers to use and perceived by them as being doable within their classrooms, (2) be easy for *both* the teacher and students to learn, (3) yield outcomes that are deemed to be meaningful in terms of real-world measures such as passing grades, (4) be sufficiently broad in its reach that it has a favorabe impact on the performance of those *without* disabilities (especially if the intervention is used in the general education classroom), and (5) be sufficiently powerful to have a favorable impact on the performance of students *with* disabilities to such a degree as to enable them to compete within the context the criterion environment (e.g., the general education classroom).

To design interventions that meet these five standards, several principles have guided KU-CRL research. First, all KU-CRL researchers are committed to designing interventions that will work within the complex realities of today's schools and classrooms. Hence, from the beginning, interventions are designed with these realities in mind so that the gap between new interventions and the realities that define practice in today's schools and classrooms and the number of times the drawing board needs to be revisited can be minimized. Second, KU-CRL researchers are committed to the principles of "participatory research" (Turnbull & Turnbull, 1989) where researchers actively team with key stakeholders (students with LD, parents, practitioners, etc.) who have important perspectives about the nature of the intervention that is being considered. Thus, the perspectives of these stakeholders are carefully considered, and input from them is gathered at all stages during the design and testing of an intervention. Third, KU-CRL researchers are committed to using sound research methodologies and designs. Hence, they work with research-design experts to help ensure that research methodologies and designs are in alignment with the nature of research question(s) being asked and the complex realities of the settings in which the studies will be conducted. Fourth, KU-CRL researchers are committed to collecting a broad array of measures that will enable consumers to have a thorough understanding of the intervention's effects at all stages during the teaching process. Thus, multiple measures that yield reliable and quantifiable results are used that, when taken as a whole, will tell a relatively complete story of the intervention's effects.

Fifth, KU-CRL researchers are committed to a field-testing process that involves several stages. Initially, a new intervention might be tested under tightly controlled conditions to determine whether the intervention is viable and worthy of testing in more authentic conditions. Ultimately, the intervention is tested under circumstances that closely approximate the complexity and unpredictable nature of actual classrooms. Sixth, KU-CRL researchers are committed to a process of continual refinement of an intervention until the magnitude of gains that meets acceptable thresholds for social significance as well as statistical significance (if possible, given the research design being used) are achieved. To meet these standards, KU-CRL researchers follow the center's motto of "being willing to go back to the drawing board." In addition, they continue to make refinements in an intervention and test it further even years after the initial research has been completed. Seventh, KU-CRL researchers are committed to translating field-test versions of interventions that have been successfully validated into instructional materials or manuals that include all the necessary supports, activities, and procedures needed by teachers to be used effectively in classrooms. The commitment to do this translation is time-consuming and resource intensive. Finally, KU-CRL researchers are committed to a process of bringing interventions to scale, that is, ensuring that schoolwide, districtwide, and national use of an intervention can take place successfully. As has been repeatedly documented (e.g., Elmore, 1996), seldom are validated educational practices brought to scale. To determine how new interventions work when they are used in schools across the nation, the KU-CRL staff has developed and maintained an international training network (ITN). The ITN currently consists of nearly 1,200 certified trainers who have been prepared to work with teachers and administrators by following known principles of professional development and school change and to assist them in successfully implementing interventions validated by KU-CRL researchers. These individuals continually provide KU-CRL researchers information about how the instructional interventions are working (or not working, as the case may be) in the nation's schools. As a result, additional adjustments can be made in the interventions and the formats of the instructional materials.

In short, these eight principles are at the heart of the intervention research that is conducted by KU-CRL researchers. These researchers believe that when these principles are applied in combination, they help to increase the level of impact that intervention research ultimately has on the performance of students with disabilities.

Indeed, these principles are especially important if researchers are to deal with the unique set of challenges that often accompany research that is conducted on students with LD—especially as these students become adolescents and move into secondary schools. Among some of the more significant challenges that need to be addressed within this research context are the following. First, sufficient numbers of certain subtypes of students (e.g., those with disabilities in math) are often difficult to find. In addition, these students often are transient or evidence high dropout rates. Therefore, locating sufficient numbers of these students to study is often difficult—especially in rigorous general education classes. As a result, researchers need to be creative in selecting and inventing new research designs that focus on small numbers of students. Second, the diversity and magnitude of problems that students experience are often greater than shown on paper. For example, many adolescents with LD demonstrate a broad array of significant personal/social problems that can have a profound influence on their overall functioning. Third, through the informed consent process, adolescents frequently choose not to participate in a study. Finally, because of the limited numbers of students available and prevailing limitations imposed by schools, randomly assigning students to groups is often not possible.

In light of these challenges and the pressing need to design interventions that will produce large effect sizes, KU-CRL researchers have employed a broad array of research designs that fully capitalize on the circumstances available to them and that compensate for the limitations that might be presented by prevailing conditions. The following sections discuss different research designs that have been used by KU-CRL researchers while developing and testing interventions that make a difference in the performance of students with LD (see Table 29.1 for a list of the designs described herein).

Single-Subject Designs

The first general type of design that has been used by KU-CRL researchers and affiliates is the single-subject design (Baer, Wolf, & Risley, 1968). This design belies its name because a methodologically sound study that employs this design must involve the inclusion of several subjects, not just a single subject. The design is especially useful with students with LD for several reasons. First, large numbers of subjects are not re-

TABLE 29.1 Example Designs Used by KU-CRL Researchers

Single-subject designs

Multiple-baseline across-students design
Multiple-baseline across-teachers design
Multiple-baseline across-skills design
Multiple-baseline across-settings design
Reversal design

Group designs

Control-group design with students
Control-group design with teachers
Comparison-group design with student
  volunteers
Comparison-group design for students with
  teacher volunteers
Comparison-group design with counterbalanced
  conditions for students
Control-group design with counterbalanced
  conditions for teachers

Combination designs

Combination designs with students
Combination designs with teachers and students

quired in this design. Because large numbers of students with LD, and especially large numbers of students with the same types of deficits (e.g., students with writing deficits), are typically not available in the same school, this design can be used quite effectively if researchers have limited access to numerous research sites or limited resources. In addition, students with LD are often available for participation in intervention studies during the time they are assigned to the resource room. Typically, just a few students are present in this setting at a time. This design is especially useful in situations in which students with disabilities are receiving the intervention in a setting with just a few other students.

In addition, this design is especially useful when researchers are interested in monitoring the progress of individual students over a time period while an intervention is being implemented to determine the effects of the intervention on each student and to determine the number of trials required by each student to reach mastery. This has been a priority for KU-CRL investigators interested in teaching skills and strategies to students with disabilities because they have been interested in developing interventions that create large gains in skills within short time periods and in ensuring that *all* students with learning disabilities benefit from the intervention. That is, instead of being interested in measuring the mean pretest and posttest scores of a large group of students who have received a short-term intervention and determining that statistically significant gains were achieved, KU-CRL researchers have been interested in monitoring the progress of each student on each practice trial and ensuring that the student is performing at or above a criterion level at the end of the study that will enable him or her to succeed in the general education curriculum. Although statistical methods can be used in conjunction with this design (e.g., Scruggs, Mastropieri, & Casto, 1987; Swanson & Hoskyn, 1998), the differences between preintervention and postintervention performance can often be seen with the naked eye if the data are displayed in graph form. Thus, this design is useful when investigators are interested in studying an intervention that takes place over an extended period requiring multiple practice trials before a student reaches mastery at a level that is substantially different than the level at which the student was performing at the beginning of the study. It enables investigators to watch each student's progress and make decisions about the time required to produce targeted gains.

This design is also especially helpful when investigators wish to monitor student progress on several measures at once. For example, if investigators wish to determine whether students can generalize the skills they are learning to different kinds of tasks, while also measuring their performance on a task on which they have had practice, this is a good design to use.

Also, this design is useful when all the students in a setting must receive the instruction. Often, school administrators are reluctant to allow researchers to do research if half of the students who will participate in the study are serving as control subjects and will not benefit. In other words, they are reluctant to give permission for students to lose valuable instructional time by participating in a study if they will not gain something from the investment of that time. With the single-subject design, all the students can potentially benefit.

Finally, this design has been useful when KU-CRL researchers have been interested in studying a new way of instructing teachers and when only a few teachers are available for participation in a study. This is often the case because just a few teachers of students with LD are employed by each school in a district. Thus, large numbers of special education teachers are often not available unless researchers have the resources to work with a large number of schools.

Multiple-Baseline Across-Students Design

KU-CRL researchers have used a variation of the multiple-baseline across-students design, called the multiple-probe across-students design (Horner & Baer, 1978), often because of the flexibility of use associated with it. Students can be taught individually or in small groups. They can be enrolled in a class in which the instruction takes place, or they can meet individually with a researcher according to their schedules. They can be enrolled in several classes across a school day or in the same class. In addition,

the design can be used to measure generalization and maintenance of a newly learned skill or strategy.

The major disadvantage associated with this design is that the same measure must be gathered on each student several times; probably the smallest number of times that might be sufficient is six. This requirement can cause problems in an instructional setting where time is at a premium and students need to be spending their time learning versus being tested. However, if the tests are short or if they are integrated into the instruction in such a way that they provide formative feedback to the student, several tests might be acceptable to school personnel.

When this design has been used by KU-CRL researchers and affiliates, all participating students are given at least three baseline "probes" or tests in order to measure their baseline performance on a type of task that they would encounter in school. When their performance across probes is stable, some of the students receive instruction; others receive additional baseline probes. These other students serve as the controls for the students receiving the instruction. Once the students who have received instruction have mastered the skill being taught, the other students then receive instruction as well. Several tiers of "other students" can be employed within the design to serve as controls for students who have received the intervention before them. Several replications of the design can be completed in order to show that there is generality across a number of subjects.

An example study in which the multiple-probe across-students design has been used is a study conducted by Bulgren, Hock, Schumaker, and Deshler (1995) on the effects of instruction in a mnemonic strategy on student test performance. In this study, a total of 12 students participated in four replications of the design (3 students participated in each replication). For each probe, the students were given information to study for a test, and on the next day they were administered the test. In some of the probes, the information to be remembered was clearly specified; in other probes, students were given written passages containing information that they had to find independently and study. There were two conditions: (1) a baseline condition in which probe tests were given before the students received instruction; and (2) a postintervention condition, which occurred after the initial instruction in the strategy. Results showed that when the students learned a strategy, called the Paired-Associates Strategy (Bulgren & Schumaker, 1996), their ability to make study cards and their scores on probe tests improved dramatically. At the end of the study, most of the students were earning probe test scores above the 80% level (the "B" level in most classes), whereas when the study began the large majority of test scores fell in the failing range.

In some other studies in which the multiple-probe across-students design was used, a third condition was included to show whether students maintained their use of a strategy over time. For example, in a study by Hughes and Schumaker (1991) in which students were taught a test-taking strategy (Hughes, Schumaker, Deshler, & Mercer, 1988), students received probe tests every 2 weeks after instruction was terminated. The results showed that they maintained their use of the strategy by earning a mean score of 85% of the points available for as many as 11 weeks after instruction had been terminated. These researchers also showed that the students' test grades in their general education classes improved. Four students' average test grades improved by one letter grade, and two students' average test grades improved by two letter grades.

In two other studies using the multiple-probe across-students design, the major target of the intervention was a decrease in errors in students' performance versus an increase in student performance as targeted in the aforementioned studies. Lenz and Hughes (1990) focused on decreasing students' errors in their oral reading of passages, and Schumaker and colleagues (1982) focused on decreasing students' errors in their written work. Both studies demonstrated that instruction in a strategy can help students reduce the number of errors they produce.

In a final variation of this design, Hock, Pulvers, Deshler, and Schumaker (2001) kept track of students' quiz and test scores in their general education classes (e.g., algebra class and biology class) while they were receiving a special type of tutoring, called Strategic Tutoring, in an after-school study club (see Study 2 in the article). What makes this study unique is that each student's test grades were monitored in relation to a different course. The study shows that the students' quiz and test scores in the targeted course dramatically increased after strategic tutoring began for five of the six students from a mean baseline test score of 50% to a mean postinstruction test score of 80% in general education classes. A mean effect size of 3.12 was achieved on student test performance, with one student's effect size as high as 10.72. A follow-up condition demonstrated that four of the six students maintained their performance levels in the targeted classes after Strategic Tutoring was discontinued.

Multiple-Baseline Across-Teachers Design

This design is similar to the design described earlier except teachers are the subjects in the design instead of students. This design has been used in studies in which teachers have been taught how to use an innovative instructional practice. In order to use the design, observers visit the participating teachers' classrooms and gather baseline data during at least three lessons in each teacher's class. Next, some teachers receive instruction in the instructional practice, whereas others do not. Once the teachers who have received instruction show that they can use the instructional technique in their classes, at least one more baseline point is gathered for the other teachers, and then they receive training and implement the instruction.

Again, the major advantage of this design is that only a few teachers are needed to complete it. This is important in today's world because teachers are busy, and they are often reluctant to add anything to their already full plates. The major disadvantage is that several observations need to be conducted in actual classrooms. Sometimes teachers are reluctant to have observers visit their classrooms several times.

An example study in which this design has been employed was conducted by Bulgren, Schumaker, and Deshler (1988). In this study, secondary general education teachers who were teaching inclusive subject-area courses were taught how to use an instructional routine—the Concept Mastery Routine—for teaching conceptual information to students. Before and after the instruction, their use of teaching behaviors associated with teaching concepts was measured through the use of observational checklists in their classes. Results showed that the teachers used a mean of 27% of the teaching behaviors before the instruction and 91% of the behaviors after the instruction. In each case, the teacher's instruction improved only after he/she attended the workshop. Concomitantly, the unit test scores of students who were enrolled in the teachers' classes also improved. Before their teachers were trained, students with disabilities earned a mean test score of 60%. After their teachers were trained, they earned a mean test score of 71%.

Another example study in which this design was applied focused on teacher implementation of the Recall Enhancement Routine in inclusive classes (Bulgren, Deshler, & Schumaker, 1997). In this study, teachers were taught how to use the routine to co-construct mnemonic devices with their students related to information that the students needed to learn. Again, the results showed that the teachers' behavior improved only after attending the workshop on the routine (see Bulgren, Deshler, Schumaker, & Lenz, 2000; Bulgren, Lenz, Schumaker, Deshler, & Marquis, 2002, for additional applications of this design).

Multiple-Baseline Across-Skills Design

Researchers at the KU-CRL have used a variation of the multiple-baseline across-skills design called the multiple-probe across-skills design. This design is appropriate when students are to be taught several skills in a sequence (not simultaneously) and when the skills are mutually exclusive (i.e., if students learn one of the skills, their behavior related to the other skills is not expected to change). When this design is used, all students participating in the study have at least three baseline probe tests on all the skills to be taught. Then all students begin instruction in the first skill to be taught at the same time. Once a student reaches the mastery criterion on the first skill to be taught, another baseline probe on the second and third skills to be taught is given to

him or her. As long as the student's performance on the second skill to be taught is stable, instruction in the second skill begins. Once the student reaches the mastery criterion on the second skill, another baseline probe is given on the third skill to be taught. As long as the student's performance on the third skill to be taught is stable, instruction in the third skill begins, and so forth for as many skills as are to be taught.

A major advantage associated with this design is that all the students can begin instruction at the same time. Some students do not need to be "waiting" for instruction to begin, and teachers need not find something else for those students to do while they wait. The major disadvantage associated with this design is that students need to take many tests, even more tests than they take with the multiple-baseline across-students design, because they have to take a test associated with each skill each time a probe is given.

One study in which this design was used was conducted by Schumaker, Deshler, Alley, Warner, and Denton (1982). In this study, the effects of instruction in the Multipass Strategy were determined. The strategy has three parts or substrategies—"Survey," "Size-up," and "Sort-out." During Survey, students spend about 3 minutes getting an overview of a textbook chapter. During "Size-up," students find the most important information in each section of the chapter and take notes on it. During "Sort-out," students review the important information for a test. Thus, the behaviors required of the students in the three parts of the strategy are mutually exclusive. The results showed that when each student learned each part of the strategy, the student's performance related to only that part of the strategy improved substantially. For example, one student performed an average of 33% of the Survey behaviors, 33% of the Size-up behaviors, and 0% of the Sort-out behaviors before instruction. After instruction in each part, he performed 100% of the required behaviors. When given a test over the information in the chapter that he studied without supervision, the student earned a score of 25% during baseline and 90% after instruction.

Another study employing this design was conducted by Clark, Deshler, Schumaker, Alley, and Warner (1984). Here, instead of using several *parts of a strategy*, the researchers used two *different strategies* to create the multiple-baseline effect. In this study, students were administered baseline probes associated with reading comprehension of two different types of reading passages: narrative and expository passages. Then they were taught the Visual Imagery Strategy (Schumaker, Deshler, Zemitzch, & Warner, 1993), which can be applied to narrative passages. Once they had mastered that strategy and their reading comprehension of narrative passages had increased, they were administered at least one probe test on an expository passage. Once their performance on this type of passage stabilized, they were taught the Self-Questioning Strategy (Schumaker, Deshler, Nolan, & Alley, 1994). Results showed that the students' reading comprehension scores increased on each type of passage only after the students had received strategy instruction related to that type of passage. For example, during baseline, the average percentage of comprehension questions the students answered correctly on a narrative passage was 55%; after instruction, the average percentage correct was 69%.

Still another study in which the multiple-baseline across-skills design was used covered writing interventions (Schmidt, 1983; Schmidt, Deshler, Schumaker, & Alley, 1989). This study focused on the instruction of four writing strategies: the Sentence Writing Strategy (Schumaker & Sheldon, 1985; Sheldon & Schumaker, 1985), the Paragraph Writing Strategy (Schumaker & Lyerla, 1991), the Error Monitoring Strategy (Schumaker, Nolan, & Deshler, 1985), and the Theme Writing Strategy (Schumaker, in press). Students were taught the strategies in sequence, and writing samples were gathered in their resource room class as well as in their English classes and social studies classes throughout the study. Each writing sample was scored for complete sentences and types of sentences, organized paragraphs, errors, and organized themes (each of these measures corresponded to one of the strategies taught). Results showed that the students' writing improved in each area after the strategy corresponding to that area was taught. In addition, five of the seven students generalized their use of all the strategies they had learned to their English

and social studies assignments without prompting. The remaining students generalized their use of the strategies after receiving generalization instruction. The four students who received instruction in all four strategies received higher scores than did the average student on the district writing competency exam. The students' skills maintained into the next school year when their English writing assignments were gathered and scored.

Multiple-Baseline Across-Settings Design

The multiple-baseline across-settings design is useful when students who fit the characteristics of the subject sample are present in several settings and when the intervention can be implemented in each of those settings. The way this design is typically used, the same student is present in all of the settings, and the intervention is applied in each setting in relation to that student across time. A requirement of the design, then, is that when the behavior of the student changes in one setting, it does not change in the other settings. KU-CRL researchers have found that this is a difficult requirement to meet because the skills and strategies that are often the focus of their interventions are taught to mastery, and students often generalize their use of the strategies to other settings without prompting. The students' spontaneous generalization of a skill thus destroys the whole purpose of the design: to show control over the dependent variable. Thus, KU-CRL researchers have rarely used this design.

Nevertheless, KU-CRL researchers have created a variation of this design. This hybrid design might be called the multiple-baseline across-settings and across-students design. In this design, the intervention is implemented in several classes (settings) by the different teachers in those classes, and the behavior of a targeted student with LD is measured in each setting. This design avoids the possible generalization effect that is probable in the multiple-baseline across-settings design when only one student takes part in each replication of the design.

One study in which this hybrid design was used is a study conducted by Lenz, Alley, and Schumaker (1987) on the use of advance organizers in secondary content classes. In this study, seven subject-area teachers and a student with LD who was enrolled in one of each teacher's classes participated. During baseline, the teachers' use of advance organizers and the students' oral reports of information they learned were measured in each lesson. Then the teachers were taught (at different times) how to use advance organizers at the beginning of each lesson. They then used advance organizers in their classes (settings). The results showed when the number of advance organizer elements used by a teacher increased in a class and when the student was taught to attend to the advance organizer elements, the number of items the student orally reported at the end of the class period also increased.

Reversal Design

The reversal design is another design that has been rarely used by KU-CRL researchers. To use this design, researchers take baseline measures, then they implement the intervention. Next, they repeat the baseline condition, then they implement the intervention for a second time, and so forth, for as many times as they wish in order to demonstrate that the intervention causes a change in the behavior. Thus, a major requirement of this design is that the behavior to be changed will "reverse" or revert to baseline levels when the baseline condition is reinstituted. Again, because KU-CRL researchers have been focused on developing interventions that cause enduring changes in behavior (note the studies mentioned earlier showing maintenance of the behavior after the intervention was discontinued), they have rarely used this design.

One way this design has been adapted by KU-CRL researchers is exemplified by a study by Bulgren and colleagues (2000) (see Study 3 in the article). The researchers were studying the effects of a teacher's use of an instructional routine in a general education science class. The instructional routine involves the use of analogies to help students understand a new concept by relating it to something they already understand. For example, a good analogy that might help students understand the functions of the parts of the eye involves showing students the parts of a camera. Bulgren et al. asked the

teacher to choose four concepts to be taught; she chose epiglottis, pancreas, alveoli, and esophagus. Each concept was taught in a separate lesson. Every other concept was paired with the teacher's use of the routine in an ABAB reversal design. The students took a test over the concept on the day following the lesson on the concept. Results showed that the students earned significantly higher scores on the tests about the concepts that were taught through the use of the routine than on the tests about the concepts that were taught with traditional means of instruction. After "epiglottis" was taught with the routine, for example, students earned an average test score of 83%. After "pancreas" was taught with traditional methods, students earned an average test score of 27%. After "alveoli" was taught with the routine, students earned an average test score of 70%. After "esophagus" was taught with traditional methods, students earned an average test score of 42%. Thus, this design can be effectively used to demonstrate experimental control when an instructional intervention can be applied to some sets of information and not applied to other sets of information in alternation to determine how well students learn that information.

Group Designs

Group designs are particularly useful in the field of education when researchers wish to compare the effects of one instructional procedure to the effects of another instructional procedure. KU-CRL researchers have often been interested in comparing the effects of an innovative instructional procedure to the effects of traditional instruction. Sometimes they have been interested in comparing the effects of a new professional development method for teachers to another method and showing that the new method produces results that are at least as good as the other method.

Usually, group designs have been used with an intervention that is relatively short in duration because the chance of getting *all* the subjects together several times is small. Students, for example, become ill, miss school, have extracurricular activities, have doctor's appointments, and have a job after school, and generally have other priorities besides participating in research studies. Teachers are often busy, too, and the likelihood of ensuring that they will get together several times is small. Thus, group designs have some limitations if an intervention takes considerable time requiring several practice trials to mastery.

Sometimes, group designs have been used by KU-CRL researchers with relatively small numbers of student or teacher subjects. Other times, KU-CRL researchers have conducted studies involving hundreds of students. They have particularly used large-group designs when they have studied interventions that are appropriate for general education classes in which large numbers of students are enrolled and which included several students with LD. Because school administrators often do not allow students to be randomly assigned to groups for experimental purposes, KU-CRL researchers have relied, for the most part, on involving schools in which students are already randomly assigned to classes or on randomly assigning intact classes to the different experimental conditions.

Sometimes teachers will not allow themselves to be randomly assigned to groups. In these cases, to move forward with a study, the researchers have allowed the teachers to assign themselves to either the experimental or the comparison group. Of course, such an arrangement makes the researchers even more responsible for showing that the two groups are equivalent at the beginning of the study. With these general considerations in mind, some of the group designs that have been used by KU-CRL researchers and affiliates are described below.

Control-Group Design with Students

In the control-group design, students are randomly assigned to one of two groups: an experimental group and a control group. The researchers need to demonstrate that the two groups are equivalent in some way, and this is typically done by having students take a pretest and showing that the students' scores on the pretest are similar. However, this is often not possible because of limitations imposed by school personnel in terms of using valuable instructional time. If giving a pretest is not possible, some

other measure might be used by the researchers to demonstrate the equivalence of the groups. Students in the experimental group receive the intervention; students in the control group do not. Except for this difference, all other conditions should be the same for both groups. For example, they should receive instruction from the same teacher, the information covered should be the same, and the same amount of instructional time should be available to both groups. As explained previously, this design has been used infrequently by KU-CRL researchers. However, it has been used in some instances when the intervention could be compressed into a block of time, like one or two class periods and when measures could be taken on the effects of the intervention immediately.

One study in which a postest-only control-group design was used focused on the effects of an advance organizer prior to student reading of a passage. In this study, Lenz (1983) recruited 46 students with learning disabilities and 51 normally achieving students to participate. Within each achievement group, students were randomly assigned to the experimental or the control group. They all took a social studies achievement test, and the researcher demonstrated that the groups were equivalent. Then all the students read three passages and took a test over each passage. Students in the experimental group received some instruction about how to attend to and use advance organizers and were given an advance organizer before reading each passage. The control group did not receive advance organizers. The results showed that the experimental students with LD answered significantly more questions about important information in the passages than the control students with LD. There were no differences between the groups of normally achieving students.

Bulgren, Schumaker, and Deshler (1994) used a variation of this design to study the effects of the Recall Enhancement Routine on the test performance of secondary students with disabilities and other students who were enrolled in general education classes. Forty-one students were recruited from two social studies classes. The students were stratified by grade level (seventh or eighth) and exceptionality (LD or non-LD).

Half the students in each stratified group were randomly selected to participate in the experimental group. The other half participated in the control group. Students in both groups received the same lecture by the same teacher. At the end of the lecture, a review period covered the information in the lecture. During the review portion of the lesson, the experimental students participated in creating mnemonic devices to help them remember some of the information in the lecture. The control students simply participated in a traditional review of the same facts (the facts were repeated). The researchers demonstrated that the groups were equivalent by showing that the two groups correctly answered about the same number of questions about facts that were not reviewed during the review period. They also showed that students with LD in the experimental group correctly answered an average of 71% of the questions about reviewed facts, whereas students with LD in the control group correctly answered an average of 42% of the questions about reviewed facts. Students without LD in the experimental group correctly answered an average of 85% of the questions about reviewed facts, whereas students without LD in the control group correctly answered an average of 54% of the questions about reviewed facts. The differences between the groups were statistically significant, and they were socially significant in that so many more students earned passing scores when the intervention was used than when it was not used.

Bulgren and colleagues (2002) used another variation of this design to study the effects of a concept comparison routine on the test performance of secondary students enrolled in five general education science classes, including students with disabilities. The teachers of each class randomly assigned the students to an experimental or a control group. The intervention was a single lesson on "Tropical Diseases" in which two diseases, malaria and snail fever, were compared and contrasted. During the lesson, experimental students, who met in one classroom during their regularly scheduled class period, received the information through the use of the new routine. Control students, who met in another classroom at the same time, received the same informa-

tion through the use of a traditional lecture. Procedural controls were in place for teacher and classroom variables. Results showed that the experimental students with disabilities and the whole group of experimental students earned significantly higher scores on a test on the information than did their counterparts in the control group. For example, experimental students with LD earned an average score of 71%, and control students with LD earned an average score of 57% on the test. Low achievers in the experimental group earned an average score of 86% and in the control group earned an average score of 63%. Normal achieving students in the experimental group earned an average score of 84% and in the control group earned an average score of 76%. Many more experimental students passed the test than control students.

Control-Group Design with Teachers

KU-CRL researchers have used the control-group design with teachers as well as students. For example, Kline, Deshler, and Schumaker (1992), as a part of a series of studies conducted to identify variables that produce implementation of empirically validated practices by teachers, conducted a study in which teachers were randomly assigned to an experimental group and a control group using a stratified method of assignment to control for the grade level at which the teachers were teaching. Both groups had received a 3-hour overview on strategy instruction and had participated in workshops on how to teach two learning strategies. As a part of this study, both groups next participated in a workshop on how to teach the FIRST-Letter Mnemonic Strategy (Nagel, Schumaker, & Deshler, 1986). The experimental teachers met in support teams once a month following the workshop. Support-team meetings were led by a school administrator. The control teachers did not participate in support-team meetings, but they had unlimited access to the administrator in charge of the training workshops and of ensuring implementation. Results showed that all the experimental teachers began the instruction, while less than half the control teachers did. The experimental teachers began the instruction within 9 days of the workshop on average, whereas the control teachers began it within 13 days. The experimental teachers taught the strategy to more students, and they proceeded further through the instruction than did the control teachers. Thus, this design can be helpful in identifying differential effects in teacher-training methods.

Comparison-Group Design with Student Volunteers

This design involves the use of two groups of students. One group receives the intervention, and the other group does not. Students volunteer to participate in the intervention. Sometimes, such a sampling method may be necessary if the intervention takes considerable time. This may be especially necessary if the students are adolescents because they often want to be involved in decisions being made about what they learn and how they spend their time. Unfortunately, this method places a limitation on the research because the students who participate in the intervention are volunteers (i.e., committed to participating in the intervention) and are possibly different from other students who might not volunteer.

An example of a study in which this design was used was conducted by Lancaster, Schumaker, and Deshler (2002). It compared the effects of live instruction to the effects of computer-based instruction in the Self-Advocacy Strategy. The point of this study was to demonstrate that the computerized instruction was as effective as live instruction from a teacher. There were three groups of students. Students volunteered to participate either in instruction in the Self-Advocacy Strategy or in a comparison group. Students who volunteered to participate in the instruction were randomly selected to participate either in the live-instruction group ($n = 8$) or in the computerized instruction group ($n = 8$). Students' use of the strategy was measured in two different ways. One measure calculated the number of responses students made to a series of questions related to individual education plans (IEPs). Prior to instruction, students in the comparison group averaged 11 responses, and students in the computerized

and live-instruction groups averaged 17 and 12 responses, respectively. The posttest was given during each student's formal IEP meeting, at which the same questions were asked. This time, students in the comparison group averaged 21 responses while students in the computerized and live-instruction group averaged 62 and 61 responses, respectively. The second measure of student use of the strategy was a calculation of the percentage of goals each student contributed to his or her IEP during the conference. This was a posttest-only measure. Students in the comparison group contributed an average of 20% of the goals found on their IEPs. Students in the computerized and live-instruction groups contributed of 66% and 79% of the goals on their IEPs, respectively. On a measure of knowledge of the Self-Advocacy Strategy, students in the live and computerized instruction groups earned average scores of 16% and 19% correct on the pretest and 94% and 97% correct on the posttest, respectively. The researchers concluded that the computerized instruction was as effective as the live instruction in the strategy in terms of knowledge of the strategy and actual performance in the IEP meeting.

Comparison-Group Design for Students with Teacher Volunteers

This design has been used by KU-CRL researchers and associates when some teachers are interested in testing an intervention by using it in their classrooms and other teachers are willing to participate in the study as comparison teachers only. Typically, the researchers have used this design in schools in which students are randomly assigned to classes. In other words, although teachers might be volunteering to use the intervention or not to use the intervention, the students in their classes have been randomly assigned into those classes and thus can be expected to be comparable samples. Of course, the researchers make sure that the student samples are truly equivalent through the use of a pretest or some other measure collected from school records.

Vernon, Schumaker, and Deshler have used this design in a series of studies focused on teaching Cooperative Thinking Strategies in inclusive general education classes. Cooperative Thinking Strategies are sets of behaviors that small groups of students can use to complete group tasks such as solving problems, deciding how to deal with a two-sided issue, and completing a large project. In many of the studies, 10 to 12 teachers volunteered to deliver the intervention (instruction in one of the Cooperative Thinking Strategies) in their classes, and another 10 to 12 teachers volunteered their classes as comparison classes. Measures taken in the classes before and after instruction included student knowledge of how to proceed on the particular type of group task, student performance of the behaviors involved in completing the group task, student performance of social skills while completing the group task, sociometric measures of student acceptance of each student in the class, and student opinions of group work. The data collected on students with disabilities was analyzed separately from the data collected on other students in the classes.

Results showed in each study that students with and without disabilities in the experimental classes knew significantly more about what they had to do and performed significantly more of the behaviors required than the students in the comparison classes after the experimental teachers implemented the instruction. For example, one study focused on teaching students a way of problem solving in groups. Twenty teachers and 392 students participated. At the beginning of the study, experimental and comparison students earned an average of 1% of the points on a test of knowledge of how to solve problems in groups. After the 10 experimental teachers taught their students a strategy for solving problems in groups, on average, the experimental students earned 75% of the points, and the comparison students earned 1% of the points on the knowledge test. Before instruction began, the student groups in the experimental and comparison classes performed an average of 34% of the problem-solving behaviors. After the instruction of the strategy in experimental classes, the experimental students performed an average of 84% of the problem-solving behaviors while the students in the comparison classes performed an average of 39% of the behav-

iors. Student groups in both sets of classes had had the same number of opportunities to practice problem solving, although the comparison classes had no instruction on the topic (Vernon, Schumaker, & Deshler, 1996).

Vernon, Schumaker, and Deshler have also used this design in a series of three studies focused on creating safe learning communities in inclusive elementary classes. The general idea associated with this work is to provide groups of students, including students with disabilities, ways to support each other during instruction. As in the Cooperative Thinking Strategies studies, two groups of teachers and their students have been involved in each community-building study. Each study has focused on one method for building a learning community. The results of the studies have been positive, showing that teacher use of the instruction leads to significant and substantial differences between experimental and comparison students with regard to their knowledge and their performance in class.

For example, one study focused on teaching students how to participate in class discussions in respectful and helpful ways. Twenty teachers and 372 students in the teachers' inclusive classes participated. The results showed that students in the experimental classes knew significantly more information about how to create a classroom community, participated more frequently, and engaged in fewer behaviors that would disrupt a discussion (e.g., yell-outs, negative comments, and laughing at speakers) than did students in the comparison classes after the experimental classes had participated in the experimental lessons. At the beginning of the study, for example, students in the experimental classes and comparison classes earned 14% and 13% of the points, respectively, on a test of their knowledge about what they should be doing in discussions and concepts related to learning community. After the instruction, experimental students earned 77% of the points, and comparison students earned 16% of the points. After the instruction, experimental students with disabilities participated a total of 289 times in the final discussion in their classes, while comparison students with disabilities participated a total of 99 times. In the first discussion, they participated a total of 121 and

108 times, respectively (Vernon, Schumaker, & Deshler, 1999). In sum, these researchers have found that they can use this comparison-group design to study the effects of interventions in inclusive classes while monitoring the performance of students with disabilities as well as other students in the classes.

Comparison-Group Design with Counterbalanced Conditions for Students

This design has been used by KU-CRL researchers to demonstrate that a particular instructional method produces learning gains for students with regard to subject-matter content (e.g., science, social studies, and literature) in inclusive general education classes. In one study in which this design was used, Bulgren and colleagues (2000) studied the effects of analogical instruction in inclusive secondary classes. Eighty-three students in eight science classes participated. The students had been randomly assigned to their classes by school personnel at the beginning of the year. The intact classes were randomly assigned to one of two experimental conditions. In one condition, students received analogical instruction related to the concept of commensalism and traditional instruction related to the concept of *pyramid of numbers*. In the other condition, students received analogical instruction related to the concept of *pyramid of numbers* and traditional instruction related to the concept of *commensalism*. All the students received traditional instruction related to the concepts of food web and heterotroph. Both groups received the instruction on all four concepts within one class period. On the next day, they took a test on the information. The results showed, for example, that the students with LD who received the analogical instruction in association with the concept of pyramid of numbers earned significantly higher scores ($M = 69\%$) than did the students who had traditional instruction on that concept ($M = 40\%$). Similar differences were found for low achievers, normal achievers, and high achievers. There were no differences between the groups on test items related to the concepts of food web and heterotroph, which indicated that the groups were equivalent.

Control-Group Design with Counterbalanced Conditions for Teachers

KU-CRL researchers have used this design to show the effects of a particular training method or condition on teacher implementation of a validated practice. For example, in one study, Kline, Deshler, and Schumaker (1992) wanted to know the effects of providing teachers with all the materials and equipment that they would need to implement an intervention. All the participating teachers attended workshops on the Word Identification Strategy (Lenz, Schumaker, Deshler, & Beals, 1984) and the Paraphrasing Strategy (Schumaker, Denton, & Deshler, 1984). The teachers were randomly divided into two groups. After the Word Identification Strategy workshop, teachers in Group 1 received all the materials and equipment needed to teach the Word Identification Strategy. Teachers in Group 2 received only the instructor's manual. After the Paraphrasing Strategy workshop, teachers in Group 2 received all the materials needed to teach the Paraphrasing Strategy. The teachers in Group 1 received only the instructor's manual. Results showed that the teachers who received the materials began the instruction sooner and taught more students the strategy than did the teachers who did not receive the additional materials.

Combination Designs

Sometimes, KU-CRL researchers have combined single-subject designs with group designs. This combination approach is especially useful when researchers want to demonstrate improved performance across time as the result of an intervention as well as compare the effects of the intervention to the effects of some other type of instruction.

Combination Designs with Students

In some studies, KU-CRL researchers and affiliates have combined the multiple-probe across-students design with the group design to determine the effects of an intervention on student performance. In the group design, students are randomly selected into one of two groups: an experimental group and a control group. In the multiple-probe design, the skills of students in the experimental group are measured across time, before and after they participate in the instructional intervention.

Van Reusen, Deshler, and Schumaker (1989) used this design to study the effects of live instruction of the Self-Advocacy Strategy (Van Reusen, Bos, Schumaker, & Deshler, 1994) on student's performance in simulated and real IEP conferences. Students with LD were randomly assigned to an experimental and a control group. All the students received at least three tests on their performance of self-advocacy skills at the beginning of the study except for one control student. Then some of the students in the experimental group received instruction in the strategy. Once their performance had improved, another group of experimental students received instruction. Once their performance had improved, a third group of experimental students received the instruction. Meanwhile, the performance of the control-group students continued to be measured. Results showed that the baseline performance levels of the two groups of students were comparable and stable. The multiple-probe design demonstrated that the performance of the experimental students improved only after they received the instruction. Students who had received the instruction made a mean of 98 relevant contributions to their IEP conferences whereas students who did not receive the instruction made a mean of 42 relevant comments. This represented a statistically significant difference. Moreover, 86% of the goals appearing in the final IEPs of students who had received the training were goals specified by the students themselves compared to 13% of the goals appearing in the final IEPs of students who had not received the instruction.

In another study in which the multiple-baseline design was combined with a comparison-group design is a study that focused on the instruction of social skills in an inclusive sixth-grade class (Vernon & Schumaker, 1993). For the comparison part of the design, a second sixth-grade class participated. Students in both classes took social skills tests before and after the experimental class received instruction in the social skills. For the multiple-baseline part of the design,

the different baselines were the four social skills taught in the experimental class. A different student in the experimental class was targeted for the measurement of each social skill in the multiple-baseline design. The intervention focused on the instruction of the four social skills *in sequence*, and the targeted experimental students' performance of the social skills was measured before and after each skill was taught. Results showed that the selected students' performance of each skill improved only after instruction in that skill had taken place. In addition, the students in the experimental class earned an average score of 45% on the social skills performance pretest and 86% on the posttest. Students in the comparison class earned average pretest and posttest performance scores of 44% and 44%, respectively.

A third study using more than one design was conducted by Schumaker and colleagues (1984). The focus of this study was teaching students a way to learn information from a textbook chapter that had been specially coded and for which a special type of audiotape had been made. Besides using a multiple-probe across-substrategies design to show that the students learned the substrategies, the researchers also used a multiple-probe across-students design to show the effects of learning the substrategies on unit test scores. They also used a reversal design to show the students' performance on unit tests when they used the special tapes versus verbatim tapes. (Prior to some unit tests, the experimental students received the specially marked textbook chapters and special audiotapes; prior to other tests, the experimental students received a verbatim audiotape of the chapter.) Finally, they used a comparison-group design to show how the experimental students performed in comparison to other students in the same general education class on the tests. The comparison students received the verbatim audiotapes. Results showed that verbatim audiotapes produced no change in the comparison students' test scores ($M = 51$%) when compared to baseline test scores ($M = 56$%). Experimental students earned substantially higher scores after using the specially designed audiotapes and marked text ($M = 91$%) than they did when they used verbatim tapes ($M = 41$%).

Combination Designs with Teachers and Students

KU-CRL researchers have used this type of design when they are interested in tracking teacher performance in the classroom while also measuring the effects of teacher performance on student performance. Sometimes, they have used a multiple-probe across-teachers design to determine teacher effects and a group design to determine student effects.

Kline, Schumaker, and Deshler (1991) used such a combination of designs to determine the effects of training on teacher delivery of feedback to students and to determine the effects of different types of feedback on student learning. Eighteen teachers were randomly assigned to one of three groups: a group that received training in a feedback routine, a group that received training in the same feedback routine plus training in how to teach students to accept feedback, and a comparison group. Participating students were randomly selected students with learning disabilities in the participating teachers' classes. All the teachers were taught to implement instruction in the Sentence Writing Strategy (Schumaker & Sheldon, 1985) in a daylong workshop. In addition, teachers in one group received explicit instruction in how to give feedback to students. Teachers in a second group received explicit instruction in how to give feedback to students and how to teach students to accept teacher feedback. Teachers in the third group (the comparison group) received consultation with regard to implementing the strategy instruction. The multiple-probe results showed that the teachers' delivery of feedback improved concomitant with instruction in how to give feedback; the group results showed that the students of teachers in the two feedback groups reached mastery in significantly fewer lessons than did students of teachers in the comparison group. In fact, they required one-third fewer practice trials (10 vs. 15), on average, representing a difference of a week of instruction. There were no differences found between the number of errors made by students of comparison teachers on practice trials 1 and 2, while there were differences between the errors made on these trials for students whose teachers received the feedback training. Moreover, 7 of 11

teachers in the feedback groups who were still in the district were teaching the strategy in the next school year, whereas none of the comparison teachers had reinitiated the instruction that year. Thus, teacher success in teaching something new to students might have a profound effect on whether teachers use that instructional practice in the future.

In another variation of the combination design, Fisher, Deshler, and Schumaker (1999) studied the effects of computerized versus live instruction on the knowledge, construction of instructional materials, and behavior of teachers in their general education classrooms. Twenty-nine of 58 preservice teachers were randomly assigned to receive instruction on how to use the Concept Mastery Routine (Bulgren, Deshler, & Schumaker, 1993) through a computerized program; the remainder were assigned to receive live instruction. These teachers took two tests before and after the instruction: a knowledge test and a test of constructing materials associated with the routine. Of eight inservice teachers, four were randomly selected to receive the computerized training, and the other four were randomly selected to receive the live instruction. These teachers took the same tests as the preservice teachers. In addition, a multiple-probe across-teachers design with three replications was used with the inservice teachers to show their performance of the routine in their classes. The results showed no differences between the groups; that is, the computerized instruction was shown to be as effective as live instruction in terms of teacher knowledge of the routine, teacher construction of materials, and teacher use of the routine.

Conclusion

Researchers at the KU-CRL and their associates have been studying the problem of educating students with learning disabilities for the past 24 years from a number of angles. They have developed and validated instructional methods for teaching these students a variety of learning strategies so that they can meet the demands associated with their required general education courses. They have developed and validated methods for teachers of general education courses to deliver the content in learner-friendly ways, ways that enable students to understand and remember the content. They have developed and validated methods for creating learning communities within classes and for teaching students how to work together in productive ways. For the most part, this research has been conducted in schools, and in many cases, regularly assigned teachers have delivered the instruction. To conduct their research under typical school conditions, KU-CRL researchers and affiliates have had to be creative in working with a variety of research designs. At times, they have had to sacrifice some of the strict rules of experimental design, like pure random assignment, to ensure that a research study was conducted. However, they have tried to substitute other types of controls within a study to help them demonstrate the effects of their intervention. They chose each design exemplified here for its fit to the problem at hand as well as its fit to the current situation in the schools. Such adaptations are needed if applied educational research is to produce outcomes and products that will be usable in today's and tomorrow's schools and that will substantially change the ways that students with disabilities are educated in the future.

Dedication

The authors wish to dedicate this chapter in honor and memory of Dr. Donald M. Baer, their teacher and supporter. His creatvity and leadership in experimental design formed the springboard from which the studies reported in this article were born. The authors are grateful for his instruction, his example, and all aspects of his beautiful mind and wonderful heart.

References

Baer, D. M., Wolf, M. M., & Risley, T. R. (1968). Some current dimensions of applied behavior analysis. *Journal of Applied Behavior Analysis, 1,* 91–97.

Bulgren, J. A., Deshler, D. D., & Schumaker, J. B. (1993). *The Concept Mastery Routine.* Lawrence, KS: Edge Enterprises.

Bulgren, J. A., Deshler, D. D., & Schumaker, J. B. (1997). Use of a recall enhancement routine and strategies in inclusive secondary classes. *Learning Disabilities Research and Practice, 12(4),* 198–208.

Bulgren, J. A., Deshler, D. D., Schumaker, J. B., & Lenz, B.K. (2000). The use and effectiveness of analogical instruction in diverse secondary content classrooms. *Journal of Educational Psychology, 92(3),* 426–441.

Bulgren, J. A., Hock, M. F., Schumaker, J. B., & Deshler, D. D. (1995). The effects of instruction in a paired associates strategy on the information mastery performance of students with learning disabilities. *Learning Disabilities Research and Practice, 10(1),* 22–37.

Bulgren, J. A., Lenz, B. K., Schumaker, J. B., Deshler, D. D., & Marquis, J. G. (2002). The use and effectiveness of a comparison routine in diverse secondary content classrooms. *Journal of Educational Psychology, 94(2),* 356–371.

Bulgren, J. A., & Schumaker, J. B. (1996). *The Paired-Associates Strategy.* Lawrence: The University of Kansas Center for Research on Learning.

Bulgren, J., Schumaker, J. B., & Deshler, D. D. (1988). Effectiveness of a concept teaching routine in enhancing the performance of LD students in secondary-level mainstream classes. *Learning Disability Quarterly, 11(1),* 3–17.

Bulgren, J. A., Schumaker, J. B., & Deshler, D. D. (1994). The effects of a recall enhancement routine on the test performance of secondary students with and without learning disabilities. *Learning Disabilities Research and Practice, 9(1),* 2–11.

Clark, F. L., Deshler, D. D., Schumaker, J. B., Alley, G. R., & Warner, M. M. (1984). Visual imagery and self-questioning: Strategies to improve comprehension of written material. *Journal of Learning Disabilities, 17(3),* 145–149

Elmore, R. F. (1996). Getting to scale with good educational practice. *Harvard Educational Review, 66(1),* 1–25.

Fisher, J. B., Deshler, D. D., & Schumaker, J. B. (1999). The effects of an interactive multimedia program on teachers' understanding and implementation of an inclusive practice. *Learning Disability Quarterly, 22(2),* 127–142.

Hock, M. F., Pulvers, K. A., Deshler, D. D., & Schumaker, J. B. (2001). The effects of an after-school tutoring program on the academic performance of at-risk students and students with learning disabilities. *Remedial and Special Education, 22(3),* 172–186.

Horner, R.D., & Baer, D.M. (1978). Multiple-probe technique: A variation of the multiple-baseline design. *Journal of Applied Behavior Analysis, 11(1),* 189–196.

Hughes, C. A., & Schumaker, J. B. (1991). Test-taking strategy instruction for adolescents with learning disabilities. *Exceptionality, 2,* 205–221.

Hughes, C. A., Schumaker, J. B., Deshler, D. D., & Mercer, C. O. (1988). *The Test-Taking Strategy: Instructor's manual.* Lawrence, KS: Edge Enterprises.

Kline, F. M., Schumaker, J. B., & Deshler, D. D (1991). Development and validation of feedback routines for instructing students with learning disabilities. *Learning Disability Quarterly, 14*(3), 191–207.

Kline, F. M., Deshler, D. D., & Schumaker, J. B. (1992). Implementing learning strategy instruction in class settings: A research perspective. In M. Pressley, K. R. Harris, & J. T. Guthrie (Eds.) *Promoting academic competence and literacy in school* (pp. 361–406. Orlando, FL: Academic Press.

Lancaster, P., Schumaker, J. B., & Deshler, D. D. (2002). The development and validation of an inactive hypermedia program for teaching a self-advocacy strategy to students with disabilities. *Learning Disabilty Quarterly, 25*(4), 277–302.

Lenz, B. K. (1983). *The effect of advance organizers on the learning and retention of learning disabled adolescents within the context of a cooperative planning model.* Unpublished doctoral dissertation, University of Kansas, Lawrence.

Lenz, B. K., Alley, G. R., & Schumaker, J. B. (1987). Activating the inactive learner through the presentation of advance organizers. *Learning Disability Quarterly, 10*(1), 53–67.

Lenz, B. K., & Hughes, C. (1990). A word identification strategy for adolescents with learning disabilities. *Journal of Learning Disabilities, 23*(3), 149–158, 163.

Lenz, B. K., Schumaker, J. B., Deshler, D. D., & Beals, V. L. (1984). *The Word Identification Strategy: Instructor's manual.* Lawrence: University of Kansas Institute for Research in Learning Disabilities.

Nagel, D. R., Schumaker, J. B., & Deshler, D. D. (1986). *The FIRST-Letter Mnemonic Strategy: Instructor's manual.* Lawrence, KS: Edge Enterprises.

Schmidt, J. (1983). *The effects of four generalization conditions on learning disabled adolescents' written language performance in the regular classroom.* Unpublished doctoral dissertation, University of Kansas, Lawrence.

Schmidt, J. L., Deshler, D. D., Schumaker, J. B., & Alley, G. R. (1988/89). Effects of generalization instruction on the written language performance of adolescents with learning disabilities in the mainstream classroom. *Reading, Writing, and Learning Disabilities, 4*(4), 291–309.

Schumaker, J. B. (in press). *The Theme Writing Strategy: Instructor's manual.* Lawrence, KS: Edge Enterprises.

Schumaker, J. B., Denton, P. H., & Deshler, D. D. (1984). *The Paraphrasing Strategy: Instructor's manual.* Lawrence: University of Kansas Institute for Research in Learning Disabilities.

Schumaker, J. B., Deshler, D. D., Alley, G. R., Warner, M. M., & Denton, P. H. (1982). Multipass: A learning strategy for improving reading comprehension. *Learning Disability Quarterly, 5,*(3) 295–304.

Schumaker, J. B., Deshler, D. D., Alley, G. R., Warner, M. M., Clark, F. L., & Nolan, S. (1982). Error Monitoring: A learning strategy for improving adolescent academic performance. In W. M. Cruickshank & J. W. Lerner (Eds.), *Best of ACLD* (Vol. 3, pp. 170–183). Syracuse, NY: Syracuse University Press.

Schumaker, J. B., Deshler, D. D., Nolan, S. M., & Alley, G. R. (1994). *The Self-Questioning Strategy: Instructor's manual.* Lawrence: University of Kansas Center for Research on Learning.

Schumaker, J. B., Deshler, D. D., Zemitzch, A., & Warner, M. M. (1993). *The Visual Imagery Strategy.* Lawrence: University of Kansas Center for Research on Learning.

Schumaker, J. B., & Lyerla, K. D. (1991). *The Paragraph Writing Strategy: Instructor's manual.* Lawrence: University of Kansas Institute for Research in Learning Disabilities.

Schumaker, J. B., Nolan, S. M., & Deshler, D. D. (1985). *The Error Monitoring Strategy: Instructor's manual.* Lawrence: University of Kansas Institute for Research in Learning Disabilities.

Schumaker, J. B., & Sheldon, J. (1985). *The Sentence Writing Strategy: Instructor's manual.* Lawrence: University of Kansas, Institute for Research on Learning Disabilities.

Scruggs, T. E., Mastropieri, M. A., & Casto, G. (1987). The quantitative synthesis of single-subject research: Methodology and validation. *Remedial and Special Education, 8*(2), 24–33.

Sheldon, J., & Schumaker, J. B. (1985). *The Sentence Writing Strategy: Student Lessons.* Lawrence, KS: Edge Enterprises.

Swanson, H.L., & Hoskyn, M. (1998). Experimental intervention research on students with learning disabilities: A meta-analysis of treatment outcomes. *Review of Educational Research, 68,* 277–321.

Turnbull, H. R., & Turnbull, A. P. (1989). *Report of consensus: Conference on principles of family research,* Lawrence, KS: Bureau of Child Research.

Turnbull, R., Rainbolt, K., & Buchele-Ash, A. (1997). *Individuals with Disabilities Education Act: Digest of significance of 1997 amendments.* Lawrence, KS: Beach Center on Families and Disability

Van Reusen, T., Bos, C., Schumaker, J. B., & Deshler, D. D. (1994). *The Self-Advocacy Strategy: Instructor's manual.* Lawrence, KS: Edge Enterprises, Inc.

Van Reusen, A. K., Deshler, D. D., & Schumaker, J. B. (1989). Effects of a student participation strategy in facilitating the involvement of adolescents with learning disabilities in the individualized educational program planning process. *Learning Disabilities, 1*(2), 23–34.

Vernon, D. S., Schumaker, J. B., & Deshler, D.D. (1993). Who benefits from social skills instruction in the mainstream classroom? *Exceptionality Education Canada, 3*(1, 2), 9–38.

Vernon, D. S., & Schumaker, J. B. (1996). *The LEARN Strategy and the THINK Strategy: Cooperative Thinking Strategies in the classroom* (Continuation Repotr No. SBIR R44MH47211-04, National Institute of Mental Healyh). Lawerence, KS: Edge Enterptrises.

30

The Methods of Cluster Analysis and the Study of Learning Disabilities

Deborah L. Speece

Since the condition of learning disabilities (LD) has been recognized, researchers have sought methods to understand the apparent heterogeneity of skills in children with the disorder. Fletcher and colleagues (1997) traced clinical interest to the late 1800s and Morris, Blashfield, and Satz (1986) attributed the first empirical effort to 1969. Both clinical/rational and empirical methods have been applied to identify homogeneous subtypes of children and there are many examples of each approach to classification research in LD (e.g., Boder, 1973; Lyon, 1985; Morris et al., 1998; Speece, McKinney, & Appelbaum, 1985; Wolf & Bowers, 1999). Although there are good reasons to approach classification from a clinical/rational perspective (Torgesen, 1982), the purpose of this chapter is to review the methods of empirical subtyping known as cluster analysis. The specific goals of this chapter are to describe the details of the method, illustrate the application of cluster analysis methods by reference to research examples in LD, assess the contribution of cluster analysis investigations to the study of LD, and suggest future directions. The examples are drawn primarily from my own work but also include research by other investigators. As

such, the review of applied work is illustrative rather than exhaustive but is designed to cover the major methodological issues germane to using cluster analysis.

Part of the appeal of applying cluster analysis techniques to the study of LD is the possibility of making sense of a field that is beset by muddled constructs and definitional conundrums. It is frequently noted that LD is a multivariate phenomenon, but distinguishing the central attributes of the condition from important correlates has proven to be a difficult task (MacMillan, 1993). An apt analogy to the situation in LD was provided by Supreme Court Justice Potter Stewart in his discussion of pornography: "I shall not today attempt to define [pornography]. . . . But I know it when I see it" (*Jacobellis v. Ohio*, 378 U.S. 184 [1964], p. 8), retrieved from http://laws.findlaw.com/us/378/184.html 10/15/2001). Similarly, there is little doubt in many minds about the existence of LD, but our ability to identify the constructs and develop a coherent classification remains a goal rather than a reality.

Of course, a statistical method can only provide some of the tools needed by investigators to develop a coherent classification, and in this chapter I present and discuss the decisions required of the investigator. Cluster analysis is not a single method but, rather, encompasses a variety of approaches (Lorr, 1994). The present discussion is limited to hierarchical agglomerative methods in which each entity (in the present case, a child) starts as his or her own cluster and successive mergers are made until all participants are in a single cluster. Thus, there are always $n - 1$ possible cluster solutions and clusters will always be obtained. The investigator must decide, among other things, what point in the hierarchy best represents the true underlying structure of the data.

Skinner (1981) provided a framework for designing and evaluating classification research regardless of whether the approach was clinical or empirical. The three major elements of the framework are theory formulation, internal validity, and external validity. Theory formulation represents a number of issues including statement of theory guiding the investigation, purpose of the classification, and selection of subjects, variables, procedures, and similarity measures, the latter pertaining to how subjects/clusters will be evaluated as similar for successive mergers to be made. Internal validity refers to the replicability of the cluster solution, and it is at this stage that cluster analysis procedures may seem to be "black magic" (Jain & Dubes, 1988). A number of procedures have been used to determine the critical questions of whether clusters exist in the data and, if so, how many. External validation is often viewed as the most interesting phase because it is here that cluster differences are assessed for usefulness and meaning. It is also the stage at which analysis returns to more familiar ground for many researchers with the use, for example, of multivariate analysis of variance (MANOVA) or analyses of variance (ANOVA) to assess cluster differences.

A cluster analysis study that addresses each aspect of Skinner's (1981) framework would include the following design features: (1) subjects are selected from a known population and selection criteria are theoretically relevant; (2) both the classification variables and external validation procedures are theoretically based; (3) hypothesized subtypes are presented and the relationship of the subtypes to external validation procedures are proposed; (4) the investigator seri-ously considers the proposition that no clusters exist in the data set; (5) sample size is large enough to test proposed cluster solutions with a split sample (cross validation); and (6) external validation results are interpretable within the theoretical model. This design may exist in the larger literature on cluster analysis, but it does not yet exist in the cluster analysis literature on learning/reading disabilities. This does not mean that classification research using cluster analysis in LD has not yielded interpretable results. Rather, the quintessential study has yet to be conducted. The issues generated by Skinner's three-stage framework are reviewed next with examples from LD research.

Theory Formulation

Specification of Theory

Even though cluster analysis is primarily an exploratory technique (Everitt & Dunn, 1983), the theoretical or conceptual basis of the study needs to be stated explicitly, as cluster analysis techniques will always yield clusters even with random data. A theoretical or conceptual framework provides the basis to develop hypothesized subtypes that should be obtained. The hypothesized subtypes can then be used as guideposts to assist in selecting possible cluster solutions, providing some confidence that the cluster solution obtained represents a meaningful, as opposed to random, partition of the data. There is no need for complete specification of the number of clusters and expected profiles because interesting, unanticipated subtypes may emerge that lead to further development of theory.

In addition to hypothesized subtypes, theory should also guide predictions about cluster differences (external validation). It is not rare for more recent investigations to offer hypothesized subtypes, but the external validation procedures are often not linked to theory on an *a priori* basis. Rather, the selection of procedures and the explanation of cluster differences have a decidedly post hoc flavor. Although this approach is often convincing, it is not a strong position. An exception to this criticism was provided by Feagans and Appelbaum (1986) in their study of oral-language subtypes of children with LD. They presented a conceptual basis for expecting a narrative language subtype and further specified that children with strong narrative skill also would exhibit better achievement, especially reading comprehension. Their hypotheses were confirmed: two narrative subtypes were identified and exhibited higher academic achievement compared to the other four subtypes across 3 years.

In a study of unselected kindergarten children, Speece, Roth, Cooper, and De La Paz (1999) hypothesized two oral-language subtypes, one representing narrative skills (based on Feagans & Appelbaum, 1986) and one representing phonological awareness skills based on the extant literature documenting the importance of this skill for early reading. They also predicted that if the subtypes were obtained, a subtype with strong phonological skills should also demonstrate better skills on word reading and spelling measures whereas a strong narrative subtype should exhibit better skills in listening comprehension. The proposed subtypes were obtained with mixed external validation results. The strong phonological subtype (which also had higher oral-language skills overall) did exhibit better reading and spelling skills compared to the other subtypes, but the strong narrative subtype had higher listening comprehension scores only in comparison to a subtype with low overall language skill. These results suggested that oral-language skills may not have a uniform influence on literacy skills, which is contrary to conventional wisdom of strong linkages between oral language and literacy.

Purpose

The purpose of a classification study guides selection of external validation procedures and is also tied to selection of subjects and classification measures. Classification systems may promote either communication with practitioners or prediction which is more related to scientific goals (Blashfield & Draguns, 1976). Blashfield and Draguns noted that these goals are in opposition because communication necessitates simplicity and ease of implementation, whereas prediction requires complexity and flexibility to examine scientific tenets. Both purposes

are equally important. The work in LD, either implicitly or explicitly, has pursued predictive purposes rather than communication. Investigations in LD usually identify multiple subtypes and explore the external validity of cluster solutions by examining cluster differences on an independent set of measures. For example, Speece and colleagues (1985) identified seven behavioral subtypes based on general education teachers' ratings and validated cluster differences on special education teacher ratings and observed classroom behavior. Morris and colleagues (1998) identified 10 cognitive/linguistic subtypes and used a variety of measures to validate them. The point is that there are usually too many subtypes identified to be useful in practice and external validation procedures are not typically related to practice.

Participants

As with any study, the issue here is the extent to which the results can be generalized to a known population. The interpretation of early classification work in LD is hampered by the use of school-identified samples, the problems of which are well known (Keogh & MacMillan, 1983; MacMillan & Speece, 1999). In some instances, the results with school-identified samples are theoretically compelling (e.g., Feagans & Appelbaum, 1986), and in others they provide hypotheses for further work (e.g., McKinney & Speece, 1986). In general, however, these types of studies demonstrate the feasibility of cluster analysis methods rather than provide generalizable classifications. One exception is the analysis of the Florida Longitudinal data set by Satz and Morris (1981). In that study an unselected group of males was used in a cluster analysis to identify subtypes with LD, thus avoiding several problems related to selection bias. Similarly, Speece and colleagues (1999) used an unselected group of kindergarten children in their study of oral-language subtypes and reading. When the goal of the study is more narrowly focused on subtypes of children with LD rather than identifying subtypes in the general population, care must be exercised in the definition and selection of subjects. Morris and colleagues (1998) used research criteria to define children as reading disabled rather than rely on school identification procedures.

Classification Measures

A problem with some cluster analysis studies is that they represent a secondary analysis of an existing database. At issue is not the secondary analysis per se but, rather, the limitations imposed on sample definition and variable selection for both classification and external validity procedures. Several studies have been designed specifically as classification investigations which provide more freedom to select a coherent set of classification variables. Speece (1987) selected classification variables using an information-processing theoretical model for a study of reading disabilities and Speece and Cooper (1990) used a multiple domain approach (achievement, behavior, intelligence, and language) to classify at-risk and normally developing children.

Another issue is the number of variables to use. More is not necessarily better. There is no rule for subject-to-variable ratios as with some statistical methods (e.g., factor analysis) but unnecessary variables may add noise to the results, making it difficult to identify the structure if there is one (Milligan & Cooper, 1987). Using a Monte Carlo comparison of clustering algorithms, Price (1993) found that increasing the number of variables decreased the detectability of clusters and advised limiting variables to the smallest set possible.

Similarity Measures and Clustering Algorithms

Skinner (1981) placed the selection of similarity measure and algorithm under the internal validation stage of a classification study. However, these decisions are placed under theory formulation for the present discussion to emphasize the point that knowledge of the conceptual basis of the study can assist in making the appropriate decisions.

Similarity measures define *how* two entities will be judged as similar, and the cluster algorithm defines *why* these mergers are made. There are hundreds of similarity measures and algorithms (Blashfield & Aldenderfer, 1988), but the discussion can be simplified to a few defining issues. Regarding similarity measures, Cronbach and Gleser (1953) demonstrated that profiles contain three pieces of information: shape (i.e., the "ups and downs" of a profile), scatter (i.e., variation among profile points), and elevation (mean level of performance across the profile). Correlational similarity measures yield clusters based on shape, whereas distance similarity measures incorporate all three pieces of information (Skinner, 1978).

Operationally, a correlation similarity measure removes the mean and standard deviation from each profile to produce "shape" clusters, whereas a distance metric uses the original form of the data, usually standardized. A problem with distance measures is that shape, scatter, and elevation are confounded and may differentially affect cluster formation. Adams (1985) suggested that correlation may be useful in situations in which the sample has relatively low (or high) performance, which may be the case for a sample with reading/learning disabilities. This approach was used in a study of children with reading disabilities (Speece, 1987) and produced six subtypes based on information-processing variables. Skinner (1978) proposed that data first be evaluated according to shape with the resulting clusters reanalyzed by including scatter and elevation to determine the relative importance of these elements. This procedure was incorporated in two studies (Speece & Cooper, 1990; Speece et al., 1999). In both cases the "shape" clusters, although internally valid, did not yield meaningful profiles, but each produced an interpretable split when scatter and elevation data were evaluated. Figure 30.1 depicts the final six-cluster solution for the Speece and Cooper study. Each pair of clusters (i.e., 1–2, 3–4, 5–6) was formed by the split of the shape clusters. Examination of the profiles for each pair shows that the shape of each profile is similar while differing on elevation across the classification variables. Clusters 2, 3, and 5 were interpreted as variations on normal performance whereas cluster 1 was indicative of an LD profile, cluster 4 was suggestive of mild mental retardation, and cluster 6 was suggestive of deficient language processing. This study is presented in more depth in a later section of the chapter.

Choice of an algorithm is closely tied to

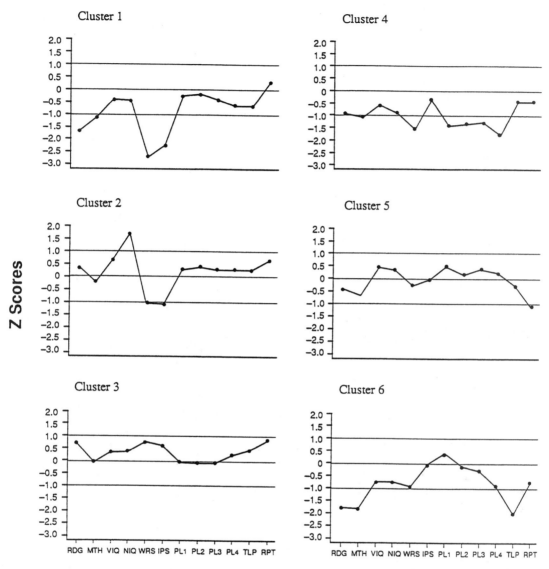

FIGURE 30.1. Mean profiles of clusters across the classification variables. RDG, reading achievement; MTH, math achievement; VIQ, verbal intelligence; NIQ, nonverbal intelligence; WRS, rating of work-related skills; IPS, rating of interpersonal skills; PL1–PL4, level of scores on Preschool Language Assessment Instrument; TLP, total prompts on Dynamic Assessment Task; RPT, residual posttest gain score on Dynamic Assessment Task. Odds ratios for Clusters 1 through 6 are 252.0, 27.0, 1.0, 43.2, 7.7, and 31.5, respectively. From Speece and Cooper (1990). Copyright 1990 by the American Educational Research Association. Reprinted by permission.

the similarity measure and Blashfield and Aldenderfer (1988) provided an extended discussion of algorithms. Applied researchers are limited generally to algorithms available in statistical software programs (e.g., SAS and SPSS), but a variety of algorithms are available and they tend to be the ones evaluated in the methodological literature. In this regard, average linkage, complete linkage, and Ward's (1963) minimum-variance algorithms are reasonable choices. The average linkage method combines entities such that members in one cluster have a greater mean similarity to each other than with all members in another cluster. With complete linkage, members of clusters are more similar to each other than to members of any other cluster. Ward's method joins members based on minimizing within cluster variance. One issue to consider is how the algorithms perform with similarity measures. With respect to recovering known structure in a data set (Monte Carlo studies), Ward's method performs best with a distance metric, whereas average linkage provides best recovery with correlation as the similarity measure (Lorr, 1983; Scheibler & Schnneider, 1985). Morey, Blashfield, and Skinner (1983) reported similar findings with a real data set with the additional finding that Ward's method with Euclidean distance provided the best discriminatory power across methods.

The careful investigator must exert some caution in using these recommendations by investigating the influence of shape, scatter, and elevation and the performance of several algorithms. This is because the recommendations by methodologists are based primarily on analyses of data sets with known structures, which is not the case in applied situations.

Internal Validity

Having addressed the multiple issues prompted by the theory formulation, the next stage of analysis requires attention to the following questions: (1) are there clusters in the data set, (2) if so, how many, and (3) can they be replicated? These questions represent the most difficult phase of cluster analysis. The reason internal validation is difficult is because there is no safety net such as an F ratio or effect size estimate to protect the investigator from drawing foolish conclusions. The importance of good internal validity procedures was illustrated by Golden and Meehl (1980). They designed a study to test cluster analysis methods by attempting to detect biological sex via MMPI responses known to provide excellent discrimination between females and males. Of the six clustering methods evaluated, only three were judged as producing accurate partitions of the data. These findings, of course, did not bode well for the method, leading the authors to call for the development of consistency (internal validation) tests.

Number of Clusters

After the publication of the Golden and Meehl (1980) study, Milligan and Cooper (1985) evaluated the effectiveness of 30 statistical stopping rules in recovering the correct number of clusters. Three of the six best performing rules are incorporated in SAS (1999) and are referred to in the SAS manual as the pseudo F statistic, the pseudo t^2 statistic, and the Cubic Clustering Criterion. These rules serve as guidance functions to determine if clusters exist and how many may be viable. The downside of these procedures is threefold. First, the evaluation was based on a simulated data set with a known structure (Milligan & Cooper, 1985). Second, the evaluation was based on clustering with Euclidean distance so performance with other similarity measures is unknown. Third, the tests are conservative; whereas significant tests provide confidence that clusters exist, nonsignificant tests do not rule out the presence of clusters (Duda & Hart, 1973; Hawkins, Muller, & ten Krooden, 1982; Sarle, 1983). Even though these stopping rules are not perfect, Duda and Hart (1973) suggested that a "suspicious test is better than none" (p. 244). Early subtyping work in learning disabilities did not incorporate these methods, but more recent applied work has taken advantage of the stopping rules (e.g., Speece & Cooper, 1990; Speece et al., 1999).

In conjunction with the stopping rules, a good practice is to analyze a data set with several algorithms to get a sense of how many clusters may be present. Ward's method, complete linkage, and average linkage typically are used. The logic underlying this procedure is that a cluster structure should not be algorithm dependent even though the algorithms use different rules for joining entities (Anderberg, 1973; Johnson & Wichern, 1982; Lorr, 1983). In practice, convergence on the number of clusters problem at this point is rare, but the procedure is helpful in narrowing the possibilities. Graphing the data is an indispensible method for examining clusters. Mean profiles across the variables used for classification can be plotted to assist in interpreting, for example, differences between a four- and five-cluster solution. Another technique is to plot cluster members (or cluster centroids) by the canonical discriminant functions derived from the data set to examine separation. Figure 30.2 represents such a plot for a three-cluster solution from the Speece and Cooper (1990) study. Morris and colleagues (1998) provided an example using cluster centroids.

After some determination is made on candidate solutions (generally several solutions are carried forward to the replication phase), it is necessary to assess correct cluster membership. Hierarchical techniques do not reassign members as the analysis proceeds, so it is possible that some members may have a better fit with another cluster. To test this possibility, a discriminant function can be derived for each cluster and the sample members can be "forcasted" into each cluster based on the fit of the data with the discriminant function. This procedure provides an index called posterior probability of membership in each cluster. Reassignment is necessary when membership probability is higher for a cluster other than for the original assignment. This general approach, outlined by Field and Shoenfeldt (1975), also has provided useful descriptive information on cluster membership of normally achieving children (Speece et al.,

1985) and longitudinal subtype stability (McKinney & Speece, 1986). Another method to determine correct membership uses the k-means iterative clustering procedure, which is a nonhierarchical technique and requires the specification of the number of subtypes. The k-means procedure uses the centroids from the hierarchical solution to form clusters and membership agreement can be assessed between the two solutions (e.g., Morris et al., 1998; Speece & Cooper, 1990).

Replication

Because of the uncertainty associated with the statistical stopping rules, replication of a cluster structure is a requirement. Two types of replication are apparent in the literature in LD: single-sample and split-sample techniques. Single-sample methods are not as powerful and are used when sample size is small. Typically, a subset of the original sample is reclustered using procedures invoked with the full sample and membership agreement between the subsample and full sample is assessed with the kappa or Rand statistic. Another technique is to add sub-

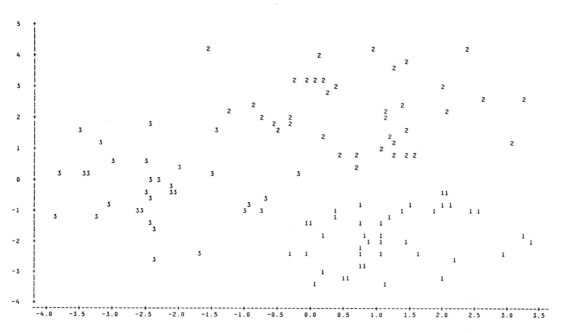

FIGURE 30.2. Two-dimensional represenation of a three-cluster solution based on performance of 112 first-grade children. From Speece (1993). Copyright 1993 by Paul H. Brookes. Reprinted by permission.

jects (e.g., normally achieving children added to original sample of children with LD) and recluster the larger sample. The addition of "noise" to the data set should not disturb the original solution if clusters are stable (Morris et al., 1998; Speece, 1987).

A powerful method of replication is to use two samples (or a split sample), each subjected to cluster analysis procedures and results for each sample compared (McIntyre & Blashfield, 1980; Morey et al., 1983). Conceptually this entails clustering samples A and B, assigning members from B to A based on A's classification functions and comparing the membership concordance between the actual and forecasted results for sample B. Applied examples of this technique can be found in the Morey and colleagues (1983) and Speece and Cooper (1990) papers. Breckenridge (1989) extended the method by recommending a double cross-validation procedure. In addition to the foregoing sequence, the results would also be examined when the order is reversed (i.e., B-A-B).

Although possibly obvious at this point, it is important to state what does not constitute evidence of internal validity: assessing cluster differences on the variables used for classification. The logic is intuitive—as cluster analysis forms groups of subjects based on similarity across the classification variables, cluster differences on these variables are a forgone conclusion. In the odd circumstance that differences are not obtained, it is safe to say the solution is not functional.

External Validity

Skinner (1981) proposed that external validation could be evaluated by three types of validity procedures: predictive (differential response to treatment), descriptive (differentiation of clusters across variables that are independent of the classification variables), and clinical (membership agreement between clusters and clinical judgment). Typically, cluster analysis studies in LD focus on descriptive validation. However, Lyon (1985) provided initial data on the validity of reading disability subtypes by examining response to instruction. Speece and colleagues (1999) examined the clinical validity of oral-language subtypes by developing

descriptive summaries of the four language profiles and asking the children's teachers to classify the children into one of the four clusters (high average, low average, high narrative, low overall). The teachers reliably classified the children, but this agreement with empirical classifications was modest. The teachers were best able to identify children in the high average cluster and, to a lesser extent, the low overall cluster but had difficulty identifying children in the other two subtypes. These clinical validity data supported the descriptive validity results that incorporated reading and spelling variables not used in the cluster analysis.

There are many examples of descriptive validation efforts in the LD literature (e.g., Feagans & Appelbaum, 1986; Lyon, Stewart, & Freedman, 1982; Morris et al., 1986, 1998). The validation procedures used by Speece and Cooper (1990) with the clusters depicted in Figure 30.1 are described in detail to provide a sense of the method.

The sample was composed of 112 first-grade children, 63 deemed at risk for school failure and 49 normally achieving children. The classification measures included reading and math achievement, teacher ratings of work-related and interpersonal skills, four levels of classroom discourse skills that represented increasing cognitive complexity, and two measures of learning potential (response to instruction) operationalized by performance on a dynamic assessment task. In this study, the external validation of the subtypes was examined by (1) comparison on a set of achievement variables not used in clustering, (2) relative risk analysis, and (3) observed classroom behavior. The analysis of the achievement variables was conducted for each pair of clusters (1–2, 3–4, 5–6) and confirmed that the profiles associated with normal performance (clusters 2, 3, 5) had significantly higher achievement than the atypical profiles. The relative risk analysis assessed the extent to which membership in a cluster was associated with elevated risk of teacher referral to a teacher assistance team, a preliminary step to referral for identification for special education services. This analysis produces an odds ratio for each cluster (reported for each cluster in the caption for Figure 30.1) and is interpreted as the increased risk, compared to cluster 3 (baseline cluster), of being referred. For example, the odds ratio (OR) of 257 associated with the LD profile (cluster 1) means that the risk of referral is 257 times that of the profile for the normal cluster (cluster 3). With the exception of cluster 5, each was significant. In addition, the risk associated with the LD profile was significantly greater than the risk for the other four clusters. Similarly, the OR for cluster 5 was significantly lower.

The children also were observed in their classrooms and two composites of classroom behavior, academic responding and inappropriate responding, were used to assess cluster differences. Here we were interested in differences among the clusters with normal variation (clusters 2, 3, and 5) and among the atypical profiles. Of most interest to the present discussion are contrasts among the atypical profiles. The LD profile (cluster 1) exhibited less academic and more inappropriate behavior than did the language disability profile (cluster 6). This may be a key to the elevated risk of referral for cluster 1 and coincides with the extremely low teacher ratings of work-related skills (WRS) and interpersonal skills (IPS) in addition to low achievement evident in the profile of classification variables. The profiles associated with mild mental retardation (cluster 4) and language disability (cluster 6) did not differ on academic responding, but cluster 4 was more inappropriate then cluster 6.

In a second study, Cooper and Speece (1990) examined a more complex rendering of observed classroom behavior and included a third cohort of children who were assigned to one of the six original clusters by the forecasting method described previously. Eight composite ecological arrangements were developed and risk for special education placement was assessed for at-risk children in each cluster and each behavioral composite. The LD profile was at significantly greater risk of placement when children received fewer opportunities to read in a small group. Two nonsignificant trends of elevated risk for this cluster were associated with higher frequencies of classroom arrangements that featured independent work. Independent of cluster membership, exposure to higher levels of independent work time was a significant risk factor for the sample. To summarize, external valida-

tion evidence for the identified clusters was obtained using an extensive and multivariate approach that included both individual differences and contextual variables.

Assessing the Contribution of Empirical Subtyping to the Study of Learning Disabilities

When I was asked by the editors to write a chapter on cluster analysis my first reaction was, "Are you sure you want one? I don't think anyone is doing it anymore." I said this despite my own recent work using the method and knowledge of the paper by Robin Morris and his colleagues (1998). To check my perception that use of cluster analysis in applied contexts had declined, I conducted some electronic searches using the PsycINFO database. The search was divided into decades (1970–1979; 1980–1989; and 1990–2001) and only journal articles were requested. Using the terms "cluster analysis" and "reading disabilities," 0, 8, and 7 articles were uncovered by decade, respectively. Broadening the parameters to cluster analysis and LD produced somewhat higher numbers: 0, 18, and 22 articles. More inclusive terms, "cluster analysis" and "learning," produced 9, 46, and 102 papers by decade. It would seem then that the use of cluster analysis, while infrequent in the reading and LD literature, has at least remained steady and increased in other educational areas. My initial perception appeared more related to the fact that my current interests in classification would be considered to be in the rational, as compared to empirical, realm (e.g., Speece & Case, 2001).

What may account for the infrequent use of cluster analysis in the LD literature? There are several possibilities. First, as is evident in this chapter, cluster analysis using hierarchical, agglomerative methods is a complicated process. Surprisingly, an advanced statistical text written by an expert in cluster analysis devoted only part of a chapter to the method (Everitt, 1996). It appears that graduate statistics courses in education and psychology may not provide detailed exposure to the method. Thus, the interested user needs to seek other means of instruction. Of course, it is possible for anyone with some knowledge of a statistical software package to produce clusters, but the use of the default methods programmed in statistical packages comes with a great deal of risk to the integrity of the results.

A second reason may be the sheer amount of work required and the uncertainty experienced particularly in the internal validation stage of analysis. Morris and colleagues (1998) described the process as requiring "painstaking scrutiny" (p. 370). Although users of cluster analysis techniques are no more noble than other researchers, competent use does require acceptance of the possibility that no clusters exist in the data, that several solutions may be plausible, and that conceptual clarity is rarely achieved.

A third reason offered by Fletcher and colleagues (1997)in their review of subtypes of dyslexia is that the work has had little impact on research in reading disabilities, a conclusion that can be generalized to work in LD. This conclusion is due to all that has been discussed in this chapter but can be reduced to the importance of a theoretical framework guiding the study. The need for a sound, theoretically driven classification model of LD is acute, but, so far, we have not been up to the task. For example, it is now clear that discrepancies between intelligence and achievement do not provide good coverage of reading disabilities (e.g., Fletcher et al., 1994; Speece & Case, 2001) but the critical classification variables have yet to be determined. Even though advances have been made in understanding early reading failure, the bulk of this evidence is limited to word reading in young children with little attention to comprehension or older readers. Part of the problem is our newness as a field. Even though interest in the study of LD has at least a 100-year history (Torgesen, 1998) progress is slow and we have had to overcome our share of false starts (Lyon, 1987).

Another possible reason for lack of impact is that researchers use methods that produce mutually exclusive clusters when overlapping cluster structure may be a better representation of the data. Lorr (1994) noted that overlap is a feature of classification in psychiatry, but this possibility has not been studied via cluster analysis in LD even though clinical experience would suggest this position is viable. Take, for example, the issue of classroom behavior and the potential correspondence with attention deficit disorder (ADD). Examination of the profile of cluster 1 in Figure 30.1 shows that, in addition to low achievement, children in this cluster also received extremely low teacher ratings on behavior (WRS, IPS). It may be that this cluster of children represents an overlap with ADD, a possibility that cannot be evaluated with the data set but should be considered in future studies. Entertaining the possibility that clusters overlap may be one method of better representing the structure of the population of children with learning disabilities. Gordon (1999) provided detail on these methods of cluster analysis.

Summary and Conclusions

Cluster analysis represents one tool needed by researchers interested in the classification of children who experience learning problems. The methods are complex and it is necessary to seek converging evidence to support the number of clusters thought to be present in the data. Although there is no definitive statistical model to guide these analyses, the methods outlined in this chapter and elaborated in the methodological literature cited can provide some confidence in the results. The applied research in the field of LD, whether within or across domains, has provided insights into the multivariate nature of LD.

However, a frank appraisal of the extant empirical subtyping research would lead to the conclusion that these studies have not had a great deal of influence on the field. In addition to the need for theory, rather than method, to drive the investigation, Skinner and Blashfield (1982) identified several other factors that may limit the impact of cluster analysis research. Two that are particularly relevant to research in LD are (1) that the research base is represented primarily by single studies rather than programmatic efforts in classification and (2) lack of integration with clinical practice.

These issues have more to do with the conceptualization of the research problem than with the method. Practitioners as well as researchers require convincing evidence that subtypes have meaning beyond the narrow boundaries drawn by users of cluster analysis. There is little research that examines the utility of a classification in terms of instructional or classroom factors (see Speece, 1993, for expansion of this idea). Predictive (response to treatment) and clinical validity efforts will need to be included in a comprehensive framework to extend the usefulness of results from cluster analysis investigations.

Efforts in this direction could be accelerated by sharing classification functions among investigators (Speece & Cooper, 1991). Because of the time required to complete a cluster analysis study and because of developmental processes, it is likely that the participants from the original sample may present different profiles by the time the cluster structure is validated descriptively. For example, the longitudinal analysis of the behavioral subtypes identified by Speece and colleagues (1985) indicated that children moved into more maladaptive subtypes over time (McKinney & Speece, 1986). Thus, further intervention validation efforts on the original sample may not be appropriate. However, another sample could be drawn, measured on the same variables or constructs, and cluster membership determined by the forecasting methods described earlier in the chapter. This approach could extend validation efforts to other investigators who may be more interested in instructional validation than in the derivation of subtypes (Speece & Cooper, 1991).

The best work in classification of LD using empirical methods is ahead of us. Careful examination of the strengths and limitations of previous work will assist in the development of coherent, relevant, and meaningful classifications.

Acknowledgment

Portions of this chapter were based on Speece (1990, 1994–95).

References

Adams, K. M. (1985). Theoretical, methodological, and statistical issues. In B. P. Rourke (Ed.), *Neuropsychology of learning disabilities: Essentials of subtype analysis* (pp. 17–39). New York: Guilford Press.

Anderberg, M. R. (1973). *Cluster analysis for applications.* New York: Academic Press.

Blashfield, R. K., & Aldenderfer, M. S. (1988). The methods and problems of cluster analysis. In J. R. Nesselroade & R. B. Cattell (Eds.), *Handbook of multivariate experimental psychology* (2nd ed., pp. 447–473). New York: Plenum Press.

Blashfield, R. K., & Draguns, J. G. (1976). Evaluative criterion for psychiatric classification. *Journal of Abnormal Psychology, 85,* 140–150.

Boder, E. (1973). Developmental dyslexia: A diagnostic approach based on three atypical reading-spelling patterns. *Developmental Medicine and Child Neurology, 15,* 663–687.

Breckenridge, J. N. (1989). Replicating cluster analysis: Method, consistency, and validity. *Multivariate Behavioral Research, 24,* 147–161.

Cooper, D. H., & Speece, D. L. (1990). Maintaining at-risk children in regular education settings: Initial effects of individual differences and classroom environments. *Exceptional Children, 57,* 117–126.

Cronbach, L. J., & Gleser, G. C. (1953). Assessing similarity between profiles. *Psychological Bulletin, 50,* 456–473.

Duda, R. O., & Hart, P. E. (1973). *Pattern classification and scene analysis.* New York: Wiley.

Everitt, B. S. (1996). *Making sense of statistics in psychology: A second-level course.* New York: Oxford University Press.

Everitt, B. S., & Dunn, G. (1983). *Advanced methods of data exploration and modelling.* London: Heinemann.

Feagans, L., & Appelbaum, M. I. (1986). Validation of language subtypes of learning disabled children. *Journal of Educational Psychology, 78,* 358–364.

Field, H. S., & Schoenfeldt, L. F. (1975). Ward and Hook revisited: A two-part procedure for overcoming a deficiency in the grouping of persons. *Educational and Psychological Measurement, 35,* 171–173.

Fletcher, J. M., Morris, R., Lyon, G. R., Stuebing, K. K., Shaywitz, S. E., Shankweiler, D. P., Katz, L., & Shaywitz, B. A. (1997). Subtypes of dyslexia: An old problem revisited. In B. Blachman (Ed.), *Foundations of reading acquisition and dyslexia* (pp. 95–114). Mahwah, NJ: Erlbaum.

Fletcher, J. M., Shaywitz, S. E., Shankweiler, D. P., Katz, L., Liberman, I. Y. Stuebing, K. K., Francis, D. J., Fowler, A. E., & Shaywitz, B. A. (1994). Cognitive profiles of reading disabilities: Comparisons of discrepancy and low achievement definitions. *Journal of Educational Psychology, 86,* 6–23.

Golden, R. R., & Meehl, P. E. (1980). Detection of biological sex: An empirical test of cluster methods. *Multivariate Behavioral Research, 15,* 475–496.

Gordon, A. D. (1999). *Classification* (2nd ed.). New York: Chapman & Hall/CRC.

Hawkins, D. M., Muller, M. W., & ten Krooden, J. A. (1982). Cluster analysis. In D. M. Hawkins

(Ed.), *Topics in applied multivariate analysis* (pp. 303–356). Cambridge, UK: Cambridge University Press.

Jacobellis v. Ohio, 378 U.S. 184, (1964), retrieved from *http://laws.findlaw.com/us/378/184.html* on 10/15/2001.

Jain, A. K., & Dubes, R. C. (1988). *Algorithms for clustering data.* Englewood Cliffs, NJ: Prentice Hall.

Johnson, R. A., & Wichern, D. W. (1982). *Applied multivariate techniques.* Englewood Cliffs, NJ: Prentice Hall.

Keogh, B. K., & MacMillan, D. L. (1983). The logic of sample selection: Who represents what? *Exceptional Education Quarterly, 4,* 84–96.

Lorr, M. (1983). *Cluster analysis for social scientists.* San Francisco: Jossey-Bass.

Lorr, M. (1994). Cluster analysis: Aims, methods, and problems. In S. Strack & M. Lorr (Eds.), *Differentiating normal and abnormal personality* (pp. 179–195). New York: Springer.

Lyon, G. R. (1985). Educational validation studies of learning disability subtypes. In B. P. Rourke (Ed.), *Neuropsychology of learning disabilities: Essentials of subtype analysis* (pp. 228–253). New York: Guilford Press.

Lyon, G. R. (1987). Learning disabilities research: False starts and broken promises. In S. Vaughn & C. S. Bos (Eds.), *Research in learning disabilities: Issues and future directions* (pp. 69–80). Boston: College-Hill Press.

Lyon, G. R., Stewart, N., & Freedman, D. (1982). Neuropsychological characteristics of empirically derived subgroups of learning disabled readers. *Journal of Clinical Neuropsychology, 4,* 343–365.

MacMillan, D. L. (1993). Development of operational definitions in mental retardation: Similarities and differences with the field of learning disabilities. In G. R. Lyon, D. B. Gray, J. F. Kavanaugh, & N. A. Krasnegor (Eds.), *Better understanding learning disabilities: New views from research and their implications for education and public policies* (pp. 117–152). Baltimore: Brookes.

MacMillan, D. L., & Speece, D. L. (1999). Utility of current diagnostic categories for research and practice. In R. Gallimore, L. Bernheimer, D. L. MacMillan, D. L. Speece, & R. R. Vaughn (Eds.), *Developmental perspectives on children with high incidence disabilities* (pp. 111–133). Mahwah, NJ: Erlbaum.

McIntrye, R. M., & Blashfield, R. K. (1980). A nearest centroid technique for evaluating the minimum variance clustering procedure. *Multivariate Behavioral Research, 15,* 225–238.

McKinney, J. D., & Speece, D. L. (1986). Academic consequences and longitudinal stability of behavioral subtypes of learning disabled children. *Journal of Educational Psychology, 78,* 365–372.

Milligan, G. W., & Cooper, M. C. (1985). An examination of procedures for determining the number of clusters in a data set. *Psychometrika, 50,* 159–179.

Milligan, G. W., & Cooper, M. C. (1987). Methodology review: Clustering methods. *Applied Psychological Measurement, 11,* 329–354.

Morey, L. C., Blashfield, R. K., & Skinner, H. A. (1983). A comparison of cluster analysis techniques within a sequential validation framework. *Multivariate Behavioral Research, 18,* 309–329.

Morris, R., Blashfield, R. K., & Satz, P. (1986). Developmental classification of learning disabled children. *Journal of Clinical and Experimental Neuropsychology, 8,* 371–392.

Morris, R. D., Stuebing, K. K., Fletcher, J. M., Shaywitz, S. E., Lyon, G. R., Shankweiler, D. P., Katz, L., Francis, D. J., & Shaywitz, B. E. (1998). Subtypes of reading disability: Variability around a phonological core. *Journal of Educational Psychology, 90,* 347–373.

Price, L. J. (1993). Identifying cluster overlap with NORMIX population membership probabilities. *Multivariate Behavioral Research, 8,* 235–262.

Sarle, W. S. (1983). *Cubic clustering criterion* (SAS Technical Report No. A-108). Cary, NC: SAS Institute.

SAS Institute (1999). *SAS/STAT User's guide: Version 8 Edition.* Cary, NC: Author.

Satz, P., & Morris, R. (1981). Learning disability subtypes: A review. In F.J. Pirozzolo & M. C. Wittrock (Eds.), *Neuropsycholoqical and cognitive processes in reading* (pp. 109–141). New York: Academic Press.

Scheibler, D., & Schneider, W. (1985). Monte Carlo tests of the accuracy of cluster analysis algorithms: A comparison of hierarchical and nonhierarchical methods. *Multivariate Behavioral Research, 20,* 283–304.

Skinner, H. A. (1978). Differentiating the contribution of elevation, scatter, and shape in profile similarity. *Educational and Psycholoqical Measurement, 38,* 297–308.

Skinner, H. A. (1981). Toward the integration of classification theory and methods. *Journal of Abnormal Psychology, 20,* 68–87.

Skinner, H. A., & Blashfield, R. K. (1982). Increasing the impact of cluster analysis research: The case of psychiatric classification. *Journal of Consulting and Clinical Psychology, 50,* 727–735.

Speece, D. L. (1987). Information processing subtypes of learning disabled readers. *Learning Disabilities Research, 2,* 91–102.

Speece, D. L. (1993). Broadening the scope of classification research: Conceptual and ecological perspectives. In G. R. Lyon, D. B. Gray, J. F. Kavanaugh, & N. A. Krasnegor (Eds.), *Better understanding learning disabilities: New views from research and their implications for education and public policy* (pp. 57–72). Baltimore: Brookes.

Speece, D. L., & Case, L. P. (2001). Classification in context: An alternative approach to identifying early reading disability. *Journal of Educational Psychology, 93,* 735–749.

Speece, D. L., & Cooper, D. H. (1990). Ontogeny of school failure: Classification of first grade children at risk. *American Educational Research Journal, 27,* 119–140.

Speece, D. L., & Cooper, D. H. (1991). Retreat, regroup or advance? An agenda for empirical classification research in learning disabilities X. In L.V. Feagans, E.J. Short, & L. Meltzer (Eds.), *Subtypes of learninq disabilities: Theoretical perspectives and research* (pp. 33–52). Hillsdale, NJ: Erlbaum.

Speece, D. L., McKinney, J. D., & Appelbaum, M. I. (1985). Classification and validation of behavioral subtypes of learning-disabled children. *Journal of Educational Psychology, 77,* 67–77.

Speece, D. L., Roth, F. P., Cooper, D. H., & De La Paz, S. (1999). The relevance of oral language skills in early literacy: A multivariate analysis. *Applied Psycholinguistics, 20,* 167–190.

Torgesen, J. K. (1982). The use of rationally defined subgroups in research on learning disabilities. In J. P. Das, R. F. Mulcahy, & A. E. Wall (Eds.), *Theory and research in learning disabilities* (pp. 111–131). New York: Plenum Press.

Torgesen, J. K. (1998). Learning disabilities: An historical and conceptual overview. In B. Y. L. Wong (Ed.), *Learning about learning disabilities* (pp. 3–34). San Diego, CA: Academic Press.

Ward, J. H. (1963). Hierarchical grouping to optimize an objective function. *Journal of the American Statistical Association, 58,* 236–244.

Wolf, M., & Bowers, P. G. (1999). The double-deficit hypothesis for the developmental dyslexias. *Journal of Educational Psychology, 91,* 415–438.

31

Neurobiological Indices of Dyslexia

Sally E. Shaywitz
Bennett A. Shaywitz

Dyslexia is characterized by an unexpected difficulty in reading in children and adults who otherwise possess the intelligence, motivation, and schooling considered necessary for accurate and fluent reading (S. E. Shaywitz, 1998, 2003). Recent epidemiological data indicate that, like hypertension and obesity, dyslexia fits a dimensional model. In other words, within the population, reading ability and reading disability occur along a continuum, with reading disability representing the lower tail of a normal distribution of reading ability (Gilger, Borecki, Smith, DeFries, & Pennington, 1996; S. Shaywitz, Escobar, Shaywitz, Fletcher, & Makuch, 1992).

Dyslexia is perhaps the most common neurobehavioral disorder affecting children, with prevalence rates ranging from 5–10% in clinic- and school-identified samples to 17.5% in unselected population-based samples (S. E. Shaywitz, 1998). Previously, it was believed that dyslexia affected boys primarily (Finucci & Childs, 1981); however, more recent data indicate similar numbers of affected boys and girls (Flynn & Rahbar, 1994; S. Shaywitz, Shaywitz, Fletcher, & Escobar, 1990; Wadsworth, DeFries,

Stevenson, Gilger, & Pennington, 1992). Longitudinal studies, both prospective (Francis, Shaywitz, Stuebing, Shaywitz, & Fletcher, 1996; B. A. Shaywitz, Holford, et al., 1995) and retrospective (Bruck, 1992; Felton, Naylor, & Wood, 1990; Scarborough, 1984), indicate that dyslexia is a persistent, chronic condition; it does not represent a transient "developmental lag" (Figure 31.1). Over time, poor readers and good readers tend to maintain their relative positions along the spectrum of reading ability (B. A. Shaywitz, Holford, et al., 1995).

Dyslexia is both familial and heritable (Pennington & Gilger, 1996). Family history is one of the most important risk factors, with 23% to as many as 65% of children who have a parent with dyslexia reported to have the disorder (Scarborough, 1990). A rate among siblings of affected persons of approximately 40% and among parents ranging from 27 to 49% (Pennington & Gilger, 1996) provides opportunities for early identification of affected siblings and often for delayed but helpful identification of affected adults. Replicated linkage studies implicate loci on chromosomes 2, 3, 6,

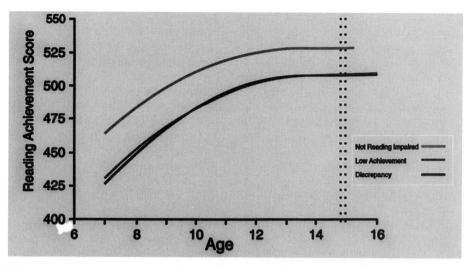

FIGURE 31.1. Trajectory of reading skills over time in readers who are nonimpaired and those who are dyslexic. Ordinate is Rasch scores (W scores) from the Woodcock–Johnson reading test (Woodcock & Johnson, 1989) and abscissa is age in years. Both readers who are dyslexic and those who are nonimpaired improve their reading scores as they get older, but the gap between the readers who are dyslexic and those who are nonimpaired remains. Thus dyslexia is a deficit and not a developmental lag. Data from Francis et al. (1996). Copyright 2002 by Sally Shaywitz.

15, and 18 (Fisher & DeFries, 2002) for the transmission of phonological awareness deficits and subsequent reading problems. Whether the differences in the genetic loci represent polygenic inheritance, different cognitive paths to the same phenotype, or different types of dyslexia is not clear.

Review of Theoretical Models

Overwhelming converging evidence from a number of lines of investigation indicates that the central difficulty in dyslexia reflects a deficit within the language system. Investigators have long known that speech enables its users to create an indefinitely large number of words by combining and permuting a small number of phonological segments, the consonants and vowels that serve as the natural constituents of the biological specialization for language. An alphabetic transcription (reading) brings this same ability to readers, but only as they connect its arbitrary characters (letters) to the phonological segments they represent. Making that connection requires an awareness that all

words, in fact, can be decomposed into phonological segments. Thus, it is this awareness that allows the reader to connect the letter strings (the orthography) to the corresponding units of speech (phonological constituents) they represent. The awareness that all words can be decomposed into these basic elements of language (phonemes) allows the reader to decipher the reading code.

To read, a child has to develop the insight that spoken words can be pulled apart into phonemes and that the letters in a written word represent these sounds. As numerous studies have shown, however, such awareness is largely missing in children and adults with dyslexia (Brady & Shankweiler, 1991; Bruck, 1992; Fletcher et al., 1994; Liberman & Shankweiler, 1991; Rieben & Perfetti, 1991; Shankweiler et al., 1995; Shankweiler, Liberman, Mark, Fowler, & Fischer, 1979; Share, 1995; S. E. Shaywitz, 1996, 1998; Stanovich & Siegel, 1994; Torgesen, 1995; Wagner & Torgesen, 1987). Results from large and well-studied populations with reading disability confirm that in young school-age children (Fletcher et al., 1994;

Stanovich & Siegel, 1994) as well as in adolescents (S. E. Shaywitz et al., 1999) a deficit in phonology represents the most robust and specific (Morris et al., 1998) correlate of reading disability. Such findings form the basis for the most successful and evidence-based interventions designed to improve reading (Report of the National Reading Panel, 2000). While children and adults with a phonological deficit represent the majority of cases of dyslexia, we note that other subtypes may, indeed, account for some cases of dyslexia, for example, surface dyslexia (Coltheart, Curtis, Atkins, & Haller, 1993; Coltheart, Masterson, Byng, Prior, & Riddoch, 1983; Coltheart, Rastle, Perry, Langdon, & Ziegler, 2001), D- and L-type dyslexia (Bakker, 1992; Bakker, Licht, & van Strien, 1991), and dyslexia resulting from deficits in naming speed in addition to phonological deficits (double-deficit hypothesis [Wolf, 1991; Wolf, Bally, & Morris, 1986; Wolf & Bowers, 1999]). Other theories of dyslexia have been proposed that are based on the visual system (Stein & Walsh, 1997) and other factors, such as temporal processing of stimuli within these systems (Talcott et al., 2000; Tallal, 2000). However, these theories have generally not received confirmatory support.

Implications of the Phonological Model of Dyslexia

Basically, reading comprises two main processes—decoding and comprehension (Gough & Tunmer, 1986). In dyslexia, a deficit at the level of the phonological module impairs the ability to segment the written word into its underlying phonological elements. As a result, the reader experiences difficulty, first in decoding the word and then in identifying it. The phonological deficit is domain specific; that is, it is independent of other, nonphonological, abilities. In particular, the higher-order cognitive and linguistic functions involved in comprehension, such as general intelligence and reasoning, vocabulary (Share & Stanovich, 1995), and syntax (Shankweiler et al., 1995), are generally intact. This pattern—a deficit in phonological analysis contrasted with intact higher-order cognitive abilities—offers an explanation for the paradox of otherwise intelligent people who experience

great difficulty in reading (S. E. Shaywitz, 1996).

According to the model, a circumscribed deficit in a phonological function blocks access to higher-order processes and to the ability to draw meaning from text. The problem is that the affected reader cannot use his or her higher-order linguistic skills to access the meaning until the printed word has first been decoded and identified. For example, an individual who knows the precise meaning of the spoken word "apparition" will not be able to use his knowledge of the meaning of the word until he can decode and identify the printed word on the page and will appear not to know the word's meaning.

The Phonological Deficit in Adolescence and Adult Life

Deficits in phonological coding continue to characterize readers with dyslexia even in adolescence; performance on phonological processing measures contributes most to discriminating and average readers and those with dyslexia, and average and superior readers as well (S. E. Shaywitz et al., 1999). Children with dyslexia neither spontaneously remit nor demonstrate a lag mechanism for "catching up" in the development of reading skills. Yet many readers with dyslexia do become quite proficient in reading a finite domain of words that are in their area of special interest, usually words that are important for their careers—for example, an individual who is dyslexic in childhood but, in adult life, becomes interested in molecular biology and then learns to decode words that form a minivocabulary important in molecular biology. Such an individual, however, while able to decode words in this domain still, exhibits evidence of his early reading problems when he has to read unfamiliar words, which he then does accurately but not fluently and automatically (Ben-Dror, Pollatsek, & Scarpati, 1991; Bruck, 1985, 1990, 1992, 1998; Lefly & Pennington, 1991; S. E. Shaywitz et al., 1999). In adolescents, the rate of reading as well as facility with spelling may be most useful clinically in differentiating average from poor readers. From a clinical perspective, these data indicate that as children approach adolescence, a manifestation of dyslexia may be a slow reading rate; in fact, children may learn to read words accurately, but they will not be fluent or automatic, reflecting the lingering effects of a phonological deficit (Lefly & Pennington, 1991). Because they are able to read words accurately (albeit very slowly), dyslexic adolescents and young adults may mistakenly be assumed to have "outgrown" their dyslexia. Data from studies of children with dyslexia who have been followed prospectively support the notion that in adolescents, the rate of reading as well as facility with spelling may be most useful clinically in differentiating average from poor readers in secondary school, and college and even graduate school. It is important to remember that these older students with dyslexia may be similar to their unimpaired peers on untimed measures of word recognition yet continue to suffer from the phonological deficit that makes reading less automatic, more effortful, and slow.

Review of the Research Literature on the Neurobiology of Reading

Anatomic Evidence

To a large degree these advances in understanding dyslexia have informed and facilitated studies examining the neurobiological underpinnings of reading and dyslexia. Historically, as early as 1891, the French neurologist Dejerine suggested that a portion of the left posterior brain region is critical for reading. Beginning with Dejerine, a large literature on acquired inability to read (alexia) describes neuroanatomic lesions most prominently centered in the parietotemporal area (including the angular gyrus, supramarginal gyrus, and posterior portions of the superior temporal gyrus) as a region pivotal in mapping the visual percept of the print onto the phonologic structures of the language system (Damasio & Damasio, 1983; Friedman, Ween, & Albert, 1993; Geschwind, 1965). Another posterior brain region, in the occipitotemporal area, was also described by Dejerine (1892) as critical in reading. More recently, a range of neurobiological investigations using postmortem brain specimens (Galaburda, Sherman, Rosen, Aboitiz, & Geschwind, 1985),

brain morphometry (Filipek, 1996), and diffusion tensor MRI (magnetic resonance imaging) (Klingberg et al., 2000) supports the belief that there are differences in the temporo–parieto–occipital brain regions between dyslexic and nonimpaired readers.

Functional Brain Imaging

Rather than being limited to examining the brain in an autopsy specimen, or measuring the size of brain regions using static morphometric indices, functional imaging offers the possibility of examining brain function during performance of a cognitive task. In principle, functional brain imaging is quite simple. When an individual is asked to perform a discrete cognitive task, that task places processing demands on particular neural systems in the brain. To meet those demands requires activation of neural systems in specific brain regions, and those changes in neural activity are, in turn, reflected by changes in brain metabolic activity, which in turn, are reflected, for example, by changes in cerebral blood flow and in the cerebral utilization of metabolic substrates such as glucose. Some of the first functional imaging studies of dyslexia used positron emission tomography ([PET] e.g., Gross-Glenn et al., 1991; Hagman et al., 1992). In practice, PET requires intraarterial or intravenous administration of a radioactive isotope to the subject so that cerebral blood flow or cerebral utilization of glucose can be determined while the subject is performing the task. Positron-emitting isotopes of nuclei of biological interest have short biological half-lives and are synthesized in a cyclotron immediately prior to testing, a factor that mandates that the time course of the experiment conform to the short half-life of the radioisotope.

Functional magnetic resonance imaging (fMRI) promises to supplant other methods for its ability to map the individual brain's response to specific cognitive stimuli. Because it is noninvasive and safe, it can be used repeatedly, properties that make it ideal for studying humans, especially children. In principle, the signal used to construct MRI images changes, by a small amount (typically of the order 1–5%), in regions that are activated by a stimulus or task. The increase in signal results from the combined effects of increases in the tissue blood flow, volume and oxygenation, though the precise contributions of each of these is still somewhat uncertain. MRI intensity increases when deoxygenated blood is replaced by oxygenated blood. A variety of methods can be used to record the changes that occur, but one preferred approach makes use of ultrafast imaging, such as echo planar imaging (EPI), in which complete images are acquired in times substantially shorter than a second. EPI can provide images at a rate fast enough to capture the time course of the hemodynamic response to neural activation and to permit a wide variety of imaging paradigms over large volumes of the brain. Details of fMRI are reviewed by Anderson and Gore (1997). Magnetic source imaging using magnetoencephalography (MEG) has emerged as a complementary functional imaging modality. It is useful in resolving the temporal sequences of cognitive processes though its spatial resolution is much less precise than PET or fMRI.

Converging evidence using functional brain imaging in dyslexic readers also shows a failure of left-hemisphere posterior brain systems to function properly during reading (Brunswick, McCrory, Price, Frith, & Frith, 1999; Helenius, Tarkiainen, Cornelissen, Hansen, & Salmelin, 1999; Horwitz, Rumsey, & Donohue, 1998; Paulesu et al., 2001; Rumsey et al., 1992, 1997; Salmelin, Service, Kiesila, Uutela, & Salonen, 1996; B. A. Shaywitz et al., 2002; S. E. Shaywitz et al., 1998; Simos, Breier, Fletcher, Bergman, & Papanicolaou, 2000; Temple et al., 2001), as well as during nonreading visual processing tasks (Demb, Boynton, & Heeger, 1998; Eden et al., 1996). In addition, some functional brain imaging studies show differences in brain activation in frontal regions in dyslexic compared to readers who are nonimpaired, in some studies readers with dylexia are more active in frontal regions (Brunswick et al., 1999; Rumsey et al., 1997; S. E. Shaywitz et al., 1998), and in others readers who are nonimpaired are more active in frontal regions (Corina et al., 2001; Georgiewa et al., 1999; Gross-Glenn et al., 1991; Paulesu et al., 1996).

The Research Program at the Yale Center for the Study of Learning and Attention

How Functional Brain Imaging Has Informed Research on Dyslexia

FUNCTIONAL MRI AND PHONOLOGICAL PROCESSING

Our research program has used fMRI to examine the functional organization of the brain for reading and reading disability. Initial studies focused on the identification of those cortical sites associated with various subcomponent operations in reading in readers who are nonimpaired. We next examined how the brain activation patterns of adults with dyslexia differed from adult readers who are nonimpaired. Most recently we have studied children with dyslexia and compared their brain imaging patterns with children who were readers who are nonimpaired. Before describing some of these results in more detail we first review the rationale for the tasks we have used and the strategy employed to analyze the results of these measures.

THEORETICAL ISSUES IN TASK DESIGN

Most functional imaging studies, whether PET or fMRI, use a subtraction methodology in attempting to isolate brain/cognitive function relations (Friston, Frith, Liddle, & Frackowiak, 1993; Petersen & Fiez, 1993; Sergent, 1994). Reading can be considered to involve three component processes: orthographic, phonological, and lexical–semantic processing. In designing tasks, it is important that the decision and response components of both the experimental and the baseline tasks be comparable. In many of our studies we used five tasks: line orientation judgment, letter case judgment, single letter rhyme, nonword rhyme, and category judgment. The five tasks are ordered hierarchically; at the lowest level, the line orientation (L) judgment task (e.g. Do [\\\V] and [\\\V] match?) taps visual–spatial processing but makes no orthographic demands. Next, the letter case judgment task (e.g., Do [bbBb] and [bbBb] match in the pattern of upper and lower case letters?) adds an orthographic processing demand but makes no phonological demands, because the stimulus items that consist entirely of consonant strings are, therefore, phonotactically impermissible. The third task, single letter rhyme (SLR) (e.g., Do the letters [T] and [V] rhyme?), while orthographically more simple than C, adds a phonological processing demand requiring the transcoding of the letters (orthography) into phonological structures, and then sufficient phonological analysis of those structures to determine that they do or do not rhyme; the fourth task, nonword rhyme (NWR) (e.g., Do [leat] and [jete] rhyme?), requires analysis of more complex structures. The fifth task, semantic category (SC) judgment (e.g., Are [corn] and [rice] in the same category?), also makes substantial demands on transcoding from print to phonology (Lukatela & Turvey, 1994; Van Orden, Pennington, & Stone, 1990) but requires in addition that the printed stimulus items activate particular word representations in the reader's lexicon to arrive at the word's meaning. In a typical set of reading tasks, the subject views two simultaneously presented stimulus displays, one above the other, and is asked to make a same/different judgment by pressing a response button if the displays are matched on a given cognitive dimension.

SEX DIFFERENCES

Our initial series of investigations focused on the identification of those cortical sites associated with various subcomponent operations in readers who are nonimpaired. Accordingly, we examined normal readers, 19 neurologically normal right-handed men and 19 women (B. A. Shaywitz, Shaywitz, et al., 1995). Of particular interest were differences in brain activation patterns during phonological processing in men compared to women. Figure 31.2, which demonstrates that activation during phonological processing in men was more lateralized to the left inferior frontal gyrus (IFG), illustrates these differences; in contrast, activation during this same task in women resulted in a more bilateral pattern of activation of this region.

These findings provide the first clear evidence of sex differences in the functional

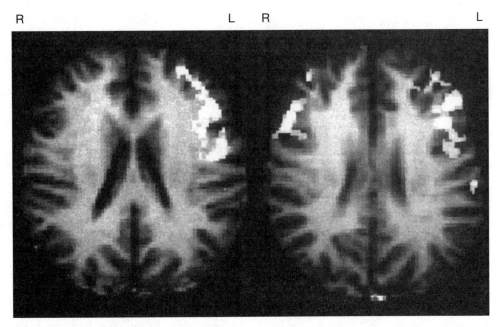

FIGURE 31.2. Sex differences in the brain during phonological processing. Composite fMRI images showing the distribution of brain activation patterns in men (left) and women (right) during, the nonword rhyming task. In men, activation is lateralized to the left inferior frontal regions but in women the same region is active bilaterally. Data from B. A. Shaywitz, Shaywitz, et al. (1995). Copyright 2002 by Sally Shaywitz.

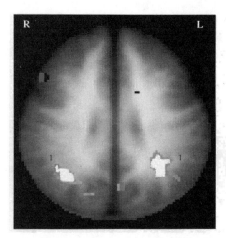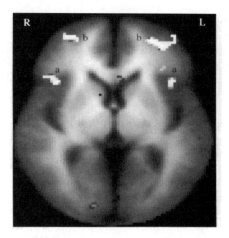

FIGURE 31.3. Composite fMRI activation maps in readers who are nonimpaired and those who are dyslexic engaged in phonological processing during the nonword rhyme task. Readers who are nonimpaired activate a large region involving the angular gyrus (1), supramarginal gyrus, and posterior portions of the superior temporal gyrus. In contrast, readers who are dyslexic demonstrate a relative underactivation in this posterior region and an increased activation in the IFG (a) and middle frontal gyrus (b) bilaterally. Data from S. E. Shaywitz et al. (1998). Copyright 2002 by Sally Shaywitz.

organization of the brain for language and indicate that these differences exist primarily at the level of phonological processing. At one level, they support and extend a long-held hypothesis that suggests that language functions are more likely to be highly lateralized in males but represented in both cerebral hemispheres in females (Halpern, 2000; Witelson & Kigar, 1992). It should be noted that while the basic sex difference in hemispheric activation in IFG appears statistically robust across investigations using large numbers of subjects, it is clear that there is much overlap between the distributions as well. For example, this effect has been replicated using different language processing tasks (Jaeger et al., 1998; Kansaku, Yamaura, & Kitazawa, 2000), yet other imaging experiments have not observed robust sex differences in lateralization (Price, Moore, & Frackowiak, 1996). As with analogous sex differences in lateralization using visual-hemifield or binaural presentation conditions in language processing tasks, given the large overlap in distribution the basic effect may not be expected to attain significance in each and every sample and for all language processing manipulations. Since our initial finding of sex differences in functional activation within IFG we have obtained three replica-

tions of the same basic sex by hemisphere pattern. In sum, the evidence from several imaging experiments involving reading seems clear—the modal pattern indicates relatively greater right-hemisphere involvement for females than for males.

FMRI IN ADULT DYSLEXIC READERS

Our aim was to use the set of hierarchically structured tasks described previously that control the kind of language-relevant coding required, including especially the demand on phonological analysis, and then to compare the performance and brain activation patterns (as measured by fMRI) of readers who are dyslexic (DYS) and readers who are nonimpaired (NI). We studied 61 right-handed subjects, 29 DYS readers (14 men, 15 women, ages 16–54 years), and 32 NI readers (16 men, 16 women, ages 18–63 years). Both groups were in the average range for IQ; DYS readers had a Full Scale IQ (mean ± *SEM*) of 91 ± 2.3 and NI readers had an IQ of 115 ± 2.2. Other than requiring that all subjects have an IQ in the average range (80 or above), we elected not to match subjects on IQ so as not to bias our sample selection in favor of less impaired readers as in dyslexia IQ is known to be influenced by reading ability. Reading performance in the DYS subjects was significantly impaired: the mean standard score on a measure of nonword reading (Woodcock & Johnson, 1989) was 81 ± 1.9 (mean ± *SEM*) in DYS readers compared to 114 ± 1.5 in NI readers, with no overlap between groups. Similarly, error patterns on the fMRI tasks revealed that DYS differed from NI most strikingly on the NWR task. Nonword reading is perhaps the clearest indication of decoding ability because familiarity with the letter pattern cannot influence the individual's response.

We focused on those brain regions that previous research had implicated in reading and language (Demonet, Price, Wise, & Frackowiak, 1994; Henderson, 1986; Petersen, Fox, Snyder, & Raichle, 1990; Pugh et al., 1996) and examined these for evidence of differences between the two reading groups in patterns of activation across the series of tasks. In this study we found significant differences in brain activation patterns between DYS and NI readers, differences that emerged during tasks that made progressive demands on phonological analysis. Thus, during NWR in DYS readers, we found a disruption in several critical components of a posterior system involving posterior superior temporal gyrus (Wernicke's area), Brodmann's area (BA) 39 (angular gyrus), and BA 17 (striate cortex) and a concomitant increase in activation in the IFG anteriorly.

Hemispheric differences between NI and DYS readers have long been suspected (Galaburda et al., 1985; Geschwind, 1985; Rumsey et al., 1992; Salmelin et al., 1996) and these were found in two regions: the angular gyrus and BA 37. Thus, there is some similarity between the fMRI data and the anatomic findings reported for the planum temporale in the superior temporal gyrus (Galaburda et al., 1985). Galaburda and colleagues (1985) noted in dyslexic brains a reversal of the usual left-hemisphere asymmetry and we found an apparent predominance of right-hemisphere activity in DYS readers in the angular gyrus and the middle and inferior temporal gyri.

FMRI IN CHILDREN WITH DYSLEXIA

In a recently completed study (B. A. Shaywitz et al., 2002) we studied 144 right-handed children, 70 DYS readers (21 girls, 49 boys, ages 7–18 years, mean age 13.3 years) and 74 NI readers (31 girls, 43 boys, ages 7–17 years, mean age 10.9 years). All children had intelligence in the average range. Criteria for DYS were met if the average of the two decoding subtests (Word Identification and Word Attack) from the Woodcock–Johnson Psycho-Educational Test Battery (Woodcock & Johnson, 1989) were below a standard score of 90 (below the 25th percentile) or 1.5 standard errors of prediction lower than the expected reading achievement score using the third edition of the Wechsler Intelligence Scale for Children (Wechsler, 1991) Full Scale IQ score. Both of these definitions validly identify children as poor readers, with little evidence for differences among subgroups of children formed with these definitions (Fletcher et al., 1994; B. A. Shaywitz, Fletcher, Holahan, & Shaywitz, 1992). To ensure good readers, and no overlap between groups, criteria for NI were reading scores above the 39th percentile.

Reading performance in the DYS children was significantly impaired: the mean standard score on a measure of pseudo-word reading (Woodcock & Johnson, 1989) (mean + *SD*) was 85.1 ± 11.0 in DYS compared to 120 ± 17.1 in NI ($p < .001$). During fMRI, significant differences between NI and DYS children were observed while the children were engaged in the tasks requiring phonological analysis, particularly NWR and semantic judgment (see earlier, CAT), and not during a task that relies primarily on visual perception and not phonology. Results were quite similar to those observed in adults, with greater activation in NI readers in anterior and posterior reading systems (see Figure 31.4).

Of particular interest was the correlation between individual differences in reading performance on standard measures of reading skill out of magnet and individual differences in brain activation patterns in left-hemisphere posterior regions. We found that performance on the Woodcock–Johnson (W-J) Word Attack test of pseudo-word reading (Woodcock & Johnson, 1989) was positively correlated with activation in posterior regions, particularly in the left occipitotemporal area. The more accurate the performance in reading, the greater the

NI vs DYS

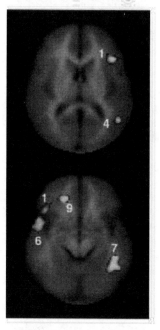

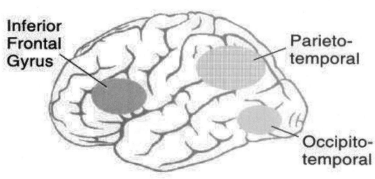

FIGURE 31.4. Composite contrast maps comparing directly the brain activation of NI and DYS children. Highlighted areas indicate brain regions that were more active in NI compared to DYS children during the nonword rhyme task. These regions involve left-hemisphere sites (the right side of the image) in the IFG, parietotemporal, and occipitotemporal regions. Data from B. A. Shaywitz et al. (2002). Copyright 2002 by Sally Shaywitz.

magnitude of the fMRI signal in these left-hemisphere regions during in-magnet reading. These findings across the full cohort of children reveals a continuum from very poor to skilled readers (S. E. Shaywitz et al., 1992) (see Figure 31.5).

In anterior regions, NI children demonstrated greater activation than did DYS children; this finding is consonant with two other reports in children (Corina et al., 2001; Georgiewa et al., 1999) as well as reports in adults (Gross-Glenn et al., 1991; Paulesu et al., 1996). At the same time, this finding contrasts with what we (S. E. Shaywitz et al., 1998) and others (Brunswick et al., 1999) have reported in adults, where DYS readers showed greater activation in the IFG. Consideration of the correlation between age and brain activation provided an explanation that could resolve these differences. Specifically, we found that during the most difficult and specific phonological task (nonword rhyming) *older* DYS readers (but not NI readers) engaged the left and

right IFG. We suggest that older DYS readers engage neural systems in frontal regions to compensate for the disruption in posterior regions.

Strengths and Limitations of fMRI

fMRI has supplanted all other kinds of functional brain imaging for the examination of cognitive systems in brain. As noted earlier, fMRI is noninvasive, does not require any intravenous injections, and does not need administration of a radioactive tracer, and thus is particularly well-suited for studies of children. For the same reasons, it is ideally suited for longitudinal studies requiring repeated fMRI in the same children, to examine, for example, the development of neural systems for reading. The user must also be aware of the limitations of the technology. One such limitation is that the subjects' complete cooperation is required. This is obvious—the investigator requires the subject to perform a particular

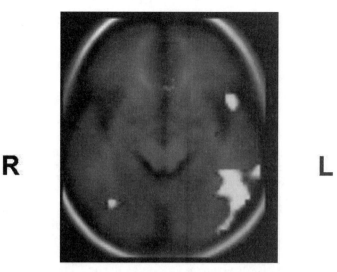

FIGURE 31.5. Correlation map between reading skill as measured by the Word Attack reading test performed out of magnet and nonword rhyme performed during fMRI for the entire group of 144 children. Highlighted areas show a positive correlation of in-magnet tasks with the out-of-magnet reading test (threshold, $p < .01$). Strong correlation was found in the occipitotemporal region in the left hemisphere. Data from B. A. Shaywitz et al. (2002). Copyright 2002 by Sally Shaywitz.

task, such as determining whether two nonwords rhyme. Given this requirement, studies using fMRI are usually limited to those children, ages 6 and older, who are able to cooperate and who will be able to perform a task while in the imager. FMRI works well for studying a process such as reading that is not taught until age 6, but investigators studying the emergence of language would find it difficult to gain the cooperation of children in late infancy and preschool, the time frame when language is developing. Another limitation of fMRI is its poor time resolution. The procedure will allow tracking events occurring over a period of seconds, but it is not possible to observe events occurring over milliseconds. Magnetoencephalography does allow resolution of events occurring over milliseconds, and the combination of fMRI and MEG would obviate the limitations of each technology. Such experiments are in process in a number of laboratories.

fMRI's Place in Complementing Traditional Comparisons between LD and Nondisabled Students.

Perhaps the most important consequence of the emerging biology of reading and dyslexia is that scientists and clinicians now have unassailable evidence that children with learning disabilities (LD) have a real disability, as real as a fractured arm or as pneumonia. No longer do parents and the children themselves have to hear critics accuse them of faking a disorder to get the assumed "perks" that go along with the diagnosis. Specifically, functional imaging studies have now converged with behavioral studies in indicating that there are important differences, here neurologically based, between LD and nondisabled individuals. Demonstration of these differences in children who are at the cusp of reading as well as in adults confirm the persistent nature of dyslexia. Studies have previously demonstrated that bright readers with dyslexia become more accurate as they mature, but they do not attain fluency or automaticity in reading. Now, functional imaging provides an explanation. Converging evidence from many laboratories implicate the left occipitotemporal region as a site for skilled, automatic reading. Failure to activate this region by readers with dyslexia explains their lack of automaticity; observation of activation of right-hemisphere frontal and posterior regions—ancillary systems for word reading—provides an explanation for accurate but not automatic reading. These secondary systems can decode the word but slowly and not with the degree of automaticity characteristic of left-hemisphere linguistically structured brain regions. These findings have important clinical implications: they confirm the biological validity of reading disability; they explain the lack of automaticity, even in those readers who develop accuracy; and they provide neurobiological evidence of the need for extra time on tests for adults who are dyslexic. In addition, the demonstration of the persistent nature of the functional disruption in left-hemisphere neural systems for reading indicates both that the disorder is lifelong and that there is no need for those who were identified as dyslexic as children to be retested as adults to have the diagnosis confirmed.

Context, Error, and Complexity in the Application of fMRI

fMRI is exquisitely context dependent in its application. For example, the neural systems activated during fMRI reflect the neural systems engaged by the task used. Thus, when we ask children to rhyme nonwords, a certain general pattern of brain activation is apparent. On the other hand, responding to whether two real words are in the same category activates some of the same neural systems as for rhyming nonwords but some different sites as well. In our studies we have modified tasks so that younger children will be able to perform the task. For example, rather than show two nonwords on a screen, our stimuli for young readers is a picture of an object (e.g., cat) and then the word "bat." The child responds yes if the word rhymes with the picture. Because both rhyming nonwords and rhyming to pictures require phonological analysis, the systems activated are similar.

Variations within fMRI Methodology

The variations within fMRI are most readily conceptualized as variations within software (i.e., paradigms, block design vs. event-related design, or methods of analyses [e.g., connectivity, and its measures]) and variations within hardware, (e.g., strength of magnetic field of imager [1.5, 3, 4, 7 T]).

First the paradigms. All the tasks that we have described are performed and analyzed using a block design, that is, a string (or block) of stimuli are shown to the subject, then a block of control tasks are shown. Data are analyzed by comparing the activations during the block of a particular task with the block of control task. The difference in activation is considered to reflect the cognitive processing of the task. In an event-related design, the subject sees a background task and then, every so often, an oddball stimulus is presented. The data are analyzed by averaging the response to all the oddball stimuli and then subtracting the activity of the background task. There are some situations in which such a paradigm is quite useful. The problem with the event-related design is that longer imaging is necessary because the stimulus of interest (the oddball) can be shown just a few times every so often; otherwise, if it is shown frequently, it is no longer perceived by the subject as an oddball. Thus, in order to collect enough data, the subject is required to stay in the imager for a longer period. Newer methods may allow for shorter imaging times (see Maccotta, Zacks, & Buckner, 2001).

As for the hardware, suffice it to say that the makers of the high field MRI units are now able to manufacture magnets with a strength two to four times the strength of current clinical imaging devices. In theory this should lead to better signal-to-noise ratio, resulting in a more sensitive measure of changes in brain blood flow. Data available from the few high field imagers currently in use indicate extraordinary resolution in brain morphology. Whether there are similar improvements in resolution of fMRI using these high field magnets remains a subject for further investigation.

Summary of Consistent Findings

Converging evidence using functional brain imaging in adults and children with dyslexia shows a failure of left-hemisphere posterior brain systems to function properly during reading (Brunswick et al., 1999; Helenius et al., 1999; Horwitz et al., 1998; Paulesu et al., 2001; Rumsey et al., 1992, 1997; Salmelin et al., 1996; B. A. Shaywitz et al.,

2002; S. E. Shaywitz et al., 1998; Simos et al., 2000; Temple et al., 2001). These findings converge with the anatomic studies, beginning with Dejerine (1891) and, more recently, a range of neurobiological investigations using postmortem brain specimens (Galaburda et al., 1985), brain morphometry (Filipek, 1996), and diffusion tensor MRI imaging (Klingberg et al., 2000) that demonstrate differences in the temporo–parieto–occipital brain regions between readers who are dyslexic and those who are nonimpaired.

Logan (1988, 1997) proposed two systems critical in the development of skilled, automatic processing, one involving word analysis, operating on individual units of words such as phonemes, requiring attentional resources and processing relatively slowly, and the second system operating on the whole word (word form), an obligatory system that does not require attention and processes rapidly. Converging evidence from a number of lines of investigation indicates that Logan's word analysis system is localized within the parietotemporal region while the automatic, rapidly responding system is localized within the occipitotemporal area, functioning as a visual word form area (Cohen et al., 2000, 2002; Dehaene et al., 2001; Moore & Price, 1999). The visual word form area appears to respond preferentially to rapidly presented stimuli (Price et al., 1996) and is engaged even when the word has not been consciously perceived (Dehaene et al., 2001). It is this occipitotemporal system that appears to predominate when a reader has become skilled and has bound together as a unit the orthographic, phonological, and semantic features of the word.

Recognition of these systems allows us to suggest an explanation for the brain activation patterns observed in DYS children. We suppose that rather than the smoothly functioning and integrated reading systems observed in NI children, disruption of the posterior reading systems results in DYS children attempting to compensate by shifting to other, ancillary systems, for example, anterior sites such as the IFG and right-hemisphere sites. The anterior sites, critical in articulation (Brunswick et al., 1999; Fiez & Petersen, 1998; Frackowiak, Friston, Frith, Dolan, & Mazziotta, 1997), may help

the child with dyslexia develop an awareness of the sound structure of the word by subvocalizing, (ie., forming the word with his lips, tongue, and vocal apparatus) and thus allow the child to read, albeit more slowly and less efficiently than if the fast occipitotemporal word identification system were functioning. The right-hemisphere sites may represent the engagement of brain regions that allow the poor reader to use other perceptual processes to compensate for his or her poor phonological skills. A number of studies of young adults with childhood histories of dyslexia indicate that although they may develop some accuracy in reading words, they remain slow, nonautomatic readers (Bruck, 1992; Felton et al., 1990) (see Figure 31.6).

Future Directions

Our research group has begun a new series of studies involving fMRI in children and young adults with dyslexia. While the cross-sectional study described earlier provided some indication of the development of skilled reading, a new longitudinal study currently in progress will allow the examination of the neural systems for reading, over time, in the same group of children, both DYS and NI readers. By carefully assessing the development of skilled reading in these children and periodically assessing the neural systems for reading, we hope to learn how the neural systems for reading develop, and how the development of these systems differ in DYS readers. At the same time, in collaboration with Michael Posner and Bruce McCandliss, we are examining how developing attentional systems relate to the development of skilled reading. Compared to reading, relatively little is known about mathematics disability, and in a series of experiments in collaboration with Stanislas Dehaene, we are examining how neural systems for mathematics develop and map onto the development of childrens' ability to calculate. The influence of a reading intervention designed to improve reading fluency on the development of neural systems for skilled reading will be examined in a project in collaboration with Robin Morris. Morris has developed an intervention that appears to be one of the

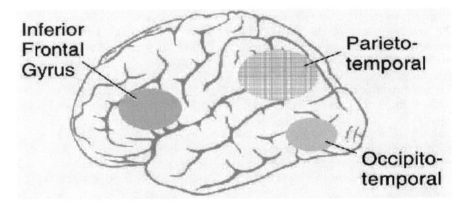

FIGURE 31.6. Neural systems for reading. Converging evidence indicates three important systems in reading, all primarily in the left hemisphere. These include an anterior system and two posterior systems: (1) anterior system in the left inferior frontal region; (2) parietotemporal system involving angular gyrus, supramarginal gyrus, and posterior portions of the superior temporal gyrus; (3) occipitotemporal system involving portions of the middle and inferior temporal gyrus and middle and inferior occipital gyrus. For details, see text. Copyright 2002 by Sally Shaywitz.

first effective interventions for improving reading fluency and by imaging children before and after that intervention we hope to demonstrate the influence of specific interventions on the neural circuitry in subtypes of poor readers. In collaboration with Robert Fulbright and Douglas Rothman we are using a new technology, magnetic resonance spectroscopy, to examine at the cellular level the basis of the disruptions noted in fMRI studies. And we continue to study a unique cohort of young adults, subjects who are participants in the Connecticut Longitudinal Study, which provides a virtually intact sample of 400 subjects who have been followed prospectively and continuously from kindergarten entry to adulthood. In particular, we will examine the influence of a full range of predictor variables (risk/protective) on an equally full range of potential outcomes. Outcome is examined from multiple perspectives, including educational, vocational, behavioral, and family and social and life satisfaction on the one hand and from the perspective of reading achievement and reading disability on the other. Here too, we will examine the neural mechanisms in a range of skilled and less skilled readers, wedding the power of epidemiology, longitudinal surveillance, and state-of-the-art neurobiology and technology.

Conclusions

Within the last two decades overwhelming evidence from many laboratories has converged to indicate the cognitive basis for dyslexia: dyslexia represents a disorder within the language system and more specifically within a particular subcomponent of that system, phonological processing. Recent advances in imaging technology and the development of tasks that sharply isolate the subcomponent processes of reading now allow the localization of phonological processing in brain and, as a result, provide, for the first time, the potential for elucidating a biological signature for reading and reading disability. Converging evidence from a number of laboratories using functional brain imaging indicates a disruption of left-hemisphere posterior brain systems in DYS readers while performing reading tasks with an additional suggestion for an associated increased reliance on ancillary systems, for example, in the frontal lobe and right-hemisphere posterior circuits. The discovery of neural systems serving reading has significant implications. At the most fundamental level, it is now possible to investigate specific hypotheses regarding the neural substrate of dyslexia and to verify, reject, or modify suggested cognitive models. From a more clinical perspective, the identification of neural systems for reading offers the promise for more precise identification and diagnosis of dyslexia in children, adolescents, and adults. Demonstration of the neural disruption in children and adults and the engagement of ancillary systems indicate the persistent nature of dyslexic throughout the lifespan and explain the observation that as dyslexics mature they become more accurate but continue to read slowly. For clinical purposes these findings strongly suggest that those with childhood diagnoses of dyslexic do not require testing as adults to confirm the diagnosis and that they do require the accommodation of extra time on their examinations.

Acknowledgments

The work described in this review was supported by grants from the National Institute of Child Health and Human Development (PO1 HD 21888 and P50 HD25802). Portions of this chapter appeared in and are similar to other reviews by us (S. Shaywitz, 1998; S. Shaywitz & B. Shaywitz, 1999; B. Shaywitz et al., 2000; S. Shaywitz et al., in press). We thank Carmel Lepore for her help in preparing the manuscript.

References

Anderson, A., & Gore, J. (1997). The physical basis of neuroimaging techniques. In M. Lewis & B. Peterson (Eds.), *Child and adolescent psychiatric clinics of North America* (Vol. 6, pp. 213–264). Philadelphia: Saunders.

Bakker, D. (1992). Neuropsychological classification and treatment of dyslexia. *Journal of Learning Disabilities, 25*(2), 1–2–109.

Bakker, D., Licht, R., & van Strien, J. (1991). Biopsychological validation of the L- and P-type dyslexia. In B. P. Rourke (Ed.), *Neuropsychological validation of learning disability subtypes* (pp. 124–139). New York: Guilford Press.

Ben-Dror, I., Pollatsek, A., & Scarpati, A. (1991). Word identification in isolation and in context by college dyslexic students. *Brain and Language, 40*, 471–490.

Brady, S. A., & Shankweiler, D. P. (Eds.). (1991). *Phonological processes in literacy: A tribute to Isabelle Y. Liberman.* Hillsdale, NJ: Erlbaum.

Bruck, M. (1985). The adult functioning of children with specific learning disabilities: A follow-up study. In I. Siegel (Ed.), *Advances in applied developmental psychology* (pp. 91–129). Norwood, NJ: Ablex.

Bruck, M. (1990). Word-recognition skills of adults with childhood diagnoses of dyslexia. *Developmental Psychology, 26*(3), 439–454.

Bruck, M. (1992). Persistence of dyslexics' phonological awareness deficits. *Developmental Psychology, 28*(5), 874–886.

Bruck, M. (1998). Outcomes of adults with childhood histories of dyslexia. In C. Hulme & R. M. Joshi (Eds.), *Cognitive and linguistic bases of reading, writing, and spelling* (pp. 179–200) Mahaw, NJ: Erlbaum.

Brunswick, N., McCrory, E., Price, C. J., Frith, C. D., & Frith, U. (1999). Explicit and implicit processing of words and pseudowords by adult developmental dyslexics: A search for Wernicke's Wortschatz. *Brain, 122*, 1901–1917.

Cohen, L., Dehaene, S., Naccache, L., Lehericy, S., Dehaene-Lambertz, G., Henaff, M., & Michel, F. (2000). The visual word form area: Spatial and temporal characterization of an initial stage of reading in normal subjects and posterior split-brain patients. *Brain, 123*, 291–307.

Cohen, L., Lehéricy, S., Chochon, F., Lemer, C., Rivaud, S., & Dehaene, S. (2000). Language-specific tuning of visual cortex? Functional properties of the Visual Word Form Area. *Brain, 125*, 1054–1069.

Coltheart, M., Curtis, B., Atkins, P., & Haller, M. (1993). Models of reading aloud: Dual-route and parallel-distributed-processing approaches. *Psychological Review, 100*, 589–608.

Coltheart, M., Masterson, J., Byng, S., Prior, M., & Riddoch, J. (1983). Surface dyslexia. *Quarterly Journal of Experimental Psychology, 35A*, 469–495.

Coltheart, M., Rastle, K. Perry, C. Langdon, R., & Ziegler, J. (2001). DRC: A dual route cascaded model of visual word recognition and reading aloud. *Psychological Review, 108*, 204–256.

Corina, D., Richards, T., Serafini, S., Richards, A., Steury, K., Abbott, R., Echelard, D., Maravilla, K., & Berninger, V. (2001). fMRI auditory language differences between dyslexic and able reading children. *NeuroReport, 12*, 1195–1201.

Damasio, A. R., & Damasio, H. (1983). The anatomic basis of pure alexia. *Neurology, 33*, 1573–1583.

Dehaene, S., Naccache, L., Cohen, L., Le Bihan, D., Mangin, J., Poline, J., & Riviere, D. (2001). Cerebral mechanisms of word masking and unconscious repetition priming. *Nature Neuroscience, 4*, 752–758.

Dejerine, J. (1891). Sur un cas de cécité verbale avec agraphie, suivi d'autopsie. *C. R. Société du Biologie, 43*, 197–201.

Dejerine, J. (1892). Contribution a l'etude anatomo-pathologique et clinique des differentes varietes de cecite verbale. *Memoires de la Societe de Biologie, 4*, 61–90.

Demb, J., Boynton, G., & Heeger, D. (1998). Functional magnetic resonance imaging of early visual pathways in dyslexia. *Journal of Neuroscience, 18*, 6939–6951.

Demonet, J. F., Price, C., Wise, R., & Frackowiak, R. S. J. (1994). A PET study of cognitive strategies in normal subjects during language tasks: Influence of phonetic ambiguity and sequence processing on phoneme monitoring. *Brain, 117,* 671–682.

Eden, G. F., VanMeter, J. W., Rumsey, J. M., Maisog, J. M., Woods, R. P., & Zeffiro, T. A. (1996). Abnormal processing of visual motion in dyslexia revealed by functional brain imaging. *Nature, 382,* 66–69.

Felton, R. H., Naylor, C. E., & Wood, F. B. (1990). Neuropsychological profile of adult dyslexics. *Brain and Language, 39,* 485–497.

Fiez, J. A., & Petersen, S. E. (1998). Neuroimaging studies of word reading. *Proceedings of the Natioal Academy of Science USA, 95*(3), 914–921.

Filipek, P. (1996). Structural variations in measures in the developmental disorders. In R. Thatcher, G. Lyon, J. Rumsey, & N. Krasnegor (Eds.), *Developmental neuroimaging: Mapping the development of brain and behavior* (pp. 169–186). San Diego,CA: Academic Press.

Finucci, J. M., & Childs, B. (1981). Are there really more dyslexic boys than girls? In A. Ansara, N. Geschwind, M. Albert, & N. Gartrell (Eds.), *Sex differences in dyslexia* (pp. 1–9). Towson, MD: Orton Dyslexia Society.

Fisher, S. E., & DeFries, J. C. (2002). Developmental dyslexia: Genetic dissection of a complex cognitive trait. *Nature Reviews, Neuroscience, 3*(10), 767–780.

Fletcher, J. M., Shaywitz, S. E., Shankweiler, D. P., Katz, L., Liberman, I. Y., Stuebing, K. K., Francis, D. J., Fowler, A. E., & Shaywitz, B. A. (1994). Cognitive profiles of reading disability: Comparisons of discrepancy and low achievement definitions. *Journal of Educational Psychology, 86*(1), 6–23.

Flynn, J., & Rahbar, M. (1994). Prevalence of reading failure in boys compared with girls. *Psychology in the Schools, 31,* 66–71.

Frackowiak, R., Friston, K., Frith, C., Dolan, R., & Mazziotta. (1997). *Human brain function.* New York: Academic Press.

Francis, D. J., Shaywitz, S. E., Stuebing, K. K., Shaywitz, B. A., & Fletcher, J. M. (1996). Developmental lag versus deficit models of reading disability: A longitudinal, individual growth curves analysis. *Journal of Educational Psychology, 88*(1), 3–17.

Friedman, R. F., Ween, J. E., & Albert, M. L. (1993). Alexia. In K. M. Heilman & E. Valenstein (Eds.), *Clinical neuropsychology* (3rd ed., pp. 37–62). New York: Oxford University Press.

Friston, K. J., Frith, C. D., Liddle, P. F., & Frackowiak, R. S. J. (1993). Functional connectivity: The principal-component analysis of large (PET) data sets. *Journal of Cerebral Blood Flow and Metabolism, 13,* 5–14.

Galaburda, A. M., Sherman, G. F., Rosen, G. D., Aboitiz, F., & Geschwind, N. (1985). Developmental dyslexia: Four consecutive patients with cortical anomalies. *Annals of Neurology, 18*(2), 222–233.

Georgiewa, P., Rzanny, R., Hopf, J., Knab, R., Glauche, V., Kaiser, W., & Blanz, B. (1999). fMRI during word processing in dyslexic and normal reading children. *NeuroReport, 10,* 3459–3465.

Geschwind, N. (1965). Disconnection syndromes in animals and man. *Brain, 88,* 237–294.

Geschwind, N. (1985). Biological foundations of reading. In F. H. Duffy & N. Geschwind (Eds.), *Dyslexia: A neuroscientific approach to clinical evaluation* (pp. 195–211). Boston: Little, Brown.

Gilger, J. W., Borecki, I. B., Smith, S. D., DeFries, J. C., & Pennington, B. F. (1996). The etiology of extreme scores for complex phenotypes: An illustration using reading performance. In C. H. Chase, G. D. Rosen, & G. F. Sherman (Eds.), *Developmental dyslexia: Neural, cognitive, and genetic mechanisms* (pp. 63–85). Baltimore: York Press.

Gough, P. B., & Tunmer, W. E. (1986). Decoding, reading, and reading disability. *Remedial and Special Education, 7,* 6–10.

Gross-Glenn, K., Duara, R., Barker, W. W., Loewenstein, D., Chang, J.-Y., Yoshii, F., Apicella, A. M., Pascal, S., Boothe, T., Sevush, S., Jallad, B. J., Novoa, L., & Lubs, H. A. (1991). Positron emission tomographic studies during serial word-reading by normal and dyslexic adults. *Journal of Clinical and Experimental Neuropsychology, 13*(4), 531–544.

Hagman, J. O., Wood, F., Buchsbaum, M. S., Tallal, P., Flowers, L., & Katz, W. (1992). Cerebral brain metabolism in adult dyslexic subjects assessed with positron emission tomography during performance of an auditory task. *Archives of Neurology, 49,* 734–739.

Halpern, D. F. (2000). *Sex differences in cognitive abilities* (3rd ed.). Mahwah, NJ: Erlbaum.

Helenius, P., Tarkiainen, A., Cornelissen, P., Hansen, P. C., & Salmelin, R. (1999). Dissociation of normal feature analysis and deficient processing of letter-strings in dyslexic adults. *Cerebral Cortex, 4,* 476–483.

Henderson, V. W. (1986). Anatomy of posterior pathways in reading: A reassessment. *Brain and Language, 29,* 119–133.

Horwitz, B., Rumsey, J. M., & Donohue, B. C. (1998). Functional connectivity of the angular gyrus in normal reading and dyslexia. *Proceedings of the National Academy of Science USA, 95,* 8939–8944.

Jaeger, J., Lockwood, A., Vanvalin, R., Kemmerer, D., Murphy, B., & Wack, D. (1998). Sex differences in brain regions activated by grammatical and reading tasks. *Neuroreport, 9,* 2803–2807.

Kansaku, K., Yamaura, A., & Kitazawa, S. (2000). Sex differences in lateralization revealed in the posterior language areas. *Cerebral Cortex, 10,* 866–872.

Klingberg, T., Hedehus, M., Temple, E., Salz, T.,

Gabrieli, J., Moseley, M., & Poldrack, R. (2000). Microstructure of temporo-parietal white matter as a basis for reading ability: Evidence from diffusion tensor magnetic resonance imaging. *Neuron, 25*, 493–500.

Lefly, D. L., & Pennington, B. F. (1991). Spelling errors and reading fluency in compensated adult dyslexics. *Annals of Dyslexia, 41*, 143–162.

Liberman, I. Y., & Shankweiler, D. (1991). Phonology and beginning to read: A tutorial. In L. Rieben & C. A. Perfetti (Eds.), *Learning to read: Basic research and its implications*. Hillsdale, NJ: Erlbaum.

Logan, G. (1988). Toward an instance theory of automatization. *Psychological Review, 95*, 492–527.

Logan, G. (1997). Automaticity and reading: perspectives from the instance theory of automatization. *Reading and Writing Quarterly: Overcoming Learning Disabilities, 13*, 123–146.

Lukatela, G., & Turvey, M. T. (1994). Visual lexical access is initially phonological: 2. Evidence from phonological priming by homophones and pseudohomophones. *Journal of Experimental Psychology: General, 123*(4), 331–353.

Maccotta, L., Zacks, J., & Buckner, R. (2001). Rapid self-paced event-related functional MRI: feasibility and implications of stimulus-versus response-locked timing. *NeuroImage, 14*, 1105–1121.

Moore, C., & Price, C. (1999). Three distinct ventral occiptotemporal regions for reading and object naming. *NeuroImage, 10*, 181–192.

Morris, R. D., Stuebing, K. K., Fletcher, J. M., Shaywitz, S. E., Lyon, G. R., Shankweiler, D. P., Katz, L., Francis, D. J., & Shaywitz, B. A. (1998). Subtypes of reading disability: Variability around a phonological core. *Journal of Educational Psychology, 90*, 347–373.

Paulesu, E., Demonet, J.-F., Fazio, F., McCrory, E., Chanoine, V., Brunswick, N., Cappa, S., Cossu, G., Habib, M., Frith, C., & Frith, U. (2001). Dyslexia-cultural diversity and biological unity. *Science, 291*, 2165–2167.

Paulesu, E., Frith, U., Snowling, M., Gallagher, A., Morton, J., Frackowiak, R. S. J., & Frith, C. D. (1996). Is developmental dyslexia a disconnection syndrome? Evidence from PET scanning. *Brain, 119*, 143–157.

Pennington, B. F., & Gilger, J. W. (1996). How is dyslexia transmitted? In C. H. Chase, G. D. Rosen, & G. F. Sherman (Eds.), *Developmental dyslexia. Neural, cognitive, and genetic mechanisms* (pp. 41–61). Baltimore: York Press.

Petersen, S. E., & Fiez, J. A. (1993). The processing of single words studied with positron emission tomography. *Annual Review of Neuroscience, 16*, 509–530.

Petersen, S. E., Fox, P. T., Snyder, A. Z., & Raichle, M. E. (1990). Activation of extrastriate and frontal cortical areas by visual words and word-like stimuli. *Science, 249*, 1041–1044.

Price, C., Moore, C., & Frackowiak, R. S. J. (1996). The effect of varying stimulus rate and duration on brain activity during reading. *Neuroimage, 3*(1), 40–52.

Pugh, K. R., Shaywitz, B. A., Shaywitz, S. E., Constable, T. R., Skudlarski, P., Fulbright, R. K., Bronen, R. A., Shankweiler, D. P., Katz, L., Fletcher, J. M., & Gore, J. C. (1996). Cerebral organization of component processes in reading. *Brain, 119*, 1221–1238.

Report of the National Reading Panel. (2000). *Teaching children to read: An evidence-based assessment of the scientific research literature on reading and its implications for reading instruction*. Bethesda, MD: National Institute of Child Health and Human Development, National Institutes of Health.

Rieben, L., & Perfetti, C. A. (1991). *Learning to read: Basic research and its implications*. Hillsdale, NJ: Erlbaum.

Rumsey, J. M., Andreason, P., Zametkin, A. J., Aquino, T., King, C., Hamburger, S. D., Pikus, A., Rapoport, J. L., & Cohen, R. M. (1992). Failure to activate the left temporoparietal cortex in dyslexia. *Archives of Neurology, 49*, 527–534.

Rumsey, J. M., Nace, K., Donohue, B., Wise, D., Maisog, J. M., & Andreason, P. (1997). A positron emission tomographic study of impaired word recognition and phonological processing in dyslexic men. *Archives of Neurology, 54*, 562–573.

Salmelin, R., Service, E., Kiesila, P., Uutela, K., & Salonen, O. (1996). Impaired visual word processing in dyslexia revealed with magnetoencephalography. *Annals of Neurology, 40*, 157–162.

Scarborough, H. S. (1984). Continuity between childhood dyslexia and adult reading. *British Journal of Psychology, 75*, 329–348.

Scarborough, H. S. (1990). Very early language deficits in dyslexic children. *Child Development, 61*, 1728–1743.

Sergent, J. (1994). Brain-imaging studies of cognitive function. *Trends in Neurosciences, 17*, 221–227.

Shankweiler, D., Crain, S., Katz, L., Fowler, A. E., Liberman, A. M., Brady, S. A., Thornton, R., Lundquist, E., Dreyer, L., Fletcher, J. M., Stuebing, K. K., Shaywitz, S. E., & Shaywitz, B. A. (1995). Cognitive profiles of reading-disabled children: Comparison of language skills in phonology, morphology, and syntax. *Psychological Science, 6*(3), 149–156.

Shankweiler, D., Liberman, I. Y., Mark, L. S., Fowler, C. A., & Fischer, F. W. (1979). The speech code and learning to read. *Journal of Experimental Psychology: Human Learning and Memory, 5*(6), 531–545.

Share, D. L. (1995). Phonological recoding and self–teaching: Sine qua non of reading acquisition. *Cognition, 55*, 151–218.

Share, D. L., & Stanovich, K. E. (1995). Cognitive processes in early reading development: Accommodating individual differences into a model of acquisition. *Issues in Education: Contributions from Educational Psychology, 1*(1), 1–57.

Shaywitz, B. A., Fletcher, J. M., Holahan, J. M., & Shaywitz, S. E. (1992). Discrepancy compared to low achievement definitions of reading disability: Results from the Connecticut Longitudinal Study. *Journal of Learning Disabilities, 25*(10), 639–648.

Shaywitz, B. A., Holford, T. R., Holahan, J. M., Fletcher, J. M., Stuebing, K. K., Francis, D., J, & Shaywitz, S. E. (1995). A Matthew effect for IQ but not for reading: Results from a longitudinal study. *Reading Research Quarterly, 30*(4), 894–906.

Shaywitz, B. A., Pugh, K. R., Jenner, A., Fulbright, R. K., Fletcher, J. M., Gore, J. C., & Shaywitz, S. (2000). The neurobiology of reading and reading disability (dyslexia). In M. Kamil, P. Mosenthal, P. Pearson, & R. Barr (Eds.), *Handbook of reading research* (Vol. III, pp. 229–249). Mahwah, NJ: Erlbaum.

Shaywitz, B. A., Shaywitz, S., Pugh, K., Constable, R., Skudlarski, P., Fulbright, R., Bronen, R., Fletcher, J., Shankweiler, D., Katz, L., & Gore, J. (1995). Sex differences in the functional organization of the brain for language. *Nature, 373,* 607–609.

Shaywitz, B. A., Shaywitz, S. E., Pugh, K. R., Mencl, W. E., Fullbright, R. K., Skudlarski, P., Constable, R. T., Marchione, K. M., Fletcher, J. M., Lyon, G. R., & Gore, J. C. (2002). Disruption of posterior brain systems for reading in children with developmental dyslexia. *Biological Psychiatry, 52,* 101–110.

Shaywitz, S. E. (1996). Dyslexia. *Scientific American, 275*(5), 98–104.

Shaywitz, S. E. (1998). Current concepts: Dyslexia. *New England Journal of Medicine, 338*(5), 307–312.

Shaywitz, S. E. (2003). *A new and complex science-based program for reading problems at any level.* New York: Knopf.

Shaywitz, S. E., Escobar, M. D., Shaywitz, B. A., Fletcher, J. M., & Makuch, R. (1992). Evidence that dyslexia may represent the lower tail of a normal distribution of reading ability. *New England Journal of Medicine, 326*(3), 145–150.

Shaywitz, S. E., Fletcher, J. M., Holahan, J. M., Shneider, A. E., Marchione, K. E., Stuebing, K. K., Francis, D. J., Pugh, K. R., & Shaywitz, B. A. (1999). Persistence of dyslexia: The Connecticut Longitudinal Study at adolescence. *Pediatrics, 104,* 1351–1359.

Shaywitz, S. E., & Shaywitz, B. A. (1999). Dyslexia. In K. Swaiman & S. Ashwal (Eds.), *Pediatric neurology: Principles and practice* (3rd ed., Vol. 1, pp. 576–584). St. Louis, MO: Mosby.

Shaywitz, S. E., Shaywitz, B. A., Fletcher, J. M., & Escobar, M. D. (1990). Prevalence of reading disability in boys and girls: Results of the Connecticut Longitudinal Study. *Journal of the American Medical Association, 264*(8), 998–1002.

Shaywitz, S. E., Shaywitz, B. A., Pugh, K. R., Fulbright, R. K., Constable, R. T., Mencl, W. E., Shankweiler, D. P., Liberman, A. M., Skudlarski, P., Fletcher, J. M., Katz, L., Marchione, K. E., La-cadie, C., Gatenby, C., & Gore, J. C. (1998). Functional disruption in the organization of the brain for reading in dyslexia. *Proceedings of the National Academy of Science USA, 95,* 2636–2641.

Shaywitz, S. E. Shaywitz, B. A., Pugh, K., Fulbright, R., Mencl, W., Constable, R., Skudlarski, P., Fletcher, J., Lyon, G., & Gore, J. (in press). The neuropsychology of dyslexia. In S. Segalowitz & I. Rapin (Eds.), *Handbook of neuropsycholology* (2nd ed., Vol. 7). Amsterdam: Elsevier.

Simos, P., Breier, J., Fletcher, J., Bergman, E., & Papanicolaou, A. (2000). Cerebral mechanisms involved in word reading in dyslexic children: A magnetic source imaging approach. *Cerebral Cortex, 10,* 809–816.

Stanovich, K. E., & Siegel, L. S. (1994). Phenotypic performance profile of children with reading disabilities: A regression–based test of the phonological–core variable–difference model. *Journal of Educational Psychology, 86*(1), 24–53.

Stein, J., & Walsh, V. (1997). To see but not to read; the magnocellular theory of dyslexia. *Trends in Neurosciences, 20*(4), 147–152.

Talcott, J., Witton, C., McLean, M., Hansen, P., Rees, A., Green, G., & Stein, J. (2000). Dynamic sensory sensitivity and children's word decoding skills. *Proceedings of the National Academy Science USA, 97,* 2952–2957.

Tallal, P. (2000). The science of literacy: From the laboratory to the classroom. *Proceedings of the National Academy of Science USA, 97,* 2402–2404.

Temple, E., Poldrack, R., Salidas, J., Deutsch, G., Tallal, P., Merzenich, M., & Gabrieli, J. (2001). Disrupted neural responses to phonological and orthographic processing in dyslexic children: An fMRI study. *NeuroReport, 12,* 299–307.

Torgesen, J. K. (1995). *Phonological awareness: A critical factor in dyslexia.* Towson MD: Orton Dyslexia Society.

Van Orden, G. C., Pennington, B. F., & Stone, G. O. (1990). Word identification in reading and the promise of subsymbolic psycholinguistics. *Psychological Review, 97*(4), 488–522.

Wadsworth, S. J., DeFries, J. C., Stevenson, J., Gilger, J. W., & Pennington, B. F. (1992). Gender ratios among reading–disabled children and their siblings as a function of parental impairment. *Journal of Child Psychology and Psychiatry, 33*(7), 1229–1239.

Wagner, R., & Torgesen, J. (1987). The nature of phonological processes and its causal role in the acquisition of reading skills. *Psychological Bulletin, 101,* 192–212.

Wechsler, D. (1991). *Wechsler Intelligence Scale for Children—Third edition (WISC–III).* San Antonio, TX: Psychological Corporation.

Witelson, S. F., & Kigar, D. L. (1992). Sylvian fissure morphology and asymmetry in men and women: Bilateral differences in relation to handedness in men. *Journal of Comparative Neurology, 323,* 326–340.

Wolf, M. (1991). Naming speed and reading: The

contribution of the cognitive neurosciences. *Reading Research Quarterly, 26*(2), 123–141.

Wolf, M., Bally, H., & Morris, R. (1986). Automaticity, retrieval processes, and reading: A longitudinal study in average and impaired readers. *Child Development, 57*, 988–1000.

Wolf, M., & Bowers, P. G. (1999). The double-deficit hypothesis for the developmental dyslexias. *Journal of Educational Psychology, 91*(3), 415–438.

Woodcock, R. W., & Johnson, M. B. (1989). *Woodcock–Johnson Psycho–Educational Battery—Revised (WJ–R)*. Allen, TX: Developmental Learning Materials.

32

What Have We Learned about Learning Disabilities from Qualitative Research?: A Review of Studies

Charles MacArthur

Qualitative methods have become increasingly common in educational research over the past two decades. For example, the *Educational Researcher* regularly publishes articles on controversies about the theoretical grounding of qualitative approaches (e.g., Peshkin, 2000). Qualitative research has had important representatives in special education as well, in particular the researchers at Syracuse University (Bogdan & Biklen, 1982; Ferguson, Ferguson, & Taylor, 1992). However, qualitative research has still not had a major impact within the field of learning disabilities (LD). One reason may be the defining focus of the field on individual differences based on neurological condition and cognition (Kavale & Forness, 1998), which is in conflict with predominant models of qualitative research that focus on understanding the influence of social context. Nonetheless, the body of qualitative research on individuals with LD has grown in the past decade.

The purpose of this review is to understand what the field has learned from qualitative research and how it might advance our understanding in the future. Rather than attempt to describe or explain qualitative methodologies, of which there are many, or enter into debates about method and epistemology, I review the research that has been done in the field using qualitative methods and attempt to answer by example the following questions:

1. What qualitative research has been done on learning disabilities? What topics, theories, and questions have been addressed?
2. What methodologies and theoretical grounding have been used, and what are the strengths and limitations of those methods?
3. What have we learned that we might not have learned using other methods? What other questions should we be asking?

The chapter begins with a brief discussion of the general characteristics of qualitative methodologies and their potential strengths and limitations. Next, I describe procedures for selection of studies for the review. The major part of the chapter consists of reviews of research addressing various topics and questions of importance to the field of LD. The first topic section reviews studies that attempted to understand the meaning of LD from the perspective of individuals with LD. The second section focuses on studies on the important policy issue of inclusion. The third section includes studies that investigated learning and instructional processes in classrooms, mostly from a sociocultural perspective. The final section considers studies that addressed issues pertaining to the education of culturally diverse students. In the conclusions, I make some general observations about the strengths and limitations of qualitative research.

Qualitative Research

Qualitative research defies concise definition because there are so many variations that differ in tradition, epistemological assumptions, theoretical background, and focal interests, as well as in specific methods. Jacob (1987) defined qualitative research in terms of core traditions that gave rise to different approaches and theoretical perspectives. Others have attempted to capture the essential features of qualitative research in general with descriptions of naturalistic inquiry (Lincoln & Guba, 1985) or interpretivist research (Ferguson et al., 1992). A lively debate continues about what counts as qualitative research and how to make theoretical and methodological progress (Putney, Green, Dixon, & Kelly, 1999).

Despite variability in theory and method, approaches to qualitative research share a set of overlapping features giving them a family resemblance. If the prototypical quantitative study is an experimental study with random assignment and quantitative measures of adequate validity and reliability designed to establish causality and/or permit prediction and control, then the prototypical qualitative study is an ethnographic investigation of a culture using participant observation, interview, and analysis of artifacts designed to understand the meaning of cultural activities to members of the culture. A few general characteristics of qualitative research stand out in most accounts.

The first characteristic is a focus on understanding people, events, and constructs in their full social and cultural context. From this commitment flows the emphasis of qualitative methods on studying phenomena in their natural setting, gathering data from as broad a range of sources as possible, and developing rich detailed descriptions of particular cases. For many qualitative researchers, this focus on context arises from an epistemological stance that reality is socially constructed (Ferguson et al., 1992; Lincoln & Guba, 1985). For others, the focus on context is a practical necessity because of the sheer complexity of factors that influence people and events (Miles & Huberman, 1984; Strauss, 1987). Experimental research is not as well suited to studying complex social settings because the experimental controls and predefined measures change the situation in ways that invalidate the findings. In this sense, qualitative research is practical because it produces findings that can be applied by practitioners in real world settings.

A second, and related, characteristic is the open-ended nature of qualitative investigations. Although researchers begin with a set of questions, they avoid *a priori* definitions of constructs, categories, hypotheses, and data sources in favor of generating them during data collection. Data collection and interpretation occur simultaneously so that initial interpretations and new questions can guide further data collection. This approach permits the development of interpretations and theories that are grounded in the particular context under study (Strauss, 1987). Thus, it is consistent with the overall goal of qualitative research to describe social phenomena in ways that capture the organization, interpretation, and meaning of the phenomena as constructed by the people involved. It also provides flexibility in examining social situations at multiple levels from the overall culture, to institutions, to group and individual behavior.

A third characteristic of much qualitative research is a focus on understanding the meaning of events and constructs from an emic, or insider, perspective. The familiar methods of participant observation, interview, and analysis of artifacts are well suited to understanding the world as experienced by the people being studied. Bruner (1990) contended that there are two irreducible ways of knowing the world, the narrative and the scientific. The scientific mode seeks explanations that are context free and can be verified by appeal to formal procedures, whereas the narrative mode seeks explanations that are particular to the context and capture the meaning of experience. According to Bruner, narrative is the primary way that people represent the world and their own identities. Qualitative research, by representing the world as experienced by the people studied, gives a voice to those people, in many cases to people such as those with disabilities who would not otherwise be heard (Pugach, 2001).

A fourth characteristic of qualitative research that separates it not from quantitative research but from other forms of narrative knowing such as literature and simple storytelling is the use of systematic procedures for gathering, analyzing, and interpreting data. Regardless of the particular methods for collecting and analyzing data, qualitative researchers stress the importance of procedures for ensuring the trustworthiness of data and checking the validity of interpretations (Lincoln & Guba, 1985; Strauss, 1987). Frequently mentioned procedures include prolonged engagement, triangulation using multiple data sources, systematic procedures for coding and organizing data, and checking interpretations with participants and other researchers. One of the potential problems in reporting qualitative research is that it is often difficult to convey in sufficient detail the procedures employed, especially in journal-length articles. Thus, it is often difficult for readers to determine whether sound research practices were followed.

A final characteristic is that qualitative research seeks understanding of particular cases in context rather than seeking to establish generalizable principles. It is not that qualitative researchers are unconcerned about whether their findings apply to other situations but that their theoretical stances and methods lead them to make claims only about the particular settings studied. Generalization is possible but only by comparing the features of the settings studied with other situations to see whether the findings might apply and by the accumulation of multiple studies. A difficulty in reporting qualitative research is the problem of communicating enough of the critical information about context to make such generalization possible.

Selection of Studies for Review

Qualitative research, as discussed previously, includes a wide range of methods and theoretical perspectives, so that any definition of qualitative methods is bound to be controversial. However, a procedural definition was necessary to select studies for the review, and a fairly inclusive definition was used. I included studies that were described using terms such as "qualitative," "ethnographic," "interpretive," and "case study," and studies that relied on analysis of field notes, interviews, or transcripts of discourse. Studies were not included if interview or observation data were reduced to quantitative categories for interpretation (e.g., surveys conducted by interview). Nor were case studies of students included in which data were primarily derived from assessments (e.g., clinical case studies or analysis of errors on assessment tasks). However, studies that combined qualitative and quantitative methods were included. In addition to fitting a definition of qualitative, reports needed to include at least some minimal description of the data collected and the method of analysis; this criterion eliminated quite a few papers that provided a narrative description of students or classroom settings without any information that would permit the reader to determine the trustworthiness of the information. Finally, studies had to include individuals with LD. Reviews of literature and theoretical papers were not included in the set of articles reviewed, though many of them are referenced as background. The selection was further limited to published journal articles, books, and chapters.

Selection of studies began with a search of the ERIC database crossing terms related to qualitative methods (e.g., "qualitative," "ethnographic," "discourse analysis," "case study," and "interpretive") with various forms of the term "learning disability" for the 11 years from 1991 to 2001. Next, one journal on special education and three specifically on LD (*Exceptional Children, Journal of Learning Disabilities, Learning Disability Quarterly*, and *Learning Disabilities Research and Practice*) were hand-searched for the same period. Finally, references in these articles were pursued. Though a systematic search was made, it is likely that some important research was missed that was published in other journals or in books.

The numbers of papers published in special education and LD journals is of some interest. All numbers are for the 11 years 1991–2001. In *Exceptional Children*, 54 articles using qualitative research were published, 5 theoretical papers and 49 research studies, including 14 on students with LD. The number of articles per year increased substantially from 2.4 (range 0–4) in the first 5 of those years to 7.8 (range 7–8) in the last 5 years. In the *Journal of Learning Disabilities*, a total of 38 articles with qualitative approaches were published, a number substantially increased by the 22 articles published as part of a series edited by Poplin (1995). Of the 38 articles, 9 were theoretical pieces and 8 were eliminated because they reported no methods, leaving 21 studies included in this review. In *Learning Disability Quarterly*, total articles using qualitative research numbered 21 with no trend over time. Omitting 5 theoretical essays and 2 studies that had no description of methods left 14 studies for the review. In *Learning Disabilities Research and Practice*, 20 articles using qualitative research were found, including 4 theoretical papers and 16 research studies. In addition, 17 papers were found in other journals or book chapters. In sum, 82 qualitative studies focusing on individuals with LD or their parents, teachers, and school programs were reviewed.

Insider View of Learning Disabilities

One of the frequently cited characteristics of qualitative research is its focus on interpreting and understanding the views of insiders to a culture (Bogdan & Biklen, 1982; Ferguson et al., 1992; Lincoln & Guba, 1985). Traditional quantitative research has investigated the views of students with LD and their teachers and parents through the use of surveys and questionnaires. Ethnographic research, in contrast, seeks understanding of the meanings ascribed to concepts and activities by prolonged engagement with individuals in their cultural settings using participant observation, interview, and artifacts as data (Bogdan & Biklen, 1982). For ex-

ample, in a classic study, Bogdan and Taylor (1982) told the life stories, from their own point of view, of two people who had been labeled retarded by the system and had lived in a variety of homes and institutions. These case histories demonstrated that persons labeled mentally retarded are individuals with a range of competencies, emotions, and needs like anyone, and that these two individuals had been damaged by the treatment they received from society. The authors rejected the concept of mental retardation as a social construction that tells little about individuals and serves to justify society in excluding the "retarded" from normal lives, warehousing them in institutions and denying them education, work, and lives in the community. The studies of individuals with LD are, perhaps, not as dramatic but nonetheless offer insights into their self-perceptions and their views on the effects of their disabilities and the impact of labeling and special education.

This category includes seven studies of the views of adults with LD, three studies of the perspectives of students on the meaning of LD, and five studies that focused particularly on students' views about inclusion. The studies of adults included vocationally successful adults, college students, recent dropouts, and teachers who themselves had LD. Gerber, Ginsberg, and Reiff (1992; Gerber & Reiff, 1991; Reiff, Gerber, & Ginsberg, 1993) studied adults who were successful vocationally to understand patterns of functioning responsible for their success. They conducted lengthy ethnographic interviews and administered measures of self-esteem, achievement motivation, and workplace relationships. Repeated interviews offered the opportunity to check emerging interpretations with the participants. In one paper (Gerber et al., 1992), they compared the responses of 46 highly successful adults with 25 moderately successful adults and found no differences on the quantitative measures. The interviews were coded and analyzed for themes that the adults believed accounted for their success. The overall theme found in the analysis was one of control, with the highly successful adults demonstrating greater goal orientation, ability to reframe their LD in positive ways, learned creativity, adaptability, persistence, and understanding of social situations. A second paper (Reiff et al., 1993) reported their analysis of a single question about the adults' definition of LD. Most of the adults provided traditional responses, such as processing difficulty, limitations in reading, or underachievement, though a few defined their problem as learning differences rather than as disabilities.

In a later study (Shessel & Reiff, 1999), 14 adults with LD representing a wide range of educational attainment (10th grade to master's degree) and age (26 to 60) were interviewed. Four negative impacts of LD were identified: problems in daily living and on the job due to limited reading, spatial difficulties, and time management; social isolation often attributed to feelings of difference developed in their school years; emotional health issues of stress, anxiety, and depression, again often attributed to negative school experiences; and the impostor phenomenon, a sense that any success was due to false impressions of competence which might be exposed as fraud. On the other hand, several respondents also discussed positive impacts, believing that their LD had made them better persons, allowed them to think creatively, increased their sensitivity and desire to help others, and improved them as helping professionals.

Three studies focused on developing a complex understanding of elementary and secondary school students' perspectives about the impact of LD. For example, Guterman (1995) studied nine high school students who had been identified as LD in elementary school and were currently placed in a mix of LD and regular classes. She interviewed them repeatedly over the course of a semester both individually and in small groups and gathered data from their files. Students also wrote autobiographies recounting their school histories. Initial interpretations were checked with the students, and another researcher audited the data. All students reported negative effects of LD on acceptance by their normally achieving peers. They felt that their peers had negative stereotypes about LD and saw them as less intelligent. Consequently, they made efforts to conceal the fact that they went to LD classes. The intensity of the interviews enabled the researcher to get beyond superficial responses. For example, students claimed that they did not internal-

ize their peers' negative stereotypes, but all remembered times they had felt they had serious personal deficiencies. Most claimed to have made peace with their LD placements, often through involvement in nonacademic activities. However, one student continued to experience painful feelings of low self-esteem and exclusion from school activities and peers. Students reported mixed feelings about the effectiveness of their LD classes. On one hand, they did not find the classes challenging and did not feel they had gained the skills they needed. On the other hand, they did not think it was reasonable to expect that teachers in regular classes could meet their needs within the regular curriculum. Given the realities of schools, they preferred to be in LD classes where they could get help and work at their own level.

Five studies focused specifically on issues related to inclusion, including students' preferences for inclusive or resource room classes, views on instructional adaptations, and grouping in inclusive classrooms. Reid and Button (1995) reported a case study of a middle school girl based on an individual interview and a group discussion on planning an essay about what it was like to have LD. They identified themes of isolation, undervaluing, and oppression by a system that was not responsive to students' needs or feelings. Albinger (1995) analyzed interviews with five elementary students in her own resource room classes. The students reported that other students called them names and it made them feel as if there was something wrong with them, though older students had a better understanding of their disabilities. Four of the five students reported fabricating stories for their peers to hide the fact that they were going to the resource room. Pugach and Wesson (1995) investigated the other side of the story, conducting interviews with students with and without LD in an inclusive fifth-grade classroom cotaught by general and special education teachers. They reported a highly positive social climate characterized by positive attitudes toward themselves and others, an acceptance of giving and receiving help from peers and both teachers, and positive images of all teachers.

A pair of studies by Vaughn, Klinger, and their colleagues (Forgan & Vaughn, 2000; Klinger, Vaughn, Schumm, Cohen, & Forgan, 1998) used a combination of quantitative and qualitative methods to analyze interviews on students' preferences for resource room or inclusive placements and grouping practices for reading instruction. For example in one study (Klinger et al., 1998), 16 students with LD and 16 without LD, who had had experience with both resource room and inclusive classroom models, were interviewed about their preferences. Responses were categorized with checks for interrater reliability, and numbers of students with LD and without giving each response were reported. Students with LD were about evenly split in overall preference for the two settings, but majorities thought that the resource room helped them learn and the inclusive class helped them make friends. No strong emotions were presented except for one LD student who disliked the resource room because his friends had teased him.

The studies included in this section relied primarily on qualitative analysis of interviews to understand the views of individuals with LD. Interview transcripts were analyzed inductively for categories of responses guided by general questions. The best of the studies, such as those by Gerber, Reiff, and their colleagues and the study by Guterman (1995), made use of repeated interviews that provided the opportunity to get to know the respondents, to pursue leads, and to check their initial interpretations with the respondents. They also gathered data from formal assessments to describe the participants. Extended interviews permit a depth of understanding of individual views that cannot be gathered in other ways. However, this methodology has limitations as well. First, the content of the interviews is subject to interviewers' biases in the course of extended interaction, as well as by the views that the respondents wish to project. For the most part, these studies did not use data from interviews with friends, parents, or teachers or from participant observation to check on the interpretations derived from the interviews. Second, generalization is problematic, especially when researchers do not explain the reasons for selection of particular cases (Reid & Button, 1995). Generalization is enhanced when researchers use purposive sampling as in the studies of successful adults (Gerber et al., 1992). Quanti-tative studies of students' perceptions can potentially claim wider generalizability, though they often do not include representative samples either.

Whatever the limitations of interviews, these studies did provide a voice for individuals with LD that is not often heard. A common theme in these studies of the insider view on LD is the emotional problems and social isolation resulting from feelings of difference and inadequacy and the attempt to conceal LD out of shame or, perhaps, a realistic expectation of discrimination. Adults (Shessel & Reiff, 1999), high school students (Guterman, 1995), and elementary school students (Albinger, 1995; Reid & Button, 1995) all reported similar experiences of negative stereotypes and exclusion by peers, in some cases balanced by a more positive acceptance of their disability and even a feeling that it had strengthened them in some way. The studies of successful adults with LD (Gerber et al., 1992; Reiff et al., 1993) focused on their ability to cope with the world after school. Of course, these adults are not representative of most graduates of special education programs. However, by highlighting the positive attributes of these individuals, the studies raised questions about whether students with LD are disadvantaged by placement in special programs that focus on their limitations rather than their strengths. Perhaps education in inclusive classrooms would help to avoid negative stereotypes and better support students' individual development. We turn now to research on inclusion.

Inclusion

In the introductory chapter to a book written with his colleagues on mainstreaming (Biklen, Bogdan, Ferguson, Searl, & Taylor, 1985), Biklen points out that the appropriate question is not whether mainstreaming is a good idea but, rather, what it means in various school contexts and what it takes to implement effective mainstreaming programs. Like many questions of school policy, inclusion of students with disabilities is a complex issue that involves principles of civil rights, cultural beliefs about disability, school funding, organizational structures, teacher and student attitudes, staff development, and classroom interactions. Qualitative methods are well suited to the study of complex issues and programs in natural settings (Miles & Huberman, 1984; Peck & Furman, 1992; Strauss, 1987). The open-ended and flexible nature of qualitative methodology permits researchers to discover the concepts, activities, and structures that are meaningful to participants in the context, to generate explanations, and to check them with further data collection.

A relatively large number of studies were found on inclusion of students with LD in general education classes. In addition to the studies of student perceptions of inclusion discussed previously, there were 22 separate studies on inclusion contained in 28 published reports. The majority of these studies described inclusion programs at the school or classroom level with a focus on describing the instruction received by students with LD. These studies covered schoolwide inclusion programs, classrooms of teachers nominated as effective at inclusion, and classrooms co-taught by teams of regular and special educators. Several studies focused on staff development or preservice training, including a series of studies on consulting teachers.

One influential study by Zigmond and Baker (Zigmond, 1995; see also Baker & Zigmond, 1995) was reported in a special issue of the *Journal of Special Education*, together with responses from seven scholars and educators. Zigmond and Baker conducted a series of case studies in five elementary schools across the country that were implementing models of full-time inclusive education. In 2-day site visits, researchers focused on the educational experiences of two target students with LD. Students were observed for 2 full days using structured field notes. Interviews were conducted with the students, their general and special education teachers, their parents, the principal, and administrators. In addition, students and their classmates completed an assessment of basic academic skills and student records and other documents were reviewed. Case studies were written for each school describing the context for inclusion, the model of inclusion, the roles of general and special education teachers and other staff, and the educational experiences of the target students. Cross-case analysis was organized around a series of questions about the meaning and practice of inclusion and its implications for personnel preparation. Though their methods did not provide sufficient length of engagement to develop an in-depth understanding of the programs studied, their study did offer a broad view of a range of programs.

Most prominently, Baker and Zigmond (1995) concluded that there was little special instruction occurring in inclusive classrooms. Some minor accommodations were made, and general education teachers implemented teaching practices recommended by special educators, such as strategy instruction, for all the students, but there was almost no "individually designed, intensive, remedial instruction of students who were clearly struggling with the schoolwork they were being given." (Baker & Zigmond, 1995, p. 178). They also noted that inclusion was defined differently across schools. For example, in some schools, it was seen as a voluntary program requiring individual commitment from teachers who chose to co-teach, whereas other schools implemented it as a schoolwide commitment. Responses to the study were divided on whether the authors thought inclusion was workable. For example, Gerber (1995) interpreted the study as evidence that inclusive education programs cannot meet the special needs of students with LD because they introduce more diversity in the classroom than teachers can manage. On the other side, Pugach (1995) argued that the cases represented only an initial effort at inclusion and that more fundamental reform of educational practice in both general and special education is needed to develop classrooms where all students can succeed.

It is important to note that qualitative studies of the instruction provided in resource room programs have not presented a more positive picture. Vaughn, Moody, and Schumm (1998) studied reading instruction in 14 elementary resource rooms, based on interviews at the beginning and end of the year and three observations. They reported that most teachers used whole-class instruction with little individualization despite a wide range of reading abilities. A follow-up with six of the teachers 2 years later (Moody, Vaughn, Hughes, & Fischer, 2000) found that teachers taught more phonics but still did not individualize instruction significantly.

Case studies of successful inclusion have focused their analysis on how inclusion can be conducted successfully. Scruggs and Mastropieri (1994b) studied three teachers recommended as successful in integrating students with disabilities into their middle school science classes. Researchers observed and videotaped instruction for several weeks at the beginning and end of the school year, interviewed the teachers and students frequently, interviewed administrators, and gathered student work. Analytic procedures included coding, member checks, and systematic search for supporting and disconfirming evidence for each claim. They reported that students with LD were able to participate in science activities successfully and received special support. They identified seven variables associated with mainstreaming success: (1) administrative support, (2) consulting support from special educators, (3) an accepting positive atmosphere, (4) appropriate curriculum with hands-on activities, (5) effective general teaching skills (e.g., structure and clarity), (6) peer assistance, and (7) disability-specific teaching skills (e.g., using explicit, concrete explanations). Based on this and other research, Scruggs and Mastropieri (1995) proposed a set of instructional features that could be used to evaluate either inclusion or resource room classes.

One model for inclusion that has been investigated in several studies is co-teaching by general and special educators. Mac-Arthur and Rozmairek (1999) reported two case studies of successful inclusion based on full-time co-teaching. In this model, teachers shared responsibility for classes of about 30 students including 6–10 students with disabilities, mostly LD. The teachers thought that co-teaching provided the level of resources necessary for intensive small-group and individual teaching for students who needed it without pulling them out of the classroom. Observations confirmed the success of the teachers in providing specially designed instruction for students with disabilities and other low-achieving students. Teachers agreed that successful co-teaching required a high degree of personal and professional compatibility and a commitment to integrate the students as fully as possible.

Walther-Thomas (1997) investigated co-teaching by 119 teachers in 18 elementary and 7 middle schools using single interviews and observations of each teacher. Rice and Zigmond (2000) used interviews and observations to investigate co-teaching by 17 secondary teachers in Australia and the United States. In both studies, teachers reported that strong administrative support, a schoolwide commitment to inclusion, adequate planning time, and personal and professional compatibility were important for success. At the secondary level (Rice & Zigmond, 2000), lack of content-area expertise by special education teachers was often a problem.

Another model for supporting inclusion is the use of special educators as consulting teachers. Gersten and his colleagues (Gersten, Darch, Davis, & George, 1991; Gersten, Morvant, & Brengelman, 1995; Marks & Gersten, 1998) developed and implemented a model of consulting teaching and conducted three intensive qualitative studies on factors that make consulting successful and on the training needed by consulting teachers. In their model, consulting teachers worked with 8 to 12 general education teachers providing recommendations for individual students, demonstration teaching, coaching, and problem solving, all focused on research-based methods for reading instruction (e.g., reciprocal teaching). One study (Gersten et al., 1995) investigated the consulting process through case studies of the coaching received by 12 general education teachers. Based on observations and audiotapes of consulting sessions, classroom observations, and regular interviews with teachers over multiple years, the researchers identified several key issues that consulting teachers needed to consider. First, the process of consulting typically resulted in uneven progress and acceptance of coaching with temporary setbacks followed by further development. Second, consulting required great sensitivity to teachers' anxiety about being evaluated. Finally, general education teachers tended to have a different perspective because they focused more on the whole class than on individuals. Another study (Gersten et al., 1991) compared two consulting teachers who had received intensive apprenticeship training with six who had received more typical training. Apprenticeship training led to dramatic differences in the amount of time spent actually advising teachers on instruction and demonstrating effective approaches. Teachers found the apprenticeship consulting teachers much more helpful. A third study (Marks & Gersten, 1998) pursued the investigation of the consulting process with a focus on factors that influenced the level of engagement of general education teachers in the process.

Looking beyond the classroom level, a pair of studies by Mamlin and colleagues (Mamlin, 1999; Mamlin & Harris, 1998) addressed school level factors that affected the success of inclusion and prereferral programs. In one detailed case study of an elementary school where inclusion was successful, Mamlin and Harris (1998) found a consistent philosophy among teachers and principal that all children were there to learn, that the staff functioned as a team, that the school was expected to be flexible in meeting students' needs, and that needs could be met without formal referral to special education except in a few cases in which more resources were needed. In contrast, a case study of a secondary school (Mamlin, 1999) found no progress toward inclusion despite a formal policy and attributed the failure to an entrenched culture of segregation and ineffective leadership from the principal.

Qualitative studies have made a significant contribution to answering the questions posed by Biklen (Biklen et al., 1985) about what inclusion means in various school contexts and what it takes to implement effective inclusion programs. Clearly, it takes a strong commitment on the part of general and special education teachers and administration (Mamlin, 1999). However, it takes much more than goodwill as demonstrated by the case studies of inclusion programs across the country in which students were not receiving instruction adapted to their needs despite teachers and administrators who supported the programs (Baker & Zigmond, 1995; Zigmond, 1995). Case studies have investigated alternative models for using special education resources in the development of inclusion programs. For example, case studies have shown the potential of co-teaching and highlighted some of the requirements for success. Another mod-

el that has been investigated intensively is to use special education teachers as consultants to general education teachers. Case studies make it clear that consulting is a demanding role requiring considerable knowledge and interpersonal skill that is best developed through apprenticeships with experienced consultants. In short, the development of effective inclusion programs is a complex undertaking. Certainly, one requirement for successful inclusion is effective teaching (Scruggs & Mastropieri, 1994a). The next section of this review focuses directly on research that attempts to understand in some detail the nature of effective instruction for students with LD.

Classroom Instructional Processes

A number of studies have used qualitative methods to understand the dynamics of instruction and learning in classroom settings. Most of these studies are based on sociocultural or social constructivist theories that emphasize the importance of social context to learning (Englert & Palincsar, 1991; Tharp & Gallimore, 1988). Sociocultural theories contend that learning and literacy are defined socially and culturally at many levels: by the society and culture as a whole, at the institutional level, in families, and in individual classrooms. Furthermore, students need to participate in meaningful literacy activities to develop an understanding of the meaning and purpose of literacy, why and when to use strategies, and how to use literacy to meet goals. Also, sociocultural theories contend that mature thought processes develop through interactions with others, particularly verbal interactions scaffolded by adults (Vygotsky, 1978). Such scaffolded instruction is extremely complex because it requires the adult to monitor the students' developing understanding and provide just the right amount of explanation, modeling, and prompting at each point in time (Pressley, Hogan, Wharton-McDonald, Mistretta, & Ettenberger, 1996). To understand learning, then, it is necessary to examine in detail the interactions that occur in classrooms and the ways that teachers and students think about the interactions as well as the larger school and societal influences (McPhail & Palincsar, 1998). Quantitative outcome measures may be used to assess learning, but qualitative methods are needed to understand the instructional interactions and the meanings ascribed to learning activities by teachers and students. Qualitative research methods have been developed that permit study of the culture of the classroom, the discourse among teachers and students, and developmental changes in groups as well as individual students.

A small but growing number of researchers are applying qualitative research methods to understand instruction for students with LD. A total of 21 studies were found in this category. One research group that has developed a systematic program of research on classroom processes from a sociocultural perspective includes Englert, Mariage, and their colleagues. They have developed programs of literacy instruction based on sociocultural principles and conducted both quantitative and qualitative research on these programs. They have used quasi-experimental methods to demonstrate the overall impact on learning (Englert, Raphael, Anderson, Anthony, & Stevens, 1991). Their qualitative studies have used discourse analysis methods (Forman & McCormick, 1995) to investigate differences between more and less effective teachers (Mariage, 1995), to describe teacher–student interactions of effective teachers (Englert 1992; Englert, Rozendal, & Mariage, 1994), and to study classroom interaction around particular literacy events (Mariage, 2000, 2001). (For further information, see Englert & Mariage, Chapter 27, this volume.)

Palincsar and various colleagues over time have also conducted a number of qualitative studies of classroom processes involving students with LD or reading problems. The initial work on reciprocal teaching (Palincsar & Brown, 1984) used quantitative measures of reading comprehension to demonstrate learning outcomes and qualitative analysis of student–teacher discourse to explain how teachers scaffolded student performance. In the period covered by the present review, she has conducted qualitative studies of literacy learning (Palincsar & Klenk, 1992; Palincsar, Parecki, & McPhail, 1995) and of inquiry approaches to science education (Cutter, Palincsar, & Magnusson, 2002; Palincsar, Magnusson, Collins, & Cutter, 2001). For example, Palincsar and colleagues (1995) conducted an exploratory case study in an elementary special education classroom of a literature unit focused on the theme of friendship. They found that students' awareness of the theme of friendship developed without explicit instruction in identifying themes and that students' conceptions of friendship grew in complexity as indicated by the language used in discussions. The work on science education is discussed later.

An important concern in the application of sociocultural theory to classroom practice and instruction is the degree of explicit instruction that is appropriate within a context of meaningful activities and social interactions. There has been a lively debate in the field of LD about the appropriate balance between explicit instruction and learning through social participation in meaningful activities (see special issues on constructivism: Harris & Graham, 1994). Some scholars have expressed the view that strategy instruction is incompatible with social constructivism (Poplin, 1988). MacArthur, Schwartz, Graham, Molloy, and Harris, (1996) conducted a case study of two teachers attempting to integrate explicit instruction in writing strategies into a language arts program described by the teachers as a reading and writing workshop based on whole-language principles. Using participant observation and interview, the research focused on the extent to which strategy instruction was consistent with teachers' prior beliefs and practices. After 4 months of strategy instruction, the teachers perceived a good fit between strategy instruction and the whole-language program, and classroom observations supported their view. First, the teachers' emphasis on authentic writing tasks provided a meaningful context for teaching strategies. Second, the teachers found that strategies offered a way to develop students' competence and increase their independence. Gains in quality and organization on quantitatively scored writing samples confirmed the teachers' assessment of improved writing performance. Third, the teachers' strong commitment to student independence led them to transfer control of strategies to students as soon as possible. Finally, their interactive teaching style and emphasis on conferencing supported effective scaffolding of the strategies. The work of Englert and her colleagues, mentioned previously, also supports the effectiveness of including self-regulated strategies in social constructivist approaches to instruction.

The studies previously mentioned have all focused on literacy learning, but qualitative methods have also been used to study learning in content-area classes. Scruggs and Mastropieri (1994a), in a case study of science instruction in an elementary special education class, focused on how students with LD would construct knowledge in an inquiry-based approach. They reported many instances of active construction of knowledge based on inquiry but also found that carefully structured teacher explanations, adaptations such as enhanced vocabulary instruction, effective behavior management, and careful coaching by teachers were necessary.

A research institute with teams from four institutions (REACH) has been conducting research on the inclusion of students with LD and other disabilities in classrooms implementing challenging curricula in science, social studies, math, and literature. Across all teams, the curricula are based on four principles: learning involves inquiry approaches using authentic tasks; cognitive strategies are integrated with instruction; learning is socially mediated through interaction with teachers and peers; and discourse is structured as constructive conversations. A variety of approaches are being used to support effective learning by students with disabilities. All teams are using a combination of quantitative and qualitative analyses to document learning outcomes and understand classroom processes that affect learning.

The REACH team at the University of Michigan led by Palincsar and Magnusson has conducted a systematic program of research on guided inquiry science instruction in elementary classrooms that includes two qualitative studies focused on inclusion of students with LD (Cutter et al., 2002; Palincsar et al., 2001). Palincsar and colleagues (2001) conducted an innovative design experiment with two phases. In the first phase, case studies of four students with LD were developed based on participant observation, videotaping, regular in-

terviews of teachers and students, and student work. Contrary to the initial beliefs of teachers, who saw small-group work as a nonproblematic way to provide peer support for low-achieving students, the case studies showed clear patterns of students with LD being subtly or not so subtly excluded from participation in the groups. In phase 2, "advanced teaching practices" to address the problems revealed by the case studies were developed collaboratively by the teachers and researchers during summer workshops, and these practices (e.g., teacher monitoring and facilitation of thinking, reading support, attention to group composition) were implemented by four teachers. In phase 2, quantitative performance assessment measures were used to compare the performance of LD, low-achieving, and high-achieving students during phases 1 and 2; all groups of students did better in the second year with the advanced teaching practices. Qualitative analyses were used to relate patterns in gains for the three groups to patterns of implementation by the teachers. Another qualitative study (Cutter et al., 2002) investigated the process of collaborative development of the advanced teaching practices during the summer workshops.

The REACH team led by Morocco has focused on implementation of schoolwide thematic studies of literature using a literacy cycle that aims to help students acquire deep understanding of literary texts and of interpretation processes through frequent opportunities to engage in authentic, meaningful reading and writing opportunities, supported by strategic thinking and constructive conversations with peers. In a case study report (Morocco, Hindin, Mata-Aguilar, & Mott, 2002), they used discourse analysis of teacher-led introductions to a new book and small-group discussions to understand how students interpreted literature in small groups, how students with disabilities were supported in those groups, and how teacher discourse mediated student learning.

The REACH team working on mathematics, led by Woodward and Baxter at the University of Puget Sound, has focused on including students with LD in classrooms that are using a math curriculum with a strong focus on problem solving. In a recent study (Baxter, Woodward, Voorhuis, & Wong, 2002), they analyzed the discourse in a fourth-grade class where the teacher conscientiously tried to include all students in the discussion. They found that discourse became markedly more student directed over time with more comments by the teacher asking for student reflections on problems, and that students progressed from reporting calculations to reporting solution strategies and justifying their claims. The students with LD were included in the discussion but often had difficulty explaining their strategies, posing a dilemma for teachers in that time spent figuring out what they meant and helping them detracted from helping the class understand a set of strategies.

The REACH team responsible for social studies, led by Ferretti, MacArthur, and Okolo at the University of Delaware, focused on the development of historical understanding and reasoning. As the culminating activity of a sixth-grade unit on immigration in the early 20th century, students debated the issue of whether immigrants should have been permitted to come to this country (MacArthur, Ferretti, & Okolo, 2002). Tests of content knowledge and interviews scored both quantitatively and qualitatively demonstrated overall gains in understanding of key concepts about immigration. Discourse analysis of a series of debates in one class was used to understand the opportunities afforded by, and the limitations of, those debates. Analyses of content and structure showed that students' discourse was influenced by the knowledge they gained during the unit, but that the rhetorical goal to defend a viewpoint about immigration led to distorted positions weakly supported with evidence, especially at first, though later rounds of the debate were more balanced and drew more on the breadth of available knowledge. Overall, the debates were more typical of everyday arguments than academic arguments. Importantly, from the perspective of special education, the debates promoted high levels of engagement and equal participation by students with and without LD as well as by boys and girls.

One interesting methodological feature of the research discussed in this section is the combination of quantitative and qualitative methods used. All these researchers made use of quantitatively scored measures of student outcomes to evaluate the effectiveness of instruction in pretest–posttest designs, quasi-experiments, or design experiments. The measures used, however, went beyond standardized measures to include authentic performance assessments, writing samples, and interviews. These researchers found no incompatibility between quantitative measures and designs and qualitative investigations of classroom discourse and group interactions based on sociocultural theories. Perhaps, this diversity of method is partially explained by the fact that most of these researchers began their careers studying learning from a primarily cognitive perspective. As their understanding of learning changed to incorporate sociocultural and sociolinguistic concepts, they found it necessary to adopt new research methods that would enable them to investigate these concepts (McPhail & Palincsar, 1998). However, they continued to recognize the importance of individual cognitive development within a social context and continued to find it appropriate to assess individual learning as well as the social dynamics of classrooms.

Qualitative research from a sociocultural perspective in the field of LD is just beginning to enhance our understanding of the dynamics of learning in classrooms. It has illustrated the importance of authentic, meaningful activities in the development of understanding. It has shown in some detail how teachers scaffold student learning through dialogue in particular classroom activities (Englert & Mariage, Chapter 27, this volume; Baxter et al., 2002) and through the ways they monitor progress and facilitate group interaction (Palincsar et al., 2001). Sociocultural theories can also be applied to collaborative work between researchers and teachers to develop instruction and change teachers' beliefs and practice (Cutter, et al., 2002). The research has also investigated the opportunities afforded by peer collaboration in activities such as literacy circles (Morocco et al., 2002) and classroom debates (MacArthur et al., 2002). Finally, the research has helped us to understand the challenges involved in supporting students with LD in general education.

Culturally Diverse Learners

Controversies about valid assessment, appropriate instruction, and overrepresentation in special education classes of racially, ethnically, and linguistically diverse learners have been prominent in the field of special education for many years (Artiles & Trent, 1994; Reschly, 1984). Reviews of the literature indicate that limited research exists to guide educational practices for English-language learners in general (Gersten & Baker, 2000) or culturally diverse learners with LD in particular (Artiles, Trent, & Kuan, 1997). Several scholars have called for a sociocultural approach to understanding the interactions of culture and disability (Bos & Fletcher, 1997; Keogh, Gallimore, & Weisner, 1997). Ethnographic methods with their primary focus on culture are well suited to developing an understanding of interactions among culture and learning. In special education, the ethnographic work of Harry (1992) with poor, Puerto Rican parents of children with disabilities demonstrates the ability of such research to capture their voices and views about disabilities and about communication with the schools. However, limited qualitative research has been done with culturally diverse students with disabilities, especially in the field of LD. A review by Artiles, Trent, and Kuan (1997) of two special education and two LD journals for a 22-year period and found only 7 qualitative studies (and only 58 quantitative studies) focused on ethnic and linguistic minorities.

The current review identified 10 studies that focused on culturally diverse students with LD. Ruiz (1995a, 1995b) reported findings from a 2-year ethnographic study of a bilingual special education classroom with 10 Latino children labeled language learning disabled (LLD). Classroom events were analyzed according to contextual features, such as grouping, topic, teacher goal, turn taking, language (Spanish/English), and linguistic features. Events were ranked for degree of formality, or structuring of rules for communication. For example, lessons for the weakest language users were relatively informal, structured around everyday communication situations, whereas lessons for higher-functioning students were characterized by formal exercises in

English usage. Sociodramatic play was highly informal. Students' language was analyzed for the degree of communicative competence displayed in each event (Cazden, 1988). Ruiz (1995a) showed that communicative competence varied with the degree of formality of the classroom event. Students who performed quite poorly under demands for correct English demonstrated greater competence in pragmatic language function, grammar, vocabulary, and confidence in informal events. Ruiz (1995b) suggested that language assessment would be more accurate if based on informal situations than on formal tests, supporting her argument with case studies of students that revealed clear differences among students in language competence with frequent communicative breakdowns by some students with severe LLD, mild problems for some other students, and language differences but not disabilities for others.

Ruiz, Rueda, Figueroa, and Boothroyd, (1995) suggested further that classroom structures characterized by informality and meaningful context would result in accelerated learning. The Optimal Learning Environments (OLE) program worked with teachers in bilingual special education classes to implement constructivist instructional approaches, such as writing workshop and reciprocal teaching (Palincsar & Brown, 1984). The process of change in teachers' beliefs and classroom practices was investigated in a series of five case studies of project teachers (Ruiz et al., 1995). Teachers' beliefs about the nature of disability and their classroom practices were placed on a continuum from reductionist to holistic/constructivist (Poplin, 1988). Teachers with the most special education training tended to hold the most reductionist beliefs about disability. Changes in beliefs about disability and in actual classroom practices over the 3 years of the project were not related to each other. These findings may be due to a conceptual flaw in the study in that a belief in the reality of individual disabilities was rated as reductionist.

Like OLE, the method of instructional conversations (IC) aims to improve student acquisition of English and literacy by structuring lessons to encourage thoughtful discussion without focusing on language form (Tharp & Gallimore, 1988). IC lessons have an instructional purpose but take the form of a natural conversation that permits students to participate at any level of language competence. Echevarria and McDonough (1995) conducted a case study of the implementation of IC in an elementary bilingual special education class. Based on extensive observation and interviews, they concluded that IC did provide a holistic context for learning, particularly through the emphasis on a central theme for discussion, and that it provided opportunities for ample student language development. However, they also noted that some adaptations, such as more concrete explanations, were needed with special education students. A small-scale quantitative study of IC with only five students (Echevarria, 1995) found that, compared to a basal approach, IC resulted in more and higher-quality talk during the discussion and more references to theme in retelling but lower scores on traditional reading comprehension measures. It may be that the focus of IC on language development did not fit these outcome measures as well as the basal approach's focus on specific story structure questions.

Clearly, a great deal more research is needed to understand how to provide effective instruction to minority students that is sensitive to differences in language and culture. The ethnographic research of Ruiz (1995a, 1995b) showed how the communicative competence of bilingual students identified as LLD varied substantially across classroom events depending on the formality of language demands. Such research provides a better understanding of the nature of language differences and disabilities and suggests types of classroom activities that might support language development. Evaluation of instructional programs for culturally diverse students should combine quantitative methods to assess learning outcomes with qualitative research to understand the classroom processes that contribute to, or limit, its effectiveness.

However, more is needed than research focused specifically on designing programs for culturally diverse students. Issues of culture should be included widely in research in special education. Qualitative researchers have a special role to play in developing the field's understanding of the impact of race, poverty, language, and culture on the lives

of children and their interactions with schools (Pugach, 2001). In addition, sociocultural factors should be considered as researchers design both quantitative and qualitative studies. There is much to recommend Bos and Fletcher's (1997) proposal that research studies routinely include information on contextual factors, such as family and community culture and teacher background, along with the student variables typically required in studies of students with LD.

Conclusions

In the foregoing sections, I illustrated the substantive contributions made by qualitative research in four areas of interest to the field of LD: the insider view on the meaning of LD and on the impact of educational programs, the implementation of models of inclusive education, the understanding of classroom instructional processes from a sociocultural perspective, and the education of culturally and linguistically diverse students with LD. We turn now to a consideration of how the distinctive characteristics of qualitative methodologies create the opportunity for addressing these and future questions.

Perhaps, the central characteristic of qualitative research is its commitment to understanding social issues in their natural context in all its complexity. From this commitment come many of the particular characteristics of various qualitative methods. First, qualitative research methods are open to the development of constructs and hypotheses as part of the research process. Because of the complexity of social contexts, it is not possible to define all the constructs of interest prior to the study. This feature gives qualitative research an exploratory nature and makes it possible to investigate unknown and unexpected phenomena. For example, the interview studies of successful adults with LD (Gerber et al., 1992) began with general questions about what LD meant to them and what made them successful, but they did not and could not know in advance what concepts and relationships among concepts would emerge from the data. Similarly, studies of the consulting teacher model (Gersten et al., 1995) began in an exploratory mode to identify features of consulting that influenced positive engagement and change by general education teachers. The features that emerged in initial analysis were then confirmed, or contradicted, by further data collection and analysis focused on those features. In the studies of how to adapt inquiry science instruction to include students with LD (Palincsar et al., 2001), research began with an open-ended exploration of barriers to full participation via case studies of individual students. These findings from case studies were then used to develop teaching practices, which were tested using a combination of quantitative and qualitative methods in the following year. This flexibility of qualitative methods makes it possible for them to discover unanticipated relationships in complex settings and to generate theories.

A second characteristic of qualitative methods important for understanding social contexts is the ability to deal with complexity. Qualitative research is able to deal with social phenomena that are organized at multiple levels because of its flexibility in determining units of analysis and analyzing interactions. For example, studies of inclusion (Baker & Zigmond, 1995; Mamlin, 1999) looked across levels of district and school administration, teacher/classroom, and individual students to understand what was happening. Thus, they could search for interactions between policies made by administrators, decisions by teachers, and impacts on students using specific methods developed for such analyses (Miles & Huberman, 1984; Strauss, 1987). Studies of classroom processes respond to another type of complexity, the complexity of multiple verbal interactions among teachers and students. For example, researchers interested in sociocultural perspectives on learning (Englert & Mariage, Chapter 27, this volume; MacArthur et al., 2002; Mariage, 2000) or in the learning of linguistically different children (Echevarria, 1995; Ruiz, 1995a) have used discourse analysis to understand the ways that teachers and students construct the meaning of classroom literacy events and the learning opportunities afforded by various discourse events.

A third characteristic is the focus on the meaning of events to participants in the culture. Within a quantitative scientific framework, one might claim to understand a con-text based on the ability to predict events or delineate causal mechanisms. However, within a qualitative or interpretive framework, one needs to understand the meaning of phenomena within the context of the culture. For example, studies of classroom processes (Englert & Mariage, Chapter 27, this volume; Morocco et al., 2002) seek to understand the meanings of classroom activities from the perspective of teachers and students because the meanings are essential to understanding how students learn. Studies of inclusion (Mamlin, 1999; Mamlin & Harris, 1998) and of consulting teacher programs (Gersten et al., 1995) found it essential to understand the educational beliefs and conceptions of teachers and principals to explain factors related to success and failure.

The focus on meanings as perceived by insiders is most obvious in studies that examined the meaning and impact of LD from the perspective of individuals with disabilities. For example, studies of adults and older students (Guterman, 1995; Shessel & Reiff, 1999) revealed their painful memories of school experiences and continuing difficulties in the social, emotional, and practical spheres of life. However, they also discovered beliefs about how the struggles with disabilities had positive effects on their coping abilities and empathy with others.

One controversial issue is whether qualitative and quantitative methods are compatible. Some in the field would deny legitimacy to interpretive methods (Kavale & Forness, 1998). Others maintain that positivist methods are based on flawed assumptions and cannot be reconciled with interpretive methods (Lincoln & Guba, 1985; Poplin, 1988). Bruner (1990) maintained that there were two fundamentally different modes of perceiving the world, the narrative and scientific, and that there was no way to evaluate the statements from one mode in terms of the other. Yet, many of the research programs discussed in this review did, in fact, combine methods that are sometimes seen as incompatible. In some cases, qualitative methods were used to enhance a basically quantitative program of research (Klinger et al., 1998). Many of the research programs focused on classroom processes were based on a sociocultural theoretical foundation often associated with qualitative research (Englert & Mariage, Chapter 27, this volume; MacArthur et al., 2002; Palincsar et al., 2001). Nonetheless, they used quantitative analysis of student outcomes to evaluate the overall effectiveness of an instructional approach in combination with qualitative methods to understand how the approach worked and how to improve it.

One argument for compatibility is that one should use whatever method is useful for the question at hand. If researchers need to demonstrate that a particular instructional approach is effective, it is not enough to show how it works or that the participants in the classroom think it works; evidence is needed that it produces some learning outcomes, and comparisons to other programs may be relevant. Another argument for compatibility is that all research, including experimental work, involves interpretive judgments that are socially constructed. If one rejects a strong positivist stance and accepts this position, then quantitative and qualitative research are compatible within a broader epistemological framework (Howe, 1988). Perhaps, as Peck and Furman (1992) suggest, the tension between qualitative and quantitative methods, or scientific and interpretive stances, is productive in stimulating the field to consider a variety of approaches to answer questions of theoretical and practical importance to the field.

References

Albinger, P. (1995). Stories from the resource room: Piano lessons, imaginary illness, and broken-down cars. *Journal of Learning Disabilities, 28,* 615–621.

Artiles, A. J., & Trent, S. (1994). Overrepresentation of minority students in special education: A continuing debate. *Journal of Special Education, 27,* 410–437.

Artiles, A. J., Trent, S. C., & Kuan, L. (1997). Learning disabilities empirical research on ethnic minority students: An analysis of 22 years of studies published in selected refereed journals. *Learning Disabilities Research and Practice, 12,* 82–91.

Baker, J. M., & Zigmond, N. (1995). The meaning and practice of inclusion for students with learning disabilities. *Journal of Special Education, 29,* 163–180.

Baxter, J., Woodward, J., Voorhuis, J., & Wong, J. (2002). We talk about it, but do they get it? *Learning Disabilities Research and Practice, 17,* 173–185.

Biklen, D., Bogdan, R., Ferguson, D. L., Searl, S. J., Jr., & Taylor, S. J. (1985). *Achieving the complete school: Strategies for effective mainstreaming.* New York: Teachers College Press.

Bogdan, R., & Biklen, D. (1982). *Qualitative research for education: And introduction to theory and methods.* Boston: Allyn & Bacon.

Bogdan, R., & Taylor, S. J. (1982). *Inside out: The social meaning of retardation.* Toronto: University of Toronto Press.

Bos, C. S., & Fletcher, T. V. (1997). Sociocultural considerations in learning disabilities inclusion research: Knowledge gaps and future directions. *Learning Disabilities Research and Practice, 12,* 92–99.

Bruner, J. (1990). *Acts of meaning.* Cambridge, MA: Harvard University Press.

Cazden, C. B. (1988). *Classroom discourse: The language of teaching and learning.* Portsmouth, NH: Heinemann.

Cutter, J., Palincsar, A. S., & Magnusson, S. J. (2002). Supporting inclusion through case-based vignette conversations. *Learning Disabilities Research and Practice, 17,* 186–200.

Echevarria, J. (1995). Interactive reading instruction: A comparison of proximal and distal effects of instructional conversation. *Exceptional Children, 61,* 536–552.

Echevarria, J., & McDonough, R. (1995). An alternative reading approach: Instructional conversations in a bilingual special education setting. *Learning Disabilities Research and Practice, 10,* 108–119.

Englert, C. S. (1992). Writing instruction from a sociocultural perspective: The holistic, dialogic, and social enterprise of writing. *Journal of Learning Disabilities, 25,* 153–172.

Englert, C. S., & Palincsar, A. S. (1991). Reconsidering instructional research in literacy from a sociocultural perspective. *Learning Disabilities Research and Practice, 6,* 225–229.

Englert, C. S., Raphael, T. E., Anderson, L. M., Anthony, H., & Stevens, D. D. (1991). Making writing strategies and self-talk visible: Cognitive strategy instruction in writing in regular and special education classrooms. *American Educational Research Journal, 28,* 337–372.

Englert, C. S., Rozendal, M. S., & Mariage, M. (1994). Fostering the search for understanding: A teacher's strategies for leading cognitive development in "zones of proximal development." *Learning Disability Quarterly, 17,* 187–204.

Ferguson, P. M., Ferguson, D. L., & Taylor, S. J. (1992). *Interpreting disability: A qualitative reader.* New York: Teachers College Press.

Forgan, J. W., & Vaughn, S. (2000). Adolescents with and without LD make the transition to middle school. *Journal of Learning Disabilities, 33,* 33–43.

Forman, E. A., & McCormick, D. E. (1995). Discourse analysis: A sociocultural perspective. *Remedial and Special Education, 16,* 150–158.

Gerber, M. M. (1995). Inclusion at the high-water mark? Some thoughts on Zigmond and Baker's case studies of inclusive educational programs. *Journal of Special Education, 29*, 181–190.

Gerber, P. J., Ginsberg, R., & Reiff, H. B. (1992). Identifying alterable patterns in employment success for highly successful adults with LD. *Journal of Learning Disabilities, 25*, 475–487.

Gerber, P. J., & Reiff, H. B. (1991). *Speaking for themselves: Ethnographic interviews with adults with learning disabilities.* Ann Arbor: University of Michigan Press.

Gersten, R., & Baker, S. (2000). What we know about effective instructional practices for English-language learners. *Exceptional Children, 66*, 454–470.

Gersten, R., Darch, C., Davis, G., & George, N. (1991). Apprenticeship and intensive training of consulting teachers: A naturalistic study. *Exceptional Children, 57*, 226–236.

Gersten, R., Morvant, M., & Brengelman, S. (1995). Close to the classroom is close to the bone: Coaching as a means to translate research into classroom practice. *Exceptional Children, 62*, 52–67.

Guterman, B. R. (1995). The validity of categorical learning disabilities services: The consumer's view. *Exceptional Children, 62*, 111–124.

Harris, K. R., & Graham, S. (1994). Constructivism: Principles, paradigms, and integration. *Journal of Special Education, 28*, 233–247.

Harry, B. (1992). *Cultural diversity, families, and the special education system.* New York: Teachers College Press.

Howe, K. R. (1988). Against the quantitative-qualitative incompatibility thesis or dogmas die hard. *Educational Researcher, 17*, 10–16.

Jacob, E. (1987). Qualitative research traditions: A review. *Review of Educational Research, 57*, 1–50.

Kavale, K. A., & Forness, S. R. (1998). The politics of learning disabilities. *Learning Disability Quarterly, 21*, 245–273.

Keogh, B. K., Gallimore, R., & Weisner, T. (1997). A sociocultural perspective on learning and learning disabilities. *Learning Disabilities Research and Practice, 12*, 107–113.

Klinger, J. K., Vaughn, S., Schumm, J. S., Cohen, P., & Forgan, J. W. (1998). Inclusion or pull-out: Which do students prefer? *Journal of Learning Disabilities, 31*, 148–158.

Lincoln, Y., & Guba, E. (1985). *Naturalistic inquiry.* Beverly Hills, CA: Sage.

MacArthur, C. A., Ferretti, R. P., & Okolo, C. M. (2002). On defending controversial viewpoints: Debates of sixth-graders about the desirability of early 20th century American immigration. *Learning Disabilities Research and Practice, 17*, 160–172.

MacArthur, C. A., & Rozmairek, D. J. (1999). Full-time collaborative teaching: Special education in an inclusive classroom. In S. Graham & K. J. Harris (Eds.), *Teachers working together: Enhancing the performance of students with special needs* (pp. 30–62). Brookline, MA: Brookline Books.

MacArthur, C. A., Schwartz, S. S., Graham, S., Molloy, D., & Harris, K. R. (1996). Integration of strategy instruction into a whole language classroom: A case study. *Learning Disabilities Research and Practice, 11*, 168–176.

Mamlin, N. (1999). Despite best intentions: When inclusion fails. *Journal of Special Education, 33*, 36–49.

Mamlin, N., & Harris, K. R. (1998). Elementary teachers' referral to special education in light of inclusion and prereferral: "Every child is here to learn . . . but some of these children are in real trouble." *Journal of Educational Psychology, 90*, 385–96.

Mariage, T. V. (1995). Why students learn: The nature of teacher talk during reading. *Learning Disability Quarterly, 18*, 214–235.

Mariage, T. V. (2000). Constructing educational possibilities: A sociolinguistic examination of meaning-making in "sharing chair." *Learning Disability Quarterly, 23*, 79–104.

Mariage, T. (2001). Features of an interactive writing discourse: Conversational involvement, conventional knowledge, and internalization in "Morning message." *Journal of Learning Disabilities, 34*, 172–196.

Marks, S. U., & Gersten, R. (1998). Engagement and disengagement between special and general educators: An application of Miles and Huberman's cross-case analysis. *Learning Disability Quarterly, 21*, 34–56.

McPhail, J. C., & Palincsar, A. S. (1998). The search for understanding of learning disabilities: A response to Kavale and Forness. *Learning Disability Quarterly, 21*, 297–305.

Miles, M., & Huberman, A. M. (1984). *Qualitative data analysis.* Newbury Park, CA: Sage.

Moody, S. W., Vaughn, S., Hughes, M. T., & Fischer, M. (2000). Reading instruction in the resource room: Set up for failure. *Exceptional Children, 66*, 305–316.

Morocco, C. C., Hindin, A., Mata-Aguilar, C., & Mott, E. A. (2002). The role of conversation in a thematic understanding of literature. *Learning Disabilities Research and Practice, 17*, 144–157.

Palincsar, A. S., & Brown, A. L. (1984). Reciprocal teaching of comprehension-fostering and comprehension-monitoring activities. *Cognition and Instruction, 1*, 117–175.

Palincsar, A. S., & Klenk, L. (1992). Fostering literacy learning in supportive contexts. *Journal of Learning Disabilities, 25*, 211–225.

Palincsar, A. S., Magnusson, S. J., Collins, K. M., & Cutter, J. (2001). Making science accessible to all: Results of a design experiment in inclusive classrooms. *Learning Disability Quarterly, 24*, 15–32.

Palincsar, A. S., Parecki, A. D., & McPhail, J. C. (1995). Friendship and literacy through literature. *Journal of Learning Disabilities, 28*, 503–510.

Peck, C. A., & Furman, G. C. (1992). Qualitative

research in special education: An evaluative review. In R. Gaylord-Ross (Ed.), *Issues and research in special education* (pp. 1–42). New York: Teachers College Press.

Peshkin, A. (2000). The nature of interpretation in qualitative research. *Educational Researcher, 29,* 5–9.

Poplin, M. (1988). The reductionistic fallacy in learning disabilities: Replicating the past by reducing the present. *Journal of Learning Disabilities, 21,* 389–400.

Poplin, M. S. (1995). Looking through other lenses and listening to other voices: Stretching the boundaries of learning disabilities. *Journal of Learning Disabilities, 28,* 292–308.

Pressley, M., Hogan, K., Wharton-McDonald, R., Mistretta, J., & Ettenberger, S. (1996). The challenges of instructional scaffolding: The challenges of instruction that supports student thinking. *Learning Disabilities Research and Practice, 11,* 138–146.

Pugach, M. C. (1995). On the failure of imagination in inclusive schooling. *Journal of Special Education, 29,* 212–223.

Pugach, M. C. (2001). The stories we choose to tell: Fulfilling the promise of qualitative research for special education. *Exceptional Children, 67,* 439–453.

Pugach, M. C., & Wesson, C. L. (1995). Teachers' and students' views of team teaching of general education and learning-disabled students in two fifth-grade classes. *Elementary School Journal, 95,* 279–295.

Putney, L. G., Green, J. L., Dixon, C. N., & Kelly, G. J. (1999). Evolution of qualitative research methodology: Looking beyond defense to possibilities. *Reading Research Quarterly, 34,* 368–377.

Reid, D. K., & Button, L. J. (1995). Anna's story: Narratives of personal experience about being labeled learning disabled. *Journal of Learning Disabilities, 28,* 602–614.

Reiff, H. B., Gerber, P. J., & Ginsberg, R. (1993). Definitions of learning disabilities from adults with LD: The insiders' perspectives. *Learning Disability Quarterly, 16,* 114–125.

Reschly, D. J. (1984). Beyond IQ test bias: The National Academy Panel's analysis of minority EMR overrepresentation. *Educational Researcher, 13,* 15–19.

Rice, D., & Zigmond, N. (2000). Co-teaching in secondary schools: Teacher reports of developments in Australian and American classrooms.

Learning Disabilities Research and Practice, 15, 190–197.

Ruiz, N. T. (1995a). The social construction of ability and disability: Optimal and at-risk lessons in a bilingual special education classroom. *Journal of Learning Disabilities, 28,* 491–502.

Ruiz, N. T. (1995b). The social construction of ability and disability: Profile types of Latino children identified as language learning disabled. *Journal of Learning Disabilities, 28,* 476–490.

Ruiz, N. T., Rueda, R., Figueroa, R. A., & Boothroyd, M. (1995). Bilingual special education teachers' shifting paradigms: Complex responses to educational reform. *Journal of Learning Disabilities, 28,* 622–635.

Scruggs, T. E., & Mastropieri, M. A. (1994a). The construction of scientific knowledge by students with mild disabilities. *Journal of Special Education, 28,* 307–321.

Scruggs, T. E., & Mastropieri, M. A. (1994b). Successful mainstreaming in elementary science classes: A qualitative investigation of three reputational cases. *American Educational Research Journal, 31,* 785–811.

Scruggs, T., & Mastropieri, M. (1995). What makes special education special? Evaluating inclusion programs with the PASS variables. *Journal of Special Education, 29,* 224–233.

Shessel, I., & Reiff, H. B. (1999). Experiences off adults with learning disabilities: Positive and negative impacts and outcomes. *Learning Disability Quarterly, 22,* 305–316.

Strauss, A. (1987). *Qualitative analysis for social scientists.* New York: Cambridge University Press.

Tharp, R., & Gallimore, R. (1988). *Rousing minds to life.* New York: Cambridge University Press.

Vaughn, S., Moody, S. W., & Schumm, J. S. (1998). Broken promises: Reading instruction in the resource room. *Exceptional Children, 64,* 211–225.

Vygotsky, L. S. (1978). *Mind in society: The development of higher psychological processes.* Cambridge, MA: Harvard University Press.

Walther-Thomas, C. S. (1997). Co-teaching experiences: The benefits and problems that teachers and principals report over time. *Journal of Learning Disabilities, 30,* 395–407.

Zigmond, N. (1995). An exploration of the meaning and practice of special education in the context of full inclusion of students with learning disabilities. *Journal of Special Education, 29,* 109–115.

Author Index

Subject Index

Page numbers followed by *f* indicate figure and *t* indicate table.